OCCUPATIONAL THERAPY WITH ELDERS

STRATEGIES FOR THE COTA

OCCUPATIONAL THERAPY WITH ELDERS

STRATEGIES FOR THE COTA

second edition

EDITORS

Sue Byers-Connon, MS, COTA/L, ROH
Formerly, Instructor
OTA Program
Allied Health Division;
Instructor, GED Program
Mt. Hood Community College
Gresham, Oregon

Helene L. Lohman, OTD, OTR/L
Associate Professor
Department of Occupational Therapy
School of Pharmacy and Health Professions
Creighton University
Omaha, Nebraska

René L. Padilla, PhD, OTR/L, FAOTA
Assistant Professor
Department of Occupational Therapy
School of Pharmacy and Health Professions
Creighton University
Omaha, Nebraska

WITH ILLUSTRATIONS BY RENÉ L. PADILLA, PhD, OTR/L, FAOTA
WITH PHOTOS BY KEVIN J. CALLAHAN, COTA/L

With 42 contributors
With 138 illustrations

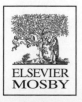

ELSEVIER
MOSBY

ELSEVIER
MOSBY

11830 Westline Industrial Drive
St. Louis, Missouri 63146

OCCUPATIONAL THERAPY WITH ELDERS
Copyright © 2004, Mosby, Inc. All rights reserved.

Library of Congress Cataloging-in-Publication Data

Occupational therapy with elders : strategies for the COTA / editors, Sue Byers-Connon,
   Helene L. Lohman, René L. Padilla ; with illustrations by René L. Padilla, with photos by
   Kevin J. Callahan.–2nd ed.
      p. ; cm.
   Includes bibliographical references and index.
   ISBN-13: 978-0-323-02430-3   ISBN-10: 0-323-02430-0 (alk. paper)
      1.Occupational therapy for the aged. 2. Occupational therapy assistants. I.
   Byers-Connon, Sue. II. Lohman, Helene. III. Padilla, René L.
   [DNLM: 1. Occupational Therapy–Aged. 2. Rehabilitation–Aged. WB 555 O1571 2004]
   RC953.8.O22O246 2004
   615.8'515'0846–dc22

                                                            2004044999

Publisher: Linda Duncan
Managing Editor: Kathryn Falk
Senior Developmental Editor: Kim Fons
Editorial Assistant: Colin Odell
Publishing Services Manager: Melissa Lastarria
Design Manager: Bill Drone

ISBN-13: 978-0-323-02430-3
ISBN-10: 0-323-02430-0

Printed in United States of America

Last digit is the print number: 9   8   7   6   5

To my husband Ron, for his support and patience. To my life-long friends; Linda, who lost her battle to cancer and Mable, a caring and giving person. To Spenser, Alex, and Avianna who make Grandparenting a joy. To all the Graduates of the OTA program at Mt. Hood Community College from 1986–2003 who helped me grow as a teacher and gave me the opportunity to share my love of the profession of Occupational Therapy.

Sue

To my parents who instilled in me the value of education, to all their friends and relatives who gave me an appreciation of their generation, and to my special Aunt Jeanne and Uncle Martin.

Helene

To all our COTA colleagues who have been a vital part of our profession for many years.

René

Shadows and Sunlight

I remember being young and wild,
Although my body forgets and betrays me.
I peer out of this aging body
With a mind that still knows
Who, when, where and how.
When did fifty
Or even sixty seem like young?
Birthdays only serve as a yardstick for the outside.
How can you measure what I feel on the inside?

My heart tears seeing friends disappear
Into places I only fear.
My memories of yesteryear seem crystal clear.
I close my eyes and feel myself running in the breeze.
The crowds along the college track applauding my triumph,
When the sound of my therapist
Cheering my toddling in a walker wakes me.
I laugh out loud
And people shake their heads as if I am half crazed.
So many losses totaling into this single moment.

The respect I had as a working man
Still fills my chest with pride.
My dearest Rosalie leaving me on Earth so quickly.
Our dreams of travel and leisurely walks are gone.
Saying goodbye to my neighborhood of 43 years,
To move into a room with a stranger.
Overhearing the hushed voices of my son and daughter
As they discuss the exorbitant costs of my care outside my door.
Then the frustrated voices in deciding who will take Dad home.

How did the tables get turned so fast?
Ironically my children become my caretakers now.
How can I express to those I love,
Do not grieve for my losses so deeply.
As I still intend to live
As best I can,
As much as you will allow me.
Keep open the windows of possibilities.
Do not shut the door of life just yet.

Yolanda Griffiths (Used by permission)

Contributors

MARLENE J. AITKEN, PhD, OTR/L
Associate Professor
Department of Occupational Therapy
School of Pharmacy and Health Professions
Creighton University
Omaha, Nebraska

TONYA BARTHOLOMEW, BSOT
Occupational Therapist
Creighton University Medical Center
Omaha, Nebraska

REBECCA BOTHWELL, OTR
Research Coordinator
Occupational Therapy Education
University of Kansas Medical Center
Kansas City, Kansas

KATHERINE (KATE) H. BROWN, PhD
Program Director
South Side Community Land Trust
Providence, Rhode Island
Formerly Associate Professor
Occupational Therapy Department
School of Pharmacy and
Health Professions;
Formerly Faculty Associate
Center for Health Policy and Ethics
Creighton University
Omaha, Nebraska

KRIS R. BROWN, BS, OTR/L
Private Practice
Sioux City, Iowa

LESLIE BRUNSTETER-WILLIAMS, BSOT
Formerly Staff Occupational Therapist
Acute Care, In-Patient, and Out-Patient Services

Rehabilitation Services Department
Trinity Lutheran Hospital
Kansas City, Missouri

SUE BYERS-CONNON, MS, COTA/L, ROH
Formerly, Instructor
OTA Program
Allied Health Division;
Instructor, GED Program
Mt. Hood Community College
Gresham, Oregon

CLAUDELLE A. H. CARRUTHERS, PhD, OTR, PT,
Adjunct Professor
MA Program in Gerontology
Bethel College
St. Paul, Minnesota;
CEO Ageless Possibilities
Minneapolis, Minnesota

BRENDA M. COPPARD, PH.D., OTR/L
Associate Professor and Chair
Department of Occupational Therapy
School of Pharmacy and Health Professions
Creighton University
Omaha, Nebraska

JANA K. CRAGG, MA, OTR
Associate Professor
Occupational Therapy Assistant Program
St. Phillip's College
San Antonio, Texas

TERRYN DAVIS, COTA
Certified Occupational Therapy Assistant
Occupational Therapy Department
San Jose State University
San Jose, California

L. Margaret Drake, PhD, OTR/L, ATR-BC, LPAT, FAOTA
Associate Professor
Department of Occupational Therapy
School of Health Related Professions
University of Mississippi Medical Center
Jackson, Mississippi

Barbara L. Flynn, PharmD, FASCP, CGP
Assistant Professor
Department of Pharmacy Sciences
School of Pharmacy and Health Professions
Creighton University
Omaha, Nebraska

Kai Galyen, OTR/L
Formerly Occupational Therapy Department
Benedictine Nursing Center
Mount Angel, Oregon

Coralie H. Glantz, OT/L, BCG, FAOTA
Co-Owner, Glantz/Richman Rehabilitation Associates
Riverwoods, Illinois

Yolanda Griffiths, OTD, OTR/L, FAOTA
Assistant Professor
Department of Occupational Therapy
School of Pharmacy and Health Professions
Creighton University
Omaha, Nebraska

LTC Karoline D. Harvey, OTR
Assistant Chief and Intern Coordinator
Department of Occupational Therapy
Walter Reed Army Hospital
Washington, DC

Jean T. Hays, COTA
Instructor/Academic Fieldwork Coordinator
Occupational Therapy Assistant
Program-Allied Health
St. Phillips College
San Antonio, Texas

Carly R. Hellen, BS, OTR/L
Dementia Care Consultant and Educator
Durham, New Hampshire

Tyrome Higgins, Master of Social Gerontology, COTA, ROH
Certified Occupational Therapy Assistant
Alamo Heights Rehabilitation Center
San Antonio, Texas

Ada Boone Hoerl, BS, COTA
Adjunct Professor
Division of Science and Allied Health
Sacramento City College
Sacramento, California

Penni Jean Lavoot, COTA, CDRS, CRC
Rehabilitation Specialist
Project Threshold
Rancho Rehabilitation Engineering Center
Downey, California

Ivelisse Lazzarini, OTD, OTR/L
Director
Allied Health Complexity Center
Edward and Margaret Doisy School of Allied
Health Professions
Saint Louis University
Saint Louis, Missouri

Helene L. Lohman, OTD, OTR/L
Associate Professor
Department of Occupational Therapy
School of Pharmacy and Health Professions
Creighton University
Omaha, Nebraska

Amy Matthews, MS, OTR/L
Instructor
Department of Occupational Therapy
School of Pharmacy and Health Professions
Creighton University
Omaha, Nebraska

Deborah L. Morawski, B.S., OTR/L
Owner, Achieving Independence
Abbey Physical Medicine & Rehabilitation
Grass Valley, California

Candice Mullendore, MS, OTR/L
Assistant Professor and Academic
Fieldwork Coordinator
Department of Occupational Therapy
School of Pharmacy and Health Professions
Creighton University
Omaha, Nebraska

Sandra Hattori Okada, MSG, OTR/L, CDRS
Gerontologist, Occupational Therapist,
Certified Driver Rehabilitation Specialist
Occupational Therapy Driving Program
Rancho Los Amigos National Rehabilitation
Downey, California

RENÉ L. PADILLA, PhD, OTR/L, FAOTA
Assistant Professor
Department of Occupational Therapy
School of Pharmacy and Health Professions
Creighton University
Omaha, Nebraska

STEVE PARK, MS, OTR/L
Associate Professor
School of Occupational Therapy
Pacific University
Forest Grove, Oregon

CLAIRE PEEL, PhD, PT
Associate Dean for Academic Affairs
School of Health Related Professions
University of Alabama at Birmingham
Birmingham, Alabama

ANGELA M. PERALTA, COTA
Certified Occupational Therapy Assistant
Occupational Therapy
Toddler & Infant Program for Special Education
Staten Island, New York
Formerly, Adjunct Instructor
Occupational Therapy Assistant Program
Touro College
New York, New York

CLAUDIA GAYE PEYTON, PhD, OTR/L, FAOTA
Director
Department of Occupational Therapy
California State University, Dominguez Hills
Carson, California

SHERRELL POWELL, MA, OTR
Professor
Natural and Applied Science
LaGuardia Community College
City University of New York
Long Island City, New York

NANCY RICHMAN, B.S., OTR/L, FAOTA
Co-Owner Glantz/Richman Rehabilitation
Associates
Riverwoods, Illinois

BARBARA JO RODRIGUES, MS, OTR/L
Occupational Therapy Program Director
Behavior Health Unit
Dominican Hospital
Santa Cruz, California

CAROL J. SCHWOPE, MA, COTA/L
Formerly Staff Therapist and Student
Coordinator
Rehabilitation Sciences
Health South at St. Mary's Hospital
Huntington, West Virginia

ELLEN SPERGEL, MEd, OTR
Professor, Coordinator of Occupational
Therapy
Occupational Therapy Assistant Program
Rockland Community College
Suffern, New York

SHARON STOFFEL, M.A., OTR/L, FAOTA
Associate Professor
Occupational Science and Occupational
Therapy
The College of St. Catherine
St. Paul, Minnesota

JEAN VANN, BS, OTR/L,
Occupational Therapist
Formerly
Legacy Visiting Nurse Association
Hospice Team
Portland, Oregon

LINDA A. WALKER, OTD, OTR/L
Assistant Professor and Academic Fieldwork
Coordinator
Department of Occupational Therapy
School of Pharmacy and Health Professions
Creighton University
Omaha, Nebraska

LISA WALKER, COTA/L, AP
Occupational Therapy Assistant
Town Center Village Rehabilitation
Portland, Oregon

Foreword

OTA students and therapists reading this second edition of *Occupational Therapy With Elders: Strategies for the COTA* will find intervention suggestions that hold potential for elders in all practice areas. Demographic projections for 2030 show those 65 and older will encompass 20% of the total elderly population. And within this sector, elders of color will reach 25.4%.[1] Readers' are reminded of this rapid graying of America's population. Text editors and chapter authors dramatically highlight the growing need for continued COTA practitioner involvement in this critical practice area.

The opening chapter identifies 'Aging Trends and Concepts' and the second chapter reviews 'Social and Biological Theories of Aging'. An introduction to the AOTA Occupational Therapy Practice Framework follows. Chapter authors' throughout the text include case examples which clearly reflect the concept and or support the theory described. Use of this narrative style facilitates better reader comprehension.

The chapter, 'The Regulation of Public Policy for Elders' describes public and private health systems, for example, Medicare, SSI, Older Americans Act, that influence COTA practice. Another chapter, 'Addressing Sexuality of Elders' presents issues which can arise in the later years. It suggests strategies whereby the COTA can better communicate about this often neglected issue.

The chapter 'Aging Well: Health Promotion and Disease Prevention' addresses the critical need for COTA interventions to incorporate a focus on health promotion and disability prevention. Readers' awareness is heightened regarding the public health goals described in the US government report, 'Healthy People 2010'.

Despite physiological change, different experiences, various financial and cultural influences, and multiple housing and treatment situations, elders can benefit from strategies which enable better management of chronic illnesses. COTAs incorporating strategies presented in the text in treatment interventions will find that elders' skill mastery can facilitate health behavior changes. Outcomes can improve quality of life for elders.

Throughout the text, authors direct readers' attention toward the critical value of client-centered interventions. COTAs recognize how this approach continues to strongly influence their clients' quality of life well into their later years. Examples included demonstrate the positive impact arising from COTA and OTR team interventions in the various practice settings. Team interventions continue to be an integral component in therapy interaction that leads to positive client and caregiver outcomes.

Readers' will find a comprehensive review of best occupational therapy practice situations across the practice continuum. Case examples include those one might find in the more traditional facilities based practice site. Equal attention is directed toward innovative options that are becoming available in the non-traditional, community-based service delivery arena.

It is a pleasure to recognize that text editors and chapter authors in, 'Occupational Therapy With Elders: Strategies for the COTA', have successfully heightened readers' knowledge of critically significant issues in the evolving aging practice arena. COTA students and practitioners reviewing the text will find useful strategies through which they can provide more effective treatment interventions. Indeed, they will also find new ideas enabling them to increase their participation in community education outreach for elders, and their informal and formal caregivers.

Anne **L. M**orris, EdD, OTR, CAPS, FAOTA
Elder Care Consulting, Springfield, Virginia
and
Adjunct Assistant Professor
NOVA Southeastern University
Online OT Doctoral Program

[1] Administration on Aging (2002).
A Profile of Older Americans: 2002.
[On-line]. Retrieved November 15, 2003 from *http://www.aoa.gov*

Preface

Certified Occupational Therapy Assistants (COTAs) continue to be the greater part of the occupational therapy workforce treating elders. A recent report states that skilled nursing facilities, which primarily service elders, continue to be the number one employer of COTAs (AOTA, 2000). This trend of working with elders is likely to continue for some time as the elder population grows. The need for COTAs to possess a strong knowledge base that will allow them to provide the best service possible and to confidently represent the profession remains as high a priority as when we prepared the first edition of this text in 1998. Therefore, we have sought to include the most up-to-date information possible in order to support COTAs as they work in this important practice area.

In this edition we retained the conceptual organization of the first edition. The first section, *Concepts of Aging*, presents foundational concepts related to the experience of elders. A general discussion of aging trends, concepts and theories is followed by a discussion of occupational therapy (OT) professional concepts, including an introduction to the recently adopted *Occupational Therapy Practice Framework* (American Occupational Therapy Association, 2002). The second section, *Occupational Therapy Intervention with Elders*, includes updated and, in some cases, new chapters with specific applications of OT strategies that take into account the principles presented in Section I. We begin Section II with issues related to all elders with such topics as cultural diversity, OT theories applied to elders, ethical aspects, and working with caregivers. We conclude Section II with chapters dedicated to strategies applicable to the work with elders who have specific medical conditions.

As we prepared this second edition we remained committed to the goals which guided us in the previous edition:

- We wanted the project to acknowledge the reality of life experience of elders and be respectful of them as occupational beings. We re-committed to the use of the term "elder" as a way to reduce these people to the stereotypical role of dependent patients and to dispel myths about aging.
- We continued to emphasize the importance of collaboration between the Occupational Therapist, Registered (OTR) and COTA. Our own collaboration as an editorial team continued to be vivid example to us of the richness of such collaboration.
- We wanted to produce a comprehensive text for both OTA students as well as practicing COTAs who wish to refresh their knowledge and for OTRs who are committed to the development of the COTA/OTR partnership.
- We wanted to highlight the important contribution COTAs make to the life of elders.
- We emphasized the illustration of principles and strategies through case studies and narratives so that the reader can easily relate their learning to real-life situations.
- We continued to ground the suggested strategies in traditional OT philosophy and practice, and emphasized the kind of reasoning that should be part of all OT intervention regardless of professional level.

It remains our hope that this text will contribute to the reader's knowledge so they can contribute to the improvement of life satisfaction of elders wherever they come into contact with them.

Sue Byers-Connon, MS, COTA/L, ROH
Helene Lohman, OTD, OTR/L
René Padilla, Ph.D., OTR/L, FAOTA

REFERENCE

The American Occupational Therapy Association (2000). 2000 compensation survey: final report. (p. 25). Bethesda, MD: Author.

The American Occupational Therapy Association (2002). Occupational therapy practice framework: Domain and process. The American Journal of Occupational Therapy (56), 6, 609-639.

Acknowledgements

It is true that writing a book is not a simple process that one person alone cannot undertake alone. We wish to acknowledge many people for their contributions to this project:

- The contributing authors, for their hard work
- The individuals who reviewed the first edition and provided feedback
- Yolanda Griffiths for the moving poem that appears at the beginning of the book
- The elders who graciously appeared in the photographs
- Kevin Callahan, COTA/L, for his photographic skill
- Kim Fons and Kathy Falk for their patience and direction
- Bruce Siebert from Graphic World Publishing Services for his direction in completing this project
- The following individuals who made contributions to updating case studies and contributions to chapters:
  Scott D. McPhee DrPH, OTR/L FAOTA
  Contributing to Chapter 8

Brian Hagen COTA/L Case study Chapter 11
Jolene Skias COTA/L Case Study Chapter 14
Erin Geissler COTA/L Contributing to Chapter 16
Tena Meehan COTA/L Case Study Chapter 17
Jodi Lane COTA/L Case Study Chapter 24

- Carol Kelly COTA/L, for sharing her experience with the Art of Movement
- Judy Bergjoid at the Creighton Health Science Library for all her help with research
- Amy Byers for her help with the Glossary
- Ann McNally for her help with the Appendix
- The administrators and faculty of the Department of Occupational Therapy, School of Pharmacy and Health Professions at Creighton University, for their encouragement.

- We would like to recognize the special contributions from Ivelisse Lazzarini for her valuable and deligent work in updating many of the chapters

Contents

CONCEPTS OF AGING

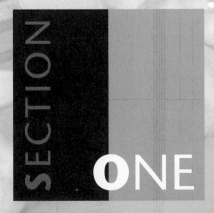

SECTION

ONE

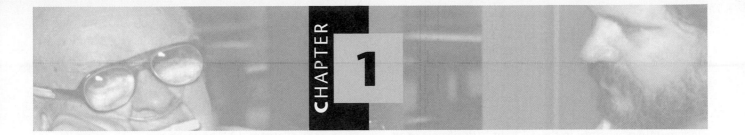

Aging Trends and Concepts

HELENE LOHMAN AND ELLEN SPERGEL

KEY TERMS

gerontology, geriatrics, cohort, health, illness, chronic illness, young old, mid old, old old, demography, trends, intergenerational, ageism

CHAPTER OBJECTIVES

1. Define relevant terminology regarding elders.
2. Describe the relation between aging and illness.
3. Discuss components of health and chronic illness.
4. Discuss a client-centred approach.
5. Describe the three stages of aging and define their differences.
6. Describe the effects of growth of the elder population on society.
7. Discuss the effects of an increasingly large number of elder women on society.
8. Describe the problems and needs of the oldest old population—that is, those elders 85 years and older, including the centenarians.
9. Describe usual living arrangements of most elders.
10. Discuss the significance of economic trends on the elderly.
11. Relate implications of demographical data for occupational therapy practice.
12. Discuss current trends impacting elders in America and implications for occupational therapy practice.
13. Describe the importance of intergenerational contact for occupational therapy treatment.
14. Describe the concept of "ageism" in today's society and the effect of the views of the American youth culture on aging.

John is a 30-year-old certified occupational therapy assistant (COTA®) practicing in a skilled nursing home facility. He provides daily occupational therapy (OT) treatment 5 days a week to elders. Most of the elders are in some stage of recovery from an acute illness and are going through OT to regain their functional abilities. Many of the elders are quite frail and some have cognitive impairments. As a student, John observed Mark, a COTA working in an independent living facility. Mark was part of a team providing wellness programming to elders.

Most of Mark's clients were quite active at the facility and in the community. On weekends, John visits his grandparents, both of whom are 75 years of age and are also independent, active members of the community. John often thinks about his grandparents, the elders at the independent living facility, and the nursing home residents. He contemplates about whom are the typical elders.

Tammy is a 20-year-old occupational therapy assistant student (OTAS) in an OTA program with a student population between the ages of 20 and 50 years. As one of her course requirements, class members participate in inter-generational book discussion groups (Lohman, Griffiths, Coppard, & Cota, 2003) at an independent living facility. The specific readings focus the book discussions on intergenerational values and beliefs. Tammy is surprised to identify generational differences and similarities. Her class members who are in their 40s and 50s discuss growing up in the 1960s and 1970s and the influence of media and the Vietnam War on their generation. The elder generations discuss the influence that World War II had on their lives. All of the generations commonly share the impact of the terrorist attacks on September 11, 2001. Tammy also notes that within each generation there are a variety of perspectives based on individual life experiences. These lively discussions have increased each participant's awareness of intergenerational commonalities and differences, as well as the individual uniqueness of each group member. The discussions have created a strong bond among the group members. Tammy feels that as a result of participating in the intergenerational book discussion group, she will be more comfortable working with elders in clinical practice.

Tammy has a strong desire to go into practice with elders. She remembers helping her grandmother recover from a stroke. When she studied the content about elders in her course work, Tammy was surprised to learn of the diversity among the elder population. She realized that just as her OTA class represents diversity among age groups and cultural groups, so does the elder population. She also recognized misconceptions she had about the elder generation. Some were based on clinical observations at a nursing home and informal observations from visits to her grandmother. One misconception was that all elders are sick and frail. Another misconception was that most elders have cognitive impairments. Through her participation in course experiences with well elders in community settings, Tammy learned that many elders are quite healthy and active, especially the younger generation of elders (those 65 to 75 years of age). Tammy also learned that moderate to severe cognitive impairment affects a small portion of the elder population, primarily the oldest of the old (those 85 years and older) (Federal Interagency Forum On Aging-Related Statistics, 2000).

COTAs may easily acquire a skewed image of the elder population, especially in a nursing home setting, which is the second largest area of practice for COTAs (The American Occupational Therapy Association, 2000). Elders in nursing homes tend to be representative of a sicker, older, and more frail elder population. Elders in nursing homes often have circulatory, cognitive, and mental disorders, and most residents require assistance with activities of daily living (ADL) (Sahyoun, Pratt, Lentzner, Dey, & Robinson, 2001). In reality, only 4.5% of all elders at any one time reside in nursing homes (U. S. Department of Health and Human Services

[DHHS], 2001). OT practice continues to change with a movement toward community-based practice, where the majority of elders reside. Therefore, COTAs must have a broader perspective about elders to work effectively with a diverse, continuously changing elder population. This chapter provides relevant background information as it relates to OT practice and to the overall elder population.

The term **gerontology** comes from the Greek terms *geron* and *lojas*, which mean "study of old men." Gerontology is often thought of as the study of the aged and can include the aging process in humans and animals. The field of gerontology is broad and includes the historic, philosophical, religious, political, psychological, anthropological, and sociological issues of the elder population. The term **geriatrics** is often used to describe medical interventions with the elderly. In OT practice, geriatrics sometimes refers to an area of clinical specialty. The term **cohort** refers to "a collection or sampling of individuals who share a common characteristic, such as members of the same age or sex group" (Potter & Perry, 2002). In gerontological literature, the elder generation may also be referred to as the *elder*, or *aged*, *cohort* compared with younger cohorts (Figure 1-1). Different terms used in this book refer to the geriatric population as the *aged*, *older*, or *the elder population*.

HEALTH, ILLNESS, AND WELL-BEING

Although **health, illness,** and **well-being** are familiar terms, they require expanded definitions for OT practice in geriatrics. One part of a definition for health is "...the absence of disease or other abnormal condition" (Potter & Perry, 2002). Few elders would be considered healthy with this general definition. However, a theory of well-being can be developed if health is considered the optimal level of functioning for a person's age and condition. Many individuals have chronic illnesses to which they

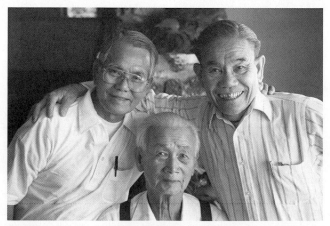

FIGURE 1-1 This group of cohorts enjoys spending time together.

have adjusted and are able to live optimally. These people could be considered to be in a state of well-being. For example, to live optimally, individuals with lifelong disabilities such as cerebral palsy and multiple sclerosis need health care system services such as OT home evaluations for environmental adaptations even though they are not ill. These individuals do not think of themselves as ill and may resent being labeled as "patients" and placed in the this role by health care professionals.

The biological systems of elders can change. Some changes that result in disease or dysfunction may be treated through medication or surgery. Other biological changes such as decreased balance can be handled with environmental adaptations such as installing brighter lights in stairwells and removing loose rugs and electrical cords from traffic areas in the home. Some sensory changes can be partially resolved with glasses and hearing aids. These biological and sensory changes should not be thought of as illnesses. They are changes that elders adjust to and incorporate into their daily lives.

Chronic Illness

Many medical conditions of elders are chronic—that is, they cannot be cured, but they can be managed. The physician may not cure heart disease, but the pain and debilitating consequences can be managed for years with medications, diet, exercise, surgery, and technology. COTAs can provide ideas to help elders manage their chronic conditions to maintain involvement in occupations (see Chapter 5). In these cases it could be said that although the disease has not been cured, the elder's life has been extended in a qualitatively meaningful way.

Most elders have a minimum of one or more chronic conditions. Recent data indicate the most prevalent conditions for elders as arthritis (49%), hypertension (36%), hearing impairments (30%), heart disease (27%), cataracts (17%), orthopedic impairments (18%), sinusitis (12%), and diabetes (10%) (DHHS, 2001). The incidence of chronic illness may be greater in minority elder groups than in white elders. In one study of elder women, black women reported having greater incidences of arthritis and hypertension than white women and other minority groups. Women of American Indian descent reported the greatest incidence of cardiovascular disease (Bierman, Haffer, & Hwang, 2001).

The following example illustrates the way one elder learns to adapt to a chronic illness. Henry has osteoarthritis and needs assistance with some ADL functions. He continues to maintain his apartment and values his independence. He takes frequent breaks to rest while doing housekeeping tasks. Because of his poor endurance, he uses a lightweight upright vacuum, which also helps to reduce upper extremity strain. Henry has an active social life outside his home. He maintains mobility in the community by taking a bus to activities. Henry has osteoarthritis, a disease

that cannot be cured. However, most COTAs would say that Henry is not sick.

Some health care practitioners may dismiss an elder's complaints with comments such as "It's your age; it's your problem; what do you expect from me? I can't cure you." They are likely to overlook important ways to treat and to reduce symptoms that may increase the length and quality of that elder's life. Generally, health professionals are educated to cure illness, and some may be less knowledgeable about illness management. Some health care practitioners feel uncomfortable treating elders who can't be cured, and thus develop a dismissive approach in response.

The alternative to a dismissive approach is a collaborative approach, or what has been referred to in OT literature as *client-centred therapy* (Law & Mills, 1998). With this approach OTs and COTAs partner with their clients to help determine therapy goals and treatment activities. They spend time getting to know clients as a people by hearing their stories through assessments such as the Canadian Occupational Performance Measure (COPM) (Law et al., 1998). Elders are central to the management of their own health and well-being. By using a client-centred approach, elders identify meaningful treatment activities and thus are more invested in treatment (Law, 2000).

A treatment partnership involves the occupational therapist, COTA, and the elder working together to help determine meaningful treatment goals that enhance the elder's quality of life. The following example illustrates this treatment partnership.

Sadie is an 86-year-old widow with arthritis living in senior citizen housing. Her daily life is a balance of self-maintenance, simple meal preparations, visits with neighbors in the community recreation room, telephone calls to family members, and watching television. Sadie has reported decreasing vision, weakness, and joint pain to her primary care physician. General anxiety and depression also appear to be features of her condition. She comments to her physician "I think that I belong in a nursing home. I'm old and I'm having difficulty taking care of myself."

Placing Sadie in a nursing home may manage some of her medical conditions, as well as provide care and social opportunities. However, the physician also can evaluate additional supports to maintain independent living in the community if that is what Sadie really desires. The physician can adjust drug dosages for management of Sadie's arthritis and order OT evaluation and treatment. The registered occupational therapist (OTR®) and COTA decide to first screen Sadie using the COPM to obtain a clearer picture of Sadie's concerns. With the COPM Sadie mentions that she would really like to remain home and identifies her main concerns as having difficulties with meal preparation and reading the newspaper. Both concerns are related to her low vision. In addition, she has difficulty getting dressed because of arthritis. On the basis of this information the OTR, COTA, and Sadie collaborate to develop the following treatment recommendations:

1. A kitchen evaluation for suggestions for low vision
2. A lighted magnifier to improve visual function with reading
3. Arthritis education that includes joint protection and mobilization, energy conservation, work simplification, and adaptive devices to improve dressing

A client-centred approach can address the elder's chronic conditions, interests, and desires. Elders with multiple chronic diagnoses that often accompany acute conditions or changes in functional status are not unusual. When managed properly, all treatments work smoothly to improve the elder's independent status and occupational well-being. The elder may need to adjust to a different status of functioning with different occupational roles. The OT treatment interventions suggested in the example may result in improved functional abilities in many areas of life and decreased anxiety about independent living. Accumulation of medical conditions does not necessarily lead to decreased function and increased disability. Despite the "graying of America," elder citizens are experiencing less disability and are living longer and better.

THE STAGES OF AGING

What age constitutes "old age"? The federally mandated age to collect Social Security is 65 years. The age that most retirement communities set as the minimum for their residents is 55 years. At age 50 years, one can join the American Association of Retired Persons. At age 40 years, Americans are protected by the Age Discrimination in Employment Act. The third stage of aging, called *senescence*, which social gerontologists define as a stage of biological decline, begins at age 30 years.

One definition of old age classifies 65 to 75 years of age as young old, 75 to 85 as mid old, and 85 and greater as old old.* This may help COTAs to think of old age in terms of occupational role performance and expectations. However, COTAs should use this classification as a guideline because every person ages differently and every elder does not fit neatly into one of these three categories. Socioeconomic factors, societal changes, and personality considerations can largely influence the way each elder approaches aging.

Young Old (65 to 75 years of age): Elders who are **young old** may be recently retired and enjoying the results of their years of employment, their essential role as grandparents, and their continuing role as parents in the growth of their adult children (Figure 1-2). They

*These classifications are an adaptation of ones developed by Lazer (1985). In his work he defined four classifications of elders as "older" (55 to 64 years), "elderly" (65 to 74 years), "aged" (75 to 84 years), and "very old" (85 years and older). Earlier, Neugarten (1974) divided elders into the "young old" (55 to 74 years) and "old old" (older than 75 years).

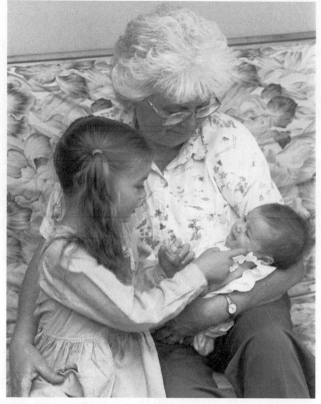

FIGURE 1-2   This newly retired elder enjoys time with her grandchildren.

have increased leisure time to pursue interests and to develop new ones. They may choose to do volunteer work with community service, return to school, and travel. Some, however, because of economic or other personal reasons, will choose to remain in the workforce. Others, because of family circumstances, may reassume the role of raising children with their grandchildren. The young old must often cope with chronic conditions such as osteoarthritis, hypertension, and cardiovascular disease. However, these chronic conditions are often managed medically and usually do not represent a major barrier to functioning or satisfactory occupational role performance. This age group may be interested in health maintenance activities (Lazer, 1985).

Mid Old (75 to 85 years of age): In the **mid old** period of life, more changes are evident. Mid old elders make modifications in their occupational role performance. They often reduce or simplify their lives in various ways, including resting during the day, volunteering less, traveling less, and limiting distance of trips. They may rely more on social systems such as Meals on Wheels, public transportation, and family for some assistance with ADL (Figure 1-3). COTAs may provide interventions when necessary. The frequent loss of significant others brings affective stressors and additional role changes (Figure 1-4; see Chapter 2

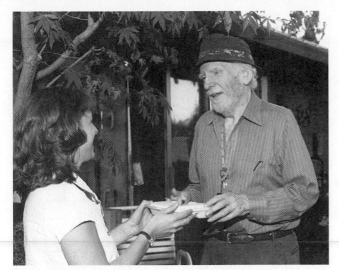

FIGURE 1-3 Some elders may use Meals on Wheels to maintain nutrition and remain in their own homes.

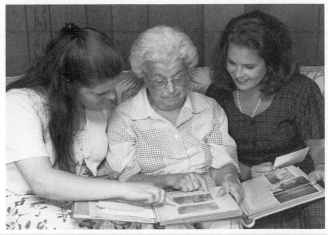

FIGURE 1-5 Elder may enjoy reflecting on life with other generations.

for a discussion of specific theories explaining the stages of aging).

Old Old (85 years of age and older): During the **old old** period of life, elders may reflect on the meaning of their lives, the quality of their relationships, and their contributions to society (Figure 1-5). They may think about the losses they are experiencing and about their own deaths. This may be a time of peace and generosity; elders in the old old period of life may find it meaningful to give valued objects to loved ones who will treasure them. Conversely, it can be a period of fear and anger resulting from unresolved conflicts. Resolution of these

conflicts can make this the most spiritual and fulfilling period for elders. Personal growth and reflection continue throughout life.

This time in an elder's life is usually a period of further systemic change affecting the sensory, motor, cardiac, and pulmonary systems. Chronic conditions impair self-maintenance capacities, and elders in the old old stage may need personal assistance with bathing, mobility, dressing, and money management that COTAs can provide. The old old may use more health support services (Lazer, 1985). If these elders live independently, they may need some family member support.

An alternative health care delivery option to help frail elders primarily in the old old age group is a national demonstration project called Program for All-Inclusive Care of the Elderly (PACE). PACE addresses elder's preventive, acute, and long-term health care needs (Alexander, 2000). It focuses on keeping these frail elders who would otherwise be in skilled nursing facilities, or possibly in hospitals, in their homes (Eng, Pedulla, Eleazer, McCann, & Fox, 1997). PACE is financially supported by monthly capitation payments from Medicare and Medicaid, or by private pay. In general, the goal of the project is to demonstrate that elders remain independent longer when their health care delivery system is sensitive and responsive to their medical, rehabilitative, social, and emotional needs. This project provides alternative models of long-term care such as adult day care, primary health care, rehabilitation, home care, transportation, housing, social services, and hospitalization. An interdisciplinary team handles case management. OTs and COTAs are important team members with their strong skills of prevention, adaptation, and restoration of function. Involvement in PACE is a good fit with the movement of OT toward community-based and wellness programming (Alexander, 2000).

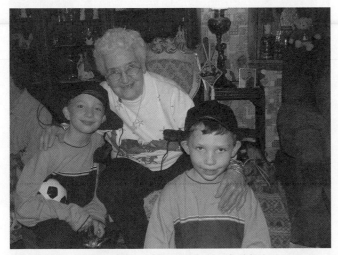

FIGURE 1-4 This elder widow in the mid old stage remains active with minimal adaptations to her lifestyle. (Courtesy Helene Lohman, Creighton University, Omaha, NE.)

PACE has been demonstrated to be a successful program meeting its goals of consumer approval, decreased institutional care, controlled usage of medical services, and decreased costs (Eng, Pedulla, Eleazer, McCann, Fox, 1997). It may be one answer to the ethical and economic dilemmas regarding ways to meet the increasing needs of elders as they live longer in a health care climate of declining resources and advancing technology.

DEMOGRAPHICAL DATA AND THE GROWTH OF THE AGED POPULATION

Demography is "the study of human populations, particularly the size, distribution, and characteristics of members of population groups" (Potter & Perry, 2002). Demographical data clearly suggest that the aged population is growing. This growth is often referred to in the literature as "the graying of America" (McLean, 1988). The portion of the elder population that consists of those 65 years or older comprises 12.4% of the total U.S. population. This population is expected to continue growing, with the "most rapid increase expected between the years 2010 and 2030 when the 'baby boom' generation will reach age 65" (DHHS, 2001). The elder generation is projected to be 20% of the total population by the year 2030 (DHHS, 2001). Minority elder populations also are growing rapidly and are projected to represent 25.4% of the elder population by the year 2030 compared with 16.4% of the elder population in 2000 (DHHS, 2001). Future generations of elders will be more ethnically and racially variant than the current elder population. By 2050, the elder white population is projected to decline from 84% to 64% of the total elder population. The growth of the minority populations will be greatest among Hispanics, who are projected to account for 16% of the elder population in 2050 (Federal Interagency Forum on Aging-Related Statistics, 2000). Many factors contribute to this significant population growth, including a declining mortality rate, advances in medicine and sanitation, improved diet, and improved technology. Figure 1-6 illustrates the growth of the elder population.

Accompanying the "graying of America" is a growth of the female aged population. For every 100 men older than 65 years, there are 143 women. This ratio increases with age. There are 117 women for every 100 men in the 65 to 69 year age group and 245 women for every 100 men in the 85 years and older age group (DHHS, 2001). Although women on average live longer than men, many function in their later years with chronic health conditions and disabilities (Bierman & Clancy, 2001), along with decreased function with ADL (Alecxih, 2001), which indicates a need for OT intervention.

About 45% of women older than 65 years are widows, and there are almost four times as many widows as widowers (DHHS, 2001); these statistics have broad sociocultural

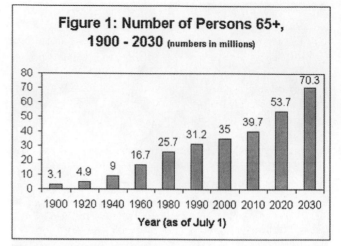

FIGURE 1-6 Number of persons 65 years of age and older: 1900 to 2030. (Adapted and reprinted with permission from the U. S. Department of Health and Human Services [DHHS]. [2001]. A profile of older Americans. Accessed September, 13, 2003. Available at http://www.hhs.gov/)

implications (Figure 1-7). A major consequence for some elder women with the loss of a spouse is an increased risk for poverty. Recent data indicate that widowed women account for approximately one third of all poor elders (Holden & Kim, 2001).

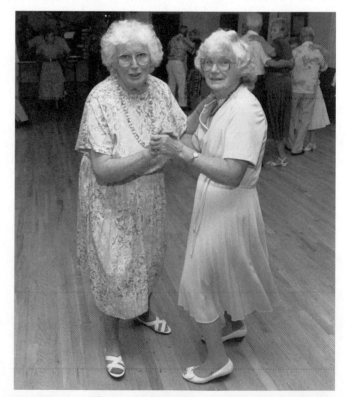

FIGURE 1-7 There are almost five times as many widows as widowers.

The Aging of the Aged Population

The fastest growing segment of the elder population is the 85 years and older cohort. As of 2000, elders older than 85 years comprised 2% of the total population and their size is projected to increase to 5% by 2050 (Federal Interagency Forum on Aging-Related Statistics, 2000). The 85 years and older cohorts have their own unique needs because they have the greatest proportion of morbidity, disability, and institutionalization of all age groups (Suzman, 2001). They are at increased risk for disabilities (DHHS, 2001) and other health problems such as cardiovascular disease and vision and hearing problems. The risk for serious injuries from falling increases as aging progresses (Tideiksaar, 2001). In addition, the risk for severe cognitive impairment is much greater in the 85 years and older age group. Approximately 33% of those 85 years and older experience moderate to severe memory impairment compared with 4.4% of elders between 65 and 69 years of age (Federal Interagency Forum On Aging-Related Statistics, 2000). Not surprisingly, the 85 years and older group uses a large amount of health, financial, and social services provided by public policies such as Medicare and Medicaid (Suzman, 2001). This large usage of federal money along with concerns about increasing costs may have future implications for continual modifications of public policies.

The 85 years and older age cohort is more likely to be institutionalized compared with their younger age cohorts. Although only 4.5% of the 65 years and older population are in nursing homes, 18.2% of those 85 years and older reside in institutional settings (DHHS, 2001). The need for long-term care is anticipated to increase as this age group grows (Alecxih, 2001; Suzman, 2001), especially for those with no living children or those living alone without other supports.

Although there are more elders among the 85 years and older population than any age cohort that lives in nursing homes and other long-term care facilities, the majority still reside in the community (Figure 1-8). Living in the community presents challenges because the need for assistance with ADL functions dramatically increases with age (Alecxih, 2001). "ADL include bathing, dressing, eating, and going around the house. Instrumental activities of daily living (IADL) include preparing meals, shopping, managing money, using a telephone, and doing housework" (DHHS, 2001).

Many elders require a support system to have assistance with ADL. Currently, more than half of those 75 years and older live by themselves in households, and only 28% of women 75 years and older live with a spouse (DHHS, 2001). Many members of this age cohort also live with family members such as adult children who provide assistance with ADL functions. The majority of care provided in the community is by family members and is an unpaid service (National Academy on an Aging Society,

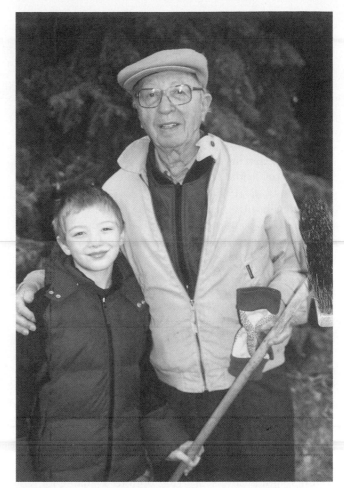

FIGURE **1-8**   This 90-year-old elder remains well and active in the community.

2000a). A future trend that may influence the type of caregiving needed for some members of the Baby Boom generation when they become the elder generation is a larger percentage of couples that are childless. Other supports such as friends or paid support will need to be accessed (Alecxih, 2001).

Another important factor to consider is that some elders, particularly the old old age group, have relatively minimal formal education (Suzman, 2001). However, the education level of all elders is increasing. The number of elders completing a high school education increased from 16% in 1970 to 70% in 2000. Approximately 16% of elders have a baccalaureate degree or higher (DHHS, 2001). Residents of nursing homes tend to have a lower education level (Spector, Fleishman, Pezzin, & Sprillman, 2000). Knowing the educational level of their clients will help COTAs adjust or determine the instruction or training.

The Oldest of the Old: The Centenarians

An even older and quickly growing group of elders are the centenarians, or those elders living beyond 100 years

(Christensen, 2001; Poone, 2002; Schneider, 2002). Researchers are now fascinated about factors contributing to this longevity. Lifestyle, genes, and socioeconomic status are researched contributors to longevity (Schneider, 2002). Of these factors, lifestyle appears to strongly impact longevity (Christensen, 2002; Poone, 2002), although further research is warranted (Poone, 2002). Some centenarians have maintained good health habits (Poone, 2002) and have been in good health throughout their lives. Centenarians mainly experience a rapid decline in health status in their final years of life (Hitt, Young-Xu, Silver, & Perls, 1999). Although more centenarians are in poorer health than the younger cohorts of elders (Poone, 2002), approximately 30% have minimal functional limitations and are quite functional (Christensen, 2002; Poone, 2002).

Living Arrangements

COTAs working in geriatric practice need to consider the elder's home environment as it is linked to finances, health status, and caregiving concerns (Federal Interagency Forum on Aging-Related Statistics, 2000). The majority of noninstitutionalized elders live in family households (Fields & Casper, 2000) and 30% live alone (DHHS, 2001). Age influences living arrangements. Elders between 65 and 74 years of age are more likely to live with a spouse. Elders, especially elder women older than 75 years, have a greater likelihood of living alone because of increased mortality with age (Fields & Casper, 2001).

There are a variety of living options available for elders. For elders with few economic resources, low-income housing is available. However, the number of units is limited and there may be long waiting lists or lottery systems for applicants. Continuing Care Residential Communities and Life-Care Community Housing are other alternatives for elders with low incomes. In some cases, residents are required to contribute all their assets. Residents have contracts for housing, supportive services, and often a continuum of services including health and nursing homes.

Assisted living facilities are a fast growing living option that has been available in the United States since the mid-1980s (Gramann, 1999). Assisted living facilities focus on frail elders or adults with disabilities. With assisted living elders receive care management and supportive services to enable maximal independence in a homelike setting. Assisted living residents need some help to remain independent but do not require the same level of 24-hour care provided in nursing home facilities (Mitty, 2001). Some elders access the additional supports of private-duty home care to remain in assisted living facilities (Gramann, 1999). Typical residents are ambulatory 80-year-old women who require help with at least two ADL (National Center for Assisted Living, 2002). Most residents use private funds to finance assisted living (Hawes, Phillips, & Rose, 2001). In some states,

elders with less income can finance assisted living with Medicaid and Social Security Income (American Association of Homes and Services for the Aging, 2002). The growth of assisted living is attributed to the increase in the aged population, the desire of elders to have their own home and not go into nursing homes, and state policies that limit access to nursing home facilities (Hawes, Phillips, & Rose, 2001). There is much variability in the types of facilities. This variability in facilities and the expensive costs for residents are areas of discussion (Hawes, Phillips, & Rose, 2001).

Board and care homes, personal care, adult day care, adult foster care, family care, and adult congregate living facilities are other alternative care options in the community. Board and care homes service elders, many of whom have been deinstitutionalized. Adult day care is a community-based group program designed to meet the needs of functionally impaired elders. This structured, comprehensive program provides a variety of health, social, and related support services in a protective setting during any part of the day but provides less than 24-hour care. Adult foster homes are family homes or other facilities that provide residential care for elderly or physically disabled residents not related to the provider by blood or marriage. Adult congregate living facilities provide seniors high-rise living accommodations with innovative service delivery options such as team laundry, cleaning, shopping, congregate meals, and home-delivered meals. Home health services also are available but are usually restricted to more acute episodic needs and require some level of homebound restrictions for reimbursement (Glantz & Richman, 1995, personal communication).

For those elders with assets, retirement communities include a variety of services such as leisure activities, congregate meals, laundry, transportation, and possibly health care. Costs have escalated in retirement communities, in some cases forcing residents to find alternative housing (Olson, 1994). In these communities, COTAs can act as activity directors, using their skills to select, analyze, and adapt activities to the abilities and interests of the residents (Glantz & Richman, 1995, personal communication) (see Chapter 8).

A new market-driven trend is the concept of "aging in place." This allows elders to receive a variety of levels of health care in the same facility. Thus, an elder might start out on an independent living unit and when function changes move to an assisted living unit and eventually to a nursing home unit or even an Alzheimer's disease unit all in the same facility (Seniorresource.com, 2002). COTAs working in these facilities can provide continuity of care as the resident's functional status changes. The concept of aging in place also can refer to elders remaining in the community with supports from services such as Senior Cents, adult day care centers, Area Agencies on Aging, and meal programs (Whitelaw, McNickle, & Blaser, 2002).

Most of these discussed living options require having adequate financial assets and good retirement planning because long-term care is costly. In 2002, the average cost for living in an assisted living apartment was $2159 per month or approximately $26,000 a year (MetLife Mature Market Institute, 2002b). Nursing home yearly costs vary across the country with an average cost of $1000 weekly or $52,000 yearly for a semi-private room (MetLife Mature Market Institute, 2002a). Medicare has never paid for long-term care, although many elders mistakenly believe this myth (Smart, 2001). Some elders have shifted their finances to qualify for Medicaid, a program for the indigent that provides some long-term care coverage. This cost shifting has stressed the program (Dychtwald, 1999) and resulted in changes to fix the loopholes.

Most federal funds for elders go toward institutional care rather than home and community services. Funding for community services for elders comes from a variety of programs such as Medicaid and the Older Americans Act (Whitelaw, McNickle, & Blaser, 2002). Long-term care insurance is an option to help people plan for their future long-term care needs. Plans differ but usually cover a variety of long-term care options such as assisted living, nursing home, Meals on Wheels, and home health. Coverage is usually based on the criteria of having difficulty with a set number of ADL. Generally, it is more financially advantageous to purchase a plan when one is younger, which results in lower premiums. Unfortunately, only 10% of elders currently have long-term care insurance (Dychtwald, 1999). Public policy efforts are being discussed to help defray the costs of long-term care insurance (Smith, 2001).

Finally, recent data on community elders suggest that 4.2% of all elders living in the community had difficulty with performing ADL and 21.6% had difficulty with one or more IADL (DHHS, 2001). These data point to one strong reason for OT intervention in any of the discussed settings.

Economic Demographics

Most elders are not impoverished. Data from 1998 suggest that medium- and high-income elders account for more than two thirds of total elders (Federal Interagency Forum on Aging-Related Statistics, 2000). Most elders are better off financially than many of the younger cohorts (Dychtwald, 1999). Elders in the medium- and high-income range will better be able to afford health services and caregiving options.

The economic status of the elder population has been variable over the past 40 years. During the 1960s and 1970s, the elder population was depicted as economically deprived (Gonyea, 1994). The poverty rate in 1966 for elders was 28.5% (Clark, 2001). During the 1990s, the elder population was presented as economically advantaged (Gonyea, 1994). The poverty rate in 1996 for elders was 11% (Clark, 2001). On the basis of current demographics,

the elder poverty rate has declined and recently stabilized (Holden & Kim, 2001). The current poverty rate for the elder population is 10.2% (DHHS, 2001), which is close to the working age population's (ages 18 to 64 years) level of poverty (Federal Interagency Forum on Aging-Related Statistics, 2000). General indicators of becoming impoverished after retirement are work history, occupational type, residence in rural areas (McLaughlin & Jensen, 2001), and preretirement income (Holden & Kim, 2001). Working in professional occupations with higher earnings and cognitive requirements may result in better retirement planning (McLaughlin & Jensen, 2001).

Elder women have a greater poverty rate than elder men. Approximately 12.2% of elder women are poor compared with 7.5% of elder men (DHHS, 2001). The economic statuses of elder men and women differ as a result of many factors. When they were younger, elder women were generally housewives or worked occasionally at paid employment. This resulted in less Social Security benefits and smaller or no pensions. When women become widowed their chances of becoming impoverished increase, especially if they lose their spouse's pension funds (Holden & Kim, 2001). Research suggests that the variables of being white and having an education beyond high school help some widows achieve more financial stability (Holden, & Zick, 1997).

Although there are differences across ethnic groups in rates of poverty, a wide economic disparity exists between white elders and elders of minority groups. Approximately 8.8% of white elders are poor, compared with 22.3% of black elders and 18.8% of Hispanic elders. Elder Hispanic women living alone have the highest poverty rate at 38.3% (DHHS, 2001).

Public policy influences the elder population's economic status. Both Social Security, which provides retirement income for elders, and Social Security Income, which provides some financial support for lower income elders (Holden & Kim, 2001), help elders. These public policies furnish approximately 50% of income for 50% of elders. Social Security has increasingly provided a greater proportion of elder income (Federal Interagency Forum on Aging-Related Statistics, 2000). Overall these public policies have proven to be antipoverty measures for elders (Koppstein, 2001).

Changes are projected to occur because of concerns related to the economic solvency of Social Security. In 2010, the young old, or those elders born between 1941 and 1945, should see a growth in retirement income. However, after 2010, there will be a slow decrease in the economic growth of retirement income, which will most affect the aged cohort born in the early 1960s (Zedlewski & McBride, 1992). According to Zedlewski and McBride (1992), this cohort may be the first to feel the full effects of the 1983 Social Security Amendments, which increased the age for those qualified to receive full retirement benefits. The current retirement age of 65 years will eventually increase to 67 years by 2027 (Rix, 2001). This change, which will be gradually phased in, is applicable to workers who are 62 years of age in the year 2000 (McBride, 1996, personal communication).

The economic solvency of Social Security is related to an increasing aging population with less tax dollars in the federal budget to pay for benefits. Discussed reforms are higher taxes, less benefits, or the privatization of retirement funds. Social Security reform will be an important discussion throughout this century (Clark, 2001). Changes in Medicare and Medicaid policy also will continue to affect the economic status of the elder population, especially if elders are required to pay more money for health care. Adding new benefits such as prescription medication may result in cutbacks in other areas of Medicare or increased costs. Finally, other factors such as the increasing costs of health care and the general state of the American economy also influence the economic status of elders. For example, after the events of September 11, 2001, the stock market took a downswing, which decreased many retirement funds (see Chapter 6 for a discussion about public policy).

Additional Trends and the Influence of Aging Trends on Occupational Therapy Practice

COTAs working with elders need to be aware of aging trends. This section discusses three additional trends that impact elders and their possible influence on COTA practice. One growing trend is elders raising grandchildren. Grandparents in a parenting role can range in age from 40 to 80 years (Dellmann-Jenkins, Blankemyer, & Olesh, 2002). Data from 1997 indicate that grandparents headed 6.7% of families with children younger than 18 years, which was an increase of 19% from 1990. Approximately 3.9 million children were being raised by grandparents (Casper & Bryson, 1999). Grandparents raising grandchildren occurs in all socioeconomic and ethnic groups (Dellmann-Jenkins, Blankemyer, & Olesh, 2002). However, families involving grandmothers solely raising grandchildren are more likely to be living in poverty (Casper & Bryson, 1998). Reasons for this phenomenon vary and can result from substance abuse, teen pregnancy, and divorce (Casper & Bryson, 1998). Grandparents raising children can experience major challenges. For example, some elders may be dealing with their own health or financial issues at the same time as the stresses of caregiving. Another challenge can be the alienation of the grandparents from family and friend supports because of their involvement in caregiving (Roe, & Minkler, 1998). However, some grandparents in a parenting role express enhanced self-worth (Dellmann-Jenkins, Blankemyer, & Olesh, 2002). COTAs working with elders in this situation need to be sensitive to the demands and enjoyment of this parenting role.

A second trend will be an increase in elders remaining in the workforce. Data from 2000 indicate that 30.3% of workers 65 to 69 years old and 12.2% of workers 70 years and older remain in the workforce (Federal Interagency Forum on Aging-Related Statistics, 2002). The percentages of elders remaining employed have varied over the past 40 years with the greatest percentage occurring in the 1960s. A gradual decrease in workforce participation took place during the 1980s (Federal Interagency Forum on Aging-Related Statistics, 2000). Since the late 1990s, the percentage of elders remaining in the workforce has gradually increased (Federal Interagency Forum on Aging-Related Statistics, 2002) and projections are for a continual growth of elders in the workforce, especially from the Baby Boomer generation (American Association of Retired Persons, 1998; Richard, D'Amico, & Geipel, 1997). Declining birth rates resulting in less available workers may influence more elders to stay in the workforce (Dychtwald, 2000). In addition, public policy such as changes in the Social Security Act from the 1983 amendments will influence the next generation of elders to remain in the workforce. These amendments allow increases in payment if retirement is delayed between the ages of 65 and 69. As discussed earlier, by 2027, full Social Security benefits will not be allowed until a person is 67 years old (Rix, 2001). The Age Discrimination in Employment Act of 1967 and its amendments along with the removal of required retirement laws also help elder workers remain in the workforce.

Currently, most employed elders work part-time or in service industries. Technology impacts most jobs (Marshall, 2001). Typical characteristics of current elder workers are being white, male, married, educated, financially secure, and healthy (National Academy on an Aging Society, 2000b). These characteristics will change with societal changes. For example, with the growth of the elder minority population, more minority elders may remain in the future workforce. The phenomenon of the elder worker, however, has not been extensively studied and many questions remain about the impact of work on elders (Marshall, 2001). The influence of an aging labor force on OT practice also remains to be seen. However, innovative therapists may identify new areas of practice to ensure continual success of elders in the workforce.

A third trend influencing elders is the increased usage of computer technology. Approximately 24.3% of elder households have a computer and 17.7% have Internet access (DHHS, 2001). The usage of computers by elders has many advantages, such as decreasing isolation and providing telemedical support (Mundorf & Brownell, 2001). Computers can assist elders with making purchases, which is a helpful benefit for those who are homebound (Figure 1-9). Adaptive computer programs aid elders with disabilities. For example, voice programs help elders with arthritis who have difficulty with keyboarding.

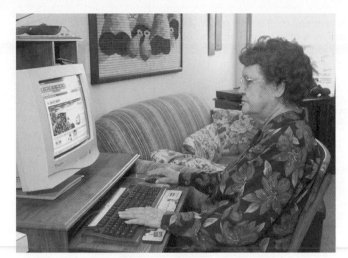

FIGURE 1-9   Elders may use computers to access the Internet to make online purchases.

Elders with low vision can benefit from many computer programs geared for their visual needs. Elders who desire more intergenerational contact can achieve this contact through discussion groups on the World Wide Web (Mundorf & Brownell, 2001). Although there are many benefits of computers, some elders are reluctant to embrace this technology or are unable to afford it. In addition, if elders do not have computer access at home, it may be difficult for some to get to public places, such as libraries, where there is free access. COTAs can suggest computer resources in the community, such as state sites supported by the Assistive Technology Act, which provide computer training, or libraries. They can suggest appropriate software to assist elders with functional concerns and can make adaptations to allow computer usage.

In summary, these three highlighted trends are examples from many trends influencing elders. As the elder generation continues to grow and as society continues to change, it will be paramount that COTAs remain aware of aging trends and consider them in terms of society and OT practice.

Implications for Occupational Therapy Practice

Because of continued growth of the elder population, the need for OTs and COTAs working with them will increase. The effects of all the demographics, issues, and trends discussed in this chapter on OT practice remain to be seen. However, it can be assumed that in the future, dilemmas related to limited resources will affect the practice arena. When the Baby Boom cohorts reach 85 years of age between the years 2032 and 2048, Manton (1991) states "it will produce a major policy challenge to provide community and institutional long term care (LTC) services to a significant portion of the U.S. population" (p. 314). At this time, no one can predict whether there will be adequate funding and social services to meet the needs of a growing elder population and whether there will be enough health care resources to address this population's health care needs. The increasing cost of health care (Holden & Kim, 2001), the ever changing economy, and the tenuous state of Social Security are current concerns that have future implications for the aged population. OT personnel will continue to be challenged to provide quality treatment in a cost-constrained environment. New models of OT geriatric care will evolve in the future, especially in community settings where the majority of elders remain. All OT personnel should be at the front end of this evolution.

INTERGENERATIONAL CONCEPTS

In today's society, same-age cohorts socialize for the most part among themselves and have minimal **intergenerational** contact. When they work in a nursing home, COTAs may have little daily interaction with well elders in the community. COTAs treat elders who are often two or three generations removed.

COTAs must be aware of generational values to better understand some elders' perceptions of treatment interventions. Some elder patients may refuse to purchase adaptive equipment because of a generational value regarding thrift that evolved from the Depression era. The exercise in Figure 1-10 demonstrates that each generation has certain values and attitudes that are influenced by similar generational experiences and historic events (Davis, 1987). Yet each person has his or her own story to tell. This exercise can be completed as a group or individually.

COTAs must have meaningful contact, either informally or formally, with both well and frail elderly to work effectively with the elder population. Many benefits are mentioned in the literature about formal intergenerational programs. Some of these benefits include a better understanding of the elder generation from a historical perspective and their values and beliefs (Lohman, Griffiths, Coppard, & Cota, 2003), mutual learning from each generation (Hirshborn & Piering, 1998/1999; Lapp, 1991), dispelling of myths (Adelman, Hainer, Butler, & Chalmers, 1998), and encouraging respect (Pine, 1997) (Figure 1-11).

AGEISM, MYTHS, AND STEREOTYPES ABOUT THE AGED

If you are a man and you are prejudiced against women, you will never know how a woman feels. If you are white and you are prejudiced against blacks, you will never know how a black person feels. But if you are young and you are prejudiced against the old, you are indeed prejudiced against yourself, because you, too, will have the honor of being old someday.

—C. Lewis, 1989

Fill in the following lifelines with significant historical and personal events about yourself, someone from the generation 10 years older than you, one of your parents, and one of your grandparents. After filling in the lifeline, answer the questions below. Refer to the following example:

Grandparent:

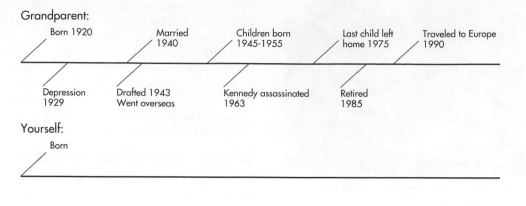

Yourself:

Born

Someone 10 years older than you:

Born

Your parent (choose one):

Born

Your grandparent (choose one):

Born

Answer the following questions:
What significant intergenerational differences did you notice between your generation, your parents' generation, your grandparents' generation, and even the generation 10 years older than you? What are some of the significant values of each generation and how were they influenced by historical events?
How might these similarities and differences between generations affect clinical treatment? *— Resist to change Must have patience fast paced*

FIGURE 1-10   Lifeline exercise. (Adapted from Davis, L. J., & Kirkland, M. [1987]. *ROTE: The role of occupational therapy with the elderly: Faculty guide.* Rockville, MD: American Occupational Therapy Association, with permission.)

"Ageism is an attitude that discriminates, separates, stigmatizes, or otherwise disadvantages older adults on the basis of chronological age" (Mosby, p. 53, 2002). **Ageism** is a form of prejudice because it promotes general assumptions, or stereotypes, about a group of people.

These assumptions are not true for all members of that group. Following are some stereotypes of ageism:

- Elders are useless because they can't see, hear, or remember.
- Elders are slow when they move about.

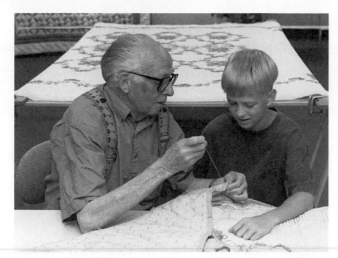

FIGURE 1-11   Older generations can give support and advice to younger generations.

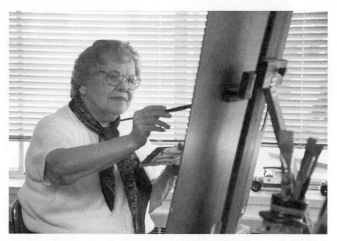

FIGURE 1-12   Contrary to myth, this elder has embraced a new occupation.

- Elders are in ill health.
- Elders cannot learn new things.
- Elders drain the economy rather than contribute to it; they are unproductive.
- Elders are too old to remain part of the workforce.
- Elders cannot perform or enjoy sexual activity.
- Elders prefer being with and talking with other elders.
- Elders are depressed and complain about all that is new.
- Elders are rich; or elders are poor.

Many of these statements have been challenged by research. With any stereotype, there may be a small amount of truth for some members of the group. For example, it is true that elders frequently need glasses as aging progresses; however, the need for glasses does not render an elder useless. An unfortunate result of these myths is that some elders may believe them. For example, whereas young persons may joke about becoming forgetful, elders may seriously question their cognitive abilities as a result of the stereotype that elders have trouble remembering (Figure 1-12).

These stereotypes may develop as a result of fear of the unknown, or from lack of contact with the aged. American culture often focuses on youth. Youth is seen as beautiful, as something to aspire to and maintain at any cost. Young is sexy, and old is not.

The medical system in the United States also has been focused on youth. The goal of this system has traditionally been to find a cure for all illnesses. This goal has prompted significant contributions to the world's health care; however, the belief in a cure for all ills may conflict with the care elder citizens need. With the United States' current technological knowledge, some chronic illnesses of old age can only be managed, not cured.

In the health care system, references to ageism often occur as a response to a medical diagnosis. OT documentation that begins, "This 91-year-old female was admitted

with the diagnosis of total hip replacement," may trigger preconceived ideas based on age bias, such as the opinion that the client is too old for treatment. Readers of this type of documentation may question the benefits versus risks of surgery or OT treatment for this elder.

In day-to-day interactions, language can encourage ageism. People working in the health care field may unintentionally be condescending when they refer to elders as "dear," "darling," or "sweetie" (French, 1990). Simply referring to a person as the older stroke patient in Room 570 dehumanizes the person. Stating that a person is incapable of doing a task because of being old or having some deficits without a true understanding of the person's functional abilities also promotes ageism. The following story illustrates this concept. At an assisted living facility there were several elders who had mild to moderate cognitive deficits. The COTA knew each elder as a human being and had an understanding of each person's identified meaningful occupations. For elders who valued cooking, the COTA organized a cooking group followed by a party. She adapted the activity so that all the elders would be successful. Before the cooking activity the team leader expressed negative feelings because she felt that the elders would be incapable of cooking. The team leader was surprised to observe that the cooking activity turned out to be beneficial and successful for the elders. The leader later honestly remarked that oftentimes her feelings of being "protective" of the residents got in her way. Feeling protective of elders does promote ageism. A protective attitude can encourage assumptions such as elders are incapable or elders are like children. Sometimes staff working with elders who have cognitive deficits and have regressed in their function can inadvertently talk to them in a childish manner. Unprofessional actions also can reflect ageism. One COTA who had a very full day skipped an appointment with an elder assuming that the elder had a cognitive

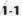

Reflection Questions about Ageism

- How did I respond to the elders I saw today?
- Am I aware of any actions or language that I used that might promote ageism?
- Am I aware of any actions or language that others used that might promote ageism?

deficit and would not remember. Later that day the elder called the COTA to inquire about what happened. The COTA learned a hard lesson from that experience about her own ageism. As these stories illustrate, reflection often helps people realize stereotypical beliefs and attitudes that they harbor. A way to be more aware of ageism and general attitudes is to record one's feeling about contact with elders in a journal. Box 1-1 provides reflection questions about ageism that COTAs should ask themselves.

Perspectives are beginning to change as reflected in initiatives such as the International Classification of Functioning, Disability and Health, or ICF (World Health Organization, 2001) and Healthy People 2010 (DHHS, 2000). The ICF "provides a unified and standardized language and framework for the description of health and health-related domains…" (World Health Organization, 2001, p. 3). It is used "to code a wide range of information about health (e.g. diagnosis, functioning, and disability, reasons for contact with health services)…" (p. 3). The ICF focuses on components that constitute health, rather than the consequences or impact of disease. The ICF considers not just the disease but also the environmental context in which people live (World Health Organization, 2001).

The Occupational Therapy Practice Framework (American Occupational Therapy Association [AOTA], 2002) reflects perspectives from the ICF. The Practice Framework considers the treatment process within the broad "domain" of occupational therapy (AOTA, 2002). Similar to the ICF, the Practice Framework takes into account the influence of context on occupation. Context includes "culture, physical, social, personal, temporal, spiritual, and virtual" (p. 612) dimensions. As Youngstrom (2002) stated, "Occupational therapists {need} to understand their role within a larger societal and health context in order to position themselves in changing traditional areas and to take advantage of opportunities in emerging areas" (p. 607). (See Chapter 7 for more information about the Occupational Therapy Practice Framework.)

Healthy People 2010 "is committed to a single, overarching purpose: promoting health and preventing illness, disability, and premature death" (DHHS, 2000, p. 1). It is based on the following two goals: (1) "increase quality and years of healthy life and (2) eliminate health disparity"

(DHHS, 2000, p. 1). Both goals impact the elder population. (See Chapter 5 for more information about Healthy People 2010.)

Many aspects of American society, including housing, employment, and recreational resources, are geared toward youth. However, that focus is slowly changing with the emergence of the senior citizen as a powerful political and economic force and with the growth of the aged population. Who knows what changes the next generation of elders, the Baby Boomers, will bring to society.

▮ CHAPTER REVIEW QUESTIONS

1 Define the terms *gerontology*, *geriatrics*, and *cohort*.
2 What is the relation between aging and illness?
3 What are the dismissal and client-centred approaches? How might they affect client care?
4 What considerations should be taken for managing clients with chronic illnesses?
5 What factors are related to the significant population growth of the elder generation?
6 What is a result of more widows than widowers among the elder population?
7 What are some of the needs of the 85 years and older generation?
8 What does the COTA need to know about the educational level of any elder for treatment interventions?
9 What age group has the highest poverty rate and why?
10 How has public policy influenced the economic status of elders?
11 What are some implications of the demographical data for future occupational therapy practice?
12 How do you think the three discussed trends (grandparents raising children, aging workforce, and increased computer usage) can impact occupational therapy practice?
13 How do you keep abreast of aging trends?
14 What is ageism? Provide examples of it in today's culture.
15 What were misconceptions you had about growth of the aged population, minority elders, the old old (85 years and older), economic demographics, and living arrangements before reading this chapter?
16 What are some of your ideas about what will happen when the Baby Boomers become the elder generation?

REFERENCES

Adelman, M. D., Hainer, J., Butler, R. N., & Chalmers, M. (1998). A well elderly program: An intergenerational model in medical communication. *The Gerontologist*, 28(3), 409-413.

Alecxih, L. (2001). The impact of sociodemographic change on the future of long-term care. *Generations*, 25, 7-11.

Alexander, T. C. (2000). Setting the PACE: The innovative program of all-inclusive care for the elderly offers a perfect fit for occupational therapists. *OTPractice, 4*, 20-22.

American Association of Homes and Services for the Aging. (2002). Discovering assisted living [WWW page]. URL http://www.aahsa.org/public/al.htm

American Association of Retired Persons (AARP). (1998). Baby Boomers envision their retirement: An AARP segmentation analysis [WWW page]. http://research.aarp.org/econ/boomer_seg_3.html

American Occupational Therapy Association. (2000). *2000 compensation survey: Final report*. Bethesda, MD.

American Occupational Therapy Association. (2002). Occupational therapy practice framework: Domain and process. *The American Journal of Occupational Therapy, 56*(6), 609-639.

Bierman, A. S., Haffer, S. C., & Hwang, Y. T. (2001). Health disparities among older women enrolled in Medicare managed care. *Health Care Financing Review, 22*, 4, 187-198.

Casper, L. M., & Bryson, K. R. (1999). Co-resident grandparents and their grandchildren: Grandparent maintained families. *International Population Reports, P23-198*, 1-10.

Christensen, D. (2001). Making sense of centenarians: Genes and lifestyle help people live through a century. *Science News, 159*(10), 156-157.

Clark, R. L. (2001). Economics. In R. C. Atchley (Ed.), *The encyclopedia of aging: A comprehensive resource in gerontology and geriatrics* (3rd ed., Vol. 2). pp. 319-321. New York, NY: Springer.

Davis, L.J., & Kirkland, M. (Eds)(1987). *ROTE: The role of occupational therapy with the elderly: faculty guide*. Module I Teaching Resources Gerontology in Theory and Practice. pp. 71-79. Rockville, MD: American Occupational Therapy Association.

Dellmann-Jenkins, M., Blankemyer, B., & Olesh, M. (2002). Adults in expanded grandparent roles: Consideration for practice policy, and research. *Educational Gerontology, 28*(3), 219-235.

Dychtwald, K. (1999). *Age power: How the 21st century will be ruled by the new old*. New York, NY: Jeremy P. Tarcher/Putnam.

Dychtwald, K. (2000). *Ken Dychtwald, author of "age power" discusses older people in the workforce* [Today Show]. New York, NY: National Broadcasting Company (NBC).

Eng, C., Pedulla, J., Eleazer, P., McCann, R., & Fox, N. (1997). Program of all-inclusive care for the elderly (PACE): An innovative model of integrated geriatric care and financing. *Journal of the American Geriatric Society, 45*, 223-232.

Federal Interagency Forum on Aging-Related Statistics. (2000). Older Americans 2000: Key indicators of well-being. *Federal Interagency Forum on Aging-Related Statistics*.

Fields, J., & Casper, L. M. (2001). America's families and living arrangements. *Current Population Reports Series, P20-537*, 1-16.

French, S. (1990) Ageism. *Physiotherapy, 76*(3), 178-182.

Glantz, C. (1996) Personal communication.

Glantz, C., & Richman N (1995) Personal comunication.

Gonyea, J. G. (1994). The paradox of the advantaged elder and the feminization of poverty. *Social Work, 39*(1), 35-41.

Gramann, D. (1999). New frontiers in integrated care. *Caring Magazine, 18*(4), 14-17.

Hawes, C., Phillips, C. D., & Rose, M. (2001). Assisted living: A new model of supportive housing with long-term care services. In R. C. Atchley (Ed.), *The encyclopedia of aging: A comprehensive resource in gerontology and geriatrics* (3rd ed., Vol. 1). New York, NY: Springer.

Hirshhorn, B. A., & Piering, P. (1998/1999). Older people at risk: Issues and intergenerational responses. *Generations*, 49-53.

Hitt, R., Young-Xu, Y., Silver, M., & Perls, T. (1999). Centenarians: The older you get, the healthier you have been. *The Lancet, 354*(9179), 652.

Holden, D. C., & Zick, C. (1997). The economic impact of widowhood in the 1990s: Evidence from the survey of income and program. *Consumer Interests Annual, 43*(34), 34-39.

Holden, K. C. A., & Kim, M. (2001). Poverty. In R. C. Atchley (Ed.), *The encyclopedia of aging: A comprehensive resource in gerontology and geriatrics* (3rd ed., Vol. 2). New York, NY: Springer.

Koppstein, R. (2001). Poverty. In M. D. Mezey (Ed.), *The encyclopedia of elder care*. New York, NY: Springer.

Lapp, C. A. (1991). Nursing students and the elderly: Enhancing intergenerational communication through human-animal interaction. *Holistic Nurse Practioner, 5*(2), 72-79.

Law, M. (2000). Identifying occupational performance issues. In V. G. Fearing & J. Clark (Eds.), *Individuals in context: A practical guide to client-centered practice* (pp. 31-45). Thorofare, NJ: SLACK Incorporated.

Law, M., Baptiste, S., Carswell, A., McCall, M.A., Polatajko, H., & Pollock, N. (1998). *Canadian Occupational Performance Measure* (3rd Ed.). Ottawa, Ontario, Canada: CAOT Publications ACE.

Law, M., & Mills, J. (1998). Client-centred occupational therapy. In M. Law (Ed.), *Client-centered occupational therapy* (pp. 1-18). Thorofare, NJ: SLACK Incorporated.

Lazer, W. (1985). Inside the mature market. *American Demographics, 48*(7), 25-43.

Lewis, C. (1989). How the myths of aging impact rehabilitative care for the older person. *Occupational Therapy Forum, 10*, 10, 11, 14, 15.

Lohman, H., Griffiths, Y., Coppard, B., & Cota, L. (2003). The power of book discussion groups in intergenerational learning. *Educational Gerontology, 29*(2), 103-116.

Manton, K. G. (1991). The dynamics of population aging: Demography and policy analysis. *Milbank Quarterly, 69*, 309-340.

Marshall, N. L. (2001). Health and illness issues facing an aging workforce in the new millennium. *Sociological Spectrum, 21*(3), 431-501.

McLaughlin, D. K., & Jensen, L. (2001). Work history and U.S. elders' transition into poverty. *The Gerontologist, 40*(4), 469-480.

McLean, C. (1988). The graying of America. *Oregon Starter, 11*. 11-17.

MetLife Mature Market Institute. (2002a). *MetLife market survey on nursing home and home care costs*. Westport, CT: Metropolitan Life Insurance Company.

MetLife Mature Market Institute. (2002b). *MetLife survey of assisted living costs 2002*. Westport, CT: Metropolitan Life Insurance Company.

Mitty, E.L., (2001). Nursing homes. In R. C. Atchley (Ed.), *The encyclopedia of aging: A comprehensive resource in gerontology and geriatrics* (3rd ed., Vol. 2). pp. 749-755. New York, NY: Springer.

Mundorf, N., & Brownell, H. (2001). Communication technologies and older adults. In R. C. Atchley (Ed.), *The encyclopedia of aging: A comprehensive resource in gerontology and geriatrics* (3rd ed., Vol. 1). pp. 224-226. New York, NY: Springer.

National Academy on an Aging Society. (2000a). Caregiving: Helping the elderly with activity limitations [Text file]. URL http://www.agingsociety.org/agingsociety/pdf/Caregiving.pdf

National Academy on an Aging Society. (2000b). Who are young retirees and older workers [Text file]. URL http://www.agingsociety.org/agingsociety/pdf/aarp1.pdf

National Center for Assisted Living. (2002). Assisted living resident profile [Text file]. URL http://www.ncal.org/about/resident.htm

Neugarten, B. L. (1974). Age groups in American society and the rise of the young-old. *Annals of the American Academy of Political and Social Sciences, 415*, 187-188.

Olson, L. K. (1994) *The graying of the world: Who will care for the frail elderly?* New York, NY: Hawthorne Press.

Pine, P.P. (1997). Learning by sharing: An intergenerational course. *Journal of Gerontological Social Work, 28*, 93-102.

Poone, L. W. (2002). Centenarians. In G. L. Maddox (Ed.), *The encyclopedia of aging: A comprehensive resource in gerontology and geriatrics* (3rd ed., Vol. 1). New York, NY: Springer.

Potter, P. A., & Perry, A. G. (2002) *Mosby medical, nursing & allied health dictionary* (6th ed.). St. Louis, MO: Mosby.

Richard J. W., D'Amico, C. D., & Geipel, G. L. (1997). *Workforce 2020: Work and workers in the 21st century.* Indianapolis, IN: Hudson Institute.

Rix, S. (2001). Employment. In R. C. Atchley (Ed.), *The encyclopedia of aging: A comprehensive resource in gerontology and geriatrics* (3rd ed., Vol. 2). New York, NY: Springer.

Roe, K. M., & Minkler, M. (1998). Grandparents raising grandchildren: Challenges and responses. *Generations, 22*, 25-32.

Sahyoun, N. R., Pratt, L. A., Lentzner, H., Dey, A., & Robinson, K. N. (2001). The changing profile of nursing home residents: 1985-1997 [Text file]. URL http://www.cdc.gov/nchs/data/agingtrends/04nursin.pdf

Schneider, J. (2002). 100 and counting. *U.S. News & World Report, 132*(19), 86.

Senior*resource*.com (2002). Aging in place [WWW page]. URL http://www.seniorresource.com/ageinpl.htm#ageinpltop

Smart, T. (2001). Long-term care: An idea coming of age? [News Bulletin]. URL http://www.aarp.org/bulletin/longterm/articles/a2003-06-23-longtermcareinsurance.html

Smith, T. (2001). Long-term care: An idea coming of age? [News Bulletin]. URL http://www.seniorresource.com/ageinpl.htm

Spector, W. D., Fleishman, J. A., Pezzin, L. E., & Sprillman, B. C. (2000). *The characteristics of long-term care users.* Rockville, MD: AHRQ.

Suzman R. M. (2001). Oldest old. In R. C. Atchley (Ed.), *The encyclopedia of aging: A comprehensive resource in gerontology and geriatrics* (3rd ed., Vol. 2). New York, NY: Springer.

Tideiksaar, R. (2001). Falls. *The encyclopedia of aging: A comprehensive resource in gerontology and geriatrics* (3rd ed., Vol. 1). New York, NY: Springer.

U. S. Department of Health and Human Services (DHHS). (2001). A profile of older Americans [WWW page]. URL http://www.hhs.gov/

U. S. Department of Health and Human Services. (2000). *Healthy people 2010: Understanding and improving health.* Washington, DC: Government Printing Office.

Whitelaw, N., McNickle, L., & Blaser, J. (2002). Expanded long-term care choices for the elderly: Aging in place [WWW page]. URL http://www.ahrq.gov/news/ulp/ltc/ulpltc8.htm

World Health Organization. (2001). *ICF: International Classification of Functioning, Disability and Health.* Geneva, Switzerland: World Health Organization.

Youngstrom, M. J. (2002). The occupational therapy practice framework: The evolution of our professional language. *The American Journal of Occupational Therapy, 56*(6), 607-608.

Zedlewski, S. R., McBride T. D. (1992) The changing profile of the elderly: Effects on future long-term care needs and financing. *Milbank Quarterly, 70*(2), 247-275.

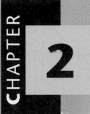

CHAPTER 2

Social and Biological Theories of Aging

MARLENE J. AITKEN

Michelle is a certified occupational therapy assistant (COTA) employed in an assisted living center that offers several levels of care. Her daily work involves treating elders who have a variety of diagnosed conditions and the planning of occupation-based activities. Michelle has observed that although many of the elders have some type of problem that requires rehabilitation, each reacts differently to illness and the aging process. At least once a week Michelle meets Kelly, a registered occupational therapist (OTR), for a supervision session, when they thoroughly discuss each person receiving OT. Michelle feels comfortable discussing almost any concern with Kelly.

After reviewing the caseload during one particular session, Michelle and Kelly began a lively discussion about the complexities of aging. Michelle noted that some of the elders who she treats as part of her caseload seem active and vigorous, whereas others seemed withdrawn and active and vigorous, whereas others seemed withdrawn and

had low energy to do therapeutic tasks. She also commented that some of the elders seemed older than their chronological age, whereas others seemed their age or younger. Kelly encouraged Michelle to review theories about aging to form a context in which to think about the elders. The next week Michelle and Kelly discussed the application of the theories to their work with elders who are part of their caseloads.

Questions like Michelle's regarding reasons for aging and the differences in aging are unanswered because aging research consists of many different studies and perspectives. COTAs need to understand the content of many theories because they help provide the scientific basis for treatment and explain, describe, and predict behavior (Holm, Rogers, & Stone, 2003). The biological theories may answer some questions about the reasons for aging. However, there have been many diverse theories proposed to account for the biological mechanisms of aging. Despite the efforts of many researchers, little progress has been made to identify a single cohesive theory of biological aging. This probably is a reflection that aging occurs in response to a variety of mechanisms.

Social theorists are concerned with the social consequences of aging and provide insight on the ways people age successfully. This chapter uses the format of current biological, social, and psychological theories to provide insight on social aspects of aging. (The physical and psychological changes that occur with the aging process are described in Chapters 3 and 4.)

BIOLOGICAL THEORIES OF AGING

The population of people older than 65 years of age is growing rapidly. This group begins to face illnesses that become more prevalent as the aging process continues. However, most studies of human aging find that no uniform rate of aging exists.

Individuals of the same age demonstrate differences in age-related variables such as vital capacity and glomerular filtration rate in the kidneys (Schneider & Reed, 1985). The major current theories that attempt to explain this differential aging fit into one of two categories: **genetic aging**, which presumes that aging is predetermined, and **nongenetic aging**, which presumes that aging events occur randomly and accumulate with time (Abrams, Beers, & Berkow, 1995). The four genetic aging theories are programmed aging, somatic mutation, free radical, and cybernetic. The nongenetic theory is the wear and tear theory.

Genetic Theories

Programmed aging

The premise of the programmed aging theories is that the human body has an inherited internal "genetic clock" that determines the beginning of the aging process. This genetic clock may manifest as a predetermined number of cell divisions, called the *Hayflick Limit*, which can occur for some individuals (Hayflick, 1987). However, the existence of a single "aging clock" that times the aging process has been questioned. Each outcome may be influenced by a wide range of factors—some are genetic, some are accidental, some vary across individuals, and some are shared but differing from person to person. Hearing loss, decreased cardiovascular endurance, cataracts, slower healing, and so on are not universal among 70-year-old people, but it is rare to find a 70-year-old person who has escaped all of these conditions, and it is equally rare to find a 20-year-old impaired by any of these conditions (Miller, 1999). If each body system had its own clock, there would be a lot of clocks to be adjusted one gene at a time, unless the genes are linked in some way.

Studies of living cells in the laboratory have shown that some cells lose the ability to replicate or divide with time.

Cells are thought to become more specialized with each turnover cycle until they can no longer replicate effectively. Some scientists believe that aging may be caused by an impairment of cells in the translation of necessary ribonucleic acid (RNA) as a result of the ineffective communication with deoxyribonucleic acid (DNA). Although the essential messages may be transcribed at all ages, the translation of these messages into functional proteins may be restricted in elders (Arking & Giroux, 2001). The cell may stop exchanging genetic information with DNA, and without genetic guidance the cell may become senescent, or old (Hayflick, 1968).

The significance of this theory continues to be debated. Studies have established that either some segments of DNA become depleted with advancing age or selected cellular structures seem to change with age so that the transcription of certain DNA is restricted.

Miller (1999) states that "the idea that aging is 'programmed in the genes' the same way development is programmed is incorrect because although natural selection affects the persistence of genetic characters that affect the development of mature adults, the decline of function that is the hallmark of aging represents an impediment and cannot be the direct outcome of an evolutionary selective process" (p. 306). In addition, heritability studies have found that more than 75% of the variation in lifespan can be explained by nongenetic factors; therefore, it is no longer reasonable to believe that longevity is "only in the genes."

Currently, there is no clear way to measure an individual's biological age. Measuring biological age would be helpful for those who wish to locate genes that influence aging, those who wish to develop antiaging interventions, and those who wish to time the aging process and link it to age-sensitive outcomes, including most important diseases.

The ongoing gene-mapping programs may help in concluding whether lifespan can be significantly altered with a variation of only a half dozen (rather than hundreds) gene locations. Additional studies will be needed to determine if the findings in the pioneering studies apply to other environments or other genetic backgrounds.

Somatic mutation theory

According to the somatic mutation theory, spontaneous unexpected chromosomal changes occur as a result of miscoding, translation errors, chemical reactions, irradiation, and spontaneous replication of errors. Mutations can occur in the tissues of aging animals. Cumulative mistakes occur not only in DNA but in RNA and enzyme synthesis. These mistakes result in progressive loss of function or feedback to the cell.

Many health problems in elders are related to immune system dysfunction, including late onset diabetes and cancer. The somatic mutation theory relates aging to the way the immune system increasingly makes mistakes by identifying the body's own cells as foreign and reacting against them. This theory is one explanation for the greater frequency of cancer in the elderly or the aging of the immune system ascribed to the elderly (Gupta & Lutz, 1999; Holliday, 2000).

Free radical theory

The free radical theory of large molecular injury looks at the products of oxygen utilization within cells. Oxidation of lipids, proteins, fats, and carbohydrates (large molecules) can result in the formation of oxygen compounds with an extra electron charge or "free radical." Additional free radicals are formed whenever metallic ions, enzymes, or cellular materials combine with oxygen. Proponents of this theory believe that low-level, free radical damage accumulates over time, resulting in age-associated decline of function in major organs such as the kidneys (Abrams, Beers, & Berkow, 1995). Environmental contaminants such as air pollutants are also related to free radical production. Free radicals act at the cell membrane level, thus interfering with the function of cells. Studies by Arking and Giroux (2001) note that exposure to the radical oxygen contaminants may help older adults develop resistance to them over time. In addition, antioxidants to protect against aging are eagerly sought by the public and form the basis for the continued financial success of products such as vitamin E and beta carotene. However, no proof currently exists that physiological aging is altered by antioxidants.

Cybernetic theory

The neuroendocrine theory of cybernetics suggests that the central nervous system is the aging pacemaker of the body (Cristofalo, 1988). According to this theory, changes in the endocrine system and hypothalamus result in some of the end organ changes seen with aging such as the rate of thyroid hormone and adrenocortical steroid production. Functional changes in this system are accompanied by a decline in functional capacity of all systems. In addition, alteration of brain dopamine levels may increase potential development of age-associated diseases such as Parkinson's disease.

Nongenetic Theory

Wear and tear theory

The wear and tear theory proposes that cumulative damage to vital parts of the body leads to the death of cells, tissues, organs, and finally, the organism. Numerous theories ascribe aging to secondary damage from toxins, cosmic rays, gravity, and so forth. These theories demonstrate the change in the length of lifespan for humans under different environmental situations (Abrams, Beers, & Berkow, 1995). Studies of identical twins indicate a genetic basis for longevity. Cases in which the time of death varies between twins indicate that environmental factors may be as important as genetic factors in determining lifespan (Bank & Jarvik, 1978).

Exposure to environmental and dietary compounds can cause changes in the characteristics of major body organ tissues such as collagen and elastin. These tissues become less pliable and less elastic, resulting in some of the gross changes associated with aging in skin, arterial blood vessel walls, the musculoskeletal system, and the lens of the eye (Cristofalo, 1988).

SOCIAL THEORIES OF AGING

Longer lifespans and an increased number of elders in U.S. society have resulted in greater attention to the aging process. Quality of life and successful aging are becoming important areas of study. The disengagement, activity, and continuity social theories each present a different process of aging and focus on different aspects of **successful aging.** The next three social theories, which consist of Erikson's and Peck's stages of psychological development and the life course, place more emphasis on the **developmental stages** of aging. The last social theory of aging, the theory of exchange, examines perceptions regarding the value of interactions and the ways these perceptions affect elders' relationships.

Researchers on the major social theories of aging, activity theory, disengagement theory, and continuity theory have not consistently demonstrated accuracy in identifying behaviors at various stages.

Disengagement Theory

Disengagement occurs when people withdraw from roles or activities and reduce their activity levels or involvement. While completing an interest checklist, an elder may indicate to the COTA former activities with various social clubs or organizations. When asked for the reason for withdrawal from these activities, the elder may state that it was because of age. On the basis of their research in Kansas City, Missouri, in the 1950s, Cumming and Henry (1961) theorized that the turning inward typical of aging people produces a natural and normal withdrawal from social roles and activities, an increasing preoccupation with self, and decreasing involvement with others. They perceived individual disengagement as primarily a psychological process involving withdrawal of interest and commitment. Social withdrawal was a consequence of individual disengagement, coupled with society's withdrawal of opportunities and interest in elder's contributions.

This disengagement theory resulted in increased research. The proposition of withdrawal being normal challenged the conventional wisdom that keeping active was the best way to deal with aging. Streib and Schneider (1971) suggested that differential disengagement was more likely to occur than total disengagement. For example, people may withdraw from some activities but increase or maintain their involvement in others. Troll (1971) found that elders often disengage into the family—that is, elders often cope with lost roles by increasing involvement with their families. People are seldom completely engaged or disengaged. Rather, they strike a balance between the two states that reflects their individual preferences, often mediated by social encouragement or discouragement from others.

The major criticism of the disengagement theory is that it does not give enough weight to the role of society's determination and initiation of disengagement. Patterns of declining interactions have been uncovered by researchers studying societal disengagement (Havighurst, Neugarten, & Tobin, 1963; Newell, 1961; Williams & Wirths, 1965). However, the decline of opportunity may not be a result of either individual disengagement or societal disengagement, but rather a combination of both (Atchley, 1991). The frequency of disengagement is very much the product of the opportunity for continued engagement. For example, elders may wish to continue many activities, but because they believe that other people may think they are "too old," they withdraw. For elders in facilities who think they are too old to continue activities, the COTA could discuss with them doing activities that would be similar to former interests. For example, if elders are interested in gardening, they could assist with the plants in and out of their residence. If elders are interested in communicating with friends, perhaps an introduction to electronic mail (e-mail) would be a meaningful activity.

Activity Theory

About the same time the disengagement theory was described, others proposed an alternative way of explaining the psychosocial process of aging. Havighurst, Neugarten, and Tobin (1963) articulated an activity theory of aging, which held that unless constrained by poor health or disability, elders have the same psychological and social needs as people of middle age. This theory emphasizes the importance of ongoing social interactions; as a result of this activity, elders maintain positive self-concepts (Cavan, 1962). This theory assumes that social activity is beneficial for elders and that it contributes to their achievement of life satisfaction. The activity theory also assumes that elders need and desire high levels of social activity and that they interpret different types of activity in the same ways as younger people. In addition, some researchers have noted that the relation between activity and well-being among elders depends on the type of activity in which they are engaged (Lemon, Bengtson, & Peterson, 1972).

The activity theory has received a great deal of criticism in that it excludes elder's physical well-being, past lifestyle, and personality attributes. It also does not account for the value or the personal meaning the elder may find in activities. Instead, it most often quantifies the number of roles and the amount of involvement in these

roles (Bonder & Wagner, 2001). In addition, the belief that it is better to be active than inactive is a bias derived from the Western culture (Bonder & Wagner, 2001). Much of OT is based on the assumption that our value of human beings comes from what we know and do, rather than on who we are and have been (Rowles, 1991). However, this perspective is changing with newer theories such as that espoused by Kielhofner (2002).

A further component of the activity theory considers the preferences of elders and the extent to which they wish to be active. Setting aside time for quiet reflection may be equally as important as more active pursuits for some elders. COTAs should remember this when attempting to get everyone involved in an activity. Some elders may welcome participation in physical activities such as bowling and walking, and others may be content with listening to quiet music and reading (Figs. 2-1 through 2-3).

Continuity Theory

The premise of the continuity theory is that elders adapt to changes by using strategies to maintain continuity in their lives. Continuity is both internal and external. **Internal continuity** refers to the strategy of forming personal links between new experiences and memories of previous ones (Cohler, 1982). **External continuity** refers to interacting with familiar people and living in familiar environments (Atchley, 1991). According to this theory,

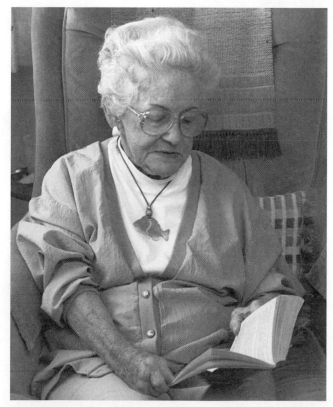

FIGURE 2-1   This elder enjoys a sedentary activity.

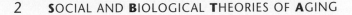

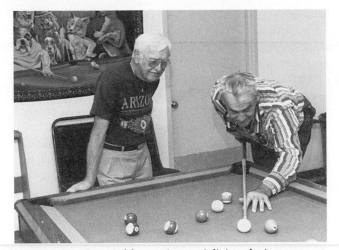

FIGURE 2-2   Some elders enjoy socializing during an active leisure activity.

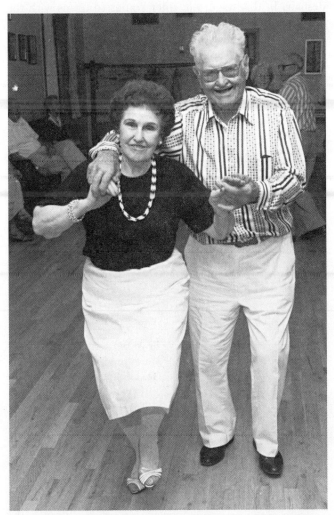

FIGURE 2-3   Through ongoing social interactions, elders can maintain a positive self-concept.

elders should continue to live in their own homes as long as possible. If this is not possible, the family should attempt to locate housing for the elder in the same general area to maintain friendships and familiar environments. Many elders continue to be independent as long as they are in familiar surroundings. Some families have noted that once they moved their elder family member from a familiar area, the elder was confused and disoriented.

Continuity of activities and environments helps the individual concentrate energies in familiar areas of activity. Practice of activities can often prevent, offset, or minimize the effects of aging. Atchley (1991) states that by maintaining the same lifestyle and residence, an older person is able to meet instrumental activities of daily living needs. Continuity of roles and activities is effective in maintaining the capacity to meet social and emotional needs for interaction and social support. Maintaining independence is important for continued good self-esteem. Continuity does not mean that nothing changes; it means that new life experiences occur and the elder must adapt to them with familiar, persistent processes and attributes. New information is likely to produce less stress when an elder has memories of similar experiences. This may be one reason new information does not have the same weight for both younger and older generations and may help to explain the reason some elders seem more conservative than others. For example, an elder may reject learning to use a computer to order home supplies and to be in contact with others despite being isolated in a rural location because the activity involves a new way of performing a task.

Because none of the three theories discussed earlier has been conclusively proven, we should not base our practice on any of them. For instance, it may be dangerous to allow an elder to withdraw by considering it a normal function of aging or to push meaningless activity with a disinterested elder. We can, however, find guidelines for our practice through aspects of any of these theories. COTAs may want to discuss with elders what activities have meaning to them. Possibly they could allow elders to reminisce about past activities, or perform client-centred assessments such as the Canadian Occupational Performance Measure (Law et al., 1998) or an interest checklist. This could give COTAs more insight into selection of activities that are most appropriate for the elders.

The activity and continuity theories are compatible with OT in that they assume that performance of meaningful activities promotes competence, independence, and well-being. Successful aging as studied by Rowe and Kahn (1998) included the importance of staying active and being productive. Kielhofner (1992) states that human beings are occupational in nature, therefore occupation is vital for our well-being. The Model of Human Occupation incorporates this assumption and is a valuable theory for OT for aging (Kielhofner, 1995, 2002).

What a person does depends on individual factors such as level of interest, values, personal causation, health, socioeconomic status, and prior occupations.

Lifespan/Life Course Theory

The lifespan, or life course, perspective is a recent approach to human development by theorists interested in the social and behavioral processes of aging (Box 2-1). **Life course** is defined by Atchley (1991) as "an ideal sequence of events that people are expected to experience and positions that they are expected to occupy as they mature and move through life." This theory was influenced by the age stratification model, which emphasizes the significant variations in elders depending on the characteristics of their birth cohort. Some researchers believe this is not actually a theory, but rather a conceptual framework for conducting research and interpreting data.

Most elders who experienced the Great Depression seem to have a different perception of the meaning of "poor." Many elders reject offers of help because they compare what little they had in the past with what they currently have, which seems sufficient. In addition, some elders who are eligible for Social Security insurance may not accept it.

Neugarten, Moore, and Lowe (1965) found considerable consensus on age-related progression and sequence of roles and group memberships that individuals are expected to follow as they mature and move through life. The stages of the adult life course as defined by this group are middle age, later maturity, and old age. Unlike Erikson's and Peck's stages, life course stages are related to specific chronological ages. Age norms generally define what people within a given life stage are "allowed" to do and be at certain ages. Many norms are established by long traditions. Others are often the result of compromise and negotiation. In addition, a series of assumptions related to the capabilities of the people in a given life stage underlies age norms. Thus, opportunities may be limited for some elders because others assume they are not strong enough or lack education or experience (Atchley, 1991). Elders who achieve greatness beyond expectations for their life stages are perceived as unique or different. Their accomplishments elicit comments about their endeavors being met by a person of "their age." Many older elders, such as the current group of centenarians, are considered pioneers because few prescribed behaviors or age norms exist for them. Havighurst (1972) suggested that people 60 years of age and older need to adjust to declining health, a life of retirement, death of spouse and friends, changing living arrangements, and increased leisure time if they want to experience life satisfaction.

Erikson's Theory of Human Development

Erik Erikson's theory of human development over the lifespan is one of the most influential descriptions of psychological change (Erikson, 1985). Erikson's stages of ego development are familiar to most students of psychology (Table 2-1).

Erikson's framework addresses the developmental tasks at each stage of the life cycle. The stage most commonly identified with aging is that of integrity versus despair. In this stage, the elder comes to terms with the gradual deterioration of the body but at the same time may reflect on the acquisition of wisdom associated with life experiences. Ego integrity involves the elders' ability to see life as meaningful and to accept both positive and negative personality traits without feeling threatened. Integrity provides a basis for approaching the end of life with a feeling of having done their best under the circumstances. Despair is the elder's rejection of self and life experiences, and it includes the realization that there is insufficient time to alter this assessment. The despairing elder is prone to depression and is afraid to die. COTAs can play a vital role in assisting elders to master this

---

BOX 2-1

Key Elements of the Lifespan Framework

- Aging occurs from birth to death.
- Aging involves biological, social, and psychological processes.
- Experiences in aging are shaped by historical factors.

From Passuth, P., & Bengtson, V. (1988). Sociological theories of aging: Current perspectives and future directions. In J. Birren & V. Bengtson (Eds.), *Emergent theories of aging*. New York, NY: Springer.

TABLE 2-1

Erik Erikson's Stage of Ego Development

Time period	Stage
Early infacy	Trust versus distrust
Later infancy	Autonomy versus shame and doubt
Early childhood	Initiative versus guilt
Childhood middle years	Industry versus inferiority
Adolescence	Ego identity versus role confusion
Early adulthood	Intimacy versus isolation
Middle adulthood	Generativity versus stagnation
Late adulthood	Ego integrity versus ego despair

From Erikson, E. (1985). *Childhood and society*. New York, NY: Norton.

developmental stage. Helping elders to develop self-empathy, the ability to bounce back from change, and a focus on the completeness of their lives supports elders' efforts to deal with this life stage.

Erikson originally proposed eight stages of psychosocial development. As Erikson himself reached later life, he noted that the predominant image of old age was quite different from when he had first formulated his theory. Because modern statistics were predicting a much longer life for the majority of older individuals, he and his colleagues contemplated adding a ninth stage of development with its own quality of experience, including some sense or premonition of immortality (Erikson, 1982; Erikson, Erikson, & Kivnick, 1986). Newman and Newman (1991) responded to the changing patterns of biological and cultural development by redefining late-life psychosocial development. They added descriptions of three additional stages, including the stage of very old age.

As increasing numbers of people reach very old age, tasks and other aspects of psychosocial development that were not systematically described in Erikson's original formulations are emerging. Newman and Newman (1991) have labeled the crisis of the old old years (age 75 years and beyond) as immortality versus extinction. The positive resolution of this crisis is the elder's confidence in the continuity of a personal contribution beyond death. For example, an elder who handcrafts rocking chairs may pass on those skills to children, who may pass them on to their children. Tasks of this stage include coping with the inevitable physical changes that accompany aging. The elder may be increasingly obliged to turn attention from the more interesting aspects of life to the demands of the body. In addition, the very old may have to shape new patterns for adapting to late life because few norms for behavior and few responsibilities are established for elders who reach very old age. Numerous articles on persons older than 100 years show a fascination with the many activities of this fastest growing age group. Most of these elders attribute their longevity to keeping their minds, not their bodies, stimulated (Stern, 1996) (Fig. 2-4).

Kishton (1994) added another task of late life, that of developing a historical perspective of the psychological events of life such as mistakes and disappointments. Kishton described this task as a process of integration of the past, present, and future. Integration of the past usually involves reconciling prior mistakes or disappointments. Reminiscence groups and other life review activities conducted as part of a treatment program by COTAs can be effective in helping elders work through this developmental task.

Peck's Stages of Psychological Development

Robert Peck (1968) believed that Erikson's eighth stage, integrity versus despair, was intended to "represent in a global, nonspecific way all of the psychological crises

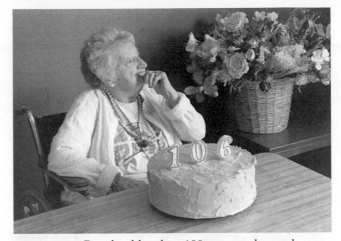

FIGURE 2-4 People older than 100 years make up the fastest growing age group.

and crisis-solutions of the last forty or fifty years of life" (p. 88). He suggested that it might be more accurate and useful to take a closer look at the second half of life and divide it into several different psychological stages and adjustments (Table 2-2).

Peck (1968) proposed four stages that occur in middle age and three stages in old age. He avoided establishing a chronological period for these stages, suggesting instead that they might occur in different time sequences for different individuals.

The first stage of old age is ego differentiation versus work-role preoccupation. The effect of retirement, particularly for men in their late 60s, is the issue at this stage.

TABLE 2-2

Robert Peck's Psychological Stages in the Second Half of Life

Time period	Stage
Middle age/First stage	Wisdom versus physical powers
Middle age/Second stage	Socializing versus sexualizing
Middle age/Third stage	Cathectic flexibility versus cathectic impoverishment
Middle age/Fourth stage	Mental flexibility versus mental rigidity
Old age/First stage	Ego differentiation versus work-role preoccupation
Old age/Second stage	Body transcendence versus body preoccupation
Old age/Third Stage	Ego transcendence versus ego preoccupation

From Peck, R. (1968). Psychological developments in the second half of life. In B. Neugarten (Ed.), *Middle age and aging*, Chicago, IL: University of Chicago Press.

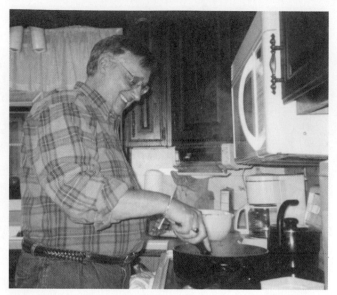

FIGURE 2-5   This retired man enjoys his new role as he prepares the family meal. (Courtesy Sue Byers–Connon, Mt. Hood Community College, Gresham, OR.)

In U.S. culture, identity tends to be tied to the individual's work role. Retiring individuals must reappraise and redefine their worth in a broader range of role activities (Fig. 2-5). Retirement also affects women, regardless of whether their careers were inside or outside the home. The housewife's work role changes drastically when the husband retires and is suddenly always in "her" domain (Fig. 2-6). With current economic and policy changes associated with the Social Security Act, this stage may move to later years as more elders remain or return to the workforce (see the discussion on elders in the workforce in Chapter 1).

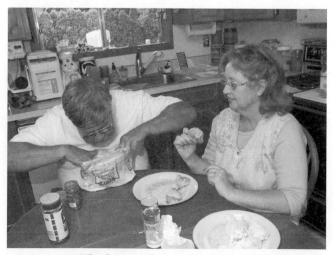

FIGURE 2-6   The housewife's work role can change when the husband retires and is suddenly in "her domain."

Peck (1968) states that a critical requisite for successful adaptation to this stage may be the establishment of varied sets of valued activities and self-attributes. These activities and attributes allow the individual to have satisfying and worthwhile alternatives to pursue. Participation in voluntary organizations can provide recreational activities and political action. Participation in the American Association of Retired Persons can be initiated as early as 50 years of age and continued after the formal work role has ended. This organization provides opportunities for travel at reduced cost. In addition, it offers medical insurance plans to supplement private insurance and Medicare and the choice to become an advocate for increased health benefits through political action committees.

Peck's second stage of old age is body transcendence versus body preoccupation. Physical decline, along with a marked decline in recuperative powers and increased body aches and pains, occurs in many elders in this stage. To those who especially value physical well-being, this may be the most difficult period of adjustment. For some elders, this adjustment means a growing preoccupation with their bodily functions. However, others have learned to define comfort and happiness in human relationships or creative mental activities. For them, only complete physical destruction can deter these feelings.

The third stage is ego transcendence versus ego preoccupation. With this stage of old age comes the certain prospect of death. Successful adaptation is not compatible with passive resignation or ego denial. It requires deep, active effort on the part of the elder to make life more secure, meaningful, and happy for those who will live after the elder's death. These elders experience a gratifying absorption in the future and are interested in doing all that is possible to make the world better for familial or cultural descendants. In practice COTAs may work with elders to do life review activities, such as developing a video to leave for future generations.

Exchange Theory

In clinical practice the OT practitioner may find it more rewarding to work with an elder who is motivated and has a "fun" personality than with an elder who does not relate well with others. COTAs may observe that the client who displays a winning personality receives more attention from everyone. This is an example of exchange theory (Fig. 2-7).

Exchange theory, as originally developed by Homans (1961), assumes that people attempt to maximize their rewards and minimize their costs in interactions with others. The major attempts to use exchange theory in work with elders are attributed to Dowd (1975, 1980). Elders are viewed from the perspective of their ongoing interactions with a number of persons. Continuing interaction is based on what the elder perceives as rewarding or costly. Elders tend to continue with interactions that

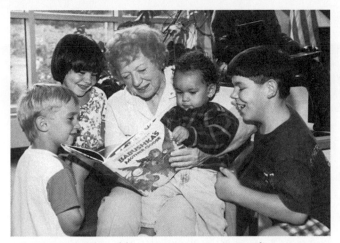

FIGURE **2-7** This elder enjoys interacting with young children.

are beneficial and withdraw from those perceived as having no benefit. Rewards may be defined in material or nonmaterial terms and could include such components as assistance, money, information, affection, approval, property, skill, respect, compliance, and conformity. Costs are defined as an expenditure of any of these.

In American culture, more emphasis is often placed on resources a person is assumed to have rather than on the actual exchange resources. The concept of ageism includes assumptions about elders, such as that elders have less current information, outdated skills, and inadequate physical strength or endurance. If elders are perceived as having few resources to contribute to a relationship, an issue over power can result, with the elder at a distinct disadvantage. Elders may be seen as powerless actors who are forced into a position of compliance and dependence because they have nothing of value to withhold to get better treatment (Atchley, 1991). Many elders accept the validity of these assumptions and fear dependency on others more than death (Aitken, 1982).

Thriving: A Holistic Lifespan Theory

For several years, gerontologists have become concerned with failure to thrive in elders, which is a sharp decline for no real physical or illness-related reason. A nursing research group was brought together to explore the phenomenon. The group broadened its vision from the syndrome failure to thrive to a more holistic lifespan concept called "Thriving." This theory seems quite applicable to our OT approach because we profess to view our clients holistically. This theory considers three interacting factors in a continuum: the person, the human environment, and the nonhuman environment. Critical to thriving are "social connectedness, ability to find meaning in life and to attach to one's environment, adaptation to physical patterns, and positive cognitive/affective function" (Haight, Barba, Tesh, & Courts, 2002, p. 22).

▮ CHAPTER REVIEW QUESTIONS

1 Scenario one: Ethel Shanas, a very famous gerontologist, once said that if you want to live a long time, you should choose your grandparents carefully. Which aging theory or theories support Dr. Shanas' suggestion?

2 Scenario two: Michelle, the COTA introduced at the beginning of this chapter, decided to include reminiscence and life review as part of her therapeutic interventions with elders in the nursing home. Which aging theory supports the selection of these activities?

3 Scenario three: The family of one of Michelle's elderly clients is upset because the elder insists on planning her own funeral and asking for specific clothes in which to be buried. In addition, she has made a list of all her furniture and other property and has designated which of her children or grandchildren are to inherit these items. Although this client has accepted her terminal illness, her family has not. Which aging theory would Michelle use to explain to the family what is happening with their relative?

4 The risk for having cancer increases significantly as people grow older. Use an aging theory to explain a possible reason for this.

5 Dr. Alex Comfort, a famous gerontologist, suggested that 2 weeks is about the ideal time to retire. What does he mean by this statement? Discuss the theory that supports your suggestion.

6 Some elder men may become extremely depressed once they retire. What could you suggest, other than antidepressant medications, that may improve their outlook on life? Discuss the theory that supports your suggestion.

7 An 80-year-old man recently made headlines because he entered the Boston marathon. Why did this make the news? How do cultural age norms influence the persistence of ageism?

8 An 85-year-old woman with severe Parkinson's disease has requested that during her activities of daily living session the COTA help her dress herself and put on makeup. Her doctor has suggested that she is "too old for rehab" and is thinking of discontinuing her OT. Justify her treatment with a theory and then explain how you would convince the doctor that it is important.

9 According to exchange theory, why does an elder feel dependent on his or her relatives?

10 Give an example of disengagement theory.

11 Give an example of activity theory.

REFERENCES

Abrams, W., and Beers, M., & Berkow, R. (1995). *The Merck manual of geriatrics.* Whitehouse Station, NJ: Merck.

Aitken, M. (1982). Self concept and functional independence in the hospitalized elderly. *American Journal of Occupational Therapy, 36*(4), 243-250.

Arking, R., & Giroux, C. (2001). Antioxidant genes, hormesis, and demographic longevity. *Journal of Anti-Aging Medicine, 4,* 125-136.

Atchley, R (1991) *Social forces and aging.* Belmont, CA: Wadsworth.

Bank, L., & Jarvik, L. (1978). A longitudinal study of aging human twins. In E. Schneider (Ed.), *The genetics of aging.* New York, NY: Plenum Press.

Bonder, B., & Wagner, M. (2001). *Functional performance in older adults.* Philadelphia: F. A. Davis.

Cavan, R. (1962). Self and role in adjustment during old age. In A. Rose (Ed.), *Human behavior and social processes.* Boston, MA: Houghton Mifflin.

Cohler, B. (1982). Person narrative and life course. In P. Baltes, & O. Brim (Eds.), *Life-span development and behavior.* New York, NY: Academic Press.

Cristofalo, V. (1988). An overview of the theories of biological aging. In J. Birren & V. Bengtson (Eds.), *Emergent theories of aging.* New York, NY: Springer.

Cumming, E., & Henry, W. (1961). *Growing old.* New York, NY: Basic Books.

Dowd, J. (1975). Aging as exchange: A preface to theory, *Journal of Gerontology, 30*(5), 584-594.

Dowd, J. (1980). Exchange rates and old people. *Journal of Gerontology, 35*(4), 596-602.

Erikson, E. (1982). *The life cycle completed.* New York, NY: Norton.

Erikson, E. (1985). *Childhood and society.* New York, NY: Norton.

Erikson, E., Erikson, J., & Kivnick, H. (1986). *Vital involvement in old age.* New York, NY: Norton.

Gupta, R., & Lutz, W. (1999). Background DNA damage from endogenous and unavoidable exogenous carcinogens: A basis for spontaneous cancer incidence. *Mutation Research, 424,* 1-8.

Haight, B., Barba, B., Tesh, A., & Courts, N. (2002). Thriving: A life span theory. *Journal of Gerontological Nursing, 28*(3), 14-22.

Havighurst, R. (1972). *Developmental tasks and education.* New York, NY: David McKay.

Havighurst, R., Neugarten, B., & Tobin, S. (1963). Disengagement, personality, and life satisfaction. In P. Hansen (Ed.), *Age with a future.* (pp. 319-324.) Copenhagen, Holland: Munksgaard.

Hayflick, L. (1968). Human cells and aging. *Scientific American, 218*(3), 32-37.

Hayflick, L. (1987). Biological theories of aging. In G. Maddox, (Ed.), *The encyclopedia of aging.* (pp. 64-68.) New York, NY: Springer.

Holliday, R. (2000). Reflections in mutation research: Somatic mutations and ageing. *Mutation Research, 463,* 173-178.

Holm, M., Rogers, J., & Stone, R. (2003). Person-task environment intervention: A decision-making guide. In E. Crepeau, E. Cohn, & B. Schell (Eds.), *Willard & Spackman occupational therapy* (10th ed.). Philadelphia: Lippincott, Williams & Wilkins.

Homans, G. (1961). *Social behavior: Its elementary forms.* New York: Harcourt Brace Jovanovich.

Kielhofner, G. (1992). *Conceptual foundations of occupational therapy.* Philadelphia: F.A. Davis.

Kielhofner, G. (1995). *A model of human occupation: Theory and application* (2nd ed.). Baltimore: Williams & Wilkins.

Kielhofner, G. (2002). *A model of human occupation: Theory and application* (3nd ed.). Baltimore: Williams & Wilkins.

Kishton, J. (1994). Contemporary Eriksonian theory: A psychobiographical illustration. *Gerontology & Geriatric Education, 14,* 81.

Law, M., Baptiste, S., Carswell, A., McColl, M. A., Polatajko, H., & Pollock, N. (1998). *Canadian Occupational Performance Measure* (3rd ed.). Ottawa, Canada: CAOT Publications ACE.

Lemon, B., Bengtson, V., & Peterson, J. (1972). An exploration of the activity theory of aging: Activity types and life satisfaction among in-movers to a retirement community. *Journal of Gerontology, 27,* 511.

Miller, R. (1999). Kleemier Award Lecture: Are there genes for aging? *Journal of Gerontology: Biological Sciences, 54*(7), B297-B307.

Neugarten, B., Moore, J., & Lowe, J. (1965). Age norms, age constraints, and adult socialization. *American Journal of Sociology, 70,* 710.

Newell, D. (1961). Social structural evidence for disengagement. In E. Cumming & W. Henry (Ed.), *Growing old.* (pp. 37-74.) New York, NY: Basic Books.

Newman, B., & Newman, P. (1991). *Understanding adulthood.* New York, NY: Holt, Rinehart & Winston.

Peck, R. (1968). Psychological developments in the second half of life. In B. Neugarten (Ed.), *Middle age and aging.* (pp. 88-92.) Chicago, IL: University of Chicago Press.

Rowe, J., & Kahn, R. (1998). *Successful aging.* New York, NY: Dell, Random House.

Rowles, G. (1991). Beyond performance: Being in place as a component of occupational therapy. *American Journal of Occupational Therapy, 45,* 265-271.

Schneider, E., & Reed, J. (1985). Modulations of aging processes. In C. Finch & E. Schneider (Eds.), *Handbook of the biology of aging.* New York, NY: Van Nostrand Reinhold.

Stern, C. (1996). Who is old? *Parade, 21,* 4.

Streib, G., & Schneider, C. (1971). *Retirement in American society.* Ithaca, NY: Cornell University Press.

Troll, L. (1971). The family of later life. *Journal of Marriage and the Family, 33,* 263.

Williams, R., & Wirths, C. (1965). *Lives through the years.* New York, NY: Atherton Press.

CHAPTER 3

Aging Process

CLAUDELLE A. H. CARRUTHERS AND LISA WALKER

KEY TERMS

function, dysfunction, primary aging, secondary aging

CHAPTER OBJECTIVES

1. Describe the aging process.
2. Explain the concepts of function and dysfunction.
3. Define and distinguish between the concepts of primary aging and secondary aging.
4. Discuss the terms *normal* and *abnormal* within the context of the aging process.
5. Apply the concepts of normal and abnormal to each of the aging changes found in cognition and in the cardiopulmonary, skeletal, muscular, neurological, integumentary, and sensory systems.
6. Explore how normal and abnormal aging changes present in patient clinical case studies.

Attempting to understand the aging process is one of the challenges of medicine. The aging process of a simple organism may be observed in a single sitting at a microscope; however, identifying the precise process in a human being is extremely difficult (Kane, Ouslander, & Abrass, 1989). Although aging is universal, it varies among people and within each organ system (Ferri, Fretwell, & Wachtel, 1997). Only at the point of death does the aging process cease (Wickens, 1993). For example, an 81-year-old elder may be physically fit, employed part-time, and an avid golfer, whereas another elder of the same age may have limited function and may find daily activities challenging (Wooten, 2002). More than 300 theories are available to explain the process of aging, which leads to the conclusion that aging has multiple causes (Avers, 2002; Blair, 1990).

Factors that affect aging include heredity, lifestyle, and environment (Hayflick, 2001). Regardless of the causes and changes experienced, people of all ages want to be functional and independent. **Function** refers to the physical ability to live in an individual's own environment (Kane, Ouslander, & Abrass, 1989). It requires the ability to perform activities of daily living (ADL) and to accurately perceive and interact with the environment. **Dysfunction** refers to the inability to live the way a person wants and possibly to an impairment that prevents independent performance of ADL (Trombly, 1995). COTAs can intervene and enhance an individual's function and independence with ADL training.

AGING CHANGES

The concepts of **primary aging** and **secondary aging** help to clarify function and dysfunction for a given individual at any age. Primary aging changes result from the aging process determined by an individual's genetic make-up. These changes do not necessarily result in dysfunction or impairment. Conversely, secondary aging changes are caused by a disease process, an impairment, or a dysfunction (Lewis, 1979). Researchers have developed criteria to distinguish a primary, or normal, aging change from a secondary, or abnormal, change.

One criteria published by Hall (1976) was named CUPID, which is an acronym denoting five possible characteristics of an aging change: cumulative, universal, progressive, intrinsic, and deleterious. A particular aging change characterized by each standard is considered a primary change. A change that cannot be categorized within each standard is a secondary aging change.

A different criteria describes primary aging changes with the "1% rule" (Kane, Ouslander, & Abrass, 1989). Most organ systems seem to gradually lose function at a rate of approximately 1% per year after the age of 30 years.

Understanding the differences between primary and secondary aging enables elders, caregivers, and COTAs to recognize a normal aging change as opposed to a disease process. This helps COTAs perform appropriate interventions and applications for meaningful client care (Dubin, 1992).

COGNITION

Cognitive aging changes relate to varied abilities and occur at different rates depending on a variety of personal characteristics. Fluid abilities are information-processing skills passively acquired through incidental learning, inductive reasoning, and daily life experiences. An elder who uses problem solving and reasoning skills to use a microwave without written or verbal instructions demonstrates fluid ability. Crystallized ability is knowledge acquired formally through experience and education such as elder hostels, conference seminars, or college classes. Crystallized ability tends to decline earlier than fluid or passive ability (Schaie, 1989a). Research has indicated that cognitive decline for most elders is selective, often ability-specific, and global rather than catastrophic (Schaie, 1984).

Often, memory loss with elders is described as problems with short-term memory. Short-term memory refers to information that is grasped momentarily to be processed and draws from sensory–perceptual stimuli in the environment or from long-term memory (Levy, 1999). Short-term memory encompasses a continuum from primary memory to working memory (Andiel & Liu, 1995). Primary memory refers to one's attention or what one can instantly remember, like immediately repeating a phone number. Working memory involves processing information like doing simple math problems (Levy, 1999). Working memory also entails doing activities that require inference such as following instructions (Andiel & Liu, 1995) or finding one's way in an unfamiliar environment (Liu, Gauthier, & Gauthier, 1991). Elders will likely have problems with working memory rather than with primary memory, which generally remains stable throughout life

(Corey-Bloom et al., 1996; Craig, Anderson, Ker, & Li, 1995; Howieson, Holm, Kaye, Oken, & Howieson, 1993). Elders with Alzheimer's disease display decline in working memory (Rochon, Water, & Caplan, 2000), which may explain why they need clear explanations for ADL that do not include inference (Andieu & Liu, 1995).

Evaluation of working memory often is neglected with memory assessments, perhaps because it is still being studied related to memory changes with aging (Andiel & Liu, 1995). However, assessing working memory is in accordance with the functional approach of occupational therapy (OT) to intervention. The Allen Diagnostic Module is an example of a cognitive assessment that includes assessment of working memory (Allen, 1999). An elder who can no longer maintain an accurate household checkbook balance because of visual loss and decreased working memory demonstrates a global cognitive decline. This loss is gradual and encompasses several cognitive processes.

Catastrophic cognitive decline that occurs with sudden onset may be a result of factors such as illness, medication side effects, poor nutritional intake, and neurological infarcts (McCloy, 2002; Cameron & Richardson, 2001-2002). An elder with a urinary tract infection may display cognitive changes. This elder could appear confused and suddenly unable to perform routine ADL. COTAs should communicate with elders and their family members and consult with members of their team to attempt to solve possible causes of the cognitive deficits. It is often impossible to differentiate the early stages of dementia vs. "benign forgetfulness."

For example, forgetting the placement of one's keys can result from simple forgetfulness or from a variety of other conditions that mimic cognitive disorders, such as depression or being overmedicated. This forgetful action also could be indicative of the early stages of dementia. However, ageism or stereotyping elders as having cognitive impairments should also be considered along with many other factors for the interpretation of this "forgetful" action. Therefore, it is important to do thorough cognitive and physical assessments to determine, if possible, the cause of cognitive problems in elders.

Both primary and secondary cognitive aging changes can be reduced. Participating in an intellectually stimulating environment, having a flexible personality style, and possessing a high cognitive status may inhibit and even reverse some primary aging effects (Gribbon, Schaie, & Parham, 1980; Schaie, 1984, 1993; Schaie & Willis, 1986) (Fig. 3-1). Secondary aging changes in cognition can be reduced if cardiovascular and other similar chronic diseases are prevented (Hertzog, Schaie, & Gibbon, 1978). COTAs can encourage elders' involvement in intellectually challenging activities such as doing crossword puzzles and participating in current event discussions and wellness activities as preventive measures for cognitive aging changes.

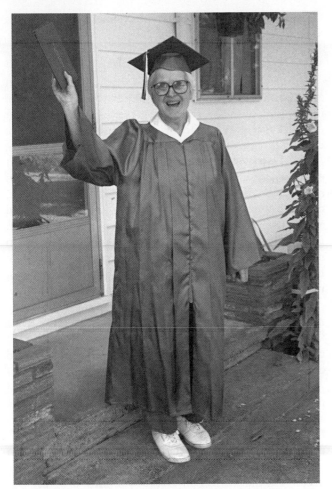

FIGURE 3-1   Elders who participate in intellectually stimulating environments may forestall some primary aging events.

INTEGUMENTARY SYSTEM

Several primary aging changes involve the skin. Wrinkles, which are one of the most noticeable changes, are often attributed to decreased blood supply and changes in collagen and elastic fiber resulting in a loss of elasticity and resilience (Vitto, 1986). Layers of subcutaneous tissue (tissue under the skin) insulate and cushion the skin against trauma. As aging progresses, the subcutaneous tissues undergo atrophic changes resulting in thinner layers of skin (Castelo-Branco et al., 1994). When these tissues atrophy, the body may have difficulty regulating temperature. Loss of subcutaneous fat and muscle may cause the face to appear thinner, eyes to appear sunken, and lips to appear larger (Buono, McKenzie, & Kasch, 1991). In the epidermis (the surface of the skin), cell replacement slows to about 50% between 30 and 70 years of age (Lyden, McGinley, & Grove, 1978). The sebaceous, or seborrheic, glands tend to decrease in function, which may lead to dry areas on the scalp and skin (Buono, McKenzie, & Kasch, 1991; Dubin, 1992).

The skin shows evidence of aging with blotches, bruising, spots, and discoloration. COTAs can be observant and, if there is an excessive amount of aging changes on the skin, may alert the interdisciplinary care team as needed. For example, excessive bruising can be a clinical sign of, among other things, a medical condition called thrombocytopenia, which can be life threatening if not identified. As the skin undergoes atrophic processes, brown and yellow discolorations occur as a result of an overall decrease in vascularity (Dubin, 1992). Red blotches on the skin are usually caused by changes in the blood vessels beneath the skin (Lyden, McGinley, & Grove, 1978). Capillaries lose the protection provided by surrounding fat, thereby possibly causing more bruising and small hemorrhagic spots in the lower extremities (Dubin, 1992) (Fig. 3-2).

Other changes occur in the tongue, gums, hair, nails, and sweat glands. The tongue and gums undergo atrophic changes and redden. Gum shrinkage around the teeth may cause difficulty with eating and dental maintenance. Hair is thickest in adulthood and decreases in diameter by as much as 20% by 70 years of age. Hair becomes thin

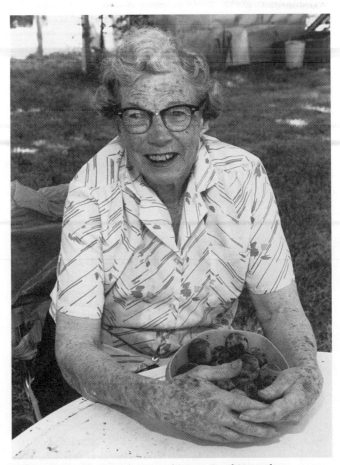

FIGURE 3-2   As people age, changes in skin such as wrinkles and bruises become evident.

and fine, and the color changes to gray or white because of a loss of pigmented cells. Besides thinning on the scalp, the hair tends to grow in a sparser pattern. The sebaceous glands attached to the hair follicles enlarge and the muscles lose their attachments to the follicles; thus pigmented hairs are more easily lost (Buono, McKenzie, & Kasch, 1991; Dubin, 1992) (Fig. 3-3). Atrophy of nail tissues causes the nails to gradually become more brittle and grow more slowly. The ability to sweat decreases as the sweat and oil glands atrophy and decrease in size and number (Dubin, 1992). As aging progresses, men and women experience changes in hormones. In men, a loss of testosterone leads to a general loss of body hair. In women, a decrease in estrogen production leads to increased facial hair (Buono, McKenzie, & Kasch, 1991).

Secondary aging changes to the skin may occur from exposure to the sun's ultraviolet rays and the inability to sweat. Regular exercise may retard the decrease in peripheral sweat gland production (Buono, McKenzie, & Kasch, 1991). Two 70-year-old individuals may have very different skin textures, which may be partially attributed to different living and work environments during preretirement years. Ultraviolet rays damage the elastic fibers beneath the skin surface and are responsible for wrinkled, dried, and tough skin textures. COTAs may suggest applying creams and lanolin, which replace natural oils, thus reducing the drying effect (Buono, McKenzie, & Kasch, 1991; Dubin, 1992). COTAs also could inform elders about sun protection tips such as use of sunscreen and wearing protective clothing to lessen the risk for skin cancer.

CARDIOPULMONARY SYSTEM

Primary aging changes of the cardiac system result in reduced cardiac output. The endocardium, which is the inner lining of the heart, thickens because of increased fat deposits that accumulate over time, possibly creating a condition known as *atherosclerosis* (Gasho, Fanelli, & Zelis, 1989). This thickened, fibrous formation around the heart causes changes to the heart's electrical system resulting in arrhythmias, or abnormal heart beats. The myocardium, or heart muscle, becomes less elastic; hence, contraction and dilation of the cardiac muscle becomes more difficult. Inside the heart, thickening occurs in the wall between the lower chambers (Kitzman, Scholz, Hagen, Ilstrup, & Edwards, 1988). The combination of a decrease in heart rate and an increase in prolonged contraction (systole) prevents elders from tolerating activity involving increased heart rates, which may result in congestive heart failure. Cardiac output declines with age as a result of changes in heart rate, peripheral vascular resistance, and coronary disease (Dubin, 1992).

Primary changes in the arterial system lead to diminished performance. General calcification within the arteries results in a diminished stress response to activities (Pierce, 1993). The aortic branches dilate, become twisted, and are less able to accommodate the changes in arterial pressure (Dubin, 1992). As vessel compliance decreases, the vessels in the extremities progressively increase resistance to blood flow (peripheral resistance), which increases systolic blood pressure (Kitzman, Scholz, Hagen, Ilstrup, & Edwards, 1988). Therefore, the response to stress is less efficient, more oxygen is needed, and the heart requires a longer period to slow down after physical stress (Blair, 1990). This diminished response also could be related to decreased cardiac output and lack of physical conditioning (Dubin, 1992).

Secondary changes include the development of atherosclerosis (lipid deposits), which makes it difficult for blood to be pumped through blood vessels (DeVries, 1970). Regular exercise and reduction in fat intake can minimize these effects (Seals, Hagberg, Hurley, Ehsani, & Holloszy, 1984).

One primary pulmonary change is a gradual decline in body fluid composition. By 70 years of age, body fluid composition may be 50% water compared with 80% water at birth. This dehydration affects the moist mucous membranes that line the nose, pharynx, trachea, bronchi, and bronchioles. Mucus may become thick and plug the tracheobronchial tree, which may lead to infections.

Other changes decrease the available oxygen supply to the body. Calcification of rib cartilage and a decline in lung tissue elasticity result in reduced compliance of the thorax. This reduced compliance causes poor gas exchange

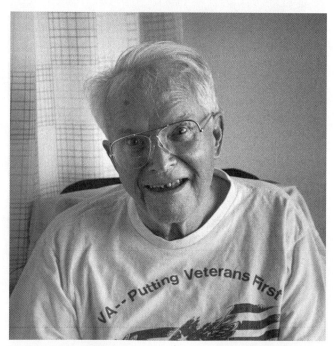

FIGURE 3-3 With aging, hair tends to grow in a sparser pattern.

and a large anteroposterior diameter (Dubin, 1992; Kuhn McGovern, 1992). Muscles that support lung function lose elasticity. Therefore, the maximum volume of oxygen that can be brought into the lungs with one deep breath decreases. Cilia, which are hairlike structures in the airways, decline in number and become less effective in removing foreign matter, thus diminishing the amount of oxygen available in the lungs and consequently raising the individual's susceptibility to secondary changes (Rockstein & Sussman, 1979).

Disease, environment, and lack of physical activity may all contribute to secondary pulmonary changes. Osteoporosis and kyphosis alter the shape of the thorax and reduce lung expansion, which may result in anatomic emphysema in elders. In addition, declining chest muscle strength impairs the effectiveness of a cough, and therefore can increase susceptibility to pneumonia and chronic bronchitis. The respiratory system suffers more from exposure to environmental pollutants and infections than any other cause (Rockstein & Sussman, 1979). Serious loss of lung function can be prevented with physical activity. Physiological reserves are so great in pulmonary function that aging alone rarely leads to significant impairment (Ham & Sloane, 1992). If COTAs notice an elder having increased coughing or difficulty clearing mucus, they should communicate their observation to members of the health care team, because this may be a sign of a serious pulmonary dysfunction. COTAs can provide information on incorporating energy conservation/work simplification techniques during ADL and instrumental activities of daily living (IADL) to maximize the elder's functional status (see Chapter 16 for a more detailed discussion).

SKELETAL SYSTEM

The primary aging changes within the skeletal system include a reduction in height, degenerative changes to joints, and a decrease in bone mass (Castelo-Branco et al., 1994). Reduction in height is caused by atrophy of the intervertebral disks and ligaments along the vertebral column. The joints of the body undergo erosion and ossification of cartilaginous joint surfaces and degenerative changes of the synovium. These processes lead to stiff joints and decreased spinal mobility (Einkauf, 1987). An increase in bone porosity causes loss of skeletal bone and elasticity.

Substantial increases in bone porosity lead to a secondary condition known as *osteoporosis* (McCloy, 2002). Approximately 44% of white women and 34% of white men who are 65 to 74 years of age have measurable osteoporosis. Osteoporosis is an increase in bone porosity that may be precipitated by a hormonal change, such as a decrease in estrogen levels in postmenopausal women. Specifically, bones become less firm and more compressed, and therefore more prone to fracture (Dubin, 1992).

Possible secondary changes related to poor posture during the individual's lifespan are calcification and eventual ossification of the ligaments (Dubin, 1992). Proper nutrition, good posture, and a daily walking program can minimize these changes (Verdote-Robertson & Reddon, 2000).

MUSCULAR SYSTEM

The primary change in the muscular system is a gradual decline of physical strength beginning around 30 years of age. In the average adult, muscle mass constitutes 43% of total body weight, whereas in elders muscle mass decreases to 25%. As the muscle fibers degenerate, they are replaced by fat cells; therefore, by 70 years of age, fat cells may constitute one third of a muscle. Some evidence shows increasing proximal muscle weakness as one ages (Serratrice, Roux, & Aquaron, 1968). Acetylcholine acts as a neurotransmitter, relaying messages between nerves that can result in movement of the muscles. With aging, the interactions between acetylcholine and the nerve endings are reduced, resulting in muscle weakness, atrophy, and hypotonia (Dubin, 1992; Hasselkus, 1974). Muscle strength also is reduced by the decreased number of capillaries per muscle fiber (Blair, 1990; Dubin, 1992).

The ability of an individual to respond to emergency situations and to perform heavy workloads declines, but the ability to perform light and moderate work is maintained. This ability to perform heavy work declines because a decrease in maximum lung capacity for oxygen occurs (Frolkis, Martynenko, & Zamostyan, 1976). A gradual loss of glycogen storage in muscles reduces a person's capacity to respond to emergency situations. In addition, the metabolic differences between fast (less oxygenated) and slow (more oxygenated) muscles begin to lessen during the aging process (Frolkis, Martynenko, & Zamostyan, 1976).

These primary changes of the muscular system can be observed in functional tasks. Muscle weakness may be evident in an elder's shorter than average step length, wider walking base, and proportionally longer time spent in the support phase versus the swing phase of the walking cycle (Dubin, 1992; Finely, Cody, & Finizie, 1969; Murray, Kory, & Clarkson, 1969). As walking speed increases, forces on the musculoskeletal system increase, and faster speeds may create levels of force that place an elder at risk for injury. Because the likelihood of injury increases with the level of force, the reduction of walking speed and length of steps reduces injury (Dubin, 1992; Hasselkus, 1974). In addition, a general slowing in reaction time and the speed of performance for completing tasks occurs (Spirduso, 1988; Welford, 1977). One secondary change in the muscular system is a decrease in muscle strength caused directly by lack of muscle use or exercise. In the aging individual, decreased muscle endurance and strength related to lack of use can be improved through activity (Fisher, Pendergast,

& Calkins, 1991). By remaining active, elders are usually able to maintain performance of functional tasks (Carruthers, 1995). COTAs can assist elders in staying active by encouraging exercise and offering suggestions on how the exercise can be incorporated during functional activities, such as gardening and home management tasks. (See Chapter 5 for further information on health promotion and disease prevention.)

NEUROLOGICAL SYSTEM

Primary aging changes affect the neurological system, which consists of the brain and spinal cord (central nervous system) and the peripheral nerves that supply the rest of the body. The brain decreases in weight by 5% to 17%—in volume and in the number of neurons (Boss, 1991; Dubin, 1992). Dubin (1992) found a decrease in the number of nerve cells in the frontal and temporal lobes. These areas influence personality, motor activity, speech, and hearing. In addition, 50% of neurons can be lost in the visual area of the occipital cortex and 33% can be lost in the sensory area of the parietal cortex without functional impairment (Blair, 1990).

Hasselkus (1974) cites changes that include a thickening of the dura mater, the material that covers the brain, excessive subarachnoid fluid under the dura, and reduction in the size of the brainstem. In addition, shortening of the spinal cord may occur; and on transection, a greatly reduced contrast in color between the white and gray matter may be evident. However, other researchers later found that white matter does not decrease (Lim, Zipursky, Watts, & Pfefferbaum, 1992). Therefore, the primary changes that result from decreased brain matter are caused specifically by a loss of gray matter.

Additional primary changes include a widening of sulci and fissures (spaces between the convolutions of the brain). The ventricles, or cavities, holding cerebrospinal fluid, which helps to cushion the brain, also widen (Boss, 1991).

These primary changes of the neurological system can be observed in an elder's performance of functional tasks. A decrease in reaction time related to muscular changes occurs with aging. Neurologically, a decrease in reaction time is a result of visual impairment, a decrease in the number of axons in the nerves, and a reduction of synthesis at nerve terminals (Boss, 1991; Dubin, 1992). In addition, sleep cycles may change such that less time is used for sleeping, with more time in light sleep and less in deep sleep (Blair, 1990; Dubin, 1992).

Secondary neurological aging changes may include a severe decrease in a neurotransmitter relaying information about an elder's surroundings. This may result in increased falls (Hasselkus, 1974) (see Chapter 16 for a more detailed discussion). These secondary changes are related to losses in proprioceptive (position of body parts in space), kinesthetic (position and balance), and visual

mechanisms (Boss, 1991). If neurotransmitters that relay information are significantly decreased, a person also may experience decreases in motor control, ability to process information, postural balance, and muscle tone (Blair, 1990; Boss, 1991).

Primary and secondary neurological changes may lead to declines in performance test measures. In general, neurological function represents an area in which test performance variability increases markedly with age, accompanied by a modest decline in function. Overall, changes, such as those indicated earlier, will affect the therapeutic clinical management of the elder (Ham & Sloane, 1992).

COTAs can help elders enhance short-term memory by encouraging visual and auditory stimulation and memory associations. COTAs could encourage the elder to use a checklist to keep track of the steps in an activity such as making tea. Timers or setting a watch with an alarm as a reminder to take medication are suggestions COTAs may recommend. (See Chapter 13 for more suggestions on cognitive adaptations with medications.) The elder can and does process new and old information. The neurological system is very complex; therefore, delineating between primary and secondary aging changes may be difficult (Blair, 1990).

COTAs working with elders may observe neurological changes during daily activities. An elder preparing a meal may have difficulty comprehending cooking instructions and may benefit from cue cards with the steps simplified to assure success. Reaching for high and low objects may cause an elder to lose balance and fall. COTAs may help elders organize their environments for safer access and minimal confusion (Beck, Doan, & Cody, 2002). Suggestions may include: storing cleaning products in an area where they are commonly used, or prepositioning supplies, equipment, and organizing work centers in the kitchen.

Changes may disrupt elders' normal routines because steps have been added or new techniques have been introduced to maintain safety. COTAs need to permit enough time for elders to process information. Writing a daily schedule may assist elders and their families in being consistent when changing a routine behavior.

SENSORY SYSTEM

The sensory system involves the processes of sensation, perception, and sensory discrimination. Sensation involves acquiring information through the sense organs. Perception is a higher sensory function, in which the information received is processed in the brain. Sensory discrimination is the minimal difference necessary for a person to distinguish between two or more sensations. Because the ability to sense is processed through the brain, the sensory systems are closely related. A general decline in the sensory system occurs in primary aging (Hooyman & Kiyak, 1988; Ordy & Brizzee, 1979).

The senses used for handling and discriminating information include gustatory, olfactory, tactile, kinesthetic, visual, and auditory visual. These sensory mechanisms enable a person to gather information and interact with the environment. (The primary aging changes related to vision and hearing are discussed in Chapters 17 and 18, respectively.)

GUSTATORY

Gustation involves the ability to discriminate and perceive the four taste qualities: sweet, sour, salty, and bitter. Two primary aging changes are decreased salivation and a lessened ability to discriminate taste. By 50 years of age, most people have lost 50% of their taste buds at the front of the tongue. Sweet and salty taste buds atrophy first. Consequently, many elders think their food tastes bitter or sour (Blair, 1990; Christianson, 1990). A diminished sense of taste may result in a decline in adequate dietary intake. COTAs may focus treatment on planning and preparing meals and encouraging elders to try good-tasting foods and to maintain a nutritional diet (McCloy, 2002).

OLFACTORY

Olfactory function declines approximately 40% with aging. Olfactory receptors are located in the upper portion of the nasal cavity. Although these receptors show some deterioration with age, a reduction in ability to smell does not necessarily occur (Blair, 1990). However, elders have difficulty distinguishing between pleasant and unpleasant odors.

COTA interventions may focus on ensuring home safety and making elders aware of their declining abilities to smell smoke, gas, and spoiling foods. Elders should be instructed to change batteries in smoke detectors regularly and check appliances visually. The "on" and "off" positions on appliances should be clearly marked using colored caulk or glue making a raised surface. Regularly cleaning the refrigerator and marking dates on leftovers may help prevent elders from consuming spoiled food. Another area of concern may be personal hygiene. A diminished olfactory sense may cause elders to be unaware of body odors. COTAs can help elders create a schedule of laundering and bathing days.

TACTILE

Reduction in tactile sensitivity in the fingertips, palms, and lower extremities is common (Verillo, 1980; Whanger & Wang, 1974). According to research, the relationship between increasing age and a decrease in tactile discrimination apparently cannot be attributed to mechanical changes of the skin, but may be a result of changes in the nervous system affecting speed, quantity, or quality of information processing (Woodward, 1993). An elder may experience a general inability to perceive heat, cold, and touch.

COTAs may address safety issues that arise from decreased sensation. COTAs can use activities such as cooking to demonstrate safety with sharp objects and stove use. The use of a bath thermometer to check water temperature may prevent burns caused by decreased sensation. The COTA may suggest a family member monitor the temperature of the hot water heater as a preventative measure.

KINESTHETIC

Kinesthesia is the sense of movement and balance. It involves the ability to perceive changes in body position and orientation. This ability decreases with age. Neurological and neuromuscular aging changes lead to disturbances in kinesthesia (Hasselkus & Shambes, 1975; Dubin, 1992). An elder experiencing a kinesthetic change has a decreased ability to determine when and in what direction the head is moving, and therefore may experience a sensation of falling (Christianson, 1990; Hasselkus, 1974). The sense of vibration in the extremities may also be lost (Birren, 1947).

Because kinesthetic decline may contribute to falls, COTAs should instruct elders, caregivers, and family members to remove rugs and clutter from walking areas and keep rooms well lit. (See Chapter 16 for a more detailed discussion on mobility and safety issues.)

CASE STUDY

Shirley is a 68-year-old woman who was admitted to a skilled nursing facility (SNF) after a 5-day hospital stay for a left hip replacement secondary to a fall in her home. Tasha is the COTA working with Shirley. On reviewing Shirley's OT evaluation, Tasha noted that Shirley had been diagnosed with multiple sclerosis (MS) approximately 20 years earlier, and Shirley was recently experiencing an increased number of falls. Shirley also had a history of osteoporosis and panic disorder. She required minimal–moderate assistance with ADL and mobility at the time of her evaluation.

Over the course of Shirley's 15-day stay at the SNF, Tasha found a client-centred approach to be helpful especially because of Shirley's increased anxiety and feelings of loss of control within the environment. Shirley was aware of having an impaired memory because of MS and asked for a cue card to be placed on the front-wheeled walker that listed the steps for incorporating total hip precautions during mobility. Based on Shirley's objective to be more independent in ADL, Tasha instructed her in the use of adaptive equipment for the lower extremity. Tasha also provided Shirley information on the county senior citizens group that furnished loaner durable medical equipment for the bathroom. Shirley called to arrange for a shower seat and bedside commode to be delivered to her home before discharge. In addition, Shirley also pursued ordering the adaptive equipment that Tasha had recommended through a local vendor and had the items sent to the SNF. As part of Shirley's plan of care to improve function in IADL, Denise established an upper extremity home exercise program for achieving optimum strength. Tasha also spent several sessions focusing on Shirleys' goal of improving function with simple meal preparation and laundry tasks. Tasha incorporated total hip precautions and energy conservation/work simplification techniques with the IADL tasks. Shirley shared with Tasha that her home was quite cluttered because of a recent move and that she had been unable to get settled before her injury. Tasha recommended a home visit to assess home safety. On her discharge from the facility, Shirley's anxiety and low frustration level had markedly diminished. She was able to progress to an independent status with ADL and ADL mobility through the use of the recommended adaptive equipment and durable medical equipment, and because she was involved in the treatment plan.

CASE STUDY REVIEW QUESTIONS

1 List the strategies used by the COTA to compensate for the primary and secondary aging process changes exhibited by the patients.

2 Identify possible negative outcomes if there had been no OT intervention.

3 What are the positive outcomes that were achieved?

4 Discuss the influence of a client-centred approach with the case study.

CHAPTER REVIEW QUESTIONS

1 Explain the differences between primary and secondary aging.

2 Summarize primary and secondary changes and describe possible functional implications of these changes for each of the following: cognition and skin, cardiopulmonary, skeletal, muscular, neurological, and sensory systems.

REFERENCES

Andiel, C., & Liu, L. (1995). Working memory and older adults: Implications for occupational therapy. *The American Journal of Occupational Therapy*, 49(7), 681-686.

Avers, D. (2002). Biological theories of aging: Implications for physical therapists. *Topics in Geriatrics 2002*, 2.

Beck. C., Doan, R., & Cody, M. (2002). Nursing assistants as providers of mental health care in nursing homes. *Generations*, 26, 66.

Birren, J. (1947). Vibratory sensitivity in the aged. *Journal of Gerontology*, 2, 267-268.

Blair, K. (1990). Aging: Physiological aspects and clinical implications. *The Nurse Practitioner*, 15, 14-28.

Boss, B. (1991). Normal aging in the nervous system: Implication for SCI nurses. *SCI Nursing*, 8, 42-47.

Buono, M., McKenzie, B., & Kasch, F. (1991). Effects on aging and physical training on the peripheral sweat gland. *Age Ageing*, 20, 439-441.

Cameron, K., & Richardson, A. (2001). A guide to medication and aging. *Generations*, 24, 8, 2001-2002.

Carruthers, C. (1995). *Functional movement themes of the elderly to transfer on and off the bed*. Unpublished doctoral dissertation.

Castelo-Branco, C., Pons, F., Gratacos, E., Fortuny, A., Vanrell, J. A., & Gonzalez-Merlo, J. (1994). Relationship between skin collagen and bone changes during aging. *Maturitas*, 18(3), 199-206.

Christianson, M. (1990). Aging in the designed environment *Physical & Occupational Therapy in Geriatrics 8*, 1.

Corey-Bloom, J., Wiederholt, W. C., Edelstein, S., Almon, D. P., Cahn, D., & Barette-Connor, E. (1996). Cognitive and functional status of the olderset old. *Journal of the American Geriatric Society*, 44, 671-674.

Craik, F. I. M., Anderson, N. D., Kerr, S. A., & Li, K. Z. H. (1995). Memory changes in normal ageing. In A. D. Baddely, B. A. Wilson, & F. N. Watts (Eds.), *Handbook of memory disorders*. West Sussex, UK: John Wiley & Sons, Ltd.

DeVries, H. (1970). Physiological effects of an exercise training regimen upon men aged 52-88. *Journal of Gerontology*, 25, 325-336.

Dial, L. (1999). *Conditions of aging*. Baltimore, MD: Williams & Wilkins.

Dubin, S. (1992). The physiologic changes of aging. *Orthopaedic Nursing*, 11, 45-50.

Einkauf, D. (1987). Changes in spinal mobility with increasing age in women. *Physical Therapy 67*, 370-375.

Ferri, F., Fretwell, M., & Wachtel, T. (1997). *Practical guide to the care of the geriatric patient*. St. Louis, MO: Mosby-Year Book.

Finely, F., Cody, K., & Finizie, R. (1969). Locomotion patterns in elderly women. *Archives of Physical Medicine and Rehabilitation*, 50, 140-146.

Fisher, N., Pendergast, D., & Calkins, E. (1991). Muscle rehabilitation in impaired elderly nursing home residents. *Archives of Physical Medicine and Rehabilitation*, 72, 181-185.

Frolkis, V., Martynenko, O., & Zamostyan, V. (1976). Aging of the neuromuscular apparatus. *Gerontology*, 22, 244-279.

Gasho, J., Fanelli, C., & Zelis, R. (1989). Aging reduces distensibility and the venodilatory response to nitroglycerin in normal subjects. *American Journal of Cardiology 63*, 1267-1270.

Gribbin, K., Schaie, K., & Parham, I. (1980). Complexities of the life style and maintenance of intellectual abilities. *Journal of Social Issues*, 36, 47-61.

Hall, D. (1976). *The aging of connective tissue*. Orlando, FL: Academic Press.

Ham, R., & Sloane, P. (1992). *Primary care geriatrics: A care-based approach*. St. Louis, MO: Mosby-Year Book.

Hasselkus, B. (1974). Aging and the human nervous system. *American Journal of Occupational Therapy*, 28, 16-18.

Hasselkus, B., & Shambes, G. (1975). Aging and postural sway in women. *Journal of Gerontology*, 30, 661-667.

Hayflick, L. (2001). Anti-aging medicine: Hype, hope, and reality. *Generations*, 25, 020. 2001-2002.

Hertzog, C., Schaie, K., & Gibbon, K. (1978). Cardiovascular disease and changes in intellectual functioning from middle to old age. *Journal of Gerontology*, 33, 872-883.

Hooyman, N., & Kiyak, H. (1988). *Social gerontology: A multi-disciplinary perspective*. Needham, MA: Allyn and Bacon.

Howieson, D. B., Holm, M. A., Kaye, J. A., Oken, B. S., & Howieson, J. (1993). Neurologic function in the optimally healthy oldest old: Neurpsychological evaluation. *Neurology*, 1882-1886.

1Up Health (n.d.) Thrombocytopenia: Symptoms and signs [WWW page]. URL http://www.1uphealth.com/health/thrombocytopenia_symptoms.html

Kane, R., Ouslander, J., & Abrass, I. (1989). *Essentials of clinical geriatrics*. New York, NY: McGraw-Hill.

Kitzman, D. W., Scholz, D. G., Hagen, P. T., Ilstrup, D. M., Edwards, W. D. (1988). Age-related changes in normal human hearts during the first 10 decades of life. Part II (Maturity): A quantitative anatomic study of 765 specimens from subjects 20 to 99 years old. *Mayo Clinic Proceedings*, 63(2), 137-146.

Kuhn, J., & McGovern, M. (1992). Respiratory assessment of the elderly. *Journal of Gerontological Nursing*, 18, 40-43.

Levy, L. L. (1999). Memory: An overview for cognitive rehabilitative intervention. *OT Practice*, CE-1-CE-7.

Lewis, S. (1979). *The mature years: A geriatric occupational therapy text*. Thorofare, NJ: Slack.

Lim, K., Zipursky, R., Watts, M., & Pfefferbaum, A. (1992). Decreased gray matter in normal aging: An in vivo magnetic resonance study. *Journal of Gerontology*, 47, B26- B30.

Liu, L., Gauthier, L., & Gauthier, S. (1991). Spatial disorientation in persons with early senile dementia of the Alzheimer type. *Journal of Occupational Therapy, 45,* 67-74.

Lyden, J., McGinley, K., & Grove, G. (1978). Age-related differences in the rate of desquamation of skin surface cells. In R. D. Adelman, J. Roberts, & V. Christafalo, (Eds.), *Pharmacological interventions in the aging process.* New York, NY: Plenum Press.

McCloy, C. (2002a). Nutritional issues of older adults: Part 1. *Topics in Geriatrics 2002,* 1-39.

McCloy, C. (2002b). Nutritional issues of older adults: Part 2. *Topics in Geriatrics 2002,* 1-24.

Murray, M., Kory, R., & Clarkson, B. (1969). Walking patterns in healthy old men. *Journal of Gerontology, 24,* 169-178.

Ordy, J., & Brizzee, K. (1979). *Sensory systems and communication in the elderly.* New York, NY: Raven Press.

Pierce, W. (1993). Aortic diameter as a function of age, gender and body surface area. *Surgery, 114,* 691-697.

Rochon, E., Water, G. S., & Caplan, D. (2000). The relationship between measure of working memory and sentence comprehension in patients with Alzheimer's disease. *Journal of Speech Language and Hearing Research, 43*(2), 395-413.

Rockstein, M., & Sussman, M. (1979). *Biology of aging.* Belmont, CA: Wadsworth.

Schaie, K. (1984). Midlife influences upon intellectual functioning in old age. *International Journal of Behavioral Development, 7,* 463-478.

Schaie, K. (1989a). The hazards of cognitive aging. *Gerontologist, 29,* 484-493.

Schaie, K. (1989b). The Seattle longitudinal studies of adult intelligence. *Am Psychol Soc, 2,* 171-175.

Schaie, K., & Willis, S. (1986). Can intellectual decline in the eld[...] be reversed? *Developmental Psychology, 22,* 223-232.

Seals, D. R., Hagberg J. M., Hurley, B. F., Ehsani, A. A., & Holloszy, J. O. (1984). Endurance training in older men and women. *Journal of Applied Physiology, 57,* 1024-1029.

Serratrice, G., Roux, H., & Aquaron, R. (1968). Proximal muscle weakness in elderly subjects. *Journal of Neurology Science, 7,* 275.

Spirduso, W. (1988). Exercise effects on aged motor function. *Annals of the New York Academy of Science, 575,* 363.

Trombly, C. (1995). *Occupational therapy for physical dysfunction* (4th ed.), Baltimore, MD: Williams & Wilkins.

Verdote-Robertson, R., & Reddon, J. (2000). Daily walking program for psychogeriatric patients: A pilot study. *Physical and Occupational Therapy in Geriatrics, 17,* 17.

Verillo, R. (1980). Age-related changes in the sensitivity to vibration. *Journal of Gerontology, 35,* 185-193.

Vitto, J. (1986). Connective tissue biochemistry of the aging dermis: Age-related alterations in collagen and elastin. *Dermatologic Clinics, 4,* 433-436.

Welford, A. (1977). Causes of slowing performance with age. *Interdisc Top Gerontol, 11,* 43-57.

Whanger, A., & Wang, H. (1974). Clinical correlates of the vibratory sense in elderly psychiatric patients. *Journal of Gerontology, 29,* 39-45.

Wickens, A. (1993). *The causes of aging.* The Netherlands: Harwood Academic Publishers.

Woodward, K. (1993). The relationship between skin compliance, age gender and tactile discriminative thresholds in humans. *Somatosensory & Motor Research, 10,* 63-67.

Wooten, A. (2002). Ability is ageless. *Generations, 26,* 31.

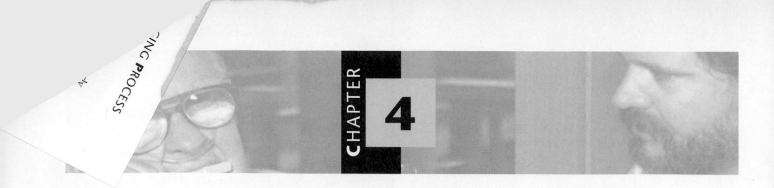

Psychological Aspects of Aging

YOLANDA GRIFFITHS

KEY TERMS

stressors, loss, coping skills, adaptations, learned helplessness, occupational shifts

CHAPTER OBJECTIVES

1. Identify myths and facts about psychological aspects of aging.
2. Identify common stressors, changes, and losses to which elders must adapt.

3. Discuss common emotional problems that may accompany losses.
4. Discuss coping skills and interventions that promote healthy transition with age.

Physical milestones measure a person's age in years, but indications of mental aging are less clear. Learning about the psychological aspects of aging enhances the certified occupational therapy assistant's (COTA's) ability to deal effectively and empathetically with elders. This chapter explores key concepts about the psychology of aging that assist in understanding elders and enhance empathy with elders.

MYTHS AND FACTS ABOUT AGING

The way elders are perceived significantly affects the way they are treated. Stereotypes are rigid concepts, exaggerated images, and inaccurate judgments used to make generalizations about groups of people. Positive and negative stereotypes create false images of aging. Western civilization often produces negative views of aging (Butler, Lewis, & Sunderland, 1991; Canja, 2001). According to Thornton (2002), current stereotypes of aging can be found in television, advertising, or popular

literature and are based on misleading information that reinforces misconceptions about elders. Advertisements often emphasize youth and sometimes use stereotypes of elders as senile, sexless, rigid, frail, unproductive, grouchy, or forgetful. Although the media have included more elders depicted as active individuals and used more models with graying hair, stereotypes of elderly persons still exist and perpetuate the faulty attitudes of others or become self-fulfilling prophecies (Thornton, 2002).

Buying into the erroneous beliefs and myths of aging produces a biased negative perception of elders and colors objectivity when working with elders. This is a form of ageism (Anderson, Keith, Novak, & Elliot, 2002; Lohman & Spergel, 1998) and deters from a realistic approach in working with elders (Cegles, 2002). Clarifying misperceptions about elders is the first step in developing effective rapport when working with this population. Consider the following myths about the psychological aspects of aging.

Myth 1: Chronological Age Determines the Way an Elder Acts and Feels

Melissa, a COTA, receives a referral to see Suzanne who is 89 years of age. Melissa has images of an elderly, cranky woman sitting in a chair with her head bowed, responding in a belligerent way about receiving treatment. Melissa enters the room of the assistive living center that Suzanne shares with her roommate, Julia. The room is filled with sports mementos, photos, and awards from both their respective grandchildren. Julia taps Melissa's shoulder and says, "If you're looking for Suzanne, she's in the sun room teaching dance lessons. You have to get up pretty early to catch up with Suzanne or she'll leave you in the dust!"

The aging process varies with each individual, and each person has different perceptions about it. Some elders do believe that their minds will deteriorate along with their bodies. Natural responses to actual losses, expected reactions to one's own aging process and death, and predictable emotional reactions to physical illness are separate aspects of aging. The truth is that elders are in a time of transition. Persons who are elderly should be treated as individuals and within their particular contexts, history, and circumstances. Refrain from generalizing that all elders approach aging in the same way.

For example, the stereotype that elders should avoid engaging in any strenuous exercise fearing their organs will fail or bones will break is pure myth. Exercise is beneficial for most and dangerous for only a few elders (Fig. 4-1). In reality, "inactivity produces muscle loss that results in limited function" (Punwar, 2000, p. 188). Elders should check with their physician for any limitations and recognize that the body does change in terms of stamina and flexibility in aging. It is not uncommon for elders to start exercising in later life even if they have been inactive for years (Tufts University, 2002). COTAs should encourage elders to take brisk walks with their grandchildren, consider new activities such as Tai Chi or water aerobics, and enjoy life (Fig. 4-2).

Myth 2: You Can't Teach an Old Dog New Tricks

The applause is thunderous as the graduates walk across the stage. It is a very special day for both Jennifer and Marion Meyer as they receive their Bachelor of Science degrees in accounting. Marion Meyer is 68 years of age. Jennifer is her 27-year-old granddaughter. Marion experienced a heart attack and her granddaughter was her caregiver during her rehabilitation. Marion often expressed regret about not going to college. Jennifer encouraged Marion to follow her dreams of furthering her education.

The ability to learn does not decline with age (Fig. 4-3). In fact, the current number of persons older than 55 years in noncredit continuing education courses is greater than ever (Cegles, 2002). According to Erp and

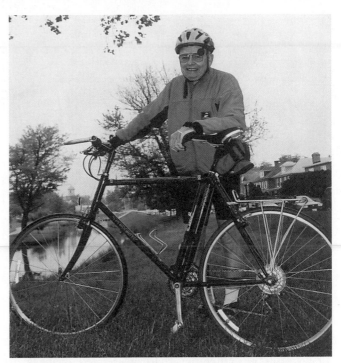

FIGURE 4-1   This elder remains physically active by regularly competing in races. (Courtesy Truby La Garde.)

Freeman (1971), adults learn differently than children because of physical characteristics, learning styles, reaction time, interests, motivation, attitudes, and values.

Horn and Cattell (1966) introduced the concepts of crystallized and fluid intelligence. Tasks involving **fluid intelligence** requiring quick reaction time decline with age (Lewis, 2003). However, performance using **crystallized intelligence** or wisdom associated with experience or education may change less throughout a

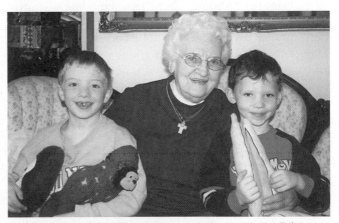

FIGURE 4-2   This elder woman remains active with her grandchildren. (Courtesy Helene Lohman, Creighton University, Omaha, NE.)

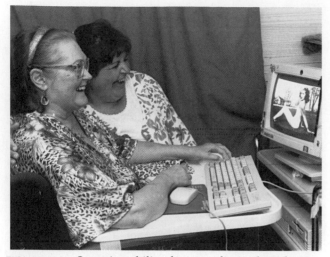

FIGURE 4-3   Learning ability does not diminish with age.

person's life or can be optimized with age (Creek, 2002; Lewis, 2002). Remember that age-related changes in learning should be considered in the context that they occur and with regard to each **individual.** Elders may take longer to learn but still do learn new ideas and skills (Creek, 2002).

Biological changes also may affect learning. For example, elders may be unable to sit for long periods because of back or hip problems. Elders may tire quickly and demonstrate decreased physical stamina. With increased use of computers, good ergonomics with regard to the computer station will decrease fatigue and neck or back stiffness associated with sustained computer use.

As a result of poor vision or hearing skills, elders may not accurately process all sensory information. Elders may need additional time to organize and process new information. People may quickly assume that an elder is confused when the information recalled seems jumbled or inaccurate. Although there may be some cognitive decline with aging because of particular medical conditions, in many ways elders may be better learners (Tufts University, 2002). Elders can integrate life experience and a broader perspective with new knowledge that younger persons often do not consider.

Elders who feel threatened by new situations may have poor self-confidence in learning situations. New situations require decision making and risk taking. Elders may avoid learning opportunities that may result in embarrassment, frustration, or conflict. In times of stress, elders may be less flexible in problem solving and rely on set ways of dealing with situations. Ultimately, the elder must want to learn, be willing to recognize any limitations, and explore other learning techniques such as keeping the brain exercised with problem-solving tasks, crossword puzzles, games, and "neurobic" exercises

(Katz, Manning, & Sutter, 1999). (See Chapter 3 for more information on cognitive changes with aging.)

Myth 3: As You Age, You Naturally Become Older and Wiser

It was most disturbing to James that he could not remember what he was doing sometimes. After all, James was a former professor of chemistry and only retired from teaching last year. Now his body seemed slower and his mind so forgetful. His forgetfulness started with little things like losing his keys and progressed to forgetting the road home after driving to the store. Finally one day, James became upset and confused in the grocery store parking lot, unable to recall the kind of car he owned. What was happening? His daughter feared that James was experiencing early stages of Alzheimer's disease. Neither James nor his daughter could understand why this was happening, especially because James had always been so active and was only 63 years of age. James has been an accomplished author and teacher and prided himself on his intellectual abilities.

Positive stereotyping can be as detrimental as negative stereotyping. Unrealistic expectations that elders can and should continue to perform as they did when they were younger may cause an elder to feel like a failure. Stating that all elders will be wiser or that all elders will become senile is not true. Mental confusion is not inevitable (Punwar, 2000). These contradictory statements prove that elders should not be lumped into one homogeneous group.

Intelligence does not decline with age. Studies done in the 1920s by Bayley and Bradway indicate that intelligence quotient (IQ) scores increase until the 20s, then level off and remain unchanged until late in life (Butler, Lewis, & Sunderland, 1991). Continued intellectual stimulation promotes successful aging. Staying active socially and engaged in activities make an elderly person less vulnerable to psychosocial situations (Lewis, 2002). With aging, it is important to determine which behaviors are caused by medical conditions versus personality traits or natural aging processes (Shrimp, 1990).

Myth 4: Elders Are Not Productive, Especially at Work

Initially, all the young employees at the local burger place called the new employment program "adopt a geezer." Paul, the manager and owner of a thriving fast food restaurant located across from the high school, often came home and complained to his wife about the unreliability of many of the youth he hired to fill the shifts. Paul said that "it was as if the kids just wanted the paycheck and had no real concern about the quality of their work."

Paul's wife, Michelle, a COTA who worked 3 days a week at the senior citizen center, suggested a mutually beneficial program that would financially help elders who were interested and capable of fulfilling a part-time position. Jim would be able to fill shifts open during the school day with steady, reliable help.

To the amazement of the young employees, the elder employees were efficient and demonstrated stamina. In fact, the young employees often remarked, "They're cool!"

According to Lewis (2002), work assists in regulating life activities and providing meaningful life experiences associated with identity, financial security, status, and opportunities for socializations. Retirement creates changes in a person's life. The psychological adaptation to the new role of retiree can be either dreaded or embraced. For some elders, retirement is anticipated as a withdrawal from traditional, stressful workday events. They are capable of learning new skills and effectively solving problems in new situations. Chronological age has little to do with being and feeling productive (Shrimp, 1990).

There will be approximately 76 million persons born in the years after World War II, known as the "Baby Boomer generation," who plan to continue working for financial, personal, or professional reasons (Canja, 2001). This includes persons engaged in both meaningful paid and unpaid work. According to the American Association of Retired Persons Work and Career Study, 60% of older persons plan to work in some capacity during their retirement years (American Association of Retired Persons, 2003) (Fig. 4-4). The study also indicates that elderly workers feel undervalued at work and want the opportunity to use their skills and talents (Fig. 4-5). With challenges in the economy about job security and possible discrimination against elders in the workplace, older workers may feel vulnerable. After retirement, elders

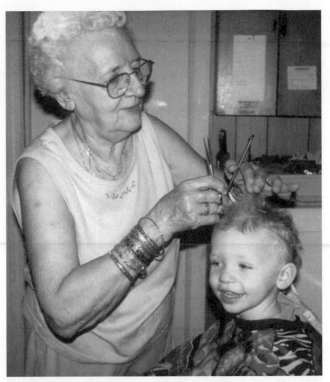

FIGURE 4-5 Some elders remain productive at work. (Courtesy Helene Lohman, Creighton University, Omaha, NE.)

often seek new areas of employment. They are capable of learning new skills and effectively solving problems in new situations (Fig. 4-5). Chronological age has little to do with being and feeling productive (Shrimp, 1990).

Retirement is sometimes a paradox when elders may have time and energy but lack financial means to be active. Conversely, when elders have the financial means and have retired from their jobs, they may desire socialization or interesting activities. According to Kielhofner (2002), elders may be challenged in their activity choices by lack of transportation, finances, companions, or self-limiting fears. COTAs can help retired elders create a plan for managing added leisure hours (Fig. 4-6). Volunteerism in the community can be a wonderful channel for leadership and organizational skills gained over a career lifetime (Canja, 2001; Cegles, 2002) (Fig. 4-7).

Myth 5: Elders Become More Conservative as They Age

Organizing a neighborhood petition to get an overpass built over the busy street next to the elementary school was the last thing Meg thought she would be doing on her 80th birthday. But here she was in the midst of neighbors and community workers stacking flyers, affixing petition forms to clipboards, and filling out a shift schedule. For years, Meg had observed many close

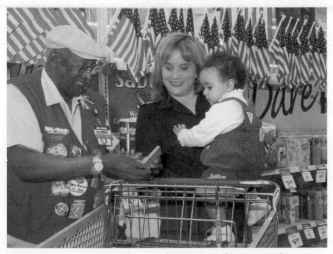

FIGURE 4-4 Many elders seek new employment after retirement.

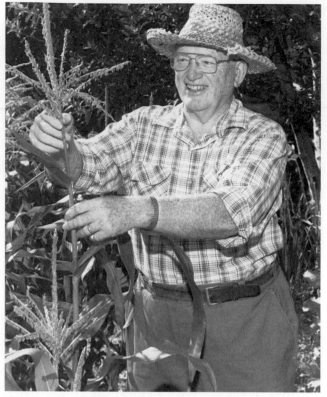

FIGURE 4-6   With added leisure hours elders must consider a new plan for managing time.

FIGURE 4-7   This retired priest volunteers in the community while remaining physically fit. (Courtesy Sue Byers-Connon, Mt. Hood Community College, Gresham, OR.)

calls when children crossing the street were almost hit by automobiles. Meg thought, "I could never forgive myself if one of those kids got hurt and I just sat here and watched from my front window."

Contrary to myth, many elders are receptive to new ideas and accept fresh roles. In fact, many elders become more politically active and even seek political office to initiate social change (Fig. 4-8). According to continuity theory, adults learn continuously from their life experiences and may pursue new interests and goals (Atchley, 1999). Even though habits and preferences contribute to a consistency in personality, developmental psychologists note that personality may be influenced as individuals deal with crisis points in each phase of life and add to their repertoires of adaptive skills. According to Canja (2001), it is untrue that elders do not want to be active contributing members of society and that the later years of life should be reserved for idleness.

Myth 6: Elders Prefer Quiet and Tranquil Daily Lives

Tim looked around the reception area of Applewood Manor on his first day of work as a COTA. Only the sounds of a television murmuring the chant of a daily

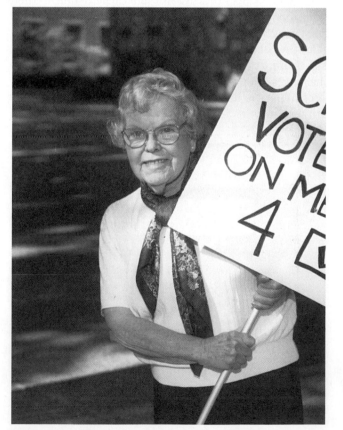

FIGURE 4-8   Many elders become politically active to initiate social change.

game show and the shuffling of residents down the hall broke the silence. The head nurse, Mrs. Kessler, walked up to Tim and said, "Isn't it wonderful how quiet and peaceful it is here? We work very hard to preserve a sense of tranquility in the sunset years of one's life."

Tim interviewed all the residents during the week to determine activities he could develop based on their interests. Not surprisingly, more than half the residents wanted less sedentary activities than they currently were experiencing. Some even wanted organized sports like tennis. Other residents wanted a piano and perhaps a jazz hour scheduled.

Another incorrect generalization is that all elders prefer a sedentary lifestyle. An elder who has experienced a rather staid and uneventful life before retirement will not necessarily continue that type of lifestyle. Elders often move in with their children's families, and their lives may become rather frenzied. Some pursue totally new interests that they may not have had time for earlier because of career and family demands. Many elders continue with vibrant lifestyles and do not sit awaiting death. Staying active is a key to healthy psychological aging (Fig. 4-9).

Myth 7: All Elders Become Senile

Harry has always been a proud, independent man. He was decorated twice during his participation in World War II. After experiencing a heart attack, Harry adjusted to the many lifestyle changes that were suggested by the health care team. Today Harry sighed as he walked with multiple pieces of paper toward the receptionist in the Occupational Therapy department. This was the third stop in a confusing, mazelike journey inside the Veterans' Administration Hospital. The hospital was under reorganization again, and procedures for appointments had changed. Previously, Harry always called for an appointment, showed up characteristically 10 minutes early, and cheerfully greeted the young COTA who assisted with the treatments. Today a young man at the front desk rattled off multiple instructions about the new procedures and handed Harry a photocopied map of the building along with a stack of new forms to be completed. Harry was still trying to understand the map when he asked the young man to slowly repeat the instructions. The young man repeated himself in a louder tone and pointed Harry in the direction of the elevators. The young man muttered, "These senile old guys..."

When elders appear confused or require more time to understand directions, misunderstandings often result. Getting older is not synonymous with feeble-mindedness or imbecility.

Brain damage may be evident as a result of physical illness. However, **senility** is a label often used inaccurately to describe specific psychosocial disorders that elders may be dealing with, such as depression, grief, anxiety, or

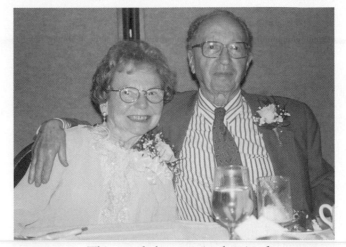

FIGURE **4-9**   This couple has remained active for more than 50 years. (Courtesy Helene Lohman, Creighton University, Omaha, NE.)

dementia. People age at different rates. Butler, Lewis, & Sunderland (1991) indicate that people become more diverse with age rather than more similar and it is inaccurate to attribute labels to all elders as a group.

STRESSORS, LOSSES, AND EMOTIONS ASSOCIATED WITH AGING

Elders often must deal with major life crises such as retirement, loss of spouse, economic changes, residence relocation, physical illness, loss of friends, and the reality of mortality. There are predictable shifts that occur in occupational patterns across the lifespan in regard to developmental processes and life stages (Royeen, 1995). The significant occupational shifts, *or changes in meaningful activities*, associated with aging may include dealing with emotional losses, variance in roles, adapting to different routines and habits, diminishing physical and mental performance, and challenges to adaptation (Levy, 1996; Royeen, 1995). Lieberman and Tobin (1983) found that "events that lead to loss and require a major disruption to customary modes of behavior seem to be the most stressful for elders." Hayslip (1983) identified the following personal factors that may influence stressors: flexibility, recognition of personal needs and limits, internal locus of control, perceived family support, and willingness to acknowledge feelings about death and dying (Box 4-1).

Christiansen (1991) indicates that certain life events are more stressful and contribute more than others to poor health. The Holmes and Rahe Social Readjustment Scale (1967) identifies life events that are ranked in terms of relative stress to an individual. Life events affect individuals differently depending on circumstance, duration, and previous coping skills, among other factors

BOX 4-1

Stressors That Affect Elders

Social stressors
Death of a loved one
Caregiving for an ill spouse
Family members moving away
Moving to live with family members
Retirement
Relocation to a nursing home because of illness
Loss of worker role

Physical stressors
Serious illness
Cumulative sensory losses
Sexual problems
Chronic conditions that reduce mobility or self-care

Cultural stressors
Negative stereotyping of elders
Health care policy management

Personal stressors
Diminished finances
Grief
Loneliness
Anger
Guilt
Depression
Anxiety
Reality of own death

Data from MacDonald, K., & Davis, L. (1988). Psychopathology and aging. In L. Davis & M. Kirkland (Eds.), *The role of occupational therapy with the elderly (ROTE)*. Rockville, MD: The American Occupational Therapy Association.

(Levy, 1996). More recent studies have attempted to measure other aspects of life events and stress levels. COTAs must consider the ways various life events affect elders to understand what motivates certain behaviors.

According to Kielhofner (2002), role changes can sometimes be involuntary, such as the unexpected death of a loved one, and elders struggle with the loss or diminishment of accompanying roles. Royeen (1995) suggests clients may be adapting to shifts in occupational patterns possibly related to atypical or unpredictable life events and developmental aging. For example, unexpected economic demise of a company may lead to the unforeseen loss of a job and retirement funds. This significantly impacts a person's occupation, inherent roles, and habits.

Need for Social Support

Levy (1996) points out that one of the best coping strategies with the changes accompanying aging and shifts

in lifestyle is social support. Although stressors may not be avoided, social support can help elders deal with losses.

The support an elder receives with the death of a loved one often diminishes to a large extent after the funeral or mourning period. The reality of the loss may not occur until later, when the elder is alone. The survivor may grieve over the loss of finances and possible change in residence, social status, or role associated with the death of the loved one. The grieving elder also may experience a form of guilt known as "death survival guilt" (Chodoff, 1963, p. 332). COTAs can assist the surviving spouse in adjusting to new roles, habits, and routines, as well as developing a strong network of social support.

Loneliness is a form of emotional isolation. Elders may experience increased social isolation with retirement, as family members relocate, or as friends move or die. Social interactions with pets, weekly church services, grocery shopping trips, or occasional visits from family members may not be emotionally fulfilling enough for an elder. COTAs can assist in exploring and structuring more frequent or new areas of social interaction in the community (Fig. 4-10). Community centers offer a variety

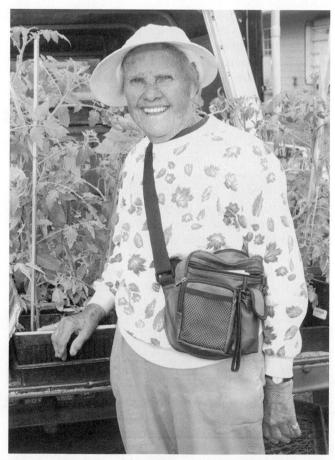

FIGURE 4-10   This elder sells tomato plants that she grows while enjoying the social interaction of others.

of activities such as cooking and art classes, trips to local attractions, and classes specifically designed for grandparents and grandchildren to attend together.

Elders may become reclusive and socially paralyzed with anxiety as a result of increasing neighborhood violence. Intensifying anger is a common emotional problem experienced by many elders as they feel a loss of control over their lives. Elders may be viewed as cantankerous or verbally aggressive when in fact they may be using angry words to express feelings of helplessness. This anger also may be founded on fear and sadness over losses.

Other changes in environment such as new living arrangements, whether imposed or by choice, also may be a challenge for elders. According to Kielhofner (2002), elders develop habits sustained over a long period often in a stable environment; when the environment changes, demands to shift habits are stressful. Or the physical or mental ability to sustain previous habits in a new environment also may be diminished.

Physical Illness

Elders may need to cope with a chronic disease or a serious physical illness. Davis (1988) notes that unexpected illness is a catastrophic stressor. The unexpected illness may be debilitating to the elder in terms of independence and self-care. A chronic illness is no less stressful; however, the elder may have adapted to the illness more gradually. Box 4-2 lists stressors associated with common physical illnesses of elders.

An elder person copes with physical illness through a psychosocial process. A negative perception of the situation and a hopeless attitude will adversely affect the way a person deals with the illness. Cohen and Larazus

BOX 4-2

Stressors Associated with Physical Illness Common to Elders

Threat to life
Loss of body integrity
Change in self-concept
Threat to future plans
Change in social roles
Change in routine activities
Loss of autonomy
Need to make critical decisions rapidly
Loss of emotional equilibrium
Physical discomfort
Monotony and boredom
Fear of medical procedures

Adapted from Davis, L. (1988). Coping with illness. In L. Davis & M. Kirkland (Ed.), *ROTE: The role of occupational therapy with the elderly*. Rockville, MD: The American Occupational Therapy Association.

pointed out that those elders who view a physical illness as a challenge cope better than those who view it as a punishment (Davis, 1988).

A grief process in dealing with any illness is to be expected. Elisabeth Kübler-Ross (1969) identified five stages to the grief process: denial, anger, depression, bargaining, and acceptance. This grief process may not be linear—that is, the elder may become depressed and then become angry or deny the situation again before accepting the illness.

An elder's ability to adapt is contingent on physical health, personality, life experiences, and level of social support (Butler, Lewis, & Sunderland, 1991; Levy, 1996; Lewis, 2002). To successfully deal with a chronic condition, an elder should adopt the following important concepts:

- Recognize permanent changes such as diet, lifestyle, work habits, or exercise that may promote recovery.
- Mentally deal with losses caused by the illness.
- Accept a new self-image.
- Identify and express feelings such as anger, fear, and guilt.
- Seek out and maintain social support from family and friends.

COTAs can help an elder deal with a chronic illness in the following ways:

- Reduce fears about the illness through education.
- Listen and be sensitive to the feelings expressed verbally and nonverbally.
- Provide encouragement.
- Assist in the development of creative yet realistic ways for elders to gain more control over their illnesses or losses associated with an illness.
- Identify ways to reduce stress and to promote social support.
- Surround the elder who has moved to a nursing care facility as a result of the illness with familiar objects, which may help maintain a sense of continuity, provide comfort and security, and aid memory.

Learned Helplessness

When elders perceive that they have no control over a particular outcome or multiple stresses in their life, they may give up hope and become dependent on others to fulfill their needs (Punwar, 2000; Seligman, 1975; Solomon, 1982, 1990). A person with an external locus of control frequently feels powerless over decisions and actions, and the more this belief is reinforced, the more likely learned helplessness occurs. Levy (1996) concludes, as a result of studies by Rodin (1986, 1989), Rowe and Kahn (1987), and Pearlin and Skaff (1995), that elders who experience a loss of control also experience diminishing coping skills and are at risk for illness. Health care workers and family members often contribute to this state of learned helplessness in the following ways:

- Expecting elders to be unable to do for themselves and completing tasks for them, thereby promoting dependence
- Imposing routines on elders for the sake of convenience, such as giving them a bath at 2:00 PM
- Showing a negative attitude by making condescending remarks about physical appearance or behaviors
- Perpetuating the sick or institutional role by validating somatic complaints or disapproving decisions

Learned helplessness often results when the elder believes a situation is permanent, and then depression and a marked lack of self-esteem follow (Barder, Slimmer, & LeSage, 1994). Elders who have already experienced multiple physical losses may feel a lack of control over their bodies and environment (Teitelman, 1990). Elders may be passive, apathetic, and depressed, and may demonstrate a lack of motivation for tasks. Increased feelings of vulnerability also contribute to learned helplessness (Foy & Mitchell, 1990). In their descriptive study, Barder, Slimmer, and LeSage (1994) indicate that elders in long-term care environments are especially vulnerable to learned helplessness.

COTAs can encourage independence and self-care activities. As elders regain a feeling of competence, learned helplessness can be reversed. Solomon (1990) suggests giving choices and options as much as possible and to challenge the client to work at a greater level than currently functioning. The concept of the client advocating for herself or himself enhances personal control in everyday life and should be integrated into daily therapy (Duncan-Myers & Huebner, 2000). This means the COTA must relinquish some of the power and control as health care advocate and empower the client to engage in independent problem solving (Cegles, 2002). One of the key concepts in preventing learned helplessness is for the COTA to be aware of his or her own beliefs about aging and mortality and to consider stereotypes that may bias attitudes toward working with elders.

CONCLUSION

Old age can be a time of self-reflection and exploration of new interests. It also can be a time of dealing with great losses and severe stress. Changes occur throughout the lifespan, and the way a person copes with changes and adapts to transitions ultimately determines his or her ability to psychologically cope with aging. Keeping active can help minimize the effects of the aging process (Cegles, 2002; Punwar, 2000). By clarifying assumptions and myths about aging, gaining awareness of the different stressors and losses associated with aging, and understanding the ways elders cope with serious illnesses, COTAs can help elders enhance quality of life as they experience aging.

CASE STUDY

Margaret, 79 years of age, sits in the sun porch clutching a pot of orchids. This is the last day she will enjoy this scene because today Margaret is moving to an assisted living facility in a town 260 miles away, which is close to her son, John. Margaret had lived in this home for almost 35 years with her husband, Andrew. When Andrew died 2 years ago of pancreatic cancer, it was a shock almost too great for Margaret to bear. Andrew had been her rock. Margaret had been Andrew's primary caretaker while he was ill. During their 40-year marriage, Margaret and Andrew had traveled all over the world and shared life-long interests including cooking, golf, and cultivating orchids in their custom built greenhouse. Margaret had been a volunteer with the children at the homeless shelter downtown until Andrew required her full-time care. The walls in their den were covered with awards and letters of appreciation for her work with the children. Now the house has been sold and many of her mementos have been packed up, sold, or given away.

Margaret had been an energetic high school history teacher and Andrew had been a chemist. They had two children, John and Karen. Karen is married and lives in London with her two daughters. Margaret and Andrew loved to travel to London to visit their grandchildren. John is recently divorced and is busy managing his new safety consulting company. Margaret has a beloved 9-year-old Labrador retriever named Henry, but she is unable to take Henry with her to the assistive living facility.

In the last 3 years, Margaret has been diagnosed with arthritis, vertigo, and early stages of dementia. Margaret fell 6 months ago and fractured her hip. She had begun to forget things such as paying bills, which caused her electricity to be turned off; leaving the stove on, which caused a small fire; and not remembering to take her medication regularly. John and Karen decided it was time to move their mother into a safer, more supervised environment. Margaret became depressed and less active after the decision was made. It seemed as if Margaret resigned herself to a situation beyond her control physically and socially. Margaret spent much of her time sleeping or sitting in the sun porch staring out the picture window. Moving to the new town meant saying goodbye to friends, relatives, and her beloved pet, as well as Andrew.

■ CASE STUDY REVIEW QUESTIONS

1 Identify the losses Margaret has experienced.
2 Describe the stressors or emotional problems that may be related to these losses. What impact would this have on her occupations? Describe shifts in occupational patterns that are linked to the changes in her life. Consider changes in roles, habits, routines, relationships, work, and leisure interests and activities.
3 Discuss what the COTA could do to help Margaret deal with these losses in terms of attitude, education, and activities.

■ EXERCISES

The following are a few activities to help the COTA gain empathy and rapport with the elderly.

INTO AGING

"Into Aging" is a commercially available game that focuses on building empathy for those who are growing old. The manual describes the game as a way for players to increase awareness of elders' problems by simulating experiences with similar problems, such as loss, isolation, powerlessness, dependency on others, and ageism. This game is available through Slack, Inc. (Thorofare, NJ).

ROLE PLAYING

Role playing is a useful activity for groups to understand aging-related issues. In preparation for the activity, each of the myths of aging discussed in this chapter should be written on index cards. Each small group will be given a set of index cards. Members of each group then enact some of the myths and stereotypes associated with the psychological aspects of aging. Each example should be followed with a discussion of feelings and thoughts about the stereotype or myth. What misconceptions did you have about aging before the activity that were subsequently clarified? What concept or concern is still puzzling or needs further exploration? How can you use the information learned in the role play in occupational therapy practice?

STEREOTYPE EXERCISE

Each member of a group should list the first six or seven images that immediately come to mind with the word *elder*. Group members should think about advertisements, movies, and personal experiences that influence their perceptions of elders. Each member should share the images with the group and explain the reasons the images are so vivid. All group members should discuss whether the images are realistic or stereotypical. Discuss how these stereotypes may bias the way a COTA would approach treatment with elders or with caregivers. Group members should brainstorm different ways to change stereotypical images to make them more realistic.

FIELD TRIP IMAGERY

Place yourself comfortably in a quiet room. You may sit in a comfortable chair or lie down. Take three deep breaths. As you exhale, clear your mind of any concerns and concentrate on the directions. Give yourself permission to use the next 10 to 15 minutes to explore what it would feel like to be 75 years old.

Pretend that you are looking into a large mirror. Imagine your physical appearance at age 75 years. What physical changes have taken place? Do you need any assistance with self-care? What emotions are you experiencing as a result of these changes?

What changes have occurred in your living arrangements? Do you live alone? Identify any changes in lifestyle as a result of finances.

What have you accomplished in your life thus far? Do you regret any events? Do you regret not achieving certain goals? Are you satisfied with your life?

Remember what you have just experienced with the visual imagery. Now slowly count to 10. As you get closer to 10, you will become more awake and tuned to the sounds of the room you are in. When you reach 10, gently open your eyes.

Free write for the next 5 minutes. It may be poetry, prose, or just phrases of what you remember of your visual imagery trip to age 75. Reflect on what key concepts of aging were apparent in the imagery. Describe your feelings.

RESOURCES

Older adult resources for mental health and wellness are available through Wellness Reproductions & Publishing, LLC (a Guidance Channel Company, 1-800-669-9208 or www.wellness-resources.com). This is a wonderful compilation of books, music cassettes, games, products, and tools to help those who work with the elderly deal with stress, aging, caregiving, and other challenges of older adults.

■ CHAPTER REVIEW QUESTIONS

1 Does chronological aging determine psychological aging? Discuss your position.
2 Identify aspects of aging that may affect learning for elders.
3 Coping with a serious illness can be especially stressful for an elder. Discuss any resulting occupational shifts and what a COTA can do to help elders understand change.
4 What is learned helplessness and what can COTAs do to help elders vulnerable to learned helplessness?

REFERENCES

American Association of Retired Persons. (2003). Staying ahead of the curve: The AARP work and career study [WWW page]. URL http://research.aarp.org/econ/multiwork.html

Anderson, D. A., Keith, J., Novak, P. & Elliot, M. (2002). *Mosby's medical, nursing and allied health dictionary*, (6th ed.). St. Louis, MO: Mosby.

Atchley, R. (1999). *Continuity and adaptation in aging: Creating positive experiences.* Baltimore, MD: Johns Hopkins University Press.

Barder, L., Slimmer, L., & LeSage, J. (1994). Depression and issues of control among elderly people in health care settings. *Journal of Advanced Nursing, 20,* 597-604.

Butler, R., Lewis, M., & Sunderland, T. (1991). *Aging and mental health.* New York, NY: Macmillan.

Canja, E. (2001). Aging in the 21st century: Myths and challenges. *Executive Speeches, 16,* 24-27.

Cegles, K. (2002). Psychological aspects of aging. In C. B. Lewis (Ed.), *Aging: The health care challenge.* Philadelphia, PA: F.A. Davis Company.

Chodoff, P. (1963). Late effects of the concentration camp syndrome. *Archives of General Psychiatry, 9*, 323.

Christiansen, C. (1991). Performance deficits as sources of stress. In C. Christiansen & C. Baum (Ed.), *Occupational therapy: Overcoming human performance deficits*. Thorofare, NJ: Slack, Inc.

Creek, J. (2002). *Occupational therapy and mental health*. Edinburgh, UK: Churchill Livingstone.

Davis, L. (1988). Coping with illness. In L. Davis & M. Kirkland (Eds.), *ROTE: The role of occupational therapy with the elderly*. Rockville, MD: The American Occupational Therapy Association.

Duncan-Myers, A. M., & Huebner, R. A. (2000). Relationship between choice and quality of life among residents in long-term-care facilities. *American Journal of Occupational Therapy, 54*, 504-508.

Erp, S. H., & Freeman, J. D. (1971). *Aging: Psychological changes*. Corvallis, OR: Continuing Education Publications.

Foy, S. S., & Mitchell, M. M. (1990). Factors contributing to learned helplessness. *Physical and Occupational Therapy in Geriatrics, 9*, 1-22.

Hayslip, B. (1983). *The aged patient: A sourcebook for the allied health professional*. St. Louis, MO: Mosby.

Holmes, T. H., & Rahe, R. H. (1967). The social readjustment rating scale. *Journal of Psychosomatic Research, 11*, 213-218.

Horn, J. L., & Cattell, R. B. (1966). Age differences in primary mental ability factors. *Journal of Gerontology, 21*, 210.

Katz, L., Manning, R., & Sutter, D. (1999). *Keep your brain alive: 83 neurobic exercises*. New York, NY: Workman Publishing, Inc.

Kielhofner, G. (2002). *A model of human occupation: Theory and application*. Baltimore, MD: Lippincott Williams & Wilkins.

Kübler-Ross, E. (1969). *On death and dying*. New York, NY: Macmillan.

Levy, L. (1996). Adaptation and the aging adult. In K. Larson, R. Stevens-Ratchford, L. Pedretti, & J. Crabtree (Eds.), *ROTE: The role of occupational therapy with the elderly*. Rockville, MD: The American Occupational Therapy Association.

Lewis, S. (2002). *Elder care in occupational therapy*. Thorofare, NJ: Slack, Inc.

Lieberman, M. A., & Tobin, S. S. (1983). *The experience of old age*. New York, NY: Basic Books.

Lohman, H., & Spergel, E. (1998). Aging trends and concepts. In H. Lohman, R. Padilla, & S. Byers-Connon (Eds.), *Occupational therapy with elders: Strategies for the COTA*. St. Louis, MO: Mosby.

MacDonald K., & Davis, L. (1988). Psychopathology and aging. In L. Davis & M. Kirkland (Eds.), *ROTE: The role of occupational therapy with the elderly*, Rockville, MD: The American Occupational Therapy Association.

Pearlin, L., & Skaff, M. (1995). Stressors and adaptation in late life. In M. Gatz (Ed.), *Emerging issues in mental health and aging*. Washington, DC: American Psychological Association.

Punwar, A. (2000). Elder care. In A. J. Punwar & S. M. Peloquin (Eds.), *Occupational therapy principles and practice* (3rd ed.). Philadelphia, PA: Lippincott Williams & Wilkins.

Rodin, J. (1986). Aging and health: Effects of the sense of control. *Science, 233*, 1271-1276.

Rodin, J. (1989). Sense of control: Potentials for intervention. *Annals of the Academy of Political and Social Science, 504*, 29-42.

Rowe, J., & Kahn, R. (1987). Human aging: Usual and successful. *Science, 237*, 143-149.

Royeen, C. (1995). The human life cycle: Paradigmatic shifts in occupation. In C. Royeen (Ed.), *The practice of the future: Putting occupation back into therapy*. Bethesda, MD: The American Occupational Therapy Association.

Seligman, M. E. P. (1975). *Helplessness*. San Francisco, CA: W.H. Freeman.

Shrimp, S. (1990). Debunking the myths of aging. *Occupational Therapy in Mental Health, 10*(3), 101-111.

Solomon, K. (1982). Social antecedents of learned helplessness in the health care setting. *Gerontologist, 22*, 282-287.

Solomon, K. (1990). Learned helplessness in the elderly: Theoretical and clinical considerations. *Occupational Therapy in Mental Health, 10*, 31-51.

Teitelman, J. L. (1990). Eliminating learned helplessness in older rehabilitation patients. *Physical and Occupational Therapy in Geriatrics, 9*, 43-54.

Thorton, J. (2002). Myths of aging or ageist stereotypes. *Educational Gerontology, 28*, 301-312.

Tufts University. (2002). You can't teach an old dog new tricks and other myths about the aging process. *Tufts University Health & Nutrition Letter, 20*, 1-3.

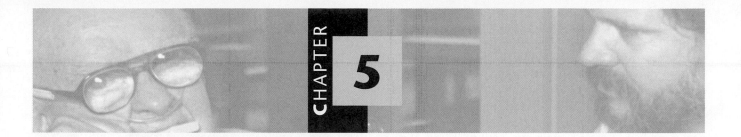

CHAPTER 5

Aging Well
Health Promotion and Disease Prevention

CLAUDIA GAYE PEYTON

KEY TERMS

health, occupation, occupational deprivation, successful aging, wellness, health promotion, occupational form, occupational performance, disuse syndrome, prevention, primary prevention, secondary prevention, health and risk screening, tertiary prevention

CHAPTER OBJECTIVES

1. Discuss the value of health and wellness promotion and disease prevention to occupational therapy (OT) practice with well and institutionalized elders.
2. Identify methods of screening and assessment used in promoting health among elders.
3. Describe health promotion activities that can be incorporated into practice with elders.
4. Describe theoretical models that emphasize the importance of occupational engagement and occupational form to the integration of healthy life patterns and performance.

5. Explain the reasons and demonstrate the ways health promotion and disease and disability prevention are instrumental in changing the future of OT practice at all levels.
6. Discuss the ways disuse syndrome contributes to the incidence and prevalence of preventable diseases and disabilities common to elderly populations.
7. Identify factors that contribute most to influencing elders to participate in wellness-focused activities.

Grow young along with me!
'Grow young along with me
The best is yet to be,
The last of life for which
The first is made.'

(Adapted from Robert Browning by Ashley Montagu, 1981)

Al is an 87-year-old man who hopes to live to be 100 years old. His wife, Irene, is 77 years of age and is content to have a few quiet hours each day to read and write letters. Al and Irene have been married for 56 years and have three adult children. They moved into a retirement housing area last year to ensure a safe living arrangement for whichever of the two lives longer. Al and Irene moved from their home of more than 40 years to this new environment with the help of a family friend.

After moving into their new home, Al and Irene often complained of feeling tired. During the next few months, they organized their lives in their new setting. They laughed and talked about getting to know some of their new neighbors. Overall, the move went well, and Al and Irene experienced the usual trials of adjusting to change.

Al and Irene are among America's fortunate well elderly. However, they are not without challenges. Al has been totally blind since he was 22 years of age. Al has survived a cranial subdural hematoma, which was removed from the left side of his brain, and was recently treated with radiation therapy for prostate cancer. Irene has experienced many surgeries during the past 15 years, including a heart double bypass, cataract surgery, a hip replacement, a rotator cuff repair, and gallbladder removal.

These two elders enjoy a remarkable level of independence, given their ages and medical histories. Some of this level of independence and relatively good health is a result of genetic endowment. In addition, lifestyle changes or other factors contributing to good health such as regular exercise and a balanced, low-fat diet have influenced independence. Historically, they have not lived without health risk. Al and Irene smoked for some time but eventually quit at 55 and 52 years, respectively. They agreed to adjust their diets on the basis of some research Al had read about the positive effects of reducing fat intake. Their dietary habits changed approximately 28 years ago. About that same time, Al began walking regularly. Initially, he experienced pain from angina, which required him to stop walking, rest, and take nitroglycerin tablets prescribed by his doctor. After several weeks of daily walking and taking the prescribed medication, Al could finally complete a trip around the block without interruption. He increased the daily walks to eventually complete 2 miles each day, which he continues to maintain. At the age of 84 years he went to guide dog training school for 3 weeks to be suited with a new guide dog because his previous dog died. His new guide dog, Chelsea, helps Al stay independent and mobile. Irene often accompanies Al and Chelsea on their daily walk (Fig. 5-1).

This story could be about anyone. The later episodes of a life story itself depend, to some extent, on the self-care choices people make along the way. As health care providers, certified occupational therapy assistants (COTAs) and occupational therapists can offer important health information and propose alternative lifestyle choices to elders. Society will increasingly look to health care providers for guidance and for models of healthful ways of living. This chapter describes the rationale for health promotion and disease or disability prevention programs that can be effective tools for use by COTAs working with elders.

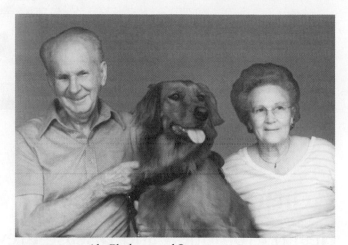

FIGURE 5-1   Al, Chelsea, and Irene.

CONCEPTS OF HEALTH PROMOTION AND WELLNESS IN OCCUPATIONAL THERAPY PRACTICE

The historic roots of occupational therapy (OT) philosophy and practice demonstrate the profession's long-standing belief in the value of occupation in promoting health and preventing functional loss caused by disease. Nelson and Stucky (1992) reviewed important OT values over the decades and wrote, "The potency of occupation in promoting health has long been recognized; this recognition is the basis for the existence of the profession of occupational therapy" (p. 22). Since the inception of OT as a profession in 1917, its premise has been to promote a healthy balance of activities for those persons who seek treatment. Activities perceived by an individual to be meaningful occupations are believed to influence the state of actual or possible health and well-being. Gilfoyle (1986) stated, "The therapeutic use of occupation to promote fullness of life is the basic value at the heart of our (professional) culture" (p. 400). The concepts of **health** and **occupation** are interrelated. Despite the various definitions and societal influences, the concept of occupation has remained centered on the value of activity to maintain enthusiasm about living. In essence, humans find meaning in what they do (Gilfoyle, 1986) (Fig. 5-2).

The value of occupation and the meaning of health are explicitly interrelated (Carlson, Clark, & Young, 1998; Jackson, Carlson, Mandel, Zemke, & Clark, 1998; Johnson, 1986; Nelson & Stucky, 1992; Riccio, Nelson, & Bush, 1990; Speake, 1987; Wilcock, 1998, 1999; Yerxa, 1993). As Nelson and Stucky (1992) described, "activation of function (occupation) is a main method of health promotion and disease prevention" (p. 21). Yerxa (1993) further described this relationship between occupation and health in her working definition of occupation:

Occupations are units of activity which are classified and named by the culture according to the purposes they serve in

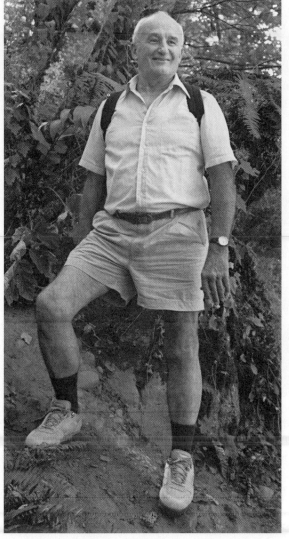

FIGURE 5-2 Activities perceived by an individual to be meaningful occupations are believed to influence the state of actual or perceived health.

enabling people to meet environmental challenges successfully[2].... Some essential characteristics of occupation are that it is self-initiated, goal directed (even if the goal is fun or pleasure), experiential as well as behavioral, socially valued or recognized, constructed of adaptive skills or repertoires,[13] organized, essential to the quality of life experienced, and possesses the capacity to influence health (p. 5).[16,17]

Richard (1991) suggested that *health* might be defined as "the ability to live and function effectively in society and to exercise self-reliance and autonomy to the maximum extent feasible, but not necessarily as total freedom from disease" (p. 79). Wilcock (1998) defined health from an occupational perspective as "the absence of illness, but not necessarily disability; a balance of physical, mental and social well being attained through socially valued and individually meaningful occupation; enhancement of capacities and opportunities to strive for individual

potential; community cohesion opportunities; and social integration, support and justice, all within and as a part of sustainable ecology" (p. 110). Wilcock (1999) advanced our perspective of the relationship between occupation and health by asserting that "occupation is clearly a prerequisite to health," (p. 195) and that major risk factors to health include problems in occupational performance such as "occupational imbalance," "occupational deprivation," and "occupational alienation" (Table 5-1).

Occupational engagement can have a profound and positive effect on the lives of elders who are well and living in the community and can improve life satisfaction among frail elders living in skilled nursing or assisted living environments. Habitual activities, those which are performed with consistency, can have a profound influence on health. "What people do is so much a part of the ordinary fabric of life that it is taken for granted and its health benefits are largely ignored" (Wilcock, 1999, p. 194). Regular participation in a balance of meaningful daily occupations can prevent the development, occurrence, and progression of most disabling conditions. However, many elders have been typecast by society and health care professionals as being unable to improve their health status. This myth is detrimental to the health and well-being of older adults and dampens motivation to try to make small changes that could provide health improvements with small investments of time and effort.

Only in recent years has the literature associated with aging focused on healthy aging and long-term survival and moved away from medically oriented disease management. Recent literature suggests changing societal views of health and longevity. Promotion of "successful aging" (Carlson, Clark, & Young 1998, p. 107) will likely replace past views of disease remediation and control. "The shifting focus from disease management and survival to health through disease prevention, health maintenance, and health promotion provides great promise for occupational therapy" (Hanft, 2002, p. 10). The prevailing diseases contributing to morbidity and mortality among elderly people can be prevented through lifestyle changes.

Although leading causes of death or mortality, these diseases are also leading causes of morbidity, or illness (Table 5-2). Morbidity can cause great suffering, occupational dysfunction, alienation, and cost. COTAs have the potential to assist patients in learning to prevent or to control the long-range and deleterious effects of prevalent hazards to health and well-being. Diet, exercise, balance, and decreased stress, along with environmental adjustment for safety and management of medications, are a few examples of minor changes that can make a long-range difference. Regardless of age, unhealthy habits and patterns of living can be changed to improve health and to enhance life satisfaction.

Carlson, Clark, and Young (1998) asserted that "potentially controllable lifestyle factors play a crucial role in

TABLE 5-1

Risk Factors to Health

Risk factors to health	Wilcock	Brownson and Scaffa
Occupational imbalance	Occurs when people engage in too much of the same type of activity, limiting the exercise of their various capacities (p. 195).	A lack of balance among work, rest, self-care, play, and leisure that fails to meet an individual's unique…needs, thereby resulting in decreased health, well-being, or both (p. 657).
Occupational deprivation	When factors beyond them limit an individual's choice or opportunity (p. 195).	Prompted by conditions such as poor health, disability, lack of transportation, isolation, unemployment, homelessness, poverty, and so forth (p. 657).
Occupational alienation	When people are unable to meet basic occupational needs, or use their particular capacities because of intervening socio-cultural factors (p. 195)	A sense of estrangement and lack of satisfaction in one's occupations. Tasks or work perceived as stressful, meaningless, or boring may result in occupational alienation (p. 657).

Data from Wilcock, A. A. (1999). The Doris Sym Memorial Lecture: Developing a philosophy of occupation for health. *British Journal of Occupational Therapy, 62*(5), 191-198; and Brownson, C. A., & Scaffa, M. E. (2001). Occupational therapy in the promotion of health and the prevention of disease and disability statement. *American Journal of Occupational Therapy, 55*(6), 656-660.

enabling people to experience healthy and satisfying lives well into old age" (p. 107). These authors proposed that an operational definition of aging in the future may in fact be the "disappearance of health" because careful living has such great potential to promote "successful aging" over a lifetime (p. 108). Research conducted by Carlson and colleagues provides insight into factors that lead to "successful aging" (p. 109) (Box 5-1). The concept that occupational therapists can "positively enhance lifestyle" (Richards, 1998, p. 299) is in line with the projected goals

TABLE 5-2

Ten Leading Causes of Death by Age Group, 2000

Cause of death	Age (yr)						
	25-34	34-44	45-54	55-64	65-74	75-84	85+
Heart	5	3	2	2	2	1	1
Cancer	4	1	1	1	1	2	2
Stroke	8	8	5	4	4	3	3
Respiratory			9	3	3	4	6
Intentional accidents	2	4	6	9			
Unintentional accidents	1	2	3	6	6	9	9
Diabetes	7	9	7	5	5	5	7
Flu and pneumonia		10			7	6	4
Alzheimer's disease						7	5
Nephritis				8	8	8	8
Assault	3	7					
Human immunodeficiency virus	6	5	8				
Congenital disorders	9						
Cirrhosis	10	6	4	7	10		
Hepatitis			10				
Septicemia				10	9	10	10

Adapted from Minino, A. M., Arias, E., Kochanek, S.L., Murphy, S. L., & Smith, B. L. (2002). Deaths: Final data for 2000. Department of Health and Human Services [DHHS], Centers for Disease Control and Prevention [CDC], National Center for Health Statistics. *50*(15), 13-15.

BOX 5-1

Factors Contributing to Successful Aging

1. Experiencing a sense of control over one's life
2. Practicing healthy habits
3. Achieving continuity with one's past
4. Performing happy activities
5. Participating in a social network of family and friends
6. Exercising regularly
7. Engaging one's mind in complex cognitive activities
8. Stopping smoking
9. Maintaining a healthy diet
10. Consuming fewer calories
11. Receiving preventative medical treatment
12. Taking aspirin and antioxidant vitamins

Adapted from Carlson, M., Clark, F., & Young, B. (1998). Practical contributions of occupational science to the art of successful aging: How to sculpt a meaningful life in older adulthood. *Journal of Occupational Science, 5*(30), 107-118.

of the U.S. Department of Health and Human Services (DHHS) for a healthy population as established in Healthy People 2010. All OT personnel need to be aware of the major public health initiatives set forth in *Healthy People 2010* (DHHS, 2000). The goals established in this document emphasize the need for increasing the quality of life of all people and prioritizing efforts leading to achievement of a longer and healthier life for all citizens. Priority goals call for the elimination of health disparities on the basis of sex, race, ethnicity, disability, sexual orientation, education, income, or residence in a rural or urban setting (p. 2). These goals fit well with the needs of the current elder population. As discussed in the document:

> The first goal of Healthy People 2010 *is to increase the quality as well as the years of healthy life. Here the emphasis is on the health status and nature of life, not just longevity.... The emphasis on functional capacity and satisfying productive life of our citizen's parallels occupational therapy's focus on enabling engagement in meaningful occupation, which supports and leads to a productive and satisfying life.*
>
> **(Brownson & Scaffa, 2001, p. 656).**

COTAs have a responsibility and an opportunity to influence change in the quality of the lives of elders by implementation of occupation-centered care. The 21st century is the time for needed health care reform, prompted by the urgency to reduce cost for care, and the time to return the responsibility for "successful aging" to the individual. Therapists should demonstrate leadership in helping individuals plan health-promoting engagement in meaningful occupations as the path to a long and healthy life. "The organizing promise of occupational

therapy emphasizes the important role of everyday activities or occupations in establishing routines and infusing meaning in daily life" (Scott et al., 2001, p. 13).

Society is now better prepared to move from a medically based model of care to a more health-centered, cost-effective approach to health care. In the medical model, the disease state has taken priority over consideration of the person as a whole being. Thus, people are often treated as an illness or a disability. For example, a hospital staff member may refer to an elder as "the total hip replacement in room 420" rather than "Mrs. Smith." Not only has the medical model reduced the value of the human spirit to the cellular or disease level, it also has contributed dramatically to the cost of health care as a result of specialization. In contrast, wellness approaches and holistic theories consider people in the context of their lives. **Wellness** has been defined as "a dynamic way of life that involves actions, values, and attitudes that support or improve both health and quality of life" (Brownson & Scaffa, 2001, p. 656). An important projected outcome of health promotion is personal wellness.

Assisting people at all ages to actively participate in taking responsibility for improving the quality of their health is not unique to OT, but it has been a prominent value held by OT personnel since the inception of the profession. Health can be enhanced and disease can be prevented through occupation. Interventions are provided at the institutional, legislative, and personal level of care, thus encouraging health at the environmental and personal level. OT personnel can be instrumental in creating healthy environments through consultation with state, city, and institutional levels of care. Political, economic, and practice environments need health professionals who understand the essential relation between occupation and health. As Mary Reilly stated in her Eleanor Clark Slagle Lecture of 1961, "man through the use of his hands as energized by mind and will, can influence the state of his own health (Reilly, 1962, p. 2). "Ultimately, health is created and lived by people within the settings of everyday life; where they learn, work, play, and love" (Wilcock, 1999, p. 195).

Health Risks and Their Effects on Occupational Engagement

Substantial research evidence supports the need for increased health promotion and disease prevention activities for elders. Hickey and Stilwell (1991) maintain that the primary goal of health promotion programs for elders should be focused on prevention of "the progression of disease and the risks of disability and death...that health promotion should be designed to help older persons maintain their functional independence and autonomy for as long as possible" (p. 828). Brownson & Scaffa (2001) define **health promotion** as "any planned combination of educational, political, regulatory, environmental, and organizational supports for actions and conditions of living conducive to the health of persons, groups, or communities, or—more simply—the process of enabling people to increase control over and to improve their health" (p. 657). Health promotion is focused on preventive efforts. The promotion of health must be considered in the contexts in which people live and relate to others. OT practitioners contribute to health promotion by first identifying those factors at the individual, group, organizational, community, and policy levels that interfere with occupational engagement.

As described by Fidler and Fidler (1978), humans develop through "doing" and through "doing" become individuals. Through occupations, people adapt in both healthy and unhealthy ways. At times through occupational patterns people learn maladaptive ways of living. In daily practice settings, COTAs meet elders who can benefit from assistance in making positive choices to improve the quality of their health. Some elders do not recognize that the quality of their lives can change with even minor adjustments in their lifestyles. During daily therapeutic interactions, COTAs have an opportunity to influence their clients' considerations of healthy lifestyles and assist them in improving the quality of their lives. Encouraging exploration of health-promoting activities and providing educational information to elders and their families may help motivate an elder to take actions that promote health and limit the potential for occupational deprivation, alienation, or imbalance associated with current habits. Elders are frequently uninformed or believe that changes later in life may offer few benefits. Helping elders understand the tremendous potential for healthy outcomes associated with small changes in daily routines can make the difference between future independence and debilitating dependence.

Nelson and Stucky (1992) suggest that "one's occupational patterns of self-care and interests comprise ... occupational situations (occupational forms) that are health promoting and disease preventing" (p. 22). The **occupational form** to which Nelson and Stucky refer includes the environmental context of the individual's life. The context is composed of physical and sociocultural characteristics that stimulate the individual to choose an **occupational performance**. For example, an elder who lives in a retirement village may choose to play golf (occupational form) because there is a golf course on the grounds (physical characteristic) and this is where most people at that village socialize (sociocultural characteristic). The value that the person places on the occupational form gives meaning and purpose to the individual's choice of actions. This sense of purposefulness is the motivator or stimulus that results in participation in activities such as playing golf. Playing golf on Thursday mornings may involve habituation of many occupational performance skills such as socialization, preparation of refreshments for

guests, and the actual performance of playing golf. This involves motor performance, cognition, and other complex functions. Activation of an interest in and performance of a cherished occupation helps the person establish a positive and continuous cycle or habit pattern. Fidler and Fidler (1978) theorize that imagery is linked with purpose. They perceive that actions related to achievement are a result of conceptualizing an image before taking action. Thus, mental imagery adds purpose to occupations. Mental images are constructed before taking action and facilitate the person's participation (Figs. 5-3 and 5-4).

The actual enjoyment of participation in chosen occupations or activities is referred to as *intrinsic motivation* (Florey, 1976). Baking a pie, walking a dog, and gardening are intrinsically motivated occupations. Actions taken toward a goal provide feedback that, if positive, may inspire continued participation in the activity or similar activities. Feedback may take the form of wonderful tomatoes from a well-nurtured garden or excitement from the completion of a small but meaningful project. Recognition from meaningful others can serve as a source of encouragement and their enjoyment may motivate continued occupational engagement. Each interaction sets up the potential for additional involvement in occupations that ultimately contribute to growth, development, self-confidence, and improved self-esteem. Conversely, negative feedback or experiences may result in a cycle of feelings of fear, helplessness, humiliation, and failure (Nelson & Stucky, 1992).

The outcome of an effective **health promotion** program is the enhancement or maintenance of function in activities of daily living (ADL) and overall life satisfaction. The need for elders to maintain functional capacity and interest and participation in meaningful occupations has been demonstrated by research findings suggesting that losses occur in the ability to perform ADL functions as a result of the disabling effects of **disuse syndrome**,

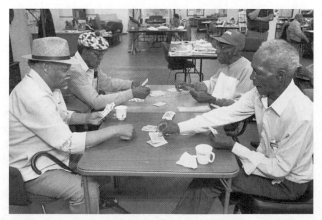

FIGURE 5-3   Purposefulness stimulates participation in activities such as the hobby of playing cards.

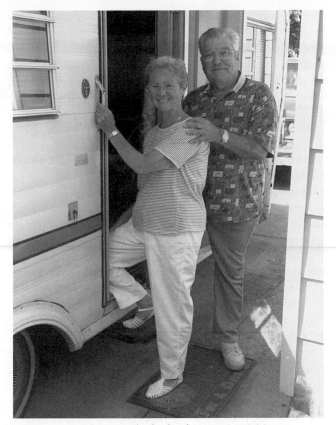

FIGURE **5-4**   This couple finds pleasure in visiting new places.

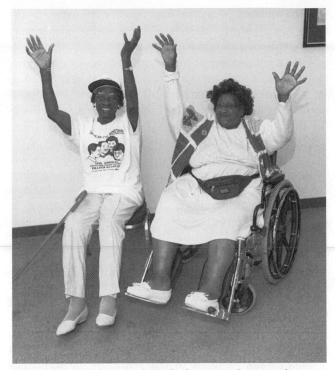

FIGURE **5-5**   Elders can benefit from regular seated exercise.

a common sequel to physical and cognitive disabilities. Approximately 14.2% of elders living in the community experience difficulty completing one or more ADL because of health-related problems. Approximately 21.6% of elders report difficulties with instrumental activities of daily living (IADL) (DHHS, 2001). Research shows that the need for assistance in completion of ADL and IADL increases with age (DHHS, 2000).

McMurdo and Rennie (1993) report that elders in nursing homes who participated in a seated exercise group for 8 weeks showed significant improvement in grip strength, chair-to-stand time, and function in ADLs, and they also experienced decreased feelings of depression. "Even very elderly residents of nursing homes can benefit from participation in regular seated exercise and can improve in functional capacity" (p. 12) (Fig. 5-5). Unfortunately, research literature indicates that "despite the known importance of and preponderance of media attention to exercise, more than 60% of women over the age of 60 participate in little or no sustained physical activity of at least moderate intensity" (Caserta & Gillett, 1998, p. 602). Studies further indicate a correlation between fear of falling and a loss of physical endurance and strength. Nuessel and Van Stewart (1999) found that "...35% of community dwelling elderly avoided doing

things they wanted to do because they were afraid of falling" (p. 4). The fear of falling impaired choices of occupation and life satisfaction. Evidence supports that exercise programs can reduce falls by increasing endurance, improving balance, and improving confidence. Rubenstein and colleagues (2000) concluded that,

> ... *a simple program of progressive resistance exercises, walking, and balance training can improve muscle endurance, and functional mobility in elderly men with chronic impairments and risk factors for falls. In addition, this study provides new evidence on the complex relationship between physical activity and falls: exercise participants significantly increased their physical activity, yet experienced fewer falls per unit of activity.*

(p. M319)

Exercise has an effect on the mind and the body. As the body grow stronger, the individual's self-confidence increases, and with positive changes come greater options for engagement in meaningful occupations.

The benefit of health promotion and disease **prevention** programs may be best understood by considering the most common risks to the health of elders. Physical and psychological risks to health and well-being, which are common to elders after retirement, are numerous. The DHHS (2001) has identified the following chronic conditions as those that most frequently "contribute to difficulty in independently performing activities of daily living (ADL) and instrumental activities of daily living

55

(IADL) functions: arthritis, hypertension, hearing impairment, heart disease, cataracts, diabetes, orthopedic impairments, tinnitus, and diabetes" (p 12).

Other authors suggest that the decline seen in aging may not be caused by age but by a condition referred to as *disuse syndrome*. This term alludes to the detrimental effects of sedentary living and limited use of capabilities in the development of chronic and debilitating conditions. Approximately 50% of symptoms currently associated with aging, such as increases in body fat and decreases in endurance, lean body mass, and strength and flexibility, are actually a result of hypokinesia, a disease of disuse (Drinkwater, 1988; Hjort, 2000; Schuster, Petrosa, & Petrosa, 1995; Smith, 1995). Experimental immobilization has been noted to cause decreases in musculoskeletal, cardiovascular, and metabolic functions similar to those seen with aging. Thus, a portion of the loss of physiological integrity in elders may be attributable to disuse syndrome (Fiatarone & Evans, 1990). According to Nied and Franklin (2002), "muscle strength declines by 15% per decade after age 50 and 30 percent per decade after age 70; however, resistance training can result in 25 to 100 percent...strength gains in older people" (p. 421). Jett and Branch (1981) conducted the "The Framingham Study of Disability" and found that 45% of elderly women aged 65 years and older and 65% of women older than 75 years cannot lift 10 pounds. Loss of strength and endurance among the elderly is most often an outcome of disuse or inactivity and is a serious impediment to daily living function and increased potential for falls.

Prevention and Health Promotion Among Elders

COTAs working with elders should be familiar with categories of prevention. Many health problems of elders are especially suited for prevention planning. Impaired mobility, injury from falls, sensory loss, adverse medication reactions, disuse syndrome, depression, malnutrition, alcohol abuse, hypertension, and osteoporosis are serious problems of the elderly that can be prevented or postponed through prevention-focused health education efforts (Webster, 1992). Brownson and Scaffa (2001) assert that "Occupational Therapy practitioners provide health promotion services, which typically involve 'lifestyle redesign' or the development of supports for healthy engagement in occupations as a means of preventing the unhealthy effects of inactivity" (p. 656).

Prevention strategies are generally organized into three categories: primary, secondary, and tertiary (Garner & Young, 1993; Webster, 1992). Primary prevention focuses on reducing the risk for disease before its onset. Primary preventive efforts with elders may consist of facilitation of lifestyle changes and use of necessary medications to reduce the development of life-threatening conditions such as cardiovascular disease and stroke. Primary prevention programs include immunization, accident prevention,

exercise, nutritional counseling, and smoking and alcohol cessation (Webster, 1992). A critical primary prevention effort should be focused on prevention of falls in elders because accidents are the sixth leading cause of death among people older than 65 years (Centers for Disease Control [CDC], 2002b).

Primary Prevention

COTAs may represent the first line of **primary prevention** for well, homebound, or institutionalized elders. Primary prevention is defined as "education or health promotion strategies designed to help people avoid the onset of unhealthy conditions, diseases or injuries" (Brownson & Scaffa, 2001, p. 657). In this capacity, COTAs have an opportunity to influence change in elders' awareness of health risks. By assisting elders to develop or return to interests that stimulate increased activity and mobility, COTAs may help reduce ill effects of a sedentary lifestyle or disuse syndrome. Many disabilities of elders start with disuse and are preventable. Studies have demonstrated the long-reaching effects of regular exercise in the prevention of weakness and fatigue, which interfere with independence in ADL functions (Butler, Davis, Lewis, Nelson, & Strauss, 1998; Fiatarone & Evans, 1990; Glantz & Richman, 1996; Lohman & Givens, 1999; McMurdo & Rennie, 1993; Rubenstein et al., 2000; Schuster, Petrosa & Petrosa, 1995). Exercise also has helped to prevent obesity, thus reducing consequent hypertension and diabetes. A daily or three times weekly exercise program or regular participation in an activity such as walking or chair aerobics can significantly reduce the potentials for falls (Rubenstein et al., 2000), which is a serious threat to the health and well-being of elder clients. In addition, exercise is related to improvements in elder's psychological well-being (Stewart et al., 1998) (Fig. 5-6).

Noteworthy outcomes exist between clients involved in rote exercise and those participating in personally meaningful occupations. Rote exercise involves the repetition of a particular movement, such as lifting a 10-lb dumbbell 10 times to develop strength, endurance, or skill. Personally meaningful occupations are intrinsically motivated—that is, characteristic of activities that have a purpose in and of themselves, such as picking up a 10-lb infant. Yoder, Nelson, and Smith (1989) found that elderly women engaged in significantly more exercise repetitions with intrinsic activities such as food preparation than with a rote exercise program. Riccio, Nelson, and Bush (1990) later found that the use of imagery as a cue facilitated more exercise repetitions than a rote exercise program. In this study, elders imagined that they were using first the right and then the left arm to pick apples and place them in a basket. In a study of elder women performing a kicking task, Thomas (1996) found that the subjects who did the task with the actual balloon performed better than those doing rote exercise or those using imagery.

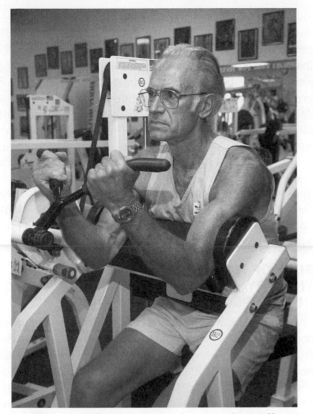

FIGURE 5-6   Regular exercise has long-reaching effects in maintaining independence.

He concludes that using actual tasks that have meaning might result in better performance. A number of other studies have investigated the effects of purposeful use of materials to facilitate movement beyond the benefits of rote exercise (Bloch, Smith, & Nelson, 1989; Heck, 1988; Kircher, 1984; Miller & Nelson, 1987; Sakemiller & Nelson, 1998; Schmidt & Nelson, 1996; Thomas & Rice, 2002; Yoder, Nelson & Smith, 1989). These studies validate OT beliefs regarding the health-enhancing value of participation in actual occupation and point to the limited effects of simulated activities. Meaningful activities important to the client help generate motivation and excitement that rote exercise cannot. Thus, clients gain more from exercises that are "embedded in meaningful, purposeful occupations" (Nelson & Stucky, 1992, p. 19) than from a rote regimen of exercise.

Fall prevention is another critical aspect of primary prevention practices that COTAs can facilitate. A home or an institutional environmental assessment may identify many fall hazards for elders (see Chapter 14). "A Matter of Balance" is a well researched fall prevention program that COTAs can implement in practice. The program utilizes a multimodel approach that addresses physical, social, and cognitive factors affecting fear of falling (Boston University Center for the Enhancement

of Late-Life Function, 2000). The use of the "Fall Risk Factor Screening Checklist" (Carlson, 1996) can contribute significant information to fall prevention (Fig. 5-7).

Secondary Prevention

Secondary prevention efforts consist of "identification and treatment of persons with early, minimally symptomatic diseases to improve outcomes and maintain health" (Garner & Young, 1993, p. 299). Secondary prevention "includes early detection and treatment designed to prevent or disrupt the disability process" (Brownson & Scaffa, 2001, p. 657). Early detection of hypertension and cancers may prevent early disability and mortality. Vision and hearing deficits are also preventable at times if detected early, as are breast and cervical cancers and depressive or substance use disorders. COTAs can contribute to early detection of serious conditions that contribute to disability and interfere with ADL and IADL functions by reminding elders of the importance of annual examinations, such as mammograms and Papanicolaou (PAP) tests. Recommendations for health and risk screening of elder populations can be different in some cases. For example, the DHHS does not provide specific suggestions for upper age limits of Pap testing but suggests recommending discontinuation after 65 if the woman's previous regular screenings were consistently normal (CDC, 2002a).

Minority group and nonambulatory elderly women are at a greater risk for serious health conditions including increased incidence of cervical cancer and cervical cancer mortality. "Women ages 35 years or older, who are racial or ethnic minorities and low income, are at increased risk for invasive cervical cancer due to lower

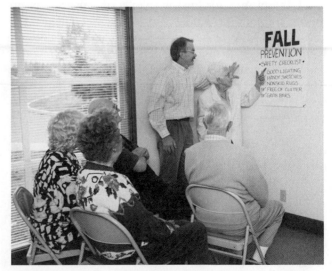

FIGURE 5-7   Fall prevention is a critical aspect of primary prevention. (Courtesy Sue Byers-Connon, Mt. Hood Community College, Gresham, OR.)

likelihood of Pap smear screen test" (Washington State Department of Health, 2002, p. 1). Reduced access to health care and to culturally appropriate health care messages has increased the risk for cervical cancers in both Hispanic and Vietnamese women in the United States. "Cervical cancer occurs most often among minority women, particularly Asian-American (Vietnamese and Korean), Alaska Native and Hispanic" (Agency for Healthcare Research and Quality, Breast and Cervical Cancer Research Highlights, 2003, p. 2).

Analysis of invasive cervical cancer incidences by age and stage at diagnosis indicated that, except for women aged 20-29 years, incidences for Hispanic women were significantly higher than those for non-Hispanic women...the incidence for Hispanic women was second only to that of Vietnamese women, which was more than twice the incidence for Hispanics.... For Hispanic and non-Hispanic women, approximately 30% of all new invasive cervical cancers diagnosed among women ages <50 years were at an advanced stage; among women who were aged 50> years, advanced stage cervical cancer represented 52% of new diagnoses.

(CDC, 2002c, p. 1068)

Iezzoni, McCarthy, and Davis (2001) found that women with lower extremity mobility difficulties are significantly less likely than other women to receive screening and preventive services such as mammograms and Pap smears. Because of the multiple and complex factors that contribute to health disparities among elderly, disabled, and minorities, health care providers at all levels should have an awareness of and a concern for the overall health of their clients. All health care providers should assume responsibility for encouraging and reminding elderly clients to schedule regular physical examinations.

Careful observation of functional capabilities may facilitate early detection of changes in elders' capabilities. COTAs can monitor loss or change of sensory capacity during routine interactions with elders (see Chapters 15 and 16). COTAs also may be instrumental in educating family members to monitor elders for changes in mood or cognitive functioning that may influence independence in ADL and IADL. Changes in mood or cognition can be associated with poor nutrition or dehydration, which can be prevented or remediated (see Chapter 21). Changes also may indicate reactions to or side effects of medications or more serious physiologic changes that require medical evaluation and attention (see Chapter 13).

Tertiary Prevention

Tertiary prevention refers to preventing the progression of existing conditions. It "relates to functional assessment and rehabilitation both to reverse and to prevent progression of the burden of illness" (Webster, 1992, p. 3). Brownson and Scaffa (2001) have defined tertiary prevention "as treatment and service designed to arrest the progression of a condition, prevent further disability, and

promote social opportunity" (p. 656). An example of tertiary prevention initiated by the COTA could be the treatment of a homebound elder who is experiencing limitations because of the pain of arthritis. The COTA would provide education about self-care activities such as joint protection and energy conservation to prevent further deterioration of arthritic joints. In addition, joint mobility can be facilitated through regular participation in a hobby within the elder's range of tolerance. Performing energy conservation activities also may assist the elder in feeling in control of his or her daily routine. Control of pain and implementation of environmental adaptations and work simplification could assist the elder and encourage greater involvement in meaningful occupations and engagement with others.

ROLE OF THE CERTIFIED OCCUPATIONAL THERAPY ASSISTANT IN WELLNESS AND HEALTH PROMOTION

COTAs play a critical role in promotion of health and prevention of disease among elders. Health education facilitates health promotion, disability reduction, and illness prevention (Pinch, 1993). Chronic illnesses that affect ADL and IADL functions are more often related to lifestyle, genetic predisposition, and environmental exposure than to age alone. Frequently, elders must change behaviors to prevent disability from developing or progressing. Professional evaluation, intervention, and educational programs implemented by COTAs can foster such life-enhancing changes. A health behavior questionnaire can determine the need for intervention through health education activities (Box 5-2). Hickey and Stilwell (1991) stated, "The overall goal of health promotion in the elderly...should be to prevent the progression of disease and the risks of disability and death" (p. 823). Health promotion should also help elders maintain functional autonomy as long as possible (Davies, 1990). Glantz and Richman (1996) proposed guidelines for the development of wellness programs for elders that emphasize goals of "optimum achievement and maintenance of competence and independence" (Box 5-3).

Hettinger (1996) developed the following *ABCs* of the wellness model in OT, which may assist COTAs in encouraging their elder clients to learn to improve and maintain their health:

*A*ttitude that includes actively pursuing wellness and ADLs that promote satisfaction and quality of life
*B*alancing productive activity, positive social support, emotional expression, and environmental interactions
*C*ontrolling health through education about behaviors that lead to wellness

This model encourages COTAs to serve as mentors, coaches, and educators (p. 12).

The American Occupational Therapy Association (AOTA) published a position statement entitled

BOX 5-2

Prevention Behavior Questionnaire

1. Name some behaviors in your life that you believe endanger or compromise your health.
2. How much control do you have to change them? (circle one)   a. some   b. little   c. none
3. Do you participate in some form of physical activity on a regular basis? (circle one)   yes   no
4. What activities do you participate in? (circle all that apply)
   a. walking   b. swimming   c. gardening   d. other _____
5. How often in a week do you engage in these activities? (circle one)
   a. daily   b. twice   c. three times   d. other _____
6. How much time do you devote to these activities? (circle one)
   a. less than 30 min   b. 1 hour   c. 2 hours   d. other _____
7. Rate the level of stress in your life (circle one):
   a. very high   b. high   c. moderate   d. occasional   e. very low
8. What do you do to relieve stress in your life? (circle all that apply)
   a. hobbies   b. exercise   c. drink alcohol   d. smoke   e. other (s) _____
9. How many meals do you eat each day? (circle one)
   a. three   b. two   c. one   d. less than one
10. Do you usually eat (circle one):   a. alone   b. with others
11. Do you consider your weight to be (circle one)   a. too high   b. average   c. too low
12. Do you monitor your daily fat intake? (circle one)   a. yes   b. no
13. How many servings do you have each day from the following food groups? (circle your answers)
    a. bread and cereal   1   2   3   4   more
    b. fruits and vegetables   1   2   3   4   more
    c. meat   1   2   3   4   more
    d. beans, peas, tofu   1   2   3   4   more
    e. milk   1   2   3   4   more
    f. dairy products   1   2   3   4   more
14. Is it necessary for you to monitor your blood cholesterol level? (circle one)   a. yes   b. no
15. Do you monitor your sodium intake? (circle one)   a. yes   b. no
16. Have you fallen (circle one)
    a. in the past week   b. in the past month   c. in the past 3 months   d. in the past 6 months
    e. in the past 9 months   f. in the past year   g. in the past 18 months
17. If so, how many times have you fallen? (circle one)   a. 1   b. 2   c. 3   d. other _____
18. Have you scalded or burned yourself recently? (circle one)
    a. in the past week   b. in the past month   c. in the past 3 months   d. in the past 6 months
    e. in the past year   f. in the past 18 months
19. Do you have arthritis? (circle one)   a. yes   b. no
20. Do you have heart disease? (circle one)   a. yes   b. no
21. Do you have cancer? (circle one)   a. yes   b. no
22. Do you have difficulty catching your breath
    a. when walking? (circle one)   a. yes   b. no
    b. when climbing stairs? (circle one)   a. yes   b. no
    c. when sitting? (circle one)   a. yes   b. no
23. Do you have asthma or emphysema? (circle one)   a. yes   b. no
24. Do you have difficulty
    a. bending over to remove items from low cabinets? (circle one)   a. yes   b. no
    b. going up or down stairs? (circle one)   a. yes   b. no
    c. getting up from a bed or chair? (circle one)   a. yes   b. no
25. Do you need assistance to walk? (circle one)   a. yes   b. no
26. What distance can you safely walk without assistance or stopping? (circle one)
    a. less than 1 block   b. 1 block   c. 1/4 mile   d. 1/2 mile   e. 1 mile   f. other _____
27. What would you like to change about your health?

Adapted from Lohman, H., & Peyton-Runyon, C. (1991). Intergenerational experiences for occupational therapy students. *Physical Occupational Therapy in Geriatrics*, 2(10), 17.

BOX 5-3

Wellness Program for Elders

Program goals
- Enhance awareness of the positive effect of wellness on health at any age
- Promote awareness of the sensory changes that occur as aging progresses
- Improve knowledge of food consumption and effects on health
- Improve decision-making skills
- Encourage self-responsibility for health
- Encourage independence and environmental mastery
- Maximize a positive focus
- Heighten awareness of behaviors that inhibit health and perpetuate disease
- Encourage independence in self-care

Possible topics
- Personal nutrition
- Exercise: sitting, standing, low-impact aerobics
- Planning of health screenings, including annual screening for cancer
- Smoking cessation
- Activities: exploring interests
- Stress and effects on the heart
- Relaxation
- Responsibility for health
- Sensory loss and safety: eliminating hazards

Adapted from Glantz, C. H., & Richman, N. (1996). The wellness model in long term care facilities. *Quest*, 7, 7.

"Occupational Therapy in the Promotion of Health and the Prevention of Disease and Disability Statement" (Brownson & Scaffa, 2001). This statement calls on OT practitioners to be involved with health promotion and disease prevention. Three main roles have been outlined: (1) promoting healthy lifestyles for all elders, (2) augmenting existing health promotion programs by including the OT perspective, and (3) focusing on intervention at the community or policy level (Brownson & Scaffa, 2001).

The *Well Elderly Study*, conducted at the University of Southern California, illustrates a successful model for OT wellness programming (Clark et al., 1997; Clark et al., 2001; Jackson, Carlson, Mandel, Zemke, & Clark, 1998; Mandel, Jackson, Zemke, Nelson, & Clark, 1999). Indications of this well designed study validate that the lives of elders living in an urban community can be enhanced through reactivation of interests and participation in meaningful occupations. The content of the program, based on the elder's input, provided detailed instructions about areas such as transportation, safety, social relationships, and finances. Interventions through education and self-discovery processes were offered in both individual and group contexts. A key outcome of this study was demonstrating the importance and health enhancing effects of reengaging elderly participants in meaningful occupations. Elderly participants assigned to the group who were facilitated by occupational therapists had better outcomes than those participants assigned to the control group or those participants of the group who were facilitated by a volunteer nonprofessional (Jackson et al., 1998). Overall, this prevention program found that occupational therapist–led groups offered a significant benefit to positive outcomes measures and that therapy helped the elders improve health and functional ability necessary for community living (Mandel et al., 1999). The results of this program have been sustained over time (Clark et al., 2001).

Health education empowers elders to take increasing responsibility for their health. COTAs have many opportunities across practice domains to provide health education programs for elders. Health promotion can occur through individual or group education efforts (Clark et al., 2001). COTAs can rely on group skills to facilitate discussion of materials and to encourage group development and cohesion. Generally, health-related topics include awareness building activities to heighten elder valuing and understanding of the benefits of exercise, cardiac risk reduction, methods of management of arthritis, stroke prevention, immunization, osteoporosis, cancer, early detection, home safety, assistive devices, and sensory changes that occur with aging (Mount, 1991). Discussion topics educate elders about leading causes of functional limitation, disability, and death, thereby facilitating the potential to change behaviors and improve quality of life.

In their research of effects of an exercise program for older adults, Hickey and Stilwell (1991) pointed out evidence to inspire COTAs to provide health-promoting activities. "The older adult responds to exercise training in the same manner as a young adult, with a 10% to 20% increase in cardiovascular fitness and strength gain of between 50% and 174% depending on the extent of reconditioning" (Hickey & Stilwell, p. 823). Such research shows that it is never too late to begin exercising.

CONCLUSION

The United States is moving into an era of health care reform that focuses on improving the quality of life for the lowest cost. The OT practitioner's role in this reform is to promote personal responsibility for health through facilitation of self-discovery activities that can enhance interest and participation in meaningful occupations. In addition, the belief that small adaptive changes can improve the quality of a person's life regardless of age or disability must be encouraged. As Ashley Montagu (1981) wrote in *Growing Young*, "…the youth of the chronologically young is a gift; growing young into what others call 'old age' is an achievement, a work of art. It takes time to grow young" (p. 194).

CHAPTER REVIEW QUESTIONS

1 Give examples of primary, secondary, and tertiary prevention functions of certified occupational therapy assistants (COTAs) working with elders.

2 Name two activity groups that could be used with each classification of prevention.

3 Explain how health and occupation are interrelated.

4 How would you define *disuse syndrome?* How does this syndrome contribute to disease and disability?

5 How can occupation be characterized as health promoting?

6 Describe the role of COTAs in wellness and health promotion program implementation.

7 How can COTAs assist elderly in preventing or overcoming occupational imbalance, occupational deprivation, and occupational alienation?

REFERENCES

Agency for Healthcare Research and Quality. (2003). Breast and cervical cancer research highlights [WWW page]. URL http://www.ahcpr.gov/research/breastca.htm

American Occupational Therapy Association (2001). Occupational Therapy in the promotion of health and the prevention of disease and disability statement. *The American Journal of Occupational Therapy, 55 (6),* 656-661.

Bloch, M. W., Smith, D. A., & Nelson, D. L. (1989). Heart rate, activity, duration, and effect in added purpose versus single-purpose jumping activity. *American Journal of Occupational Therapy, 43,* 25-30.

Boston University Center for the Enhancement of Late-Life Function (2000). Fear of falling: An emerging health problem. *Roybal Program Brief,* pp. 1-6. Retrieved on December 22, 2003 from http://www.applied-gerontology.org/BUBrief.pdf.

Brownson, C. A., & Scaffa, M. E. (2001). Occupational therapy in the promotion of health and the prevention of disease and disability statement. *American Journal of Occupational Therapy, 55*(6), 656-660.

Butler, R. N., Davis, R., Lewis, C. B., Nelson, M. E., & Strauss, E. (1998). Physical fitness: How to help older patients live strong and longer. *Geriatrics, 53*(9), 26-8, 31-2, 39-40.

Carlson, A. (1996). Fall prevention in Hilo, Hawaii. *OT Week, 10*(36), 14-15.

Carlson, M., Clark, F., & Young, B. (1998). Practical contributions of occupational science to the art of successful aging: How to sculpt a meaningful life in older adulthood. *Journal of Occupational Science, 5*(30), 107-118.

Caserta, M. S., & Gillett, P. A. (1998). Older women feelings about exercise and their adherence to an aerobic regimen over time. *Gerontologist, 38*(5), 602-609.

Centers for Disease Control [CDC] (2002a). Cervical cancer and Pap test information. *The National Breast and Cervical Cancer Detection Program* [WWW page]. URL http://www.cdc.gov/cancer/nbccedp/info-cc.htm

Centers for Disease Control [CDC] (2002b). Deaths: Final data for 2000. *National vital statistics reports, 50*(15), 1-120.

Centers for Disease Control [CDC] (2002c). Invasive cervical cancer among Hispanic and non-Hispanic women—United States, 1992-1999. *Morbidity and Mortality Weekly, 51*(47), 1067-1070.

Clark, F., Azen, S. P., Carlson, M., Mandel, D., LaBree, L., Hay, J., Zemke, R., Jackson, J., & Lipson, L. (2001). Embedding health promoting changes into the daily lives of independent-living older adults: Long-term follow-up of occupational therapy intervention. *Journals of Gerontology-Series B: Psychological Sciences and Social Sciences, 56B*(1), P60-63.

Clark, F., Azen, S. P., Zemke, R., Jackson, J., Carlson, M., Mandel, D., Hay, J., Josephson, M. D., Cherry, B., Hessal, C., Palmer, J., & Lipson, L. (1997). Occupational therapy for independent-living older adults: A randomized control trial. *Journal of the American Medical Association, 278*(16), 1321-1326.

Davies, A. M. (1990). Prevention in aging. In R. L. Kane, J. G. Evans, & D. MacFadyen (Eds.), *Improving health of older people.* New York, NY: Oxford University Press.

DeKuiper, W. P., Nelson, D. L., & White, B. E. (1993). Materials based occupation versus imagery-based occupation versus rote exercise: A replication and extension. *Occupational Therapy Journal of Research, 13*(3), 183-197.

Drinkwater, B. L. (1988). Exercise and aging: The female master athlete. In J. Puhl, C. Brown, & R. O. Voy (Eds.), *Sports science perspectives for women: Proceedings from the Women and Sports Conference.* Chicago, IL: Human Kinetics Books.

Fiatarone, M. A., & Evans, J. E. (1990). Exercise in the oldest old. *Topics in Geriatric Rehabilitation, 5*(2), 63-77.

Fidler, G. S., & Fidler, J. W. (1978). Doing and becoming: Purposeful action and self-actualization. *American Journal of Occupational Therapy, 32*(5), 305-310.

Florey, L. (1976). Development through play. In C. Schaefer (Ed.), *The therapeutic use of child's play.* New York, NY: Jason Aronson.

Garner, D. J., & Young A. A. (Eds.) (1993). *Women and healthy aging: Living productively in spite of it all.* New York, NY: The Haworth Press.

Gilfoyle, E. M. (1986). The future of occupational therapy: An environment of opportunity. In S. E. Ryan (Ed.), *The certified occupational therapy assistant.* Thorofare, NJ: Slack, Inc.

Glantz, C. H., & Richman, N. (1996). The wellness model in long term care facilities. *Quest, 7,* 7-11.

Hanft, B. (2002). Promoting health: Historical roots-renewed vision. *OT Practice, 2,* 10-15.

Heck, S. H. (1988). The effect of purposeful activity on pain tolerance. *American Journal of Occupational Therapy, 42,* 577-581.

Hettinger, J. (1996). The wellness connection. *OT Week, 10,* 12-13.

Hickey, T., & Stilwell, D. L. (1991). Health promotion for older people: All is not well. *Gerontologist, 31*(6), 822-828.

Hjort, P. F. (2000). Physical activity and health in elderly—walk on. *Tidsskr Nor Laegeforen, 120*(24), 2915-2918.

Iezzoni, L. I., McCarthy, E. P., & Davis, R. B. (2001). Use of screening and prevention services among women with disabilities. *American Journal of Medical Quality, 16*(4), 135-144.

Jackson, J., Carlson, M., Mandel, D., Zemke, R., & Clark, F. (1998). Occupation in lifestyle redesign: The well elderly study occupational therapy program. *American Journal of Occupational Therapy, 52*(5), 326-334.

Jett, A. M., & Branch, L. G. (1981). The Framington disability study: ii. Physical disability among the aging. *American Journal of Public Health, 71,* 1211-1216.

Johnson, J. A. (1986). *Wellness: A context for living.* Thorofare, NJ: Slack, Inc.

Kircher, M. A. (1984). Motivation as a factor of perceived exertion in purposeful versus nonpurposeful activity. *American Journal of Occupational Therapy, 38,* 165-170.

Lohman, H., & Givens, D. (1999). Balance and falls with elders: Application of clinical reasoning. *Physical and Occupational Therapy in Geriatrics, 16,* 17-32.

Mandel, D. R., Jackson, J. M., Zemke, R., Nelson, L., & Clark, F. A. (1999). *Lifestyle redesign: Implementing the well elderly program.* Bethesda, MD: The American Occupational Therapy Association.

McMurdo, M. E., & Rennie, L. (1993). A controlled trial of exercise by residents of old peoples' homes. *Age-Ageing, 22*(1), 11-15.

Miller, L., & Nelson, D. L. (1987). Dual purpose activity versus single purpose in terms of duration on task, exertion level, and affect. *Occupational Therapy in Mental Health, 7,* 55-67.

Minino, A. M., Arias, E., Kochanek, S. L., Murphey, S. L., & Smith, B. L. (2002). Deaths: Final Data for 2000. Department of Health and Human Services [DHHS]. Centers for Disease Control and Prevention [CDCa], National Center for Health Statistics, 50, 15, 13-15.

Montagu, A. (1981). *Growing young.* New York, NY: McGraw-Hill.

Mount, J. (1991). Evaluation of a health promotion program provided at senior centers by physical therapy students. *Physical and Occupational Therapy in Geriatrics, 10*(1), 15-25.

Nelson, D. L., & Stucky, C. (1992). The roles of occupational therapy in preventing further disability of elderly persons in long-term care facilities. In R. A. Levine & J. Rothman (Eds.), *Prevention practice: Strategies for physical therapy and occupational therapy.* Philadelphia, PA: WB Saunders.

Nied, R. J., & Franklin, B. (2002). Promoting and prescribing exercise for the elderly. *American Family Physician, 65,* 419-426.

Nuessel, F., & Van Stewart, A. (1999). Literary exemplars of illness: A strategy for personalizing geriatric case histories in clinical settings. *Physical and Occupational Therapy in Geriatric Medicine, 16,* 33-46.

Pinch, W. J. (1993). Health promotion and the elderly. *NSNA/Imprint, 40*(2), 83-86.

Reilly, M. (1962). Occupational therapy can be one of the great ideas of 20th century medicine: Eleanor Clarke Slagle lecture. *American Journal of Occupational Therapy, 16,* 1-9.

Riccio, C. M., Nelson, D. L., & Bush, M. A. (1990). Adding purpose to the repetitive exercise of elderly women through imagery. *American Journal of Occupational Therapy, 44,* 714-717.

Richard, B. (1991). Workplace Literacy Technology for Nursing Assistants. *Journal of Health Occupations Education, 6*(1), 73-85.

Richards, S. E. (1998). The Carson Memorial Lecture 1998: Occupation for health—and wealth? *British Journal of Occupational Therapy, 61*(7), 294-300.

Rubenstein, L. Z., Josephson, K. R., Trueblood, P. R., Loy, S., Harker, J. O., Pietruszka, F. M., & Robbins, A. S. (2000). Effects of a group exercise program on strength, mobility, and falls among fall-prone elderly men. *Journal of Gerontology Series A, Biological Sciences and Medical Sciences, 55A*(6), M317-M321.

Sakemiller, L. M., & Nelson, D. L. (1998). Eliciting functional extension through the use of a game. *American Journal of Occupational Therapy, 52*(2), 150-157.

Schmidt, C. L., & Nelson, D. L. (1996). A comparison of three occupational forms in rehabilitation patient's receiving upper extremity strengthening. *Occupational Therapy Journal of Research, 16*(3), 200-215.

Schuster, C., Petrosa, R., & Petrosa, S. (1995). Using social cognitive theory to predict intentional exercise in post-retirement adults. *Journal of Health Education, 26,* 1-14.

Scott, A. H., Butin, D. N., Tewfik, D., Burkhardt, M. A., Mandel, D., & Nelson, L. (2001). Occupational therapy as a means to wellness with the elderly. *The Hayworth Press,* 3-22.

Smith, M. T. (1995). Implementing annual cancer screening for elderly women. *Journal of Gerontological Nursing, 2*(7), 12-17.

Speake, D. L. (1987). Health promotion activity in the well elderly, *Health Values, 11,* 6-25.

Stewart, A. L., Mills, K. M., Sepsis, P. G., King, A. C., McLelland, B. Y., Roitz, K., & Ritter, P. L. (1998). Evaluation of CHAMPS: A physical activity program for older adults. *Annals of Behavior and Medicine, 19*(4), 353-361.

Thomas, J. J. (1996). Materials based, imagery based and rote exercise and occupational forms: Effects on repetitions, heart rate, duration of performance and self perceived rest periods in well elderly women. *American Journal of Occupational Therapy, 50*(10), 783-789.

Thomas, J. J., & Rice, M. S. (2002). Perceived risk and its effect on quality of movement in occupational performance of well-elderly individuals. *Occupational Therapy Journal of Research, 22*(3), 104-110.

U.S. Department of Health and Human Services. (2000). *Healthy People 2010: Understanding and improving health.* Washington, DC: U.S. Government Printing Office.

U.S. Department of Health and Human Services. (2001) A profile of older Americans [WWW page]. URL http://www.hhs.gov

Washington State Department of Health. (2002). Early cervical cancer detection important for women of color and women living in rural areas [WWW page]. URL http://www.doh.wa.gov/Publicat/2002_News/02-06.htm

Webster, J. R. (1992). Prevention, technology, and aging in the decade ahead. *Topics in Geriatric Rehabilitation, 7,* 4.

Wilcock, A. A. (1998) Occupation for health. *British Journal of Occupational Therapy, 61*(8), 340-345.

Wilcock, A. A. (1999). The Doris Sym Memorial Lecture: Developing a philosophy of occupation for health. *British Journal of Occupational Therapy, 62*(5), 191-198.

Wilcox, A. A. (1995). The occupational brain: A theory of human nature. *Journal Occupational Science Australia, 2*(1), 68-73.

Yerxa, E. J. (1993). Occupational science: A new source of power for participants in occupational therapy. *Journal of Occupational Science, 1,* 1-3.

Yoder, R. M., Nelson, D. L., & Smith, D. A. (1989). Added-purpose versus rote exercise in female nursing home residents. *American Journal of Occupational Therapy, 43,* 581-586.

CHAPTER 6

The Regulation of Public Policy for Elders

CORALIE **H**. **G**LANTZ AND **N**ANCY **R**ICHMAN

KEY **T**ERMS

Omnibus Budget Reconciliation Act of 1987, Medicare, Medicaid, managed care, F tags, Minimum Data Set, triggers, Resident Assessment Protocols, care planning, Prospective Payment System, skilled services, unskilled services, Outcome and Assessment Information Set, Older Americans Act, Olmstead Act, Social Security Insurance, advocacy

CHAPTER **O**BJECTIVES

1. Describe public and private health systems in the United States that influence practice.
2. Clearly define the role of the certified occupational therapy assistant (COTA) within Omnibus Budget Reconciliation Act regulations.
3. Learn ways the input of the COTA in the Resident Assessment Instrument is valuable in the integrated team approach.
4. Increase knowledge about Medicare eligibility, guidelines, and regulations.

5. Describe the Prospective Payment System and COTA practice within that system.
6. Describe the influence of public policy regulations on Home Health Care.
7. Describe how Social Security insurance and the Older Americans Act influence COTA practice.
8. Increase awareness of trends in the regulation of public policy.
9. Learn the importance of advocacy for the occupational therapy profession.

Marie is a certified occupation therapy assistant (COTA) who was invited to speak to a class of occupational therapy assistant (OTA) students about public policy. Marie began her lecture by stating, "Today we are going to discuss the influence of public polices such as Medicare and Medicaid on occupational therapy practice."

Marie scanned the faces of the students. They appeared to look disinterested. She observed students looking out the window, using their laptops to access the Internet, and a few stifling yawns. "Okay," Marie slowly stated as she reorganized her thoughts, "I have decided to first share my story. In 1998 I was working for a rehabilitation company that contracted at several skilled nursing facilities in the area. I was making a very high salary—over $50,000 a year for a COTA just out of school! I didn't think to question where that salary came from. Later I realized that to pay my salary the contract company must have been getting money from somewhere and that money possibly came from charging large amounts to Medicare for patient treatments. You see, Medicare was paid retrospectively based on what was charged after treatments. Today, as you will learn, cost measures have been established called 'prospective payment,' or payments paid ahead of time based on preestablished amounts. Anyway, one day your instructor Sally brought the OTA students to observe patients at the facility where I was employed. During a free moment Sally asked me if I had considered the impact of the Balanced Budget Act on my practice. 'No,' I responded. 'I assume that my contract company will take care of me.' You see, I never paid much attention to public policy. I found that subject far removed from my life and frankly I was not interested. My ignorance about public policy ended up affecting me personally, as in 1999, soon after the new law became instituted in skilled nursing facilities, I lost my job. The contract company reorganized because of the changes and I was among several rehabilitation personnel who lost their jobs. In a blink of an eye I went from earning $50,000 a year to being on unemployment, which was difficult as a single mother." Marie paused and looked around the classroom and observed a group of attentive students gazing back at her. Marie continued, "I found myself reflecting about my career. What was I going to do? Should I enter another area of practice? The more I thought about it I realized that my passion was in working with elders. So I did a huge amount of networking and within 3 months I was lucky to be hired by a skilled nursing facility as an in-house staff therapist. Practice had changed so I had to learn the Prospective Payment System. It was difficult at first but eventually I adjusted."

"Now I pay close attention to policy trends, I have become involved in the state and national occupational therapy organizations, and I try to influence change by writing letters and making phone calls to the senators and congress people from this district. I even visited my representative while attending a conference in Washington, D.C. I never again want to be uninformed about public policy and its impact on practice." As Marie continued with her lecture the class was attentive.

Public policy develops from legislation at the federal and state levels and represents society's values (MacClain, 1996, personal communication). For example, the Medicare Act, which resulted in a national health insurance plan for elders, was enacted in 1965. Medicaid, a combined federal and state insurance program that addresses the health care needs of the indigent, was enacted in 1966.

Both measures were enacted at a time when civil rights was valued by society and was reflected in many government acts that passed around that time such as the Developmental Disabilities Act and the Vocational Rehabilitation Act. The language of public policies is meant to be general. The specifics about each public policy are in its regulations, which COTAs need to comprehend because they directly impact occupational therapy (OT) practice. COTAs working in a skilled nursing facility (SNF) should understand the **Omnibus Budget Reconciliation Act (OBRA) of 1987** and the **Prospective Payment System (PPS)** resulting from the Balanced Budget Act (BBA) of 1997 to provide appropriate care and be effective treatment team members. COTAs also must have a direct understanding of **Medicare** and **Medicaid** to ensure that treatment they provide is reimbursed by third-party payers. In addition to knowledge of reimbursement sources, COTAs should know about community resources funded by public policy. For example, a COTA working in home health may recommend that an elder receive Meals on Wheels or other services from the Area Office on Aging, which is funded by the **Older Americans Act (OAA).** In addition, the **Olmstead Act** of 2001 helps elders with disabilities with community living. Although all these public policies are positive for practice with elders, if funding is threatened, effects on practice may be extremely negative.

Medicare, Medicaid, OBRA, the Olmstead Act, and OAA are examples of public policy that can affect health care for elders. This chapter discusses the influence of these acts on OT practice and concludes with suggestions for the COTA on ways to promote changes in public policy and advocate for elder rights.

HEALTH CARE TRENDS IN THE UNITED STATES

Health care in the United States is transforming rapidly as a result of a quickly changing society. A knowledge of these health care trends helps with understanding policies that develop. Previously, the family physician was the sole provider of health care. The physician knew individuals throughout their lives and treated them as whole people rather than as illnesses or diseases. Recently, the health care industry has undergone an extensive period of fragmented approaches to service delivery. The current trend, especially for elders, is toward comprehensive, cost-effective health care. Consumers want simplified access to a range of services with predictable costs. This has led to the emergence and growth of various public and private sources of health coverage that are often called **Managed Care,** although this is a general term for all types of integrated delivery systems. The following sections describe public and private systems (Managed Care) that are influenced by public policy.

PUBLIC SOURCES

Public sources include Medicare, Medicaid, federal and state employee health plans, the military, and the Veterans Administration. The public sources of Medicare and Medicaid, which are often accessed by the elder clients that COTAs treat, are discussed in the following sections.

Medicare

Medicare, or Title 18 of the Social Security Act, was first implemented in 1966. As part of the Social Security Amendment of 1965, the Medicare program was created to establish a health insurance program to supplement retirement, survivors, and disability insurance benefits. Originally, Medicare covered most people 65 years of age and older. However, since then the program policy has expanded to cover other groups of people, including those entitled to disability benefits for at least 24 months, those with end-stage renal disease, and those who elect to buy into the program. Qualified disabled and working individuals who lose Medicare benefits because of a return to work are allowed to purchase Medicare Part A and Part B insurance (Centers for Medicare & Medicaid Services [CMS], n.d.(d); Lubarsky, Swerwan, Schroeder, and Duffy, 1995).

Medicare+Choice Program

The Medical+Choice (M+C) program, created by the BBA of 1997, was a Congressional effort to provide a wide choice of private health plans to Medicare beneficiaries. But 5 years later the number of plans available had in fact declined, and those remaining had made significant changes to their benefit packages. The BBA of 1997 and federal budget constraints limit M+C payment rates, whereas health care costs are increasing and providers are more aggressive in their contract and price negations with these plans. As a result, beneficiaries looking to Medicare HMOs as an affordable supplemental insurance option are being asked to pay more for fewer benefits (CMS, n.d.[d], 2002b; Department of Health and Human Services Centers for Medicare & Medicaid Services, 2002b).

Medicaid

As described by CMS (2003, b),

[Medicaid, or] Title XIX of the Social Security Act, is a program which provides medical assistance for certain individuals and families with low incomes and resources. The program became law in 1965 as a jointly funded cooperative venture between the Federal and State governments to assist States in the provision of adequate medical care to eligible needy persons. Medicaid is the largest provider of medical and health-related services to America's poorest people. It is designed to benefit those whose health and disability status has resulted in low income or high expenses. It does not have an age requirement, although the elder population often receives a larger portion of funds than other age groups. Within broad national guidelines which the Federal government provides, each of the States: establishes its own eligibility standards; determines the type, amount, duration, and scope of services; sets the rate of payment for services; and administers its own program [p .1].

States must provide basic health services, including inpatient and outpatient hospital services, laboratory and x-ray examinations, nursing facility services, physician and nurse practitioner services, and family planning services. State administrations have the option to cover any of 30 or more specific services, including OT. States also have been required to ensure that descriptions of their services meet federal guidelines and that all Medicaid recipients are treated equally (Sommers, Browne, & Carter, 1996). In most states, Medicaid provides home health care coverage to Medicaid beneficiaries who are also eligible for care in an SNF. OT is considered an optional service in home health. Unlike Medicare, the requirement for one of the qualifying services such as nursing, physical therapy, or speech and language pathology as a prerequisite for OT services *may* not exist. In some states, the client does not have to be homebound to qualify for these home health care benefits.

Medicaid reimbursement is considerably less than Medicare and in some states requires prior approval. In many states the Medicaid program is administered as a managed care plan. Medicaid pays a high percentage of nursing care expenditures in the nursing home industry. Because of funding restrictions, Medicaid places an emphasis on institutional care rather than other options that might permit elders to remain in their communities. However, the degree of emphasis varies among states because some have waiver programs and demonstration projects that involve broader funding for innovative programs and nontraditional care management. As Evashwich (1996) states, "An extremely important feature of the public long-term care system is the lead role that state governments have in shaping the characteristics of local financing and delivery systems for long-term care services" (p. 203). Thus, the Medicaid program varies considerably from state to state and within each state over time. Because of these variances, the COTA must have access to local information and be an advocate for OT on a local and national level.

Medicaid Managed Care and Managed Care

In June of 2002, the Bush Administration released final regulations implementing patient protections for Medicaid beneficiaries enrolled in managed care. These include protections such as requiring that beneficiaries have a choice of at least two plans and access to an adequate network of providers, establishment of an internal appeals process, and adoption of the **"prudent layperson"** standard for emergency care. The regulations provide regulatory guidance to states, managed care organizations, and beneficiaries on the important statutory changes made by the BBA of 1997. The regulations are important because 58% of Medicaid beneficiaries are enrolled in managed care. Because there can be policy decisions on a state level, beneficiaries and their advocates need to work with state governments to make sure the regulations are implemented in ways that ensure high-quality health care services. Advocates also will need to be aware of the protections afforded by the new rules. For example, a plan to allow states to limit emergency room access was rescinded. Finally, it is important to remember (as the preamble to the regulations points out) that these rules represent a *floor* or a minimum: States are permitted to enforce more stringent consumer protections should they wish to enact them (DHHS, 2002a).

Elders also may be receiving care from managed care organizations. These organizations manage the care given to consumers and often involve the entire range of utilization control tools applied to manage the practice of physicians and others, regardless of practice setting. The growth in these organizations reflects the trend of the one-stop, cost-effective care. With Medicare, elders are encouraged to enroll in managed care plans, which involve forfeiting traditional benefits. Managed care systems often advertise the inclusion of services beyond the basic Medicare plan, such as prescription and dental plans. The provision of rehabilitation services with some plans is different from traditional Medicare, and elders who require extensive rehabilitation may not have access to the level of care provided by Medicare. Many elders have gone back to traditional Medicare plans when they realize how their care is compromised. Some plans have closed in some parts of the country, which has left members with no insurance plan.

Reimbursement rates to managed care providers are capitated, meaning that a set rate is provided either per treatment or per condition. This payment may not be enough to include extensive therapy. A capitated system provides financial incentive for physicians to refrain from referring clients to services such as OT. This trend toward managed care affects delivery of OT services to elders. The occupational therapist (OTR)/COTA team needs to continue emphasizing the functional treatment they provide and advocate for services.

FEDERAL PUBLIC POLICIES AND CERTIFIED OCCUPATIONAL THERAPY ASSISTANT PRACTICE: OMNIBUS BUDGET RECONCILIATION ACT

F Tags

The federal government "**F tags**" (that is, F followed by a number) refer to specific regulations in the OBRA law. For example, the F tag dealing with the rehabilitation services states: "Provision of services: If specialized

rehabilitation services such as, but not limited to physical therapy, speech-language pathology, occupational therapy, and mental health rehabilitative services for mental illness and mental retardation, are required in the resident's comprehensive plan of care, the facility must (1) Provide the required services; or (2) Obtain the required services from an outside resource from a provider of specialized rehabilitative services" (HCFA, p. 156, 1995).

OBRA, a landmark act of Congress, is not influenced by budgetary concerns. This act focuses on elders' rights, quality of care, and quality of life in the nursing home setting. OBRA went into effect in October 1990, and was revised with final rules published in 1995. Compliance with the OBRA regulation is necessary for a nursing facility to receive reimbursement from Medicare or Medicaid. This discrepancy between what is required for good care, rehabilitation, and dignity and what is funded can cause ethical and moral dilemmas for COTAs. Knowledge of the regulations that govern care can help the COTA advocate for the services the patients need.

Scope of Omnibus Budget Reconciliation Act

OBRA (HCFA, 1995) was designed as a regulatory framework, which includes a comprehensive assessment, the Resident Assessment Instrument (RAI), as the foundation for planning care delivery to nursing home residents. The OBRA law focuses not only on quality care but also on function and quality of life. It addresses residents' rights, including the right to "...services to attain or maintain the highest practicable physical, mental, and psychosocial well-being, in accordance with the comprehensive assessment and plan of care" (F309) (HCFA, p. 83, 1995). This includes activities of daily living, as stated in F310, "A resident's abilities in activities of daily living do not diminish unless circumstances of the individual's clinical condition demonstrate that diminution was unavoidable," (HCFA, 1995) and in F311, "A resident is given the appropriate treatment and services to maintain or improve his or her abilities" (HCFA, 1995). Other categories of residents' rights address freedom from restraint and opportunity to participate in social, religious, and community activities. Many categories and guidelines of residents' rights included in the OBRA law have implications for OT practice.

The Resident Assessment Instrument

To understand the COTAs role in the provision of OBRA, OT practitioners must first learn about the RAI (HCFA, 1995). The RAI, which is the comprehensive assessment required by OBRA, must be completed for all residents residing longer than 14 days in specific nursing facilities. The three components of the RAI are: (1) **Minimum Data Set (MDS)**, (2) **Triggers**, and (3) **Resident Assessment Protocols (RAPs)** and the RAP summaries. Completion of these components leads directly to the care plan process.

The RAI first addresses the problem identification process. After a resident's problems are recognized, a **care plan** is created to identify sound clinical interventions and treatment goals. This care plan becomes each resident's unique path toward achieving or maintaining a maximal level of well-being. The RAI considers the resident as an individual with strengths in addition to functional limitations and health problems.

Federal regulations require that the RAI be conducted or coordinated with the participation of appropriate health professionals. Although not required, completion of the RAI is best accomplished by an interdisciplinary team. Team members' combined experience and knowledge enable a better understanding of the strengths, needs, and preferences of each resident, thereby ensuring the best possible quality of care. Facilities have flexibility in determining the participants in the assessment process as long as it is accurately conducted. A facility may assign responsibility for completing the RAI to a number of qualified staff members, including the COTA. In most cases, participants in the assessment process are licensed health professionals.

Minimum data set

The MDS (HCFA, 1995) is a screening tool in which strengths and deficits are recognized and triggered for further assessment. Many sections of the MDS address areas within the scope of OT practice, including cognition, communication, vision, mood and behavior problems, psychosocial well-being, physical functioning and structural problems, continence, various disease diagnoses and health conditions, oral and nutritional status, activity pursuits, special treatment and procedures (including therapy), and discharge potential. An OT practitioner usually fills out the section on physical functioning (Fig. 6-1).

COTA involvement in completion of sections of the MDS can be beneficial. Because the initial MDS does not have to be completed until the fourteenth day after admission, the resident often has been evaluated and is being treated by the OTR/ COTA team. If this is the case, COTAs can use the OT evaluation and knowledge gained in treating the resident to accurately fill out the MDS. Under the regulations for the PPS, a system that regulates Part A payments in SNFs, the MDS is also used to determine Medicare payment for those residents that meet the eligibility qualifications. OT treatment influences that payment system and COTAs may be responsible for tracking minutes of treatment for sections of the MDS.

Even if no treatment has taken place, the data collection and resident interview may help COTAs give the necessary information to others on the interdisciplinary team. In some situations, COTAs complete the "Physical Functioning and Structural Problems" section for all newly admitted residents. COTAs also may be required to complete the same MDS section for later resident reviews. Completion of a new MDS is required when significant changes in the resident's status have occurred. (The Appendix contains information on obtaining a copy of guidelines for the MDS.)

COTAs should also be familiar with the actual OBRA Final Rules, Enforcement Requirements, Survey Procedures, and Interpretive Guidance. COTAs completing any portion of the MDS assessment must certify accuracy of the section(s) they complete by noting their credentials and the date and indicating the portion of the assessment completed. The signature of a registered nurse is required to certify completion of the assessment.

Triggers and Resident Assessment Protocols

After completion of the MDS, those areas that have been triggered, or identified, as needing further assessment are reviewed with RAP guidelines. The triggers identify MDS responses specific to a resident. They alert the assessor to residents who either have or are at risk for development of specific functional problems and require further evaluation using the RAPs. The RAP guidelines "present comprehensive information for evaluating factors that may cause, contribute to, or exacerbate the triggered condition" (Morris, Murphy, & Nonemaker, p. 4-5, 1995). RAPs also examine guidance for further assessment and possible interventions for resolution to problems. COTAs can write meaningful RAP summaries by collecting data from the resident's records, family members, and staff members.

"If the condition is found to be a problem for the resident, the RAP Guidelines will assist the interdisciplinary team in determining if the problem can be eliminated or reversed, or if special care must be taken to maintain a resident at his or her current level of functioning" (Morris, Murphy, & Nonemaker, Chapter 4, p. 4, 1995). Using the RAP guidelines, the COTA can complete this further exploration and review of the problem area with a summary that includes: (1) the nature of the condition (may include presence or lack of objective data and subjective complaints), (2) complication and risk factors that affect the decision to proceed to care planning, (3) factors that must be considered in developing the individualized care plan interventions, and (4) the need for referrals and further evaluation by appropriate health professionals. This documentation should support the decision to proceed (or not proceed) with a care plan to address the problem (HCFA, 1995; Health Care Financing Administration [HCFA], 1995) (Box 6-1).

Care Planning

Care planning in SNFs is based not only on identified resident problems but also a resident's unique characteristics, strengths, and needs. The individual resident's characteristics are measured by using standardized MDS items and the RAP process. The care plan must be oriented

SECTION G. PHYSICAL FUNCTIONING AND STRUCTURAL PROBLEMS

1. (A) ADL SELF-PERFORMANCE—(*Code* for resident's **PERFORMANCE OVER ALL SHIFTS during last 7 days**—*Not including setup*)

0. *INDEPENDENT*—No help or oversight—OR—Help/oversight provided only 1 or 2 times during last 7 days

1. *SUPERVISION*—Oversight, encouragement or cueing provided 3 or more times during last 7 days—OR—Supervision (3 or more times) plus physical assistance provided only 1 or 2 times during last 7 days

2. *LIMITED ASSISTANCE*—Resident highly involved in activity; received physical help in guided maneuvering of limbs or other nonweight bearing assistance 3 or more times—OR—More help provided only 1 or 2 times during last 7 days

3. *EXTENSIVE ASSISTANCE*—While resident performed part of activity, over last 7-day period, help of following type(s) provided 3 or more times:
—Weight-bearing support
—Full staff performance during part (but not all) of last 7 days

4. *TOTAL DEPENDENCE*—Full staff performance of activity during entire 7 days

5. *ACTIVITY DID NOT OCCUR* during entire 7 days

(B) ADL SUPPORT PROVIDED—(*Code for MOST SUPPORT PROVIDED OVER ALL SHIFTS during last 7 days; code regardless of resident's self-performance classification*)

0. No setup or physical help from staff
1. Setup help only
2. One person physical assist   4. ADL activity itself did not
3. Two+ persons physical assist   occur during entire 7 days

			(A) SELF-PERF	(B) SUPPORT
a.	BED MOBILITY	How resident moves to and from lying position, turns side-to-side, and positions body while in bed.		
b.	TRANSFER	How resident moves between surfaces—to/from: bed, chair, wheelchair, standing position (EXCLUDE to/from bath/toilet).		
c.	WALK IN ROOM	How resident walks between locations in his/her room.		
d.	WALK IN CORRIDOR	How resident walks in corridor on unit.		
e.	LOCOMO-TION ON UNIT	How resident moves between locations in his/her room and adjacent corridor on same floor. If in wheelchair, self-sufficiency once in chair.		
f.	LOCOMO-TION OFF UNIT	How resident moves to and returns from off-unit locations (e.g., areas set aside for dining, activities, or treatments). **If facility has only one floor,** how resident moves to and from distant areas on the floor. If in wheelchair, self-sufficiency once in chair.		
g.	DRESSING	How resident puts on, fastens, and takes off all items of **street clothing,** including donning/removing prosthesis.		
h.	EATING	How resident eats and drinks (regardless of skill). Includes intake of nourishment by other means (e.g., tube feeding, total parenteral nutrition).		
i.	TOILET USE	How resident uses the toilet room (or commode, bedpan, urinal); transfers on/off toilet, cleanses, changes pad, manages ostomy or catheter, adjusts clothes.		
j.	PERSONAL HYGIENE	How resident maintains personal hygiene, including combing hair, brushing teeth, shaving, applying makeup, washing/drying face, hands, and perineum (EXCLUDE baths and showers).		

FIGURE 6-1 Example of the Physical Functioning and Structural Problems section of the Minimum Data Set.

(*Continued*)

			(A)	(B)
2.	**BATHING**	How resident takes full-body bath/shower, sponge bath, and transfers in/out of tub/shower (EXCLUDE washing of back and hair). ***Code for most dependent*** in self-performance and support. **(A)** BATHING SELF-PERFORMANCE codes appear below 0. Independent—No help provided 1. Supervision—Oversight help only 2. Physical help limited to transfer only 3. Physical help in part of bathing activity 4. Total dependence 5. Activity itself did not occur during entire 7 days (*Bathing support codes are as defined in* ***Item 1, code B above***)		
3.	**TEST FOR BALANCE** **(see training manual)**	(*Code for ability during test in the* ***last 7 days***) 0. Maintained position as required in test 1. Unsteady, but able to rebalance self without physical support 2. Partial physical support during test; or stands (sits) but does not follow directions for test 3. Not able to attempt test without physical help		
		a. Balance while standing		
		b. Balance while sitting—position, trunk control		

				(A)	(B)
4.	**FUNCTIONAL LIMITATION IN RANGE OF MOTION** **(see training manual)**	(*Code for limitations during* ***last 7 days*** *that interfered with daily functions or placed resident at risk of injury*) **(A)** *RANGE OF MOTION* **(B)** *VOLUNTARY MOVEMENT* 0. No limitation 0. No loss 1. Limitation on one side 1. Partial loss 2. Limitation on both sides 2. Full loss			
		a. Neck			
		b. Arm—Including shoulder or elbow			
		c. Hand—Including wrist or fingers			
		d. Leg—Including hip or knee			
		e. Foot—Including ankle or toes			
		f. Other limitation or loss			

5.	**MODES OF LOCOMOTION**	(***Check all that apply*** *during* ***last 7 days***) Cane/walker/crutch — **a.** Wheeled self — **b.** Other person wheeled — **c.**	Wheelchair primary mode of locomotion — **d.** *NONE OF ABOVE* — **e.**	
6.	**MODES OF TRANSFER**	(***Check all that apply*** *during* ***last 7 days***) Bedfast all or most of time — **a.** Bed rails used for bed mobility or transfer — **b.** Lifted manually — **c.**	Lifted mechanically — **d.** Transfer aid (e.g., slide board, trapeze, cane, walker, brace) — **e.** *NONE OF ABOVE* — **f.**	
7.	**TASK SEGMENTATION**	Some or all of ADL activities were broken into subtasks during **last 7 days** so that resident could perform them 0. No 1. Yes		
8.	**ADL FUNCTIONAL REHABILITATION POTENTIAL**	Resident believes he/she is capable of increased independence in at least some ADLs — **a.** Direct care staff believe resident is capable of increased independence in at least some ADLs — **b.** Resident able to perform tasks/activities but is very slow — **c.** Difference in ADL Self-Performance or ADL Support, comparing mornings with evenings — **d.** *NONE OF ABOVE* — **e.**		
9.	**CHANGE IN ADL FUNCTION**	Resident's ADL self-performance status has changed as compared with status of **90 days ago** (or since last assessment if less than 90 days) 0. No change 1. Improved 2. Deteriorated		

FIGURE **6-1** cont'd

BOX 6-1

Certified Occupational Therapy Assistant's Sample Resident Assessment Protocol on Activities of Daily Living Function and Rehabilitation Potential

Resident has exhibited problems in dressing and use of the toilet. Resident's difficulty with putting on clothing is related to weakness in the left upper extremity and possible perceptual problems. Resident needs both physical assistance and verbal instructions. Independent toileting is restricted because of unsafe transfers to the toilet and the inability to handle clothing. Resident is at risk for falls when transferring. Frustration is noted by verbal sighs when attempting to dress. Unsafe ADL techniques have been noted with dressing and transferring. Resident appears to be able and motivated to learn. These problems should be addressed in the resident's plan of care, and this resident should be referred to occupational therapy for further evaluation and treatment.

toward prevention of declines in functional levels, management of risk factors, and building of strengths. It also should reflect standards of current professional practice. Care planning should include treatment objectives with measurable outcomes and should reflect the resident's goals and wishes, especially if a resident wishes to refuse treatment. The planning also should include the facility's efforts to find alternative means to address the problem. OT interventions included in the care plan should identify the importance of occupational performance and roles to the individual. The process should incorporate interdisciplinary expertise to develop a care plan to improve a resident's functional abilities and should involve residents, family members, and others close to the elder (Morris, Murphy, & Nonemaker, 1995).

The certified occupational therapy assistant's role in care planning

COTAs can contribute to the care planning process by providing insight on identified resident problems. This input may include discussion of the deficits and interventions recognized from OT evaluation and treatment and information for other staff members about the components involved in functional deficits. COTAs can communicate their knowledge and make intervention suggestions at the care plan conference, which is usually attended by an interdisciplinary team.

Quality indicators and measures in skilled nursing facilities

Public policy regulates quality care in nursing home facilities. As the discussion below indicates, regulation

addressing quality starts with the MDS, the screening document from the OBRA regulations.

The Quality Indicators (QIs) of the CMS National Reporting System allows surveyors and facilities access on the Internet to data generated by the MDS in each facility. It allows for the identification of potential problems, measures of facility care, outcomes, and comparisons with other facilities. When a problem with quality of care exists, it will flag the issues involved. Many of the problems of potentially poor care practices identified by QIs are appropriate interventions for OT. Proactive attention to these identified deficits can change life for the residents and improve the survey process for the SNF (Center for Health Systems Research and Analysis, 1999) (Box 6-2).

In the Fall of 2002 the Centers for Medicare & Medicaid Services (CMS), known previously as the Health Care Financing Administration (HCFA), initiated a new program designed to give consumers correct information about SNFs. The data from the MDS are converted into information to make individuals aware of how performance differs across nursing homes, to allow Medicare beneficiaries to make placement decisions, and for the facility to improve their quality of care in specific areas. The facility admission profile takes into consideration those facilities that specialize in treating specific diagnoses or conditions and therefore have a greater incidence of those conditions—that is, facilities with wound care programs would have a greater incidence of pressure sores. This is an additional focus for OT intervention (Box 6-3) (DHHS, 2002d).

MEDICARE
Medicare Part A Prospective Payment System

The PPS was established with the BBA of 1997 (Pub.L.105-33). These regulations were created to control increasing costs of health care with Medicare A in SNFs. As the name implies, reimbursement occurs prospectively on the basis of a level of care or an anticipated level of care rather than retrospectively on the basis of what was charged. The final rule governing PPS was published in July 1999 (HCFA, 1999). Under this rule there were significant reimbursement changes in SNFs, and the impact on the delivery of therapy services was monumental.

PPS regulations include specific time guidelines to review the status of each resident, called assessment reference dates. For example, treatment given or ordered during Days 1 through 5 determines the patient's status for the first payment period of 14 days. Grace days are provided so that rehabilitation can begin when a patient is medically stable (CMS, 2001b). The MDS, a mandated assessment instrument under the OBRA regulations, was used to determine clinical care before it became the reimbursement tool under the PPS. Listed on the MDS is the amount of

BOX 6-2

Quality Indicators

Accidents
- Incidence of new fracture
- Prevalence of falls

Behavior/emotional patterns
- Prevalence of symptoms of depression

Clinical management
- Use of nine or more different medications

Cognitive patterns
- Incidence of cognitive impairments

Elimination/Incontinence
- Prevalence of bladder or bowel incontinence
- Prevalence of occasional or frequent bladder or bowel incontinence without a toileting plan
- Prevalence of indwelling catheters

Infection control

Nutrition/eating
- Prevalence of weight loss
- Prevalence of tube feeding
- Prevalence of dehydration

Physical functioning
- Prevalence of bedfast residents
- Incidence of decline in late loss activities of daily living
- Incidence of decline in range of motion

Psychotropic drug use

Quality of life
- Prevalence of daily physical restraints
- Prevalence of little or no activity

Skin care
- Prevalence of stage 1-4 pressure ulcers

Data from Center for Health Systems Research and Analysis (CHSRA). (1999). Facility guide for the nursing home quality indicators [WWW page]. URL http://cms.hhs.gov/medicaid/mds20/qifacman.pdf

BOX 6-3

Quality Measures

Measures for chronic resident
- Late loss activities of daily living decline
- Prevalence of infections
- Inadequate pain management
- Pressure-sores prevalence without faculty admission profile (FAP)
- Pressure sores prevalence with FAP
- Use of physical restraints

Postacute care measures
- Prevalence of delirium without FAP
- Prevalence of delirium with FAP
- Pain management
- Improvement in walking
- Incidence of decline in range of motion

Psychotropic drug use

Quality of life
- Prevalence of daily physical restraints
- Prevalence of little or no activity

Skin care
- Prevalence of stage 1-4 pressure ulcers

Data from U.S. Department of Health & Human Services Centers for Medicare & Medicaid Services. (2002). *Quality measures for national public reporting: User's manual*. Cambridge, MA: ABT Associates, Inc.

TABLE 6-1

Resource Utilization Groups— Rehabilitation Categories

Rehabilitation categories	Discipline and minutes in the last 7 days
Ultra High	720 minutes from at least two disciplines, one for at least 5 days
Very High	500 minutes from at least one discipline for at least 5 days
High	325 minutes from at least one discipline for at least 5 days
Medium	150 minutes from any combination of the three disciplines
Low	45 minutes for at least 3 days by any combination of the three disciplines and two or more nursing rehabilitation services for at least 15 minutes for 6 more days

Data from Health Care Financing Administration (1998, May 12). Federal register: Medicare program: Prospective payment system and consolidated billing for skilled nursing facilities; final rule. Retrieved from http://cms.hhs.gov/providers/snfpps/fr12ma98.pdf on May 20, 2003.

minutes of therapy services, both anticipated and delivered, which is one factor in determining the daily rate the SNF receives for the care of the resident.

The PPS is based on resources used by the patient and is divided into Resource Utilizations Groups (RUGs). Five of the RUGs—Rehabilitation Ultra High, Rehabilitation Very High, Rehabilitation High, Rehabilitation Medium, and Rehabilitation Low—are associated with the amount and type of therapy services (Table 6-1). The highest rehabilitation RUG level (ultra high) requires at least two therapy disciplines to deliver treatment. For the 5-Day MDS Assessment, the highest two levels (Ultra High, Very High) require actual minutes of therapy delivered. For the first assessment period, the other three levels of rehabilitation can be attained by either delivered therapy or by anticipating the number of minutes of all therapy services combined that will be delivered in the first 15 days after admission. For all subsequent assessment periods, payment for the RUG rehabilitation levels is based on actual minutes of therapy delivered. Other RUG levels are based on medical acuity and additional issues that determine the resources needed by the patient (CMS, 2001b).

COTAs need to keep careful records of the time spent with patients and be aware of what can and cannot count toward therapy minutes. The initial evaluation and any documentation of treatment responses cannot count toward therapy minutes. Evaluation procedures that are done in conjunction with therapy delivery are included in the calculation of minutes (CMS, 2001b). Group therapy with four or fewer patients who have similar diagnoses and goals counts toward therapy minutes. The minutes provided in a group setting may not equal more than 25% of therapy time (HCFA, 1999). The 25% is calculated for each discipline separately. Group therapy can be an effective way to provide treatment and at the same time help with productivity standards (Zellis, 2001).

The decisions on the type and amount of therapy services to be provided are determined by an interdisciplinary team that should include the physician, therapists, and nurses. This clinical decision making then needs to be evaluated and reconciled with the payment system time frames and regulations. The financial issues should not compromise the clinical evaluations and recommendations. Accuracy and efficiency in the evaluation and treatment regimens and in clinical and record keeping documentation become significant under this system. Thorough knowledge of all the factors that impact reimbursement, not just therapy services, will make the COTA a more valuable part of the interdisciplinary team. As COTAs follow public policy trends, they may find future changes in any of these regulations. PPS changed payment for services, but the established Medicare Rules for eligibility, certification, duration, and frequency of treatment remain the same (see discussion in the following sections).

Eligibility for Medicare Part A in a Skilled Nursing Facility

Eligibility for Medicare Part A services in an SNF is determined by an entitled person (one who carries a Medicare card) who has stayed in the hospital for the required 3 consecutive days. The client's health condition must necessitate **skilled services** that can only be provided in a skilled care facility within 30 days of hospital discharge or within 30 days of the last covered SNF stay. Skilled service are those performed by qualified technical or professional health personnel and must be provided under the general supervision of skilled nursing or rehabilitation personnel to ensure client safety and achievement of the desired medical result. A physician must certify the necessity for skilled services, and the client must have Medicare benefit (days) available (HCFA, 1987). The COTA must understand Medicare rules and regulations. Because COTAs participate in the screening process to determine appropriate candidates for OT services, they may be asked to verify the client's current or potential Medicare status.

Rehabilitation services

SNF rehabilitation services are covered if the following factors are met:

1. The client requires skilled nursing services or skilled rehabilitation services.
2. The client requires these services daily. In the case of therapy services, they can be provided 5, 6, or 7 days per week, using a combination of disciplines. Under the PPS an individual can qualify for skilled coverage with therapy intervention 3 days per week with the low rehabilitation category of the RUGs.
3. Considering economy and efficiency, the daily skilled services can be provided only on an inpatient basis in an SNF.
4. These skilled services must be furnished pursuant to a physician's order.
5. The services are necessary for the treatment of a client's illness or injury and must be of reasonable duration and quantity (CMS, 1987).

Coverage Concepts: Skilled Medicare

A screening assessment to determine Medicare eligibility is performed before admission to an SNF. Clients may be eligible for Medicare reimbursement for many reasons, including the following skilled nursing services: intravenous or intramuscular medications or feedings, nasogastric feedings, and treatment for stage III or IV decubitus ulcers (CMS, 1987). If the placement is for skilled nursing services rather than skilled therapy services, the OT department should be consulted to determine whether the client also needs skilled OT services. It is sometimes financially advantageous for the patient to have a nonrehabilitation RUGs level, but this should not exclude needed therapy intervention. The therapeutic intervention will be less intense but still provided. This is most often the case during the first assessment reference date period. Under the PPS system, some funding is included in the skilled nursing categories for needed therapy services. This is often misunderstood and therapy services are not used. Under OBRA regulations, the facility cannot deny therapy services to the patient when there is an identified medical necessity for therapy services.

The concept of skilled and unskilled therapy must be understood to obtain reimbursement from Medicare for OT treatment. Skilled care includes teaching and assessing safety factors in relation to modification of the environment or approaches to increase function, modifications of techniques to reduce pain and enhance function, and any other changes that increase functional responses from the patient (CMS, 2002) (Table 6-2). Unskilled services would be exercises that are repetitive in nature, passive exercises to maintain range of motion or strength, and positioning in bed without reference to specific complications (CMS, 2002). Although a client's diagnosis is a valid factor in deciding the need for skilled services, it should never be the only factor considered. The key issue is whether the skills of a therapist are needed for the required services (CMS, 2002; HCFA, 1987). Skilled therapy services cannot be denied on the basis of diagnosis. This was clarified in a CMS Program Memorandum as it relates to therapy services needed by individuals with a diagnosis of Alzheimer's disease or other dementias (CMS, 2001a). Before this memorandum there had been many denials on the basis of having the diagnosis of Alzheimer's disease.

In some cases, people can become qualified for skilled services if a medical complication exists that requires skilled personnel to perform or supervise the service or to monitor the person. For example, range of motion by itself is usually not considered a skilled service. However, if the person has severe osteoporosis and is at risk for breaking bones, therapy should be furnished by a skilled therapist. Table 6-3 provides examples of OT services that may be furnished by nonskilled personnel and are therefore not reimbursed.

Justification for occupational therapy intervention

COTAs must recognize and understand criteria for OT intervention (Table 6-4). Professional therapy intervention in the SNF should be developed according to resident needs relative to the complexity and intensity of required treatment. Treatment plans should be based on function and must address integration to the COTA plan of care. Treatment should be reinforced by other disciplines such as skilled nursing. The resident's prior level of function, mobility, and safety in addition to self-care deficits are primary and essential indicators for professional intervention and must be reflected in assessments (Lubarsky, Swerwan, Schroeder, and Duffy, 1995). The OTR and COTA should maintain communication with employees of local intermediaries because they serve as resources for documentation and billing questions.

Eligibility and Entitlement for Medicare Part B

With Medicare, Supplementary Medical Insurance (Part B) is a voluntary program. Part B is available to individuals (including disabled persons) entitled to Part A, U.S. residents who are legal citizens older than 65 years, and aliens lawfully admitted for permanent residence who have resided in the United States for 5 consecutive years (CMS, n.d.[e]). The program requires enrollment and the payment of a monthly premium. In most states, elders who receive Medicaid benefits are reimbursed for the Medicare Part B premium.

Part B services include physician, outpatient, and home health services in addition to services furnished by rural clinics, ambulatory surgery centers, and comprehensive outpatient rehabilitation. Part B Medicare also covers

TABLE 6-2

Skilled Occupation Therapy Services	
Example	**Reasons**
Linferd: An 89-year-old client who recently had a stroke. Because of hemianopsia and problem-solving difficulties, Lingerd requires moderate assistance with ADL functions that require use of upper and lower extremities. He is motivated to do OT treatment.	Recent condition Identifiable functional deficits in performance areas
Gertrude: A 72-year-old client who recently had a total hip replacement. She is unable to safely dress and requires education in hip safety precautions. The COTA provides instructions for lower extremity dressing and other ADL functions. Treatment includes teaching safety precautions.	Recent condition (hip surgery) Safety concerns Identifiable functional deficit
Fred: A 92-year-old client who recently sustained a right wrist fracture. He is right hand dominant. The client was independently performing ADL functions before his wrist was fractured. He now requires moderate assistance with ADL functions because of decreased ROM in the right upper extremity. The COTA provides a home ROM program and instruction in ADL functions.	Recent injury Functional deficits with ADL caused by difficulty with the performance component of ROM Prior level of independence Skilled expertise of the COTA needed to teach home ROM program

ADL, activities of daily living; COTA, certified occupational therapy assistant; OT, occupational therapy; ROM, range of motion.

TABLE 6-3

Nonskilled Occupational Therapy Services	
Example	**Reasons**
Gwendolyn: A 69-year-old client diagnosed with right cerebral vascular accident. Previously, she performed all ADL functions independently. On initial evaluation, Gwendolyn was able to perform ADL functions independently but slowly. Her status on initial evaluation was independent with ADL, although performance was slow.	Slow performance with ADL functions is not significant enough to require the intervention of a skilled practitioner. The client will likely improve on her own over time without treatment intervention.
Sebastian: A 75-year-old client diagnosed with rheumatoid arthritis. OT was ordered to provide an adapted pencil gripper to assist with writing. The COTA provided the gripper.	Treatment does not require the skilled expertise of the COTA. Anyone could provide an adapted pencil gripper.
Bob: A 74-year-old client diagnosed with Alzheimer's disease. He is dependent in feeding. The COTA monitors feeding 3 times/wk for 2 weeks.	The client's condition is chronic and has not shown significant improvement. Treatment is routine, therefore not requiring the skilled expertise of the COTA.

ADL, activities of daily living; COTA, certified occupational therapy assistant; OT, occupational therapy.

TABLE 6-4

Justification for Professional Therapy Service	
Example	**Reasons**
Hilde was admitted into an SNF to recuperate from hip replacement surgery. In addition, she was to learn to ambulate with a walker and independently perform ADL functions, particularly her own dressing. Once Hilde learned these skills, she might return to her retirement home apartment and receive home health care to ensure her continued progress and safety.	The immediate or short-term potential for progress toward a less intensive or lesser skilled service area exists.
Hilde was depressed and the COTA primarily treated her for depression rather than the total hip replacement. However, intervention may be considered skilled if the COTA could demonstrate that the treatment was directly related to motivating the client to safely perform ADL functions.	The philosophy and plan of treatment must realistically focus on achievement of outcomes for the specific phase of rehabilitation, such as being an inpatient in a skilled facility.
The COTA focuses on Hilde's treatment on going home with safety considerations.	Treatment also must focus on the plan for the next expected phase such as outpatient or home care.
During treatment, the COTA should address short-term deficits in safely performing ADL functions. The OT treatment should also take into account the performance component of the client's difficulty with problem solving.	Treatment is expected to address the type and degree of deficits and effects of other problems in relation to the short-term or interim goals.
The COTA would thoroughly document changes in Hilde's status and her motivational level.	The therapist must emphasize variances in the elder's response to treatment and new developments.

ADL, activities of daily living; COTA, certified occupational therapy assistant; OT, occupational therapy; SNF, skilled nursing facility.

various ancillary services, such as OT (CMS, 2003b). Medicare Part B OT services include inpatient and outpatient therapy services furnished by an SNF or under contract arrangements, which means the SNF contracts for provision of therapy services. For OT treatment to qualify for reimbursement under Medicare Part B, a physician must certify that the therapy services are required and a plan for furnishing the services is established by the physician and the OTR. Services are furnished while the client is under the physician's care. The plan of care must be developed and certified at least once every 30 days. If the physician has not seen the client within 30 days, the OTR or the COTA is responsible for contacting the physician and arranging for the plan of care to be signed. The services must be directly identifiable to individual clients and a result of specific medical needs. Part B coverage is provided after the 100 days of coverage under Part A are exhausted or if the client should not remain under Medicare Part A for the 100 days as determined by standard guidelines. Part B coverage can be provided to clients located in a non-Medicare–certified bed within the SNF. Part B covers only 80% of the allowable charges. The remaining 20% is billed to the client or to coinsurance. COTAs must be aware of this fact to educate clients about Medicare billing costs and to get informed consent for treatment and payment.

All Part B services for therapy are billed to Medicare using Physician's Current Procedural Terminology codes. Codes are revised annually and the amount of reimbursement is calculated on the basis of a number of factors, including the established relative value of the procedure, practice expenses, and malpractice costs with an adjustment for a specific geographical area. COTAs in collaboration with the OTR decide how to code delivered treatment. Codes describe outcomes. They may be service codes that are billed only once per day regardless of the amount of time spent in delivering the procedure. Service codes include evaluation, reevaluation, splint application, and most modalities. Timed codes are the majority of the codes applicable to treatment provided by the COTA. Multiple units of timed codes can be delivered during a day of treatment. They are based on 15-minute units and Medicare Regulations guide how to calculate units (Box 6-4) (CPT, 2002).

Medicare Coverage for Home Health

The BBA of 1997, as amended by the Omnibus Consolidated and Emergency Supplemental Appropriations Act of 1999, called for the development and implementation of a PPS for Medicare home health services. The following discussion overviews the Medicare regulations for the home health system.

Eligibility for Medicare Part A in home health care

Eligibility for Medicare Part A home health services does not require a 3-day hospital stay. However,

---

BOX 6-4

Calculating Time for Billing: Physician's Current Procedural Terminology Codes

Example:

97530 therapeutic activities, each 15 minutes

1 unit ≥ 8 minutes to < 23 minutes
2 units ≥ 23 minutes to < 38 minutes
3 units ≥ 38 minutes to < 53 minutes
4 units ≥ 53 minutes to < 68 minutes
5 units ≥ 68 minutes to < 83 minutes
6 units ≥ 83 minutes to < 98 minutes
7 units ≥ 98 minutes to < 113 minutes
8 units ≥ 113 minutes to < 128 minutes

Therapists should not bill for services performed for less than 8 minutes. The expectation is that a provider's time for each unit will average 15 minutes in length. If therapists have a practice of billing less than 15 minutes for a unit, these situations will be highlighted by the intermediary for review.

The above schedule of times is intended to provide assistance in rounding time into 15-minute increments. It does not imply that any minute until the eighth should be excluded from the total count as the timing of active treatment counted includes time.

The beginning and end of the treatment should be recorded in the patient's medical record along with the note describing the treatment. (The total length of the treatment to the minute could be recorded instead.) If more than one Current Procedural Terminology code is billed during a calendar day, then the total number of units that can be billed is constrained by the total treatment time. For example, if 24 minutes of 97112 and 23 minutes of 97110 were furnished, then the total treatment time was 47 minutes, so only 3 units can be billed for the treatment. The correct coding is 2 units of 97112 and one unit of 97110, assigning more units to the service that took more time.

Data from Centers for Medicare and Medicaid Services. (2001). Medical Intermediary Manual: Part 3—Claims process. Medicare Transmittal 1828 [Text file]. URL http://cms.hhs.gov/manuals/pm_trans/R1828A3.pdf)

---

the elder must be homebound, have a physician's referral, and require skilled services. *Homebound* means the elder is unable to leave the home without considerable effort and assistance. The elder does not have to be bedridden (CMS, 1997). Visiting a physician is an example of a legitimate reason to leave the home. A client does not qualify for Part A home health services based solely on the need for OT. Nursing, physical therapy, or speech-language pathology must first open the case. However, OT may be introduced along with these other services and may continue after the other services have ended (Youngstrom, 1995). Currently, the legislative attempts to change these qualification regulations have been unsuccessful.

Medicare Part B in home health care

OTRs working in their own private practice who are certified as Medicare Part B providers may bill home health visits under Part B. They must follow all required billing and reimbursement procedures and need to bill both Medicare for 80% of the fee and the client's supplemental insurance for the 20% coinsurance. The client does not need to be homebound for therapy to be covered under Medicare Part B, regardless of whether billing is done by a Home Health Agency (HHA) or an OT in private practice. Because of variations in billing processes, many HHAs do not choose to bill under both plans. The majority of agencies bill primarily under Part A (Youngstrom, 1995).

Conditions of participation for therapy services in home health

The regulations for HHAs are, of course, quite extensive. The following are the *Conditions of Participation for Therapy Services* as established by CMS (CMS, 1997):

> Any therapy services offered by the Home Health Agency (HHA) directly or under arrangement are given by a qualified therapist or by a qualified therapy assistant under the supervision of a qualified therapist and in accordance with the plan of care. The qualified therapist assists the physician in evaluating level of function, helps develop the plan of care (revising it as necessary), prepares clinical and progress notes, advises and consults with the family and other agency personnel, and participates in in-service programs. Services furnished by a qualified physical therapy assistant or qualified occupational therapy assistant may be provided under the supervision of a qualified physical or occupational therapist. A physical therapy assistant or occupational therapy assistant performs services planned, delegated, and supervised by the therapist, assists in preparing clinical notes and progress reports, and participates in educating the patient and family, and in in-service programs. Specific instructions for assistants must be based on treatments prescribed in the plan of care, patient evaluations by the therapist and accepted standards of professional practice. The OTR evaluates the effectiveness of the services provided by the assistant. Documentation in the clinical record should show that communication and supervision exist between the assistant and the therapist about the patient's condition, the patient's response to services furnished by the assistant and the need to change the plan of care.
>
> **(p. 54-55).**

Treatment in home health care

From the initiation of treatment, patients must be informed of their rights and therapists need to be aware of these rights, such as the right to be informed in advance about the care to be provided and of any changes in the care. In addition, patients should participate in the care planning process, be informed about the confidentiality of the clinical records, and be advised of the availability of the toll-free HHA hotline in their state.

Orders for therapy services include the specific procedures and modalities to be used and the amount, frequency, and duration. With assessment, the **Outcome and Assessment Information Set (OASIS)** is a key component of Medicare's partnership with the home care industry to foster and monitor improved home health care outcomes and is an integral part of the Conditions of Participation for Medicare-certified HHAs. It represents core items of a comprehensive assessment for an adult home care patient and forms the basis for measuring patient outcomes for purposes of outcome-based quality improvement. Most data items in the OASIS were developed as systems of outcome measures for home health care. The items have use for outcome monitoring, clinical assessment, care planning, and other internal agency-level applications. OASIS data items encompass sociodemographic, environmental, support system, health status, and functional status attributes of adult patients. In addition, selected attributes of health service use are included (CMS, n.d.[b]).

The plan of care is developed in consultation with the agency staff and covers all pertinent diagnoses, including mental status, types of services and equipment required, frequency of visits, prognosis, rehabilitation potential, functional limitations, and activities permitted. It also describes nutritional requirements, medications, and treatments; any safety measures to protect against injury; instructions for timely discharge or referral; and any other appropriate items (CMS, n.d.[b]).

COTAs assist in preparing clinical notes and progress reports. A clinical note is a notation of a contact with a patient that is written and dated. It describes signs and symptoms, treatment and patient's reaction, and any changes in physical or emotional condition. The progress report summarizes facts about care furnished and the patient's response during a given period. All personnel furnishing services must maintain liaisons to ensure that their efforts are coordinated effectively and support the objectives outlined in the plan of care

SUPPLEMENTARY SECURITY INCOME PROGRAM

The Supplementary Security Income program, which was enacted in 1972, is a federal assistance program that increased the money available for the needy elder, blind, and disabled individuals who did not qualify for Social Security benefits. This amendment to the Social Security Act established a minimum income program fully funded by the federal government. Unlike Social Security, Supplementary Security Income is not a retirement program (Rich & Baum, 1984). Elders who did not work long enough to receive reasonable Social Security benefits are the primary recipients. States supplement the federal assistance with their own benefits, which accounts for the differences in monthly payments among states.

Despite increases in public programs, some elders remain below the poverty level. In 35 states the criteria for receiving Supplementary Security Income determines Medicaid eligibility (Rich & Baum, 1984).

The recipient is eligible for food stamps. The states must permit the individual to deduct medical expenses in determining income and to establish Medicaid eligibility by "spending down." Spending down implies reducing one's financial assets to meet the eligibility standards in effect since 1972. More than one million eligible people do not participate in the program, possibly because they associate the program with welfare (Evashwick, 1996).

Many individuals who qualify for Supplementary Security Income have the same types of problems as institutionalized elders. Their needs for therapy often go unidentified because they live in social environments rather than medical environments such as an SNF. These social environments may be substandard and provide no case management unless individuals are involved with community-based health programs. These individuals often do not have access to Medicare Part B services because they may not have the resources to buy into the voluntary program. The need for OTR and COTA collaboration and development of services for these individuals is clear, but therapists need to find creative ways to fund programs and advocate for the needed care. Appropriate services from therapists may reduce the need for institutionalization.

OLDER AMERICANS ACT

In 1965 the OAA was enacted to provide services for elders. The premise of OAA was that services provided to elders at least 60 years of age would enable them to remain in their homes and communities. Funding was established for nutrition programs, senior centers, transportation, housing, ombudsman, and legal services. Differences in these programs exist among states because administration is at the state level. In addition, more opportunity for OT involvement exists in some regions than in others. The OAA was designed to foster independence, but rehabilitative services were not included. The act established the Administration on Aging, an agency specifically responsible for developing new social services for elders.

OAA was reauthorized in 1992 (OAA, 1992) and additional funding was added for resource centers to promote links among acute care, rehabilitative services, and long-term care systems. Some limited references to preventative health services include home injury control services, programs relating to chronic disabling conditions, and provision of information concerning diagnoses. Other limited resources include prevention, treatment, and rehabilitation of age-related diseases and chronic disabling conditions. Resources such as homemakers, chore workers, home-delivered meals, and community-based programs provide respite for caretakers of dependent relatives and friends. Goals to establish OAA-coordinated programs for elders were not reached. The act was reauthorized again in 2000. In 2003, many of the Area Agencies on Aging responsible for the administration of these services have had significant budget cuts, impacting the scope and breadth of programs.

OLMSTEAD ACT

An Executive Order (13217, 2001) was signed on June 18, 2001, that allowed and encouraged the promotion of community-based alternatives for individuals with disabilities, such as accommodations that meet needs of these individual, available caregivers to provide assistance, transportation programs, and in some cases employment options. Federal agencies can assist states to meet challenges of this order and these efforts are to be coordinated by the Health and Human Service (HHS). This presents opportunities for COTAs to become involved in new and different forms of rehabilitation, environmental modification, and advocacy. Further information about this act can be obtained from state Medicaid agencies, state Developmental Disabilities Councils, or the American Occupation Therapy Association Federal Affairs Department.

TRENDS WITH FEDERAL HEALTH CARE POLICIES

Predictions of the effects of governmental change on Medicaid and Medicare laws, funding, and therapy coverage for OT are difficult. With the "graying of America," costs for programs that serve this population will continue to increase, thereby justifying close scrutiny. The trend to encourage Medicare recipients to obtain Medicare Managed Care plans is a result of cost-containment efforts. To contain costs and to prevent abuse of Medicare, CMS has placed "CAPS" on OT and other rehabilitation services that Medicare beneficiaries can receive in a calendar year. The use of "CAPS" is strongly opposed by the American Occupational Therapy Association, which suggests that other cost-control measures would not have the adverse affects of the "CAPS" on Medicare beneficiaries (American Occupation Therapy Association, 2003).

Another trend is the incorporation of concepts of function in any payment reform. The reformed Medicaid system in some states is based on the OBRA/MDS assessment using a system called resource-related groups (RRGs). The RRG system considers many factors, including the client's functional limitations in addition to medical, restorative, and functional needs. In October of 2002, government Medicaid payment rates decreased in SNFs. Many administrators in SNFs believe this diminution in payment rates will imperil the financial stability of facilities. Changes in reimbursement practices are likely to continue and evolve for many years.

Financial concerns motivate the shift from entitlement programs, or government programs with specific guidelines for eligible beneficiaries, to policies based on need rather than age (Binstock, 1994). Currently, **Social Security Insurance** and Medicare benefits are structured according to age, with no restriction based on income level. The Social Security program was established in 1935 by the U.S. government to ensure payment for survivor's insurance, contributions to state employment insurance, old age assistance, and Medicare and Medicaid benefits (Binstock, 1994). The trend to emphasize economic status rather than age criteria has been reflected in legislation. The Social Security Reform Act of 1983 (Binstock, 1994) authorized taxing of Social Security benefits for individuals and couples with a certain level of annual income. The trend to raise the eligibility age for old age benefits is likely to continue because it is a cost-saving measure. Social Security insurance will remain a much debated topic in the legislature until there is more control over its economic solvency.

ADVOCACY

Health care is in a state of flux that will directly affect OT practice. Involvement of COTAs in advocacy for elders and the OT profession can make a difference. Eleanor Roosevelt once stated, "Every person owes a portion of his time and talent to the up building of a profession to which he/she belongs" (Scott & Acquaviva, 1985). Every COTA and OTR must encourage the benefits of OT and establish the role of the profession within society. COTAs must stay informed about all government decisions regarding health care (Box 6-5). The rapidly changing face of today's health care economy demands innovative and progressive responses from individuals.

OTs and OTAs must be strong advocates for their profession and the clients that benefit from OT treatment by adjusting to change and adapting to new ways to deliver treatment. The following statement from Tom Scully, Administrator from CMS, resulted from the advocacy efforts of a therapist who persevered to get the clarification on coverage for patients with the diagnosis of Alzheimer's disease:

> Our technical clarification to Medicare contractors regarding payment for therapies for Alzheimer's patients reinforces our commitment to making sure that all beneficiaries receive the care to which they are entitled to under Medicare Advances in medical science are helping physicians diagnose Alzheimer's Disease at its earliest stages. Depending on a beneficiary's medical condition, the Centers for Medicare & Medicaid Services believes that certain specific therapies can be helpful in slowing a beneficiary's decline due to this terrible illness

(CMS, 2002b, p. 1).

BOX 6-5

Ways for Certified Occupational Therapy Assistants to Become Involved with Public Policy

Be able and ready to articulate a clear definition of occupational therapy (OT) for the public; be visible.

Regularly access the American Occupational Therapy Association (AOTA) web site to keep abreast of public policy trends.

Serve on OT task forces and committees on a state or national level.

Become involved in the state OT associations legislative committee.

Volunteer for community committees that advocate for elders, such as an Alzheimer's association.

Read public and OT literature as much as possible to keep up on trends.

Write and submit articles to professional and consumer publications about OT practice.

Find a mentor who understands public policy.

Write letters or visit important people such as legislators, managed care and corporate executives, third-party payers, and case managers.

Learn the legislative process in your state and testify for relevant issues at public hearings.

If questions or concerns cannot be answered or addressed on a local level, network with the legislative division of AOTA.

In response to advocacy concerns that Medicare contractors were increasingly denying services to Medicare beneficiaries on the sole basis of being diagnosed with Alzheimer's disease, CMS issued a memorandum to clarify existing reimbursement policies (Box 6-5). The September 2001 instructions (CMS, 2001a) directed Medicare contractors not to install system edits that would automatically deny Medicare-covered services based only on claims for dementia. These actions clarify that Medicare would provide payment for specific speech, occupational, and rehabilitation therapies. More specifically, Medicare may pay doctors and other health care providers for neurodiagnostic testing, medication management, and psychological therapy when provided to patients with Alzheimer's disease.

Thus, advocacy efforts do work, for as Tom Scully stated: "Alzheimer's advocates came to us with what seemed to be a significant problem for Alzheimer's patients. Intuitively, this longstanding approach appeared to discriminate against Alzheimer's patients, and we were happy to fix it" (CMS, 2002b, p. 5).

CHAPTER REVIEW QUESTIONS

1 What are the eligibility requirements for Medicaid?

2 In what aspects of Omnibus Budget Reconciliation Act can occupational therapy (OT) can be involved?

3 Can a certified occupational therapy assistant (COTA) complete the Minimum Data Set?

4 What is a Resident Assessment Protocol?

5 What is the Prospective Payment System and how does it influence therapy practice?

6 What qualifies a person for Medicare Part A OT coverage in a skilled nursing facility?

7 What is required for OT services in home health care?

8 What is the current assessment system in home health care?

9 What is Social Security insurance and who can benefit from it?

10 What are some of the federal health policy trends that influence practice?

11 How can COTAs be advocates for the OT profession?

REFERENCES

American Occupational Therapy Association. (2003). OTs/OTAs: Work for cosponsors on bills to repeal Medicare outpatient caps [WWW page]. URL http://capwiz.com/aota/issues/alert/?alertid=1097601

Binstock, R. H. (1994). Changing criteria in old-age programs: The introduction of economic status and need for services. *Gerontologist, 34*(6), 726.

Center for Health Systems Research and Analysis (CHSRA). (1999). Facility guide for the nursing home quality indicators [WWW page]. URL http://cms.hhs.gov/medicaid/mds20/qifacman.pdf

Centers for Medicare & Medicaid Services (CMS). (1987). Coverage of services, skilled nursing facility manual [WWW page]. URL http://www.cms.hhs.gov/manuals/12_snf/sn201.asp

Centers for Medicare & Medicaid Services (CMS). (1997). Conditions of participation: Home health agencies. In Interpretive Guidelines—Home Health Agencies [WWW page]. URL http://www.cms.hhs.gov/oasis/intguide.pdf

Centers for Medicare & Medicaid Services (CMS). (2001a). Program memorandum intermediaries/carriers: Medical review of services for patients with dementia [WWW page]. URL http://216.239.37.100/cobrand?q=cache:X6jarCShA2sJ:cms.hhs.gov/manuals/pm_trans/AB01135.pdf+Alzheimer%27s+Disease+&hl=en&ie=UTF-8

Centers for Medicare & Medicaid Services (CMS). (2001b). Skilled nursing facility prospective payment system refinements and consolidated billing quick reference guide [WWW page]. URL http://www.cms.hhs.gov/medlearn/refsnf.asp

Centers for Medicare & Medicaid Services (CMS). (2002a). Medicare program integrity manual [WWW page]. http://cms.hhs.gov/manuals/108_pim/pim83c06.pdf

Centers for Medicare & Medicaid Services (CMS). (2002b). Statement of Tom Scully, administrator centers for Medicare & Medicaid services on therapy coverage of Alzheimer's disease patients [WWW page]. URL http://www.hcanys.org/dementia/AlzheimerScully4-1.PDF

Centers for Medicare & Medicaid Services (CMS). (2003a). Medicare & you 2003 [WWW page]. URL http://www.medicare.gov/Publications/Pubs/pdf/10050.pdf

Centers for Medicare & Medicaid Services (CMS). (2003b). Overview of the Medicaid program [WWW page]. URL http://www.cms.hhs.gov/medicaid/mover.asp

Centers for Medicare & Medicaid Services (CMS). (n.d.[b]). OASIS regulations [WWW page]. http://www.cms.hhs.gov/oasis/hhregs.asp

Centers for Medicare & Medicaid Services (CMS). (n.d.[c]). The home health prospective payment system (PPS) [WWW page]. http://www.cms.hhs.gov/providers/hhapps/default.asp

Centers for Medicare & Medicaid Services (CMS) (n.d.[d]). What is Medicare? [WWW page]. http://www.medicare.gov/Basics/WhatIs.asp#PartA

Centers for Medicare & Medicaid Services (CMS) (n.d.[e]). Your Medicare Benefits. Retrieved on July 21, 2003 from http://www.medicare.gov/Choices/overview.asp

CPT Expert Ingenix (November 2002). Salt Lake City Utah, 290-291Exec. Order No. 13217, 3 C.F.R. 33155.

Department of Health and Human Services Centers for Medicare & Medicaid Services. (2002). Payment to home health agencies. *Federal Register, 67,* 125.

Evashwick, C. J. (1996). *The continuum of long-term care.* Albany, NY: Delmar Publishers.

Health Care Financing Administration. (1987). *Coverage of services, Medicare regulations.* Baltimore, MD: The Administration.

Health Care Financing Administration. (1995a). *Omnibus Budget Reconciliation Act (OBRA).* Baltimore, MD: The Administration.

Health Care Financing Administration. (1995b). *State operations manual: Provider certification* (Appendix R, pp. R-41-42) (DHHS Publication No. HCFA-7). Baltimore, MD: The Administration.

Health Care Financing Administration (1998, May 12). Federal register: Medicare program: Prospective payment system and consolidated billing for skilled nursing facilities; final rule. Retrieved from http://cms.hhs.gov/providers/snfpps/fr12ma98.pdf on May 20, 2003.

Health Care Financing Administration. (1999). Medicare program, prospective payment system and consolidated billing for skilled nursing facilities—Update final rule and notice. *Federal Register, 64*(146), 41643-41683.

Lubarsky, J. M., Swerwan, J.R., Schroeder, E.L., & Duffy, J. L. (1995). *Medicare resource manual: A guide through the critical steps.* Hindsale, IL: Life Services Network of Illinois.

Morris, J. N., Murphy, K., & Nonemaker, S. (1995). *Resident assessment instrument (RAI) user's manual.* Baltimore, MD: Health Care Financing Administration.

Older Americans Act (1992). 45 CFR 1321.

Rich, B. M., & Baum, M. (1984). *The aging: A guide to public policy.* Pittsburgh, PA: University of Pittsburgh.

Scott, S. J., & Acquaviva, J. D. (1985). *Lobbying for healthcare.* Rockville, MD: Government and Legal Affairs Division, American Occupational Therapy Association.

Sommers, F. P., Browne, S., & Carter, M. E. (1996). *Medicaid: Current law and issues in reform proposals.* Bethesda, MD: American Occupational Therapy Association.

U.S. Department of Health & Human Services Centers for Medicare and Medicaid Services. (2002a). *Medicaid managed care final regulations.* Baltimore MD: Centers for Medicare and Medicaid Services.

U.S. Department of Health & Human Services Centers for Medicare and Medicaid Services. (2002b). *Medicare managed care manual.* Baltimore, MD: Centers for Medicare and Medicaid Services.

U.S. Department of Health & Human Services Centers for Medicare and Medicaid Services. (2002c). *Survey procedures for the application of conditions for participation for home health agencies interpretive guidelines.* Baltimore, MD: Centers for Medicare and Medicaid Services.

U.S. Department of Health & Human Services Centers for Medicare & Medicaid Services. (2002d). *Quality measures for national public reporting: User's manual.* Cambridge, MA: ABT Associates, Inc.

U.S. Department of Health and Human Services Centers for Medicare and Medicaid Services. *Provider Reimbursement Manual* (PRM) Part I Section 2203.2. Baltimore, MD: Centers for Medicare and Medicaid Services.

Youngstrom, J. J. (1995). *Reimbursement for home health services: Guidelines for occupational therapy in home health.* Bethesda, MD: Commission on Practice Home Health Task Force.

Zellis, S. (2001). Occupational therapy and PPS: Let's take another look. *Gerontology Special Interest Section Quarterly, 24*(4), 1-3.

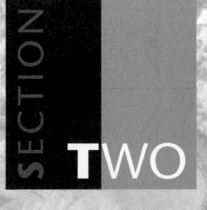

OCCUPATIONAL THERAPY INTERVENTION WITH ELDERS

SECTION **T**WO

CHAPTER 7

Occupational Therapy Practice Models

RENÉ PADILLA

KEY TERMS

clinical practice models, values, dysfunction, skills, occupation, function, assessment,
task, roles, performance, culture, environment, self-care, work, play and leisure,
treatment, context, cognition, maturation, motor action, subsystem, habits

CHAPTER OBJECTIVES

1. Explain the importance and use of practice models in occupational therapy intervention with elders.
2. Briefly summarize the Occupational Therapy Practice Framework and three occupational therapy practice models as they relate to aging, including Facilitating Growth and

Development, Cognitive Disabilities, and the Model of Human Occupation.
3. Demonstrate the ways certified occupational therapy assistants can incorporate theoretical principles into practice with elders.

Deepak was admitted to the rehabilitation center with a severe infection in the left knee that had been replaced just 3 months earlier. Deepak had been looking forward to his recent retirement. As an executive for a large firm, he and his family had lived in 10 different countries around the world. Now that all his children had graduated from college, he was planning a peaceful life in a small town by the ocean where he and his wife could play golf every day, attend cultural events in a nearby city, and occasionally go deep-sea fishing. A few days after he was admitted to the rehabilitation center he received news that his wife had fallen and fractured a hip. While preparing her for surgery at a different hospital, the doctors had discovered that she had a very aggressive cancer that had metastasized throughout her body. There was no hope for recovery, and she was discharged home under the

care of her daughter and a hospice service. Deepak spoke to his wife on the telephone twice a day, and often was tearful during his conversations with her. The purpose of Deepak's hospitalization was that he become independent in his self-care and in his mobility while not bearing any weight on his left leg. The weight-bearing restrictions were expected to be necessary for at least 10 weeks while his infection cleared and his knee was replaced again.

Martha is a small, frail woman in her late sixties who has been living in a skilled nursing facility for more than a year. When she was in her late twenties her automobile had been hit by a train and she sustained a head injury that resulted in her inability to speak and left hemiplegia. She had regained the ability to do her self-care and to walk without assistance, although over the years she had suffered many falls because of poor balance. For more than 40 years she had lived with her sister. When her sister died, Martha attempted to live on her own for some time, but became ill with pneumonia. Her relatives insisted she live at a skilled nursing facility because they were not able to care for her. Because of another bout with pneumonia, Martha is very weak and is unable to bathe and dress herself without assistance. She is also not able to walk.

Ursula was recently referred to an adult day care center in the downtown area of a large city. Her Alzheimer's disease has progressed to the point where she needs supervision 24 hours a day. Ursula's husband has been working at a local bookstore to make some money to supplement his retirement income. Ursula and her husband were prisoners in a Nazi concentration camp in their youth, and in the last month Ursula has seemed to be reliving that experience, often becoming quite agitated and isolative at the center.

Carlos immigrated to the United States from Cuba nearly 30 years ago. Although he is in his late sixties, he continued to work running a family-owned restaurant until 5 days ago when he had a stroke. Because of his stroke, Carlos seems unable to understand and speak in English, and continually repeats the same two lines of a Spanish song whenever he does speak. He also is unable to hold himself in midline and does not seem aware of one side of his body. Nearly every day his room in the acute care hospital has been full of relatives and friends, many of whom bring food. Carlos has a fever, and the doctors suspect he is having difficulty swallowing.

Deepak, Martha, Carlos, and Ursula represent the diversity of people who seek occupational therapy (OT) intervention because they are not able to carry out the activities that are important to them in their daily lives. The certified occupational therapy assistant (COTA) needs tools to address all these unique needs according to basic OT philosophy and theoretical principles. The OT programs for these individuals must not only consider the physical and cognitive limitations that affect their ability to care for themselves. These programs must also take into account the whole history of these individuals and the adjustments that are needed because of dramatic changes in their environments. Deepak's wife is dying and his children no longer live at home. Martha has been moved against her will from her familiar home to a skilled nursing facility where she knows no one. Carlos has gone from spending nearly all his waking hours at his business to a hospital room, and Ursula's mind has gradually replaced her physical surroundings for dreadful ones that reside in her memory. Although these OT programs must maintain a common thread that identifies them as "occupational therapy," they also should be flexible enough to provide individual meaning for each client. OT clinical practice models are intended to connect professional philosophy and theory with daily practice.

OVERVIEW OF PRACTICE MODELS

This chapter provides an overview of several conceptual models in which occupation is described as the principal feature of any OT treatment. First, the Occupational Therapy Practice Framework (American Occupational Therapy Association [AOTA], 2002) is reviewed, which articulates the general domain and process of intervention of the OT profession and gives the broadest look at how we might go about understanding Deepak's life and current needs. Second, an overview of Llorens' Facilitating Growth and Development model (1976) is provided, which, although published nearly three decades ago, is still the only conceptual model that emphasizes a developmental perspective in the practice of OT with adult clients. This model can help us to understand Martha's stage in life. Third, the Cognitive Disabilities Model (Allen, 1985; Allen, Earhart, & Blue, 1992, 1995) is described, which helps us to understand how cognitive process affects the performance of occupation and will be particularly useful in working with elders such as Ursula, although it certainly also has applications for Deepak, Martha, and Carlos. Finally, the Model of Human Occupation (Kielhofner, 2002) is discussed as a model that makes an effort to assist practitioners to consider clients holistically. This model will help us to understand elders like Carlos as people with dynamic abilities and needs who actively interact with their environments.

The common link among all forms of OT intervention cannot be overemphasized. The philosophy of OT practice includes values, beliefs, truths, and principles that should guide the general practice of the profession. One tenet of this philosophy is that the human being is inherently active and can influence self-development, health, and environment with purposeful activity. Thus the human is able to adapt to life's demands and become self-actualized. Dysfunction occurs when the human being's ability to adapt is impaired in some way. OT intervention seeks to prevent and remediate dysfunction and facilitate maximal adaptation through the use of purposeful activities (AOTA, 1995). The use of purposeful activity, or occupation, is the common thread for every OT intervention.

Since the OT profession began, the term "occupation" has described the individual's active participation in self-care, work, and leisure (AOTA, 1993), which constitute the ordinary, familiar things people do every day (AOTA, 1995). The person must use combinations of sensorimotor, cognitive, psychologic, and psychosocial skills to perform these occupations (AOTA, 1994). Specific environments and different stages of life influence these occupations. Kielhofner (1995) defines *occupation* as "doing culturally meaningful work, play or living tasks in the stream of time and in the contexts of one's physical and social world" (p. 3).

To understand the concepts of occupations and use them to facilitate function and adaptation, COTAs must have broad knowledge of the biological, social, and medical sciences in addition to OT theoretical premises. OT practice models provide organized frameworks for that knowledge, which allows the therapist to apply pertinent information to a specific client's problem. Thus practice models guide the therapist in creating individual treatment programs that are culturally meaningful and age-related and that facilitate development of sensorimotor, cognitive, psychological, and psychosocial skills. By using a practice model for guidance, the four COTAs assisting the patients discussed earlier can ensure professional treatment programs that are tailored to meet the needs of each client.

OT practice models do not offer concrete plans for improvement of function. Instead, these models suggest use of various graded occupations that demand development of performance abilities, thereby improving function. COTAs may use the information in the practice models to formulate questions to assess the client's needs, interests, and meanings; select assessment tools; and accordingly design a unique intervention strategy. COTAs should be familiar with several practice models because each model usually has a specific focus and does not address all dimensions of occupational functioning.

Occupational Therapy Practice Framework

The *Occupational Therapy Practice Framework: Domain and Processes* (referred to subsequently simply as "the Framework"; AOTA, 2002) represents the latest effort of the AOTA to articulate language with which to describe the profession's focus. As such, the Framework is intended to help occupational therapists (OTRs) and occupational therapy assistants (OTAs) analyze their current practice and consider new applications in emerging areas. In addition, the Framework was developed to help the external audience (physicians, payers, community groups, and others) understand the profession's emphasis on function and participation in social life.

The domain of concern of a profession refers to the areas of human experience in which practitioners of the profession help others. According to the Framework, the focus of the OT profession is "on assisting people to engage in everyday life activities that they find meaningful and purposeful" (AOTA, 2002, p. 610). For OT, the breadth of meaningful everyday life activities is captured in the notion of "occupation." OTRs and OTAs help people perform meaningful occupations that affect their health, well-being, and life satisfaction. These occupations permit participation in desired roles and life situations in the home, school, workplace, and community. Notably, personal meaning is emphasized as the central characteristic of occupation. The degree to which personal meaningfulness is decreased may render a therapeutic intervention as merely purposeful (i.e., achieving a goal a client understands but in which he is not particularly invested) or simply inconsequential.

According to the Framework, meaningfulness of occupation is tightly intertwined with the contexts in which the person lives. Further, the Framework recognizes that "engagement in occupation includes both the subjective (emotional or psychological) aspects of performance and the objective (physically observable) aspects of performance" (AOTA, 2002, p. 611). Thus, all aspects of engagement (physical, cognitive, psychosocial, and contextual) should be addressed in OT treatment (Fig. 7-1).

The Framework has organized the many occupations in which an individual, group, or population may engage into broad categories called "areas of occupation" (Table 7-1). Engagement in these performance areas requires particular clusters of performance skills (Table 7-2). For example, to tie one's shoes (a "dressing" activity within the ADL performance area) one must, among many things, maintain erect posture while bending and reaching one's foot, and then one must manipulate the laces and pull on them with sufficient force to tighten them but not enough to break them (all examples of motor skills). This sequence of actions is carried out by one's ability to plan and sequence events (examples of process skills). A fascinating feature of human occupation is that many combinations of performance skills are choreographed into automatic or semiautomatic patterns that enable one to function on a daily basis without demanding undue attention. After one has tied one's shoes with sufficient frequency, one can often do it without thinking or looking at the laces while one does it because it has become a habit. Broader habits can be said to become organized into routines (e.g., one might dress in a certain way and take a particular route to get to work), and frequently routines correspond to the variety of roles in which one functions (e.g., because one is the supervisor of an office, one might routinely meet with employees each morning at a certain time). The Framework describes useful habits (support performance in daily life), impoverished habits (which are not completely established or need practice to improve), and dominating habits (which are so demanding that they interfere with daily life).

As stated earlier, the Framework emphasizes the importance of considering the context or contexts in which a person engages in occupation. Context refers to the "variety of interrelated conditions within and surrounding the client that influence performance" (AOTA, 2002, p. 613). This definition implies that some contexts are external to the person (e.g., physical, social, and virtual), whereas others are internal (e.g., personal and spiritual), and yet others have a combination of external and internal features (e.g., culture). These contexts offer opportunities for occupational engagement, but at the

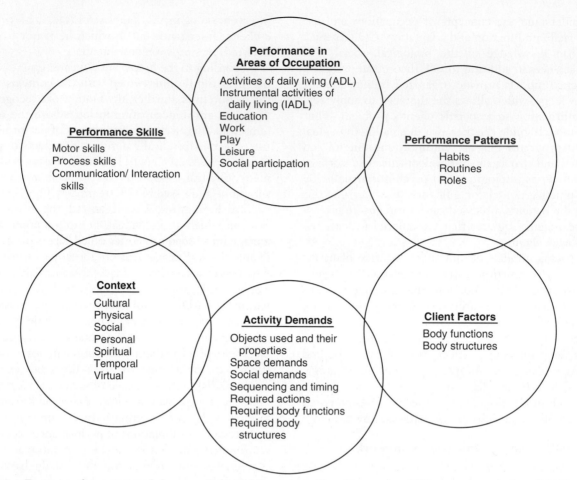

Performance in Areas of Occupation
Activities of daily living (ADL)
Instrumental activities of daily living (IADL)
Education
Work
Play
Leisure
Social participation

Performance Skills
Motor skills
Process skills
Communication/ Interaction skills

Performance Patterns
Habits
Routines
Roles

Context
Cultural
Physical
Social
Personal
Spiritual
Temporal
Virtual

Activity Demands
Objects used and their properties
Space demands
Social demands
Sequencing and timing
Required actions
Required body functions
Required body structures

Client Factors
Body functions
Body structures

FIGURE 7-1   Domain of occupational therapy. (Adapted from American Occupational Therapy Association. [2002]. Occupational therapy practice framework: Domain and processes. *American Journal of Occupational Therapy, 56,* 609-639.)

same time they restrict it; for example, a theater may offer an elder the opportunity to watch a theatrical performance, but not to swim or ride a horse, whereas a swimming pool may offer the opportunity to swim, but not to watch a theatrical performance.

Two other elements may affect how a person engages in occupation. A person may not be able to meet the demands inherent in an activity (e.g., without a fair amount of conditioning, an elder might not be able to climb up a mountain), or the person may find the demands too low (e.g., a champion chess player may find it quite boring to play Tic Tac Toe). Activity demands include such things as the objects used in the activity and the characteristics of these objects, space and social demands, required actions, and required body functions and structures. For example, the activity of playing golf requires balls and golf irons; takes place on a golf course; is often played with others, and therefore requires taking turns; involves a sequence of tasks from placing the ball, hitting it, and then locating it in the distance; and the

bodily functions of joint mobility and muscle power to swing the iron while not letting the iron fly away and harming someone standing nearby. Furthermore, playing golf involves the person's cardiovascular system while walking, vestibular functions while turning one's trunk and following through with the swing, and a variety of other body structures and functions. Interestingly, engagement in occupation is not only affected by these functions and structures, it may affect them in turn; for example, an elder's cardiovascular and neuromuscular functions become conditioned while gradually increasing the time spent walking in a golf course.

The Framework describes the OT process as consisting of three dynamic and interactive phases: evaluation, intervention, and outcome. Evaluation consists of the initial step of obtaining the client's occupational profile and a second step of analysis of the client's occupational performance. The occupational profile is focused on the person's history, experiences, daily living patterns, values, needs, beliefs, and so on. The profile consists,

86

TABLE 7-1

Areas of Occupation

Activities of daily living	Instrumental activities of daily living
Bathing/showering	Care of others
Bowel and bladder management	Care of pets
Dressing	Child rearing
Eating	Communication device use
Feeding	Community mobility
Functional mobility	Financial management
Personal device care	Health management and maintenance
Personal hygiene and grooming	Home establishment and management
Sexual activity	Meal preparation and cleanup
Sleep/rest	Safety procedures and emergency responses
Toilet hygiene	Shopping

Education	Work
Formal educational participation	Employment interest and pursuits
Exploration of informal personal educational needs or interests (beyond formal education)	Employment seeking and acquisition
	Job performance
	Retirement preparation and adjustment
Informal personal education participation	Volunteer exploration
	Volunteer participation

Play	Leisure
Play exploration	Leisure exploration
Play participation	Leisure participation

Social Participation
Community
Family
Peer, friend

Adapted from American Occupational Therapy Association. (2002). *Occupational therapy practice framework: Domain and processes. American Journal of Occupational Therapy, 56,* 609-639.

essentially, of understanding what the person finds important and meaningful and, therefore, of high priority. Although obtaining contextual information is important throughout the whole intervention process, it is particularly essential at this stage because it will provide the foundation for specific evaluation of occupational performance, and certainly for the selection of intervention strategies later in the OT process. For example, if an elder who has had a mild stroke states that he has assembled and collected fishing flies his whole life, a detailed assessment of fine motor skills may be indicated to ascertain whether he has the necessary motor skills to manipulate the small pieces used in this meaningful occupation. Likewise, an analysis of any other areas of occupational performance that may negatively influence the person's engagement in meaningful occupation should be performed. Notably, barriers to participation in occupation may not necessarily reside in the client, but may be located in the client's context. For example, although an elder may like to tie fishing flies, his family may not make the materials available to him because they cannot imagine him going fishing any time soon. In this case, they may not understand the meaningfulness of the occupation of fly tying, and therefore create a barrier for his participation in the occupation.

The occupational profile and analysis of occupational performance guide the identification of OT treatment goals and intervention strategies. Thus, the intervention phase is centered around what the client finds most meaningful in life and of greatest priority. An intervention plan will include strategies to address performance skills, patterns, contexts, activity demands, and client factors that may be hindering performance. An ongoing collaboration among the OTR, OTA, and client is indispensable to assure that goals, treatment strategies, and progress are continually evaluated and adapted to meet the client's priorities.

According to the Occupational Therapy Practice Framework, "the important dimension of health that OTRs and OTAs target as the profession's overarching outcome is 'engagement in occupation to support participation'" (AOTA, 2002, p. 618). This means that it is the responsibility of OT practitioners to assure that their interventions lead to actual participation in life situations and not simply to improvement in performance skills. In the earlier example of the elder who found tying fishing flies meaningful, it is not sufficient to help him develop the motor skills necessary to maintain this interest. The ultimate goal of OT is for the elder to actually engage in fly tying in the most natural context possible. Thus, instructing the elder to exercise his fingers with elastic bands may contribute to his skills, but cannot be the limit of OT intervention. Likewise, using fly fishing to develop dexterity can be considered insufficient intervention if the elder never has the opportunity to use the product of his hands in a meaningful way.

Deepak: The framework in use

The Framework can help us to understand Deepak's life situation and plan intervention that best supports his participation in all areas of life. According to the Framework, the initial phase of evaluation should involve obtaining an occupational profile. By asking Deepak about his current concerns related to engaging in occupations

TABLE 7-2

Performance Skills		
Motor skills*	**Process skills***	**Communication/interaction skills***
■ Posture (stabilizes, aligns) ■ Mobility (walks, reaches, bends) ■ Coordination (coordinates, manipulates, flows) ■ Strength and effort (moves, transports, lifts, calibrates, grips) ■ Energy (endures, paces)	■ Energy (paces, attends) ■ Knowledge (chooses, uses, handles, heeds, inquires) ■ Temporal organization (initiates, continues, sequences, terminates) ■ Organizing space and objects (searches/locates, gathers, organizes, restores, navigates) ■ Adaptation (notices/responds, accommodates, adjusts, benefits)	■ Physicality (contacts, gazes, gestures, maneuvers, orients, postures) ■ Information exchange (articulates, asserts, asks, engages, expresses, modulates, shares, speaks, sustains) ■ Relations (collaborates, conforms, focuses, relates, respects)

Adapted from American Occupational Therapy Association. (2002). Occupational therapy practice framework: Domain and processes. *American Journal of Occupational Therapy, 56,* 609-639.
*Skills listed as verbs to denote they imply action.

and daily life activities, as well as about his work history, life experiences, family traditions, and other personal facts, we find out that he has relied heavily on his wife to help with the family's transition from country to country. Deepak now has a great sense of debt toward her and some guilt for having spent much time working away from home. The physician has recommended that Deepak not put any weight on his left leg for 6 weeks. Deepak's main concern is that because of his left knee infection he will not be able to be of any assistance to his wife in her last weeks of life.

Understanding Deepak's main concern will help us to establish a collaborative relationship with him while we evaluate his skills and environment. If, for example, we had proceeded to evaluate his ability to dress and bathe himself and assessed his endurance and joint range of motion without knowing about his concerns, we might have further reinforced his sense of uselessness and limited potential for social participation. Instead, we can now identify which activities he believes would be the most important for him to be able to do to convey caring for his wife. For Deepak, these include being able to help her move in bed, get in and out of a bed and a chair, run errands for her and, if necessary, help her eat. Thus, we can proceed by evaluating his endurance, balance, and strength, all needed to help his wife move in bed or get in and out of a chair. We can help adapt the environment and teach him body mechanics in order to have the maximum leverage while moving his wife. We can further evaluate his ability to complete activities of daily living, because he will need to be dressed to run errands outside of the home.

Naturally, there are many other areas for assessment and treatment with Deepak. However, the above illustrates how the central concern for him is related to an area of occupation rather than to a body structure. OT intervention can still be organized to address many client factors, but the treatment is not likely to seem meaningful unless Deepak is able to understand that it contributes to his main concern.

Facilitating growth and development

The Facilitating Growth and Development Model views the OT practitioner's role as one "concerned with facilitating or promoting optimal growth and development in all ages of man" (Llorens, 1976). An individual's growth and development may be threatened by disease, injury, disability, or trauma. The OT practitioner may be required to assist the individual in coping with illness, trauma, or disability, or to help with rehabilitation. The OT practitioner also may seek to prevent maladaptation and promote health maintenance.

This model requires the OT practitioner to understand the developmental tasks and adaptive skills that are usually mastered at different ages. The model describes the belief that the human being "develops simultaneously in the areas of neurophysiological, physical, psychosocial and psychodynamic growth, and in the development of social language, daily living, socio-cultural, and intellectual skills during the life span" (Llorens, 1976, p. 2). The way the individual integrates and organizes these areas of development to perform in work, education, play, self-care, and leisure activities during each stage of life is of primary concern to OT. In addition to understanding the individual's development, the OT practitioner must understand the ways illness, disease, trauma, and disability may threaten that development. Finally, OT addresses the environmental variables necessary to support the development and maintenance of the important adaptive skills cited by Llorens (1976).

The Facilitating Growth and Development Model synthesizes the work of numerous authors who have contributed to the understanding of human maturation (Llorens, 1976). The model includes descriptions of the adaptive skills mentioned during each life stage, including infancy to age 2 years, ages 2 to 3 years, ages 3 to 6 years, ages 6 to 11 years, adolescence, young adulthood, adulthood, and maturity. Each stage is built on the foundation of the stages the person has completed (Table 7-3). This text, however, focuses on the last stage.

During the OT process, the OTR and COTA assess the client's development and determine potential disruptions in each adaptive skill area. The OTR and COTA analyze this information to determine the effects on age-appropriate occupational performance in the areas of work, education, self-care, and play and leisure. The OTR

and COTA may then devise intervention strategies that facilitate development of a specific skill needed for successful occupational performance (Table 7-4). Matching the client's needs with the right therapeutic activities requires careful analysis of inherent requirements of each activity.

Depending on the client's needs, selected activities may include sensory, developmental, symbolic, and daily life tasks. These activities are combined with the social interaction that is most beneficial for the client. Sensory activities are those that primarily influence the senses through human action, such as touching, rocking, running, and listening to sounds. Developmental activities involve the use of objects such as crafts and puzzles in play, learning, and skill development situations. The client develops specific performance skills by engaging in

TABLE 7-3

Characteristics of Maturity

Neurophysiologic and physical development
Possible alterations in sensory functions (visual, auditory, tactile, kinesthetic, gustatory, and olfactory), motor behavior (coordination of extremities), information processing (higher level integration, including conceptualization and memory), and physical endurance

Psychosocial—ego integrity and maturity
Acceptance of life experiences and the life cycle

Psychodynamic
Coping with continued growth after middle age, decision making regarding growth or death (giving up on life), dealing with insincerity of friends and acquaintances, inner life trends toward survival, possible decrease in efforts to maintain false pride, often a reduction in defenses, more suspiciousness, and necessity of dealing with psychological deterioration

Sociocultural
Group affiliation: family, social, interest, civic

Social language development
Predominantly verbal use, some use of nonverbal behavior to communicate

Activities of daily living and developmental tasks
Adjustment to decreasing physical strength and health, adjustment to retirement and reduced income, adjustment to death of spouse, adjustment to one's own impending death, establishment of affiliations with own age group, and meeting of social obligations.

Ego-adaptive skills
Ability to function independently; ability to control drives and select appropriate objects; ability to organize stimuli, plan, and execute purposeful motion; ability to obtain, organize, and use knowledge; ability to participate in primary group; ability to participate in a variety of relationships; ability to experience self as a holistic, acceptable object; ability to participate in mutually satisfying relationships oriented to sexual needs

Intellectual development
Possible neurophysiologic and physical development alteration and return of egocentrism

Adapted from Llorens, L. A. (1976). *Application of a developmental theory for health and rehabilitation.* Rockville, MD: American Occupational Therapy Association.

TABLE 7-4

Activity Analysis
Sensory aspects How much touch and movement does the activity require? To what extent are visual perception skills used in the activity? Does the activity require auditory perception and discrimination? Are perception and discrimination of smells and taste involved in the activity?
Physical aspects How much does the activity require bilateral movements of arms and legs? Does the activity require the use of both hands at the same time? Can the activity be completed with one hand? How much muscle strength and joint range of motion does the activity require? How much sitting, standing, and variability in position is necessary to complete the activity? Does the physical performance require much thought organization? Which fine and gross motor movements does the activity require? How much eye–hand coordination is needed for the activity? How much time and what equipment is needed for the activity?
Psychodynamic aspects Does the activity permit expression of feelings, thoughts, original ideas, and creativity? Is there opportunity for the constructive expression of hostility, aggression, expansiveness, organization, control, narcissism, expiation of guilt, dependence, and independence? How does the activity permit or require sex role identification?
Social aspects How much contact and guidance from others is required to complete the activity? How much does the activity require the person to work alone or with others? How much socialization does the activity permit?
Attention and skill aspects How much initiative and self-reliance does the activity require? Does the activity require technical skills? Are manipulative and creative abilities needed? Does the activity require persistence to complete? How much repeated motion is needed?
Practical aspects How much noise and dirt are created during the activity? What materials and equipment are used and what are their costs? Can waste or scrap material be used?

Data from Llorens, L. A. (1976). *Application of a developmental theory for health and rehabilitation*. Rockville, MD: American Occupational Therapy Association.

these types of activities. Symbolic activities are designed to help the client satisfy needs and elicit and cope with emotional responses. Examples include gouging wood and kneading clay, which may release muscle tension and help process anger. Another example of a symbolic activity is leading a group in a task. This activity may satisfy the client's need to be heard and feel competent. The emotional response from leading a group may be improved self-esteem. Daily life tasks, also called *activities of daily living*, include tasks such as brushing teeth, getting dressed, cooking, and cleaning. Finally, social interaction includes participation in dyads with the therapist or another person and groups. These activities encourage development of sociocultural competence and language and intellectual skills.

According to the Facilitating Growth and Development Model, OT intervention should continue until the client reaches sufficient competence in performing the skills and activities described as developmentally appropriate.

The OTR and COTA continually monitor and reevaluate the client's progress in improving, maintaining, or restoring areas of occupational performance and therefore clearly know when the client no longer requires specialized OT services.

Martha: The model in use

Llorens' (1976) developmental model can help give us a more complete picture of Martha's life and occupational needs. She has lived for more than half her life with the disability that resulted from her head injury. However, she has been relatively healthy and independent. She now is facing the neurophysiologic and physical alterations that are normal with maturity, but that seem to compound the occupational performance challenges brought by her disability. Her bouts with pneumonia have left her debilitated and she has been moved to a skilled nursing facility.

According to Lloren's developmental model (1976), a life priority for Martha is to accept life experiences and the life cycle, not to distinguish which of her problems are caused by her age and which by her head injury. Of great importance will be for her to continue developing coping skills to deal with both her limitations in function and the changes in her environment now that she no longer lives with her sister. She has the opportunity to participate in a variety of relationships with fellow patients and staff. Finally, of great importance will be to stimulate her continued intellectual development. Although her ability to bathe and dress herself independently are important, that need should not overshadow the other needs she has as a developing human being.

Cognitive Disabilities

As its name indicates, the Cognitive Disabilities Model is concerned with OT services that are designed for clients with cognitive impairments. These impairments may be the result of psychiatric illness, medical diseases, brain traumas, or developmental disorders. Psychiatric illnesses such as depression and schizophrenia have associated cognitive impairments. Alzheimer's dementia and cerebrovascular accidents are examples of medical conditions that result in cognitive impairments, and closed head injuries are an example of trauma to the brain that can also result in a brain disorder. Brain dysfunction also may result from use of prescribed medications or other drugs. The cognitive impairment that results from these conditions may be short term or long lasting.

Assertions of the Cognitive Disabilities Model are based on information from neuroscience, biology, psychology, and traditional OT theory (Allen, Earhart, & Blue, 1995). According to this model, occupation is synonymous with voluntary motor action. Observing voluntary motor actions such as dressing, completing a craft, or preparing a simple meal is of primary interest to the OT practitioner because of the inferences that can be made about brain function. Voluntary motor actions are "behavioral responses to a sensory cue that are guided by the mind" (Allen, 1985, p. 6). That is, voluntary motor actions occur as a consequence of the relation among the external physical environment of matter, which provides sensory cues; the internal mind, which provides purpose; and the body, which produces behavior in the form of motor activity. Observing a person's voluntary motor action gives the OT practitioner insight into the relation among these three domains. Each domain is further described by subclassifications.

Based on extensive research, the Cognitive Disabilities Model proposes a categorization of six cognitive levels that describe the way an individual relates matter, behavior, and mind as demonstrated in performance of voluntary motor actions (Allen, 1985; Allen, Earhart, & Blue, 1995) (Table 7-5). Level 1 represents the greatest degree of impairment, and level 6 represents normal performance.

As this model has evolved, each cognitive level has been expanded to include several subcategories or "modes." Only the global characteristics of each level are described in this text. This practice model may be used to describe client performance and to guide selection of activities or tasks that permit the client to function consistently at the greatest possible level. (Other chapters in this text describe conditions associated with elders for whom application of the cognitive disabilities model may be appropriate, including the aging process in Chapter 3; side effects of medication in Chapter 13; malnutrition and dehydration in Chapter 18; strokes in Chapter 19; Alzheimer's dementia in Chapter 20; depression, schizophrenia, and drug addiction in Chapter 21; and brain tumors in Chapter 25.)

Observing clients perform activities and tasks that are part of their daily routines is ideal during assessment because these activities are usually important to the client and caregivers. These activities also allow the OTR and COTA team to separate issues related to learning a new activity, which might not accurately convey the client's current cognitive performance. Consequently, task assessment should be preceded by information obtained from the client and caregivers regarding the client's most familiar tasks. After observing the client, the OTR and COTA team can compare the performance with the characteristic behaviors for each cognitive level. The OTR and COTA must remember that a client may function at a variety of levels depending on familiarity with the task and the time of day. Knowledge of the client's optimal functional level helps the OTR and COTA team design intervention strategies that maximize the client's abilities.

Several standardized tests may be used to determine cognitive level, including the Expanded Routine Task Inventory (RTI) (Allen, 1985) and the Allen Cognitive Levels Test (ACL) (Allen, Earhart, & Blue, 1995). The RTI evaluates the individual's ability at each of the six levels to complete a variety of routine tasks along a physical scale, such as grooming, dressing, bathing, walking, exercising, feeding, toileting, taking medication, and using adaptive equipment; a community scale, such as housekeeping, obtaining and preparing food, spending money, doing laundry, traveling, shopping, telephoning, and taking care of a child; a communication scale, such as listening, talking, reading, and writing; and an employment scale, such as maintaining pace and schedule, following instructions, performing simple and complex tasks, getting along with coworkers, following safety precautions and responding to emergencies, and supervising and planning work. The ACL test helps to determine cognitive level by assessing response to verbal instructions and problem-solving techniques when a client is presented with a leather lacing project (Allen, 1985). The large ACL was developed to compensate for visual loss in the elder population, and

TABLE 7-5

Allen Cognitive Levels

	Level 1 Automatic actions	Level 2 Postural actions	Level 3 Manual actions	Level 4 Goal-directed actions	Level 5 Exploratory actions	Level 6 Planned actions
Matter						
Sensory cues	Awareness is at threshold of consciousness	Responds to proprioceptive cues	Responds to tactile cues	Follows visible cues	Follows related cues	Follows symbolic cues
Perceptibility	Attends to cues that penetrate subliminal state	Aware of own body and objects that come into contact with it	Aware of immediate external surfaces	Aware of concepts of color and shape of objects	Aware of concepts of space and depth	Aware of intangible concepts
Setting	Mainly internal	Within range of motion	Within arm's reach	Within visual field	Restricted to task environment	Expanded to potential task environments
Sample	Responds to alerting stimuli	Copies demonstrated body action	Identifies material objects	Makes exact match of sample	Conceives tangible possibilities of variations	Conceives hypothetic ideas
Behavior						
Motor actions	Actions are habitual and automatic and have little thought	Spontaneous actions are postural (bending and stretching)	Hands are used to manipulate material objects repetitively	Actions are goal directed but restricted to tangible environment	Possibilities are explored through motor action that causes a visible effect	Actions are preceded by pause to think and plan
Tool use	Needs stimulation to use body parts in habitual tasks	Uses body parts spontaneously	Uses found objects by chance; success is accidental	Uses hand tools as a means to a concrete end	Uses hand tools to vary means and end	Creates tools; uses power tools

Number	Completes one action at a time	Completes one action at a time	Completes one action at a time	Completes one step of task at a time	Completes several steps at a time	Completes indefinite steps
People	Attends to those who shout or touch	Attends to those who move	Attends to the object manipulation of others	Shares goals with others	Shares exploration with others	Shares plans and recognizes autonomy
Directions	Understands single verbs; physical contact is needed for action	Understands pronouns and names of body parts; gross motor and guided movements	Understands names of material objects and actions on an object	Understands adjectives and adverbs; must see each step in a series	Understands prepositions and explanations; each step and potential errors must be demonstrated	Understands conjunction and conjectures; demonstration is not necessary
Mind						
Attention	Attention is focused on subliminal cues; external attention is very transient	Attends to proprioceptive cues, to own body, and to movement	Attends to tactile cues, focuses attention on the immediate effects of own actions	Attends to clearly visible cues; focuses attention to complete a task, end product sustains attention	Attends to related visual cues; may seek novelty through variation, but must see effects first	Attends to symbolic cues, thinks before testing results
Goal attainment	Is awake; completes very habitual behaviors (eating and drinking)	Chance body movement creates interesting results that may be repeated	Chance movement creates visible results that are repeated many times	Uses several movement schemes to achieve an end goal	Becomes aware of problems when they become visible; uses trial and error approach	Problems are solved covertly; images are used to test solutions
Time	Attention is maintained for seconds at a time	Attention is directed for minutes at a time	Attention is directed for half an hour at a time	Attention is maintained for an hour at a time	Attention is maintained and goals are remembered for weeks at a time	Sense of past, present, and future is maintained

Data from Allen, C. (1985). *Occupational therapy for psychiatric diseases: Measurement and management of psychiatric diseases*. Boston, MA: Little, Brown & Company.

the Cognitive Performance Test was developed to provide a standardized, ADL-based instrument for the assessment of functional level in Alzheimer's dementia.

Once the client's cognitive level has been determined, the OT intervention goals must be considered (Allen, Earhart, & Blue, 1992). Allen (1985) states that participation in an occupation does not necessarily mean the client will improve. This assumption fails to recognize other possible reasons for recovery, including that the client may recover spontaneously without any treatment. Consequently, the purpose of OT intervention should be to document alterations and improvements in functional abilities, sustain current performance, and reduce pain and distress associated with the symptoms. Goals are not intended to improve cognitive level but to ensure consistency of performance at the safest and least restrictive level. The case of Ray illustrates this point. Ray is a 70-year-old man with Alzheimer's dementia. An OTR and COTA team determined that he is currently functioning at cognitive level 4. This means that Ray can spontaneously complete tasks when cues are clearly visible. A goal for Ray to live independently would not be appropriate because he does not deal with cues that are not within his field of vision and consequently can easily place himself in danger. Appropriate OT goals for Ray according to this model may include consistent initiation of daily self-care routines, initiation of laundry washing, consistent monitoring of Ray in unfamiliar environments, and provision by his caregivers of appropriate cues to maximize his performance.

Once the client's goals have been determined, the COTA may select a variety of activities that match the characteristics of the matter, mind, and behavior domains appropriate to the client's cognitive level. The COTA must be adept at analyzing a task to know precisely the way it requires matter, mind, and behavior to interact for the client to successfully perform a voluntary motor action. Tasks are selected by the degree of demand on the client to perform consistently at a particular cognitive level. The OTR and COTA team evaluated Ray and determined he was at cognitive level 4. Consequently, he can understand basic goals of activities, can purposefully use objects placed within his field of vision, and is able to match examples of tasks demonstrated to him. To reinforce his ability to maintain a sense of accomplishment, the COTA may select a simple woodworking project for Ray. The COTA can place all materials for this project on a table in front of Ray and instruct him to sand the wooden pieces. Telling him to pick up the sandpaper, hold it so the grain comes in contact with the wood, and rub it against the wood is unnecessary. These steps would be obvious to Ray because the materials are in his field of vision. Once Ray completes the sanding, the COTA may instruct him in a similar way to glue the pieces together as shown in the sample, stain the stool, and varnish it.

Ray lacks the foresight to plan for potential problems; consequently, the COTA should demonstrate the amount of glue, stain, and varnish needed in addition to the application procedures.

Once the client is performing at a level that most consistently demonstrates remaining task abilities and the environment has been structured to compensate for the client's limitations, skilled OT services should be discontinued. Discharge considerations are made from the beginning of OT intervention. The cognitive disabilities model specifically focuses on preparing the client for discharge to the least restrictive environment (Allen, Earhart, & Blue, 1995). Therefore, the COTA must observe voluntary motor actions to understand the way each client interacts with the environment. The COTA and OTR should recommend that the client be discharged to the setting that best supports the client's task abilities.

Ursula: The model in use

Ursula's Alzheimer disease has progressed to the point where there is a clear cognitive deficit. Therefore, the Cognitive Disabilities Model is ideal to help us develop a suitable treatment plan. The first step is to determine the cognitive level at which Ursula is functioning. During the RTI, Ursula shows that she performs at cognitive level 4. This is consistent with her husband's report, who states that at home Ursula follows his visible cues and only seems to pay attention to objects within her immediate visual field. He notes that she does not seem able to find items she needs even though they are in plain view in the room. However, once she finds the item, she is able to use it correctly.

The OT program for Ursula should consist of activities at level 4 that encourage her to complete steps of repetitive tasks after they have been demonstrated for her. For her safety, the environment should be structured so that all the items she needs are in plain view in front of her. She should be given one instruction at a time, and instructions should focus on the motor actions rather than on the abstract goal of projects. Examples of suitable projects include simple printing or painting tasks, woodworking kits with few and large pieces, and simple food preparation tasks that do not require use of a stove or other potentially dangerous appliance. For her safety, Ursula should never be left alone or unattended.

Model of Human Occupation

The Model of Human Occupation was designed for use with any individual experiencing difficulties in performing occupation. This model evolved from earlier research by Reilly (1962) on occupational behavior. Using concepts from General Systems Theory, Open Systems Theory, and Dynamical Systems Theory, this model gives an explanation for the way occupation is motivated, organized, and performed, thereby emphasizing the human system's spontaneous, purposeful, tension-seeking properties and acknowledging its creative properties (Kielhofner, 2002). In addition, this model provides a view of the degree of intimacy between the environment and the performance of occupation.

Human beings maintain constant interaction with the environment and receive many types of input such as olfactory and sensory stimulation and behavior expectations. The individual uses that input in many ways (e.g., food becomes energy; sensory stimulation may translate to touch, pain, or temperature; and words are interpreted). This process is known as throughput. Part of the result of the process of input and throughput is that a behavior, or output, is produced. Finally, as the person performs the behavior, the experience of doing it and any results from it form the process of feedback, which becomes a new source of input into the system. The Model of Human Occupation explains occupation as the cumulative and highly dynamic expression of this process. For example, in meal preparation, the cook sees the food items (input), considers what recipe to use (throughput), prepares the food items (output), feels arm movement, and sees the result of the preparation (feedback). While seeing that feedback, the cook notices that the food is beginning to turn brown (input), decides it is burning (throughput), removes the pan from the stove (output), and experiences moving the pan until it is off the stove (feedback). To further explain this dynamic interaction between the individual and the environment from which the occupation arises, the Model of Human Occupation describes external and internal environments of the human being as composed of several subsystems.

According to this model, the external environment offers opportunities for certain behaviors while requiring others. For example, the institution of school offers the teacher a room in which to walk around, speak, write on the chalkboard, and sit in a chair. At the same time, the school requires from the teacher the behavior of instructing the students. The teacher will be fired if those requirements are not met. Providing opportunity and requiring behavior is a complementary relationship. The influence of this relationship comes from several sources in the environment, including the physical realm, such as objects and built or natural structures; the social realm, which includes the tasks deemed appropriate and desirable and the social groups sanctioning the behavior; the settings in which occupation occurs, such as home, neighborhood, school, workplace, and gathering, recreation, and resource sites; and the overall culture, such as values, norms, and customs, which affects the individual's life (Fig. 7-2).

The earlier example of meal preparation can be used to elaborate on these external environment concepts. To perform this occupation, the cook requires several objects, including food ingredients and seasonings, a knife, some

pans, and the stove. The processes of dicing, chopping, stirring, and frying the food are all tasks recognized as cooking. Because of health concerns, the cook may choose to prepare a meal consisting only of vegetables for his or her family (social group). The setting of the meal is the cook's home, where he or she can exercise creativity in preparing and seasoning the food and presenting the meal. In addition, the choice of vegetables only may be influenced by a cultural value that an athletic body is preferable to an obese one. If the cook were performing the occupation of cooking as the main task of his or her job at a restaurant, however, the objects, tasks, social group, setting, and possibly cultural expectations may present completely different opportunities and behavior expectations. There he or she might use industrial size knives and tools, prepare large amounts of fried fish, be part of a team of cooks, and work in a restaurant that specializes in ethnic food.

The Model of Human Occupation describes the individual's internal environment as composed of subsystems (Fig. 7-3). The volition subsystem is responsible for guiding the individual through occupation choices throughout the day. According to this model, occupation choice is influenced by the individual's disposition about expected outcome and by self-knowledge, or awareness of the self as an active participant in this world. Both these influences determine the way the individual anticipates, chooses, and experiences occupation. These concepts are illustrated by George and Pam, an elder couple residing in a senior housing community. Every Saturday night they dress in their best clothes and walk to the common hall to play bridge with other members of their community. They choose to do this because they anticipate the pleasure of friends' company and because they believe they are capable bridge players. Helen, who lives in the same community as George and Pam, chooses not to play bridge. Although she is a champion player, she anticipates feeling out of place because she is a widow and does not have a regular partner.

The volition subsystem is composed of personal causation, values, and interests. Personal causation refers to the awareness individuals have of their abilities (i.e., knowledge of capacity) and to individuals' perceptions that they have control over their behavior (i.e., sense of efficacy). An individual is more likely to engage in an occupation he or she feels capable of doing. Values refer to the convictions people have that help them assign significance and standards of performance to the occupations they perform. Each individual has values that form the individual's views of life. These values elicit a sense of obligation to do what one believes is right. Finally, interests refer to the desire to find pleasure, enjoyment, and satisfaction in certain occupations. Interests may also be attractions people feel toward certain occupations and preferences regarding ways occupations are performed. For example, George, Pam, and Helen each have a sense

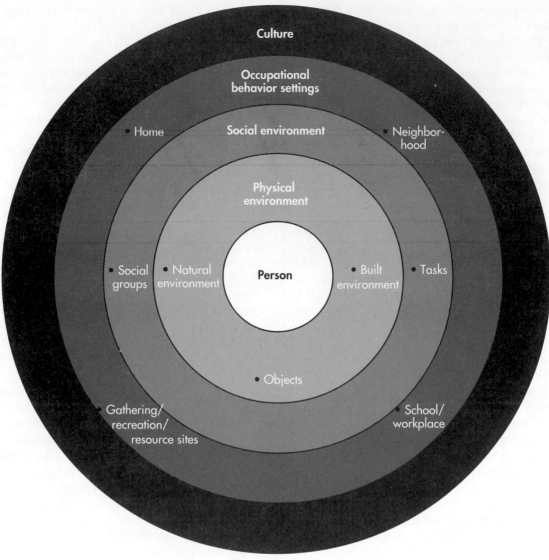

FIGURE 7-2   External environment layers.

of themselves as good or effective bridge players (personal causation). This sense was developed over time, so that after playing as partners for more than 30 years, George and Pam have a specific playing style (preference) and are attracted to the opportunity to play bridge on Saturday nights rather than staying home and watching television. Although Helen may have developed the same interest and personal causation, she believes that playing bridge is most meaningful with your spouse as your partner. Because she has no spouse, this value is sufficient to deter her from participating in the Saturday night games at the senior housing community.

In contrast to the volition subsystem, which has to do with conscious choice of occupation, the habituation subsystem has to do with the routine activities of daily life. These routines require little deliberation because they are built on repetition. The habituation subsystem is composed of habits and internalized roles. Habits have to do with the typical way an individual performs a particular occupation and organizes it within a typical day or week, and the unique style the individual brings to performance. For example, going to the common hall on Saturday night to play bridge is part of George and Pam's weekly routine. While playing bridge, both drink coffee. George typically puts one teaspoon of sugar in his cup before pouring in the coffee, and Pam pours her coffee first and then mixes in the sugar. During the game, George is talkative and Pam is quiet, but both break into song when they win the game.

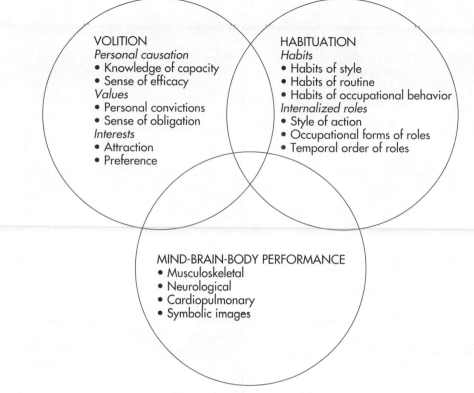

FIGURE 7-3 Internal organization of the human being.

Internalized roles refer to typical ways in which an individual relates to others. Roles are the identities and behaviors people assume in various social situations. These roles are based on the individual's perceived expectations of others. Thus, roles involve obligations and rights of the individual in the various social contexts. According to the Model of Human Occupation, the specific occupational behaviors that encompass a role, the style in which actions in a role occur, and the way an individual's roles are prioritized are of particular interest to the OT practitioner. George, Pam, and Helen each have an image of the role of bridge player. For George and Pam, this role includes the occupations of dressing nicely, walking to the common hall, playing by the rules, and sitting around a table conversing with others. Helen may view the role in a similar way, but she has the additional sense that the role of bridge player requires having one's spouse as partner. Because she is a widow, Helen has abandoned the role of bridge player. Conversely, George and Pam routinely enter this role on Saturday nights.

The final subsystem of the human being's internal environment is the mind–brain–body performance subsystem. As its name implies, this subsystem represents the complex interplay among the musculoskeletal, neurological, perceptual, and cognitive abilities required to actually perform an occupation or enact a behavior. Interaction

with the environment occurs through this subsystem. The individual perceives challenges and opportunities in the environment through the perceptual system and processes this information in the brain. According to the meaning ascribed to the perception, the brain plans an action, which is carried to the muscles, joints, and bones of the limbs that perform the action. Whereas an occupation's meaning is ascribed by the volition subsystem and the social context is determined by the habituation subsystem, the related actions are created by the performance subsystem. George and Pam like to play bridge (volition subsystem) and do so every Saturday night (habituation subsystem). During the bridge game, George and Pam keep in mind the rules and play accordingly. They sit with others around a table and maintain a grasp on the cards (performance subsystem). The complex interplay between mind, brain, and body inherent in the performance of any occupation occurs through specific skills, including motor skills, process skills, and communication–interaction skills (Table 7-6).

A strength of the Model of Human Occupation is the holistic view it provides of any dysfunction. Traditional health practice often focuses on one or two particular traits of a dysfunction rather than on all the contributing factors. All the effects of dysfunction on an individual's life are rarely fully explored (Kielhofner, 2002). This lack

TABLE 7-6

Performance Skills

Motor domains and skills
Posture
Stabilizes
Aligns
Positions

Mobility
Walks
Reaches
Bends

Coordination
Coordinates body parts
Manipulates
Uses fluent movements

Strength and effort
Moves objects
Transports objects
Lifts objects
Calibrates force, speed, and movement

Energy
Endures
Paces work

Communication and interaction domains and skills
Physicality
Gestures
Gazes

Approximates body appropriately
Postures
Contacts

Language
Articulates
Speaks
Focuses speech
Manages
Modulates

Relations
Engages
Relates
Respects
Collaborates

Information exchange
Asks
Expresses
Shares
Asserts

Process domains and skills
Energy
Paces
Attends

Knowledge
Chooses tools and materials
Uses tools and materials appropriately

Handles tools and materials appropriately
Heeds directions
Inquires for directions

Temporal organization
Initiates
Continues
Sequences
Terminates

Organization
Searches and locates
Gathers
Organizes
Restores
Navigates

Adaptation
Notices and responds
Accommodates
Adjusts
Benefits

Social interaction domain and skills
Acknowledging
Turns body or face toward others
Looks at partner
Confirms understanding
Touches others appropriately

Sending
Greets
Answers
Questions
Complies
Encourages
Extends
Clarifies
Sets limits
Thanks

Timing
Times response
Speaks fluently
Takes turns
Times duration
Completes

Coordinating
Approaches
Places self at appropriate distance
Assumes position
Matches language
Disclosure
Expresses emotion

---

of understanding the whole situation may be particularly detrimental to the elder. For example, Calvin is a 78-year-old man recently admitted to the hospital after falling and fracturing his left femur. On admission, an x-ray examination was done, Calvin was taken to surgery, and an open reduction of the fracture was performed. A cast was put on Calvin's leg and he was referred to physical and OT for a brief rehabilitation course. The physical therapist focused rehabilitation on getting in and out of bed and walking with the reduced weight-bearing guidelines recommended by the physician. The OTR evaluated Calvin and identified difficulties in dressing and toileting because of the cast and weight-bearing precautions. The OTR asked the COTA to train Calvin to dress and toilet with adaptive equipment, to which Calvin easily complied. Calvin was discharged to return home in 2 days, at which time the OTR and COTA team documented that Calvin was independent in dressing and toileting with necessary equipment and was aware of home modifications needed to avoid further falls. Unfortunately, nobody on the health team carefully investigated the reason Calvin fell. Although he can care for himself, he finds living alone unbearably lonely. In addition, three of Calvin's lifelong friends died in the past year. Thus, Calvin has a deep sense of hopelessness. He occasionally tries to alleviate his feelings of loneliness and despair by drinking alcohol. He fell after one of these drinking episodes. When the admitting health worker at the hospital asked him if he consumed alcohol, Calvin responded truthfully that he did so only occasionally. During his hospital stay Calvin appeared bright and friendly because he received much desired social contact. A more systematic evaluation of Calvin's life would have revealed a deeper problem related to his volition and habituation subsystems. Instead, the OTR and COTA team focused on the obvious performance subsystem problem, which actually was only a symptom of a more complex issue. The team's care also should have addressed Calvin's feelings of hopelessness (volition) and the reduced number of roles he has to help him organize his days (habitation). Furthermore, the COTA and OTR should have helped Calvin explore community resources.

According to the Model of Human Occupation, any traditional OT tool is valid for assessment and treatment. Not one single assessment or treatment tool can completely address the complexity of the individual. Some suggested evaluation tools include the Assessment of Communication and Interaction Skills (Salamy, Simon, & Kielhofner, 1993), the Assessment of Motor and Process Skills (Fisher, 1999), the Assessment of Occupational Functioning (Watts, Hinson, Madigan, McGuigan, & Newman, 1999), the Occupational Case Analysis Interview and Rating Scale (Kaplan & Kielhofner, 1989), and the Occupational Performance History Interview (Kielhofner et al., 1997). Interest and role checklists, activity configurations, manual muscle tests, range of motion tests, and cognitive tests are among the many tools that may be used to evaluate each subsystem. Ultimately, data should be gathered regarding all subsystems of the individual's internal and external environments. Once problems are identified, intervention is prioritized according to all subsystems that are interdependent. In Calvin's case, if the volition and habituation issues had been identified, OT intervention could have focused on helping Calvin find other meaningful activities and resources for continued social contact in addition to addressing his dressing and toileting needs.

Carlos: The model in use

Because Carlos is unable to speak, an observational assessment tool should be used to describe a baseline of occupational functioning. An Assessment of Motor and Process Skills (Fisher, 1999) can help us see that although Carlos is unable to speak, he is able to perform fairly complicated motor tasks. As part of the Assessment of Motor and Process Skills, Carlos was asked to make a fruit salad. Carlos positioned his body appropriately for the task, stabilized all objects, including the fruit and knife, maintained a secure grasp on the objects, chose the right tools, sequenced the task correctly, and cleaned the workspace without being asked to do so. This demonstrated that Carlos continued to consider his role as cook as very important and that he was motivated to remain active. When tasting the fruit salad, there was no coughing, and it became apparent that part of his problem may have been that his family was feeding him while he was in bed. By making the fruit salad, Carlos demonstrated to his family that he was not an invalid and that he was motivated to be upright and active. This allowed the family to step back and encourage him to increase his level of activity rather than overprotect him as they had been

doing. In 2 days Carlos' fever was gone and he was developing a system to communicate with his family members through gestures and pictures.

CONCLUSION

Building on the use occupation as a common thread for any OT intervention, each of the practice frameworks or models provides a unique way to organize and think about information regarding the individual's function. In addition, each model guides the selection of treatment strategies appropriate for the specific needs of the individual. Finally, the use of practice models assists the COTA in looking beyond the obvious functional deficits, thereby ensuring a more holistic approach to care of complexities of an elder's life.

▌ CHAPTER REVIEW QUESTIONS

1 Explain the meaning of occupation and why this concept should be at the core of any occupational therapy intervention.

2 Describe at least two ways in which a practice model can help the certified occupational therapy assistant work with elders.

3 Explain why it is important to consider context in an elder's occupational performance.

4 Considering Llorens' developmental model, explain the social interaction needs an elder is likely to have when placed in a long-term care facility.

5 You have planned a task group for psychiatric clients during which you plan to carve pumpkins for Halloween. Using the Cognitive Disabilities Model, describe how you would modify the activity if the members of the group are functioning at a cognitive level 4.

6 Using the language of the Model of Human Occupation, explain how you would prioritize treatment for an elderly Native American elder who was admitted to the hospital after a car accident in which his wife and adult son died. He has severe fractures in all extremities, and there is the possibility of a mild head trauma. When you approach this gentleman, he refuses to speak and remains staring out the window.

REFERENCES

Allen, C. (1985). *Occupational therapy for psychiatric diseases: Measurement and management of cognitive disabilities.* Boston: Little, Brown, and Company.

Allen, C., Earhart. C. & Blue, T. (1992). *Occupational therapy treatment goals for the physically and cognitively disabled.* Rockville, MD: The American Occupational Therapy Association.

Allen, C., Earhart, C., & Blue, T. (1995). *Understanding cognitive performance modes.* Ormond Beach, FL: Allen Conferences.

American Occupational Therapy Association (1993). Position paper: purposeful activity. *American Journal of Occupational Therapy, 47,* 1081.

American Occupational Therapy Association (1994). Uniform terminology for occupational therapy—third edition. *American Journal of Occupational Therapy, 48,* 1047.

American Occupational Therapy Association (1995). The philosophical base of occupational therapy. *American Journal of Occupational Therapy, 49,* 1026.

American Occupational Therapy Association (2002). Occupational therapy practice framework: Domain and processes. *American Journal of Occupational Therapy, 56,* 609-639.

Fisher, G. (1999). *Assessment of motor and process skills* (3rd ed.). Ft. Collins, CO: Three Star Press.

Kalplan, K., & Kielhofner, G. (1989). *The occupational case analysis and interview and rating scale.* Thorofare, NJ: Slack.

Kielhofner, G. (1995). *A model of human occupation: Theory and application* (2nd ed.). Baltimore, MD: Williams & Wilkins.

Kielhofner, G. (2002). *A model of human occupation: Theory and application* (3rd ed.). Hagerstown, MD: Lippincott Williams & Wilkins.

Kielhofner, G., Mallison, T., Crawford, C., Nowak, M., Rigby, M., Henry, A., & Walens, D. (1997). *A user's guide to the Occupational Performance History Interview II (OPHI-II)* (version 2.0). Chicago, IL: Model of Human Occupation Clearinghouse, Department of Occupational Therapy, College of Applied Health Sciences, University of Illinois at Chicago.

Llorens, L. (1976). *Application of a developmental theory for health and rehabilitation.* Rockville, MD: The American Occupational Therapy Association.

Reilly, M. (1962). Occupational therapy can be one of the great ideas of 20th century medicine. *American Journal of Occupational Therapy, 16,* 1-9.

Salamy, M., Simon, S., & Kielhofner, G. (1993). *The assessment of communication and interaction skills* (research version). Chicago, IL: University of Illinois.

Watts, J., Hinson, R., Madigan, M., McGuigan, P., & Newman, S. (1999). The assessment of occupational functioning: Collaborative version. In B. Hempill-Pearson (Ed.), *Assessments in occupational therapy in mental health.* Thorofare, NJ: Slack.

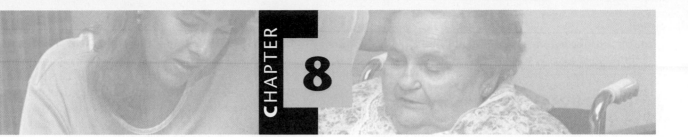

CHAPTER 8

Opportunities for Best Practice in Various Settings

SUE BYERS-CONNON AND STEVE PARK

KEY TERMS

client-centred practice, COTA/OTR partnership, occupational therapy practice framework, service competency, continued competency, underutilized, overutilized, geropsychiatric unit, inpatient rehabilitation, adult foster home, skilled nursing facility, assisted living, home health agency, community center, adult day care, emerging practice

CHAPTER OBJECTIVES

1. Illustrate certified occupational therapy assistant (COTA) practice in typical and emerging practice settings.
2. Become familiar with the occupational therapy practice framework.
3. Understand need for service competency and continued competency.
4. Appreciate the COTA/occupational therapist registered (OTR) partnership.
5. Value the importance of client-centred practice.

Occupational therapists and occupational therapy assistants assist individuals to link their ability to perform daily life activities with meaningful patterns of engagement in occupations that allow participation in desired roles and life situations in home, school, workplace, and community.

(American Occupational Therapy Association [AOTA], 2002a, p. 611)

Marta works with elders in a geropsychiatric unit, assisting elders and families to manage daily life activities at home. Arianna works with elders in an adult foster home, helping the elders to engage in leisure and social activities throughout their week. Rachel works in an inpatient rehabilitation unit, helping elders to regain their independence in basic activities of living daily. Jean works as a resident services coordinator at an assisted living facility, overseeing the quality delivery of resident services. Drew works with elders in a skilled nursing facility (SNF), facilitating their ability to participate in basic and instrumental daily activities and regain former roles. Amanda works for the local chapter of Parkinson's Society, leading movement groups for elders. Manisha works in home health, helping elders to engage in a routine of needed and desired daily life activities within their homes. Carlos works at an adult day care center, assisting elders to engage in a routine of productive and leisure activities and achieve life satisfaction.

The above certified occupational therapy assistants (COTAs) recently attended a reunion for all graduates from the Occupational Therapy Assistant (OTA) program at Blue Lake Community College, established 20 years ago. Of the 150 COTAs who attended, the majority work with elders in one capacity or another. Some work in more typical settings, such as an SNF or geropyschiatric unit, others work in emerging practice settings, such as adult foster homes and assisted living facilities. Despite working in different settings, the common thread is that the COTA is assisting elders to engage in daily *activities* and meaningful *occupations*. Although the settings differ, the focus and process of delivering occupational therapy (OT) services is similar.

This chapter addresses the role of COTAs, emphasizing the similar focus and process of OT service delivery with elders across different practice settings, using the Occupational Therapy Practice Framework (AOTA, 2002a) as a guide.* Other initial concepts presented are the importance of the COTA/occupational therapist registered (OTR) partnership, service competency, continued competency, and practice issues. A series of vignettes follow that illustrate best practice for COTAs and that describe their work with elders in specific settings.

OCCUPATIONAL THERAPY COLLABORATIVE PARTNERSHIPS

To support elders to achieve health, well-being, and life satisfaction through participation in meaningful activities, the COTA/OTR team provides valuable OT services. Even though OTRs assume responsibility for supervising COTAs, both should understand that the delivery of occupational services occurs collaboratively between the two partners (AOTA, 2002a). According to AOTA (2002b), supervision is defined as "a cooperative process in which two or more people participate in a joint effort to establish, maintain, and/or elevate a level of competence and performance" (p. 9). This supervisory relationship is necessary to both ensure the safe and effective delivery of OT services and foster the professional development of the COTA. OT service provision should be done in accordance with national and state regulations and laws (AOTA COP, 1998).

Together, the COTA/OTR partners should develop and document a supervisory plan that details how often they will meet, what type of supervision is applicable,

*Throughout this chapter, terms from the Occupational Therapy Practice Framework are identified in italics.

and what areas should be addressed. For example, a COTA/OTR team works in an SNF and meets once a week for an hour to review and discuss their client's concerns and status. In addition, they discuss specific ways to foster the COTA's professional expertise, such as developing advanced therapeutic skills when working with elders experiencing depression and better ways to incorporate the teaching–learning process when working with an elder's family members, significant others, and caregivers. In other settings, such as home health, the COTA and OTR meet face-to-face once a month for an hour; however, during the work week, they keep in frequent contact through telephone calls and electronic mail (e-mail) messages. Although these contacts focus primarily on clients, they also discuss areas for professional development. The frequency, methods, and focus of supervision varies according to the skills of the COTA and OTR, the needs and complexity of clients, and each setting's unique needs and requirements (AOTA, 2002b).

The COTA and OTR need to value the skills and knowledge each brings to the partnership, and the expertise of each partner should be used effectively (Black, 1996). A respectful relationship occurs when both partners communicate openly, trust each other, share their knowledge, and are willing to learn from each other. Sue, a COTA, worked at a rehabilitation unit for 3 years when Steve, an OTR and recent graduate, joined the team. Steve appreciated Sue's expertise to identify, plan, and adapt therapeutic activities related to elders' specific interests and needs, particularly leisure, household, and community activities. Sue appreciated the way Steve fostered her understanding of elders' specific health conditions and how to apply this knowledge during evaluation and intervention. Sue taught Steve new and different ways of engaging clients in activities while Steve modeled a **client-centred** approach when interacting with elders. Steve trusted Sue to carry out interventions and share her thoughts and professional opinion, and Sue felt comfortable asking Steve for supervision when needed. Both Sue and Steve were respectful of each other without it being a hierarchical relationship.

Establishing a strong collaborative **COTA/OTR partnership** is an ongoing process that requires active participation by both the COTA and OTR to identify the partnership's strengths and areas for improvement. To assist with the process, COTAs and OTRs should identify each other's competencies, as well as the common knowledge and skills they share. This requires a comprehensive understanding of the role and responsibilities of both COTAs and OTRs during the evaluation and intervention planning process. To understand this, the Occupational Therapy Practice Framework (AOTA, 2002a) and its relation to the COTA/OTR team process is presented in the following section.

OCCUPATIONAL THERAPY PRACTICE FRAMEWORK

...health is supported and maintained when individuals are able to engage in occupations and in activities that allow desired or needed participation in home, school, workplace, and community life situations.

(AOTA, 2002a, p. 611)

In 2002, AOTA introduced the *Occupational Therapy Practice Framework: Domain and Process*, a document designed to assist both OTRs and COTAs to more clearly affirm and articulate OT's unique focus on *occupation* and daily life *activities* and to illustrate an intervention process that facilitates clients' engagement in occupation to support their participation in life (AOTA, 2002a). Following is a brief overview of the two major areas of the document—(1) *Domain of Occupational Therapy* and (2) *Process of Occupational Therapy: Evaluation, Intervention, and Outcome*—that COTAs and OTRs should be familiar with when working with elders. Occupational therapy practitioners* are encouraged to obtain a copy of the *Occupational Therapy Practice Framework: Domain and Process* because the following sections only focus on highlights from the document.

Domain of Occupational Therapy

Occupational therapy practitioners assist people to engage in those everyday life *activities* that they find meaningful and purposeful, helping people to perform needed or desired activities (AOTA, 2002a). Through "improvement" in the performance of everyday life activities, people are better able to engage in meaningful *occupations* that influence their *health, well-being,* and *life satisfaction.*

When a person considers a particular everyday life *activity* as meaningful and purposeful, the specific activity is viewed as an *occupation* (AOTA, 2002a). Specific activities in which a person engages that possess central importance and meaning and from which a person derives a sense of competence, identity, accomplishment, satisfaction, or fulfillment, are considered *occupations* for that person (AOTA, 2002a). For example, an elder enjoys creating wooden toys in his workshop for his granddaughter, deriving pride in his skill as a craftsman and from the pleasure the toys bring to his granddaughter. For another elder, that same activity may not hold the same meaning. In fact, some elders may view making wooden toys as a chore or childish. If so, then making wooden toys would be considered merely an *activity*, one without the meaning that would make it a personal *occupation.*

---

*The term "occupational therapy practitioners" will be used to denoted both occupational therapists and occupational therapy assistants.

The distinction between *activities* and *occupations* is not always clear in everyday life, but occupational therapy practitioners recognize the value that *activities* and *occupations* both play during the process of OT (AOTA, 2002a). For elders, both *activities* and *occupations* need to be addressed during OT evaluation and intervention. If only an elder's *occupations* are considered during therapy, there may be important *activities* in the elder's life that are not adequately addressed. For example, when using the toilet, it may be important for an elder to assist to the best of his or her ability to reduce the physical and emotional stress on the caregiver. If an occupational therapy practitioner ignores toileting because the elder doesn't think it's important to become as independent as possible, then both the elder and the caregiver are at risk for physical injury and emotional distress. However, if an occupational therapy practitioner focuses solely on an elder's performance in *activities* and ignores the elder's engagement in meaningful *occupations*, an important contribution to the elder's health, well-being, and life satisfaction may be ignored. For example, focusing therapy on increasing an elder's independence in dressing when he or she does not find much personal meaning in this objective may not only damage the therapeutic relationship, but the occupational therapy practitioner may miss an opportunity to enhance the elder's health, well-being, and life satisfaction by assisting the elder to engage in *occupations* of meaning. Enhancing the elder's performance in *occupations* that have greater meaning to him or her, such as tending to tomato plants, walking his or her dog around the block twice a day, or washing the dishes after a meal his or her spouse has prepared, may be of greater benefit to the elder than achieving "independence" in dressing. The important aspect is that all *activities* and *occupations* addressed during OT intervention consider the *contexts* in which the elder lives, works, and plays.

With a primary focus on a person's engagement in everyday life activities and occupations, the framework outlines six major elements that constitute the primary domain of OT (Table 8-1). No one element is considered more important than the other. Occupational therapy practitioners need to consider all elements when focusing on the targeted outcome of OT intervention: a client's quality of *engagement* in occupation (AOTA, 2002a).

The first element, *Performance in Areas of Occupation*, identifies the primary categories of *occupations* that occupational therapy practitioners consider when working with individuals, groups, or populations (AOTA, 2002a). These categories represent the primary focus of OT: a person's *engagement* in activities of daily living (ADL), instrumental ADL, education, work, play, leisure, and social participation. Depending on the specific setting in which a COTA works, some areas may be emphasized

TABLE 8-1

Domain of Occupational Therapy

Performance in areas of occupation	Activities of daily living: basic or personal
	Instrumental activities of daily living
	Education
	Work
	Play
	Leisure
	Social participation
Performance skills	Motor skills
	Process skills
	Communication/interaction skills
Performance patterns	Habits
	Routines
	Roles
Context	Cultural
	Physical
	Social
	Personal
	Spiritual
	Temporal
	Virtual
Activity demands	Objects used and their properties
	Space demands
	Social demands
	Sequencing and timing
	Required actions
	Required body functions
	Required body structures
Client factors	Body functions
	Body structures

Based on data from American Occupational Therapy Association (AOTA). (2002). Occupational therapy practice framework: Domain and process. *American Journal of Occupational Therapy, 56*(6), 609-639.

more than others. For example, after an acute care hospitalization for pneumonia, it is important for elders to be able to manage their personal ADL when they return home. Although this may be a major area of concern for discharge, the framework prompts occupational therapy practitioners to also address other potential areas of concern to the elder, such as leisure activities and social participation, issues that may be equally important to an elder after discharge.

The second element, *Performance Skills*, identifies the small units of performance a person uses while performing everyday life *activities* and *occupations* (AOTA, 2002a). Occupational therapy practitioners use their observation skills to identify those *motor*, *process*, and *communication/interaction skills* that are effective or ineffective when

a person is performing everyday life *activities* and *occupations*. For example, a COTA and an elder are in a pharmacy where the COTA is primarily interested in the elder's communication/interaction skills while picking up a prescription. Throughout the process, the COTA observes the elder's skill to project his voice to the pharmacist behind the counter and effectively ask questions about a medication's side effects.

The third element, *Performance Patterns*, outlines the *habits*, *routines*, and *roles* adopted by persons as they carry out their daily life *activities* and *occupations* (AOTA, 2002a). An important element of OT is for clients not just being able to perform an activity once but being able to engage in a series of *activities* and *occupations* over time that sustains a person's health, well-being, and life satisfaction. For example, a COTA working with an elder experiencing mild memory loss might assist the elder to develop a consistent routine to safely prepare toast and coffee each morning. The fourth element, *Context*, refers to the varied conditions and surroundings under which people engage in *activities* and *occupations*. The performance of any one *activity* or *occupation* is influenced by the *cultural, physical, social, personal, spiritual, temporal,* and *virtual contexts* in which the *activity* or *occupation* is performed. For example, a cultural norm that a family values and follows forbids female individuals from providing personal, intimate care for male elders, such as bathing, toileting, or dressing.

The fifth element, *Activity Demands*, illustrates a key skill that occupational therapy practitioners possess: the ability to analyze activities. Each *activity* or *occupation* "possesses" specific demands—some activities require a large outdoor physical environment, such as a lawn to play croquet, whereas other activities require a relatively quiet indoor environment that promotes conversation, such as a living room where coffee and pastries can be served for church members. Furthermore, each activity will "demand" more or less of a specific *body function* or *structure*—some require more fine motor coordination, such as needlepoint, whereas others require greater strength, such as vacuuming. The sixth element, *Client Factors*, is based on the *World Health Organization International Classification of Functioning, Disability, and Health* (World Health Organization [WHO], 2001) and represents those physical, cognitive, and psychosocial factors (*body structures* and *functions*) that influence a person's ability to perform everyday life *activities* and *occupations* (AOTA, 2002a).

Process of Occupational Therapy: Evaluation, Intervention, and Outcome

Understanding the client as an occupational human being for whom access and participation in meaningful and productive activities is central to health and well-being is a perspective that is unique to occupational therapy.

(AOTA, 2002a, p. 613)

Occupational therapy practitioners view *occupation* as both the means and end of OT intervention. With this in mind, the process of service delivery begins with an evaluation of a client's *occupational* needs, problems, and concerns. It continues with an intervention process that emphasizes the therapeutic use of *occupations* and *activities*. The process ends with a review of *outcomes* to identify if the client's occupational needs, problems, and concerns were resolved over the course of OT intervention (AOTA, 2002a). The framework contains three major elements that represent the process of delivering OT services.

The first element, *Evaluation*, represents the first stage of the process and focuses on understanding what the client wants and needs to do with respect to everyday life *activities* and *occupations* and identifies factors that act as supports or barriers to the client's performance in *activities* and *occupations* (AOTA, 2002a). To do so, occupational therapy practitioners must consider those elements identified in the domain of OT—*performance skills, performance patterns, activity demands, contexts,* and *client factors*—and how they influence the performance of *activities* and *occupations* identified as concerns by the client.

The evaluation process is divided into two steps: (1) creating an *occupational profile* and (2) *analyzing occupational performance*. Using a client-centred approach, occupational therapy practitioners gather information to understand what is important and meaningful to a client and identify the client's goals and priorities that are important to him or her (AOTA, 2002a). The process of creating a client's *occupational profile* will vary depending on the client and the setting but the focus remains the same: What are the client's current and potential problems relative to engaging in *occupations* and everyday life *activities*? Information from the occupational profile guides the next stage in the evaluation process: *analysis of occupational performance*. Once a client's concerns are identified with respect to specific *occupations* and *activities*, occupational therapy practitioners conduct *performance analyses*. This involves observing clients engage in daily *activities* and *occupation* and requires an understanding of the complex and dynamic interaction between the specific *activities* and *occupations*, the client's *performance skills* and patterns, the *contexts* in which the *activities* and *occupations* need to occur, the *demands* of the activities and occupations, and *client factors*. To analyze a client's performance, specific *occupations* and *activities* (and the context in which they take place) are identified, and then the client is observed performing those activities and occupations. During this process, the occupational therapy practitioner notes the effectiveness of the client's *performance skills* and *patterns*. Then using other information gathered during the evaluation process, the occupational therapy practitioner interprets the data to identify what supports and/or hinders the client's performance. OTRs are ultimately responsible

for initiating and completing the intervention plan. COTAs, supervised by an OTR, assist during the evaluation process according to skill level and service competency (AOTA, 2002b) (Table 8-2).

The second element, *Intervention*, consists of three steps: (1) *developing the intervention plan*, (2) *implementing the plan*, and (3) *reviewing the intervention*. Although OTRs are ultimately responsible for developing the intervention plan, COTAs may assist with the plan's development (AOTA, 2002b). The intervention plan, developed in collaboration with clients, should create or promote, establish or restore, maintain, or modify clients' performance of everyday life *activities* and *occupations*. This is done to support engagement and participation in life or to prevent future problems with engagement in everyday *activities* and *occupations*, or both (AOTA, 2002a). Another essential element of the intervention plan is the collaboration between clients and occupational therapy practitioners to identify and set goals for intervention that focus on those activities and occupations that could "improve" or be "maintained" over the course of intervention.

Interventions are then implemented to address those *performance skills, patterns, contexts, activity demands,* and *client factors* that hinder the client's engagement in desired activities and occupations (AOTA, 2002a). Again, this is a collaborative process between clients and occupational therapy practitioners. This process focuses on facilitating a change in the *activity demands*, the *context, client factors*, and/or a client's *performance skills* and *patterns* that directly result in a client's improved or maintained performance of everyday life *activities* and *occupations*. Throughout *intervention implementation*, the process is monitored for its effectiveness and progress toward the identified goals and may be modified accordingly.

The final element, *Outcomes*, focuses on identifying the "success" of the intervention (AOTA, 2002a). Did intervention foster an "improvement" with a client's performance in desired and needed *activities* or *occupations*? Were future problems with a client's performance prevented? To do so, methods to evaluate *outcomes* should be used during the initial evaluation process and throughout intervention to identify what progress, if any, a client is making toward the goals and priorities identified at the beginning of OT intervention. As with evaluation and intervention, COTAs and OTRs work collaboratively to monitor intervention *outcomes*.

Certified Occupational Therapy Assistant/Occupation Therapist Registered Competencies with Evaluation, Intervention, and Outcome Process

All occupational therapy practitioners should be competent and provide intervention on the basis of current best practice. A unique aspect within the COTA/OTR partnership is the establishment of service competency for

TABLE 8-2

Certified Occupational Therapy Assistant/Occupational Therapist Registered Responsibilities During Process of Occupational Therapy Service Delivery

COTA	Framework	OTR
	Evaluation	
• Contributes to evaluation process	Occupational profile	• Responsible for evaluation process, coordinating with COTA
• Administers specific assessments after establishing service competency	Analysis of occupational performance	• Initiates and completes the evaluation
• Shares assessment information with OTR		• Interprets data with input from COTA
	Intervention	
• Provides input to intervention plan	Intervention plan	• Responsible for developing intervention plan collaboratively with clients and COTA
• Provides intervention appropriate to skill level and service competency	Intervention implementation	• Responsible for intervention, coordinating with COTA
• Provides information to assist with intervention review	Intervention review	• Responsible for intervention review, coordinating with COTA
	Outcomes	
• Understands client's targeted outcomes		• Responsible for selection and measurement of outcomes, coordinating with COTA
• Provides information to OTR related to outcome achievement		

Based on data from American Occupational Therapy Association (AOTA). (2002). Roles and responsibilities of the occupational therapist and the occupational therapy assistant during the delivery of occupational therapy services. *OT Practice*, 7(15), 9-10; and American Occupational Therapy Association Commission on Practice (AOTA COP). (1998). *Standards of practice for occupational therapy.* Bethesda, MD: The Association. COTA, certified occupational therapy assistant; OTR, occupational therapist.

COTAs. **Service competency** is the process by which COTAs collaborate with OTRs to demonstrate that they can perform tasks in a similar manner as the OTR and achieve the same results (AOTA, 1999). For example, to establish service competency, an OTR may observe a COTA administer the Canadian Occupational Performance Measure (COPM) (Law, et al., 1998) several times with different elders. If the COTA consistently administers the COPM according to the manual's instructions and the OTR concurs that the results are accurate with each administration, then the COTA has demonstrated service competency to perform this specific assessment. From then on, the COTA may independently perform the assessment (Black, 1996) and share the results with the OTR. In essence, with the establishment of service competency, less direct supervision is required. Documentation of service competency is recommended (AOTA, 2002b).

Demonstration of **continued competency** is a requirement of most regulatory boards, employers, accrediting bodies, and consumers (Stancliff, 1996). Establishing professional competency is ongoing and may involve various methods, such as pursuing continuing education, establishing a plan for professional development activities, engaging in a peer review process, and receiving on-the-job training. The knowledge and skills gained must be directly applicable to practice (Thomson, et al., 1995). For example, Rachel attended a workshop specifically for COTAs that focused on incorporating a neurodevelopmental approach when providing OT services for elders with strokes. After returning to the rehabilitation center, she directly applied the knowledge and skills from the workshop with elders who had experienced a stroke (see Chapter 19). One elder, Elmer, liked to restore vintage cars and Rachel asked his wife to bring one of their cars to the rehabilitation center. While Elmer polished the car, Rachel worked with him and his wife so that Elmer could learn how to incorporate more normal movement patterns and inhibit muscle tone.

When reentering the workforce or changing practice areas, the demonstration of continued competency is important (Stancliff, 1996). For example, Drew had worked in a school setting for 1 year. He always had an interest in working with elders and accepted a job offer from an SNF. Before he began work, he attended a workshop to become familiar with Medicare guidelines and the perspective payment system (see Chapter 6). He also attended a study group with three other COTAs who worked in SNFs, where they focused on specific skills, such as transfer techniques, use of adaptive equipment, and application of hip precautions during ADL. In doing this, Drew was actively demonstrating continued competence relevant to his new area of practice.

After COTAs work in the field for a time, the distance increases between the knowledge they learned in school and the current knowledge that should be used to ensure best practice (Reed, as cited in Stancliff, 1996). COTAs need to be responsible to the elders for whom they provide services and *continued competency* is a way that the public can determine if the COTA is aware of new intervention ideas and trends and not working solely from the information he or she received during his or her initial education (Reed, as cited in Stancliff, 1996).

After graduating from an accredited OTA program, graduates are initially certified by the National Board of Certification in Occupational Therapy (NBCOT). This initial certification is valid for 3 years (Truby LeGarde, personal communication, August, 2003). After 3 years, COTAs may choose to recertify and continue to use the letter "C" in their title (COTA), designating that they are certified by NBCOT. The recertification process requires participation in professional development activities, such as: (1) attending workshops and seminars, (2) participating in a mentoring relationship, (3) providing in-service training, (4) reading peer reviewed professional articles, (5) volunteering in community and professional organizations, and (6) supervising level II fieldwork students (NBCOT, 2002). Practitioners are also asked to complete a questionnaire related to illegal, unethical, and incompetent behaviors. The NBCOT initial and continuing certification program serves the public interest by "attempting to assure that occupational therapy practitioners engage in the safe, proficient, and competent practice of occupational therapy by meeting ethical and professional standards prior to entering the profession as well as on a continuing basis" (NBCOT, 2002, p. 10). State regulatory bodies and other agencies or associations may also require the demonstration of continued competency.

Issues related to certified occupational therapy assistant practice

Both overuse and underutilization of COTAs in the workplace may occur. COTAs may be underused when employers, as well as supervising OTRs, do not understand a COTA's degree of skill and knowledge. Restricting a COTA to tasks below his or her skill level, such as those performed by a restorative aide, does not allow COTAs to work to their greatest potential. Tasks such as transporting and scheduling patients, keeping inventory of bath equipment, and assisting patients to eat meals do not reflect the greater knowledge and skills that COTAs acquire during their education. COTAs are **underused** when they are not permitted to fully contribute throughout the entire spectrum of OT services. COTAs are qualified to gather initial information related to the elder's interests, values, needs, and patterns of daily living; to administer standardized assessments; to assist with planning intervention; to implement intervention; and to assist with monitoring outcomes under the general supervision of an OTR (AOTA COP, 1998).

Overuse may occur when COTAs are asked to contribute to the OT process in areas beyond the scope of their education and qualifications. Accepting referrals, conducting initial OT evaluations, and interpreting data are examples of tasks that are specifically designated for an OTR to complete (AOTA, 2002b; Black, 1996). In some instances, this may occur when COTAs are encouraged to take on tasks beyond the legal and ethical scope of practice. For example, an OTR may say "I don't have time to see the client. Why don't you start the initial evaluation?" In other instances, COTAs may be asked to perform these tasks when there is inadequate supervision or not enough practitioners to provide OT services (Black, 1996). For example, the facility administrator may ask the COTA to complete the discharge summaries because he or she only want to employ an OTR 4 hours a week. In these cases, the COTA needs to advocate for proper use of COTAs and discuss the issues with the OTR and others who need to understand the legal, ethical, and professional responsibilities of a COTA/OTR partnership.

CERTIFIED OCCUPATIONAL THERAPY ASSISTANTS WORKING WITH ELDERS IN VARIOUS SETTINGS

During the class reunion, Chris Henson, the OTA instructor for the adulthood and aging course, invited graduates to share their work experience with the OTA students during a series of class presentations. She was particularly interested in graduates who worked in both typical and emerging practice settings. A synopsis of each of the presentations is presented and integrates concepts from the Occupational Therapy Practice Framework (AOTA, 2002a).

Geropsychiatric Unit

Marta has worked at a 15-bed **geropsychiatric** unit in a small urban town for 7 years. She enjoys the challenges she faces everyday working with elders admitted with varied psychiatric diagnoses such as dementia, bipolar disorder, and schizophrenia. Although most elders are admitted from their homes, typically for behaviors with which their family members can no longer cope, such as aggression and confusion, Marta doesn't let these behaviors become the focus of her practice. Instead, she views each elder as a unique *occupational* being, focusing on those daily life *activities* and *occupations* of priority and concern to elders and their family members. Marta recently worked with one elder, José, a 62-year-old former migrant farm worker born and raised in Mexico who was admitted to the unit with suspected early-onset dementia. After she and Noel, the OTR with whom she collaborates, discussed the information from José's *occupational profile*, they realized that José no longer walked to and visited with friends within the local Hispanic community, one of his most meaningful *occupations*. José's family had become increasingly concerned about his memory loss and confusion and was afraid to let him leave the house for fear he would become lost or have an accident. Furthermore, they wanted to preserve José's dignity and did not want his friends and acquaintances to know about his increasing confusion and memory loss. Although José was admitted to the unit for suspected early-onset dementia, Marta viewed José as an *occupational* being who was experiencing the loss of meaningful *occupations*, rather than as a confused old man who was becoming a burden to his family.

With Marta's 9 years of experience as a COTA, the staff relies on her judgment to identify those daily *activities* and *occupations* in which elder patients can successfully engage and which aspects of their daily *routine* present additional challenges and require additional support and assistance. Marta said that the elders "often look okay and say that they don't have any problems but the reality is they get into trouble carrying out simple daily life tasks, if they chose to do them at all." To promote more successful engagement in routine activities, Marta relies on her skill to analyze an elder's performance of *activities* and *occupations*, identifying those factors that support or hinder the elder's successful engagement in *activities* and *occupations*. Although Noel works with the elders during the morning, Marta works from 2:30 to 8:00 PM during the week, providing her with opportunities to observe elders during their early evening routine of eating dinner, undressing, bathing, toileting, and preparing for bed. Marta acknowledges the importance of *performance patterns* to support successful engagement in activities and works closely with families and staff to establish consistent *routines* and *habits* for elders on the ward, focusing on creating a physical and social environment that promotes success and decreases confusion. With José, she and Noel worked closely with his family so they could create a *routine* of *activities* and meaningful *occupations* when he returned home to help reduce the confusion José was experiencing and his verbal outbursts.

Because Marta begins her workday at 2:30 PM and Noel ends his at 4:30 PM, they have little scheduled time for consultation and supervision. Both agree, though, that this time is essential, not only to meet regulatory statues in their state, but also to ensure that patients receive quality OT intervention. After her meeting with Noel, Marta leads group activities at 3:30 in the afternoon. Depending on the needs of the group of elders at any one time, Marta will lead groups that focus on life skills, such as task, craft, or cooking groups. Because of the elders' short stay on the unit, often less than 2 weeks, Marta finds that engaging them in activities that are familiar and not too challenging helps them to make sense of their daily life in the unit. Marta particularly enjoys leading the reminiscence group activity where she engages elders with the use of familiar scents, pictures, and objects, encouraging them to interact and share their personal stories (Fig. 8-1). The gardening group activity is particularly enjoyable because Marta can adjust the challenge of the activity to each elder's capability (Fig. 8-2). For those elders who may experience difficulty potting a plant on their own, Marta decreases the *activity demands*, such as asking an elder to help scoop dirt out of the bag or holding a pot while someone else scoops in the dirt. For others, merely sitting at the table and smelling the flowers is enough of a challenge. Those elders who are more able can choose what they would like to plant and carry out the process more independently, often sharing their own gardening expertise with Marta and other elders. No matter what capacity an elder may possess, Marta always ensures that all elders have a potted plant at the end of the group activity that they can give to a family member or friend during evening visits.

After leading groups in the afternoon and completing her notes on each elder's participation, Marta works with the unit staff during the evening dinner hour, observing

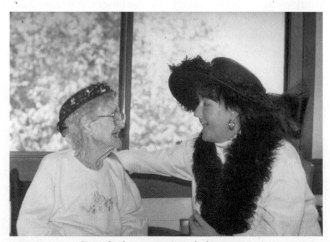

FIGURE 8-1 Certified occupational therapy assistants should actively participate in the activity along with elders.

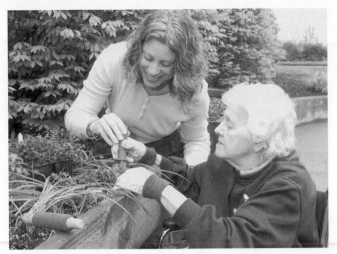

FIGURE 8-2   Certified occupational therapy assistants are skilled at ensuring all elders are able to participate in desired activities.

each elder's ability to eat meals. As Marta and Noel have determined that Marta has achieved service competency to manage eating and feeding problems with elders, Marta is responsible for identifying successful strategies to encourage elders to eat their meals and conveys those strategies to staff members for all meals and snacks. As needed, she will suggest and monitor the use of adaptive equipment. Although it can be quite challenging at times, Marta also works to create a pleasant and supportive environment during the dinner hour in which elders can successfully interact with family members when they chose to visit.

Because Marta works a later shift, she is responsible for meeting with family members and educating them not only about the elder's diagnosis, but about what level of care they currently require. She is particularly adept at identifying what aspects of activities each elder can do on his or her own and what aspects with which he or she requires assistance. Occasionally, family members may want to protect and help the elder too much and Marta works with them to preserve the elder's independence and dignity while teaching family members to provide the right amount of support.

Although Marta relies primarily on informal observation to gather important information about the elders, she occasionally administers the Allen Cognitive Level (ACL) screening tool (Allen, Earhart, & Blue, 1992) for which she has established service competency. She shares the results with Noel and together they interpret the results to share with other team members. This information is useful because it provides insight into an elder's cognitive abilities and his or her capacities in specific tasks or groups. Most of the time, though, Marta relies on her skills to analyze an elder's performance of activities

during groups and the evening routine. The information from these informal observations provides her with the valuable information that she needs to help the elders and their family members plan to return to their own homes.

Inpatient Rehabilitation

After graduating from Blue Lake Community College 5 years ago, Rachel moved to a large metropolitan city and began full-time work at an **inpatient rehabilitation** facility. She and Beth, the OTR with whom she works, share a caseload of 12 patients, the majority of whom are elders who have experienced a cerebrovascular accident (CVA). Rachel, who does not consider herself a "morning" person, nonetheless arrives at work Monday through Friday at 7:30 AM. She starts her day working with patients in their rooms, assisting them to achieve greater independence and satisfaction with their morning personal ADL, such as eating, grooming, dressing, toileting, and bathing (Fig. 8-3). One of her favorite elders was Glen, with whom she had worked after he had experienced a CVA. When Rachel was assisting Glen in the mornings to get ready for the day, Glen would become frustrated because he could never find his hearing aide. One day it would be in the drawer under his clothes and the next it would be under the bed sheets. Rachel communicated with the evening nursing staff to ensure that Glen always put his hearing aide in the top right drawer before he went to bed. Although this seemed like such a small thing to do, Glen was much happier each morning because he could easily locate his hearing aide. Rachel works extra hard to establish routines for elders on the ward, knowing that establishing

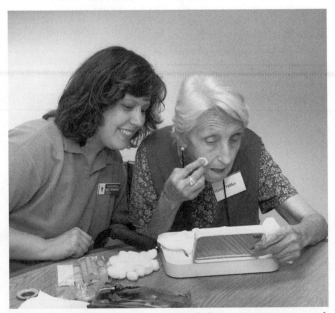

FIGURE 8-3   Certified occupational therapy assistants work with those personal activities of importance to the elder.

performance patterns is particularly important for elders when they are away from their usual home environment.

During the initial OT evaluation, Glen raised a concern that he did not want to be a burden on his wife when he returned home. During Glen's short 12-day admission, Rachel worked diligently to ensure that Glen's wife would be comfortable and safe assisting Glen at home. Thus, although "independence" with toileting, dressing, and bathing was not the ultimate goal, during Glen's morning routine Rachel and Beth focused on developing Glen's *performance skills* so it would easier for both Glen and his wife when Glen returned home. While Glen was not pulling up his pants on his own by discharge, Rachel had worked out a system whereby Glen was able to stand upright on his own and safely *stabilize* himself on a solid counter while his wife pulled up his pants and fastened them for him.

After morning ADL and during the remainder of the day, Rachel and Beth work together to help the elders reach their goals, collaborating to share the responsibility for gathering initial *evaluation* information, implementing *intervention*, and evaluating *outcomes* (Fig. 8-4). During her level II fieldwork, Rachel had observed her supervisor administer the COPM (Law et al., 1998), although Rachel had never done it herself. Because the COPM is an open-ended interview requiring the OT practitioner to solicit the *occupational performance* issues of concern to the client, Rachel and Beth developed a plan for Rachel to become comfortable and achieve service competency to administer the COPM and other standardized assessments.

When Rachel interviewed Glen using the COPM (Law et al., 1998), Glen identified that he still wanted to be able to take care of his 5-year-old grandson, Brandon, because Glen and his wife provide child care 3 days a week. As this was a priority for Glen, several OT sessions a week were devoted to help Glen develop the *performance skills*

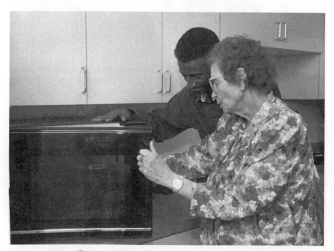

FIGURE 8-4 Instrumental activities of daily living are often important for elders for when they return home.

needed for Glen to play catch and read story books with Brandon. Rachel worked with Glen to develop the specific *motor skills* necessary to play catch, such as *bending* and *reaching* for a ball on the ground and *grasping* and *lifting* the ball with his affected arm and hand. Rachel also worked with Glen on skills necessary to read story books, such as *manipulating* the pages and *coordinating* his affected arm with his other arm to hold the book. On the basis of the *occupational profile* completed during the initial evaluation, Rachel knew that Glen enjoyed challenging physical activities because he considered himself a sportsman. She particularly enjoyed working with Glen to identify various physical activities, both within the OT department and outside the hospital, that would further develop his *motor* skills to help him reach his personal goals. Rachel was able to draw on Glen's strengths, specifically his relatively good *communication/interaction skills* (the skills to convey intentions and needs and coordinate social behavior) and *process skills* (the skills to organize actions to safely and effectively perform daily tasks), to help Glen improve his ability to perform daily life activities.

An important aspect of Rachel's work, although not her favorite, is documentation. To demonstrate the need for OT intervention, Rachel and Beth have worked together to develop their documentation skills. They have attended conferences and met with local insurance representatives to explain the focus of OT and to understand the insurance representative's point of view. Rachel and Beth share responsibility to write progress notes for their caseload. Although the OTR is responsible for documenting changes between initial evaluation and discharge (AOTA COP, 1998), Rachel contributes to the process, sharing her knowledge about patient *outcomes*. Because Beth and Rachel agree it is important that clients also express their views regarding their progress, Rachel often readministers the COPM (Law et al., 1998) with patients before discharge. Although Glen did not make much progress with his morning ADL in terms of physical independence, the use of the COPM revealed that he was more satisfied with his performance because he believed that he was no longer as much of a burden to his wife. Although he did not believe he was entirely able to take care of his grandson, he did believe he was far better than he was when first admitted to the rehabilitation unit. By using a standardized assessment such as the COPM, Rachel and Beth have more credible evidence to document an elder's progress and communicate the *outcomes* and benefit of OT services to help elders achieve their personal goals.

Adult Foster Home

After graduating 2 years ago, Arianna reflected about what aspects of OT practice she liked. She decided she liked working with elders and particularly enjoyed group activities. Arianna also realized that she preferred more nontraditional settings because she had the opportunity during her professional education to explore settings that were not typical of a medical model. During her course on adulthood and aging, she spent time at a local senior center where she helped with the local Arthritis Foundation program titled People With Arthritis Can Exercise (PACE) (Arthritis Foundation, 2003). This program combines exercise, joint protection techniques, and information about the pain cycle. Elders learn relaxation techniques and ways to incorporate joint protection within everyday tasks such as opening medications, cutting food, and taking care of indoor plants. Arianna also taught the elders about energy conservation and how to incorporate these principles into their daily routine.

Part of her level I fieldwork was spent at an assisted living center where she spent time running groups with the activity director. She was able to incorporate the skills and knowledge she learned in her OTA classes, such as designing and organizing groups, leadership strategies, group dynamics, and stages of group process, as well as meeting the individual needs of the group participants (Howe & Schwartzberg, 2001).

She noticed an **adult foster home** in her neighborhood and approached the owners, Elizabeth and Danny, about providing group activities for the elders. Arianna knew, per state regulations where she lived, that adult foster homes are required to provide 6 hours of activities a week for each resident, not including television and movies. Because the state requires the activities to be of interest and meet each elder's abilities, her COTA skills to identify, adapt, and implement appropriate activities for elders were exactly what the owners needed. Arianna talked about her experience working with elders and her abilities to develop and lead group activities. She explained to the owners that although she was a COTA, the services she would provide would not be considered OT. She would use expertise that did not require OTR supervision, such as making sure that elders were seated securely with their feet flat on the floor and using activities that incorporated full range of motion. Elizabeth and Danny were interested because they had been trying to provide activities without any outside help. After clarifying her intent with the state licensing board, Arianna began working, providing 2 half days of activity programming and consultation per week.

Most of the seven elders at the adult foster home were ambulatory; only one elder used a wheelchair. Anthony and Florence were legally blind, Maria had a severe hearing loss, Alfred used oxygen 24 hours a day for his chronic obstructive pulmonary disease, Herbert had Parkinson's disease, and Leona and Alfonso had dementia. Arianna met with each elder individually to get to know them and identify their activity interests. She used her COTA skills to develop an *occupational profile* that noted each elder's interests and dislikes, as well as information related to

medical needs, such as dietary restrictions, allergies, and "do not resuscitate" status. She also developed a form to document the type of group activity, the length of time each elder participated, the degree of participation, how each elder responded during the activity, and if he or she declined to participate that day. This form was left at the adult foster home at the end of the month for the owners and served the purpose of documenting participation, as well as serving as a time sheet for her hours worked. Elizabeth and Danny employed other people so a payroll tax system was in already place. Because her husband's employer provided health insurance coverage for spouses, Arianna was fortunate in not having to worry about this.

Arianna organized and implemented a variety of activities, following Howe and Schwartzberg's (2001) guidelines for group process, to provide a solid basis while designing each group activity. Arianna began each group with small talk, encouraging each resident to share talking about current events. Arianna would then incorporate warm-up activities to encourage movement, such as telling a story with the elders acting out the movements. Activities such as marching in a parade or playing balloon volleyball were popular with the elders. Then the main activities would occur, focusing on those activities of interest to the elders, such as preparing the salad for the evening meal, planting herbs in pots, making place mats for holiday meals, and learning new card games. Each group activity closed by asking the elders to plan the next activity.

As with well designed groups, the elders would often "direct" the activities themselves. For example, while making strawberry shortcake, Leona began reminiscing about growing up in an area where there were many berry farms (Fig. 8-5). She lamented that a community college and housing development now occupy the berry fields. Others joined in and talked about how they had to pick berries to earn money to buy their school clothes. Despite her significant memory loss, Leona shared her mother's favorite jam recipe and asked if the group could make the jam at the next meeting. During another activity, Florence shared how she used to enjoy playing Bingo but is currently not able to get out to games and cannot see the cards well enough to play. Arianna took note and another activity was designed where the elders made Bingo cards with large black numbers so that everyone could see and participate. Arianna also purchased poker chips to cover the numbers because Herbert had trouble picking up small discs. The elders' favorite activities, though, were ones that included cooking or baking. They took pride in preparing meals and inviting family members. Even Alfred, who "never cooked a meal in his life," participated and took pride in telling his daughter that he made the cornbread by himself (even though he did require some help!). The majority of time, Arianna planned activities for all residents to participate. She also made

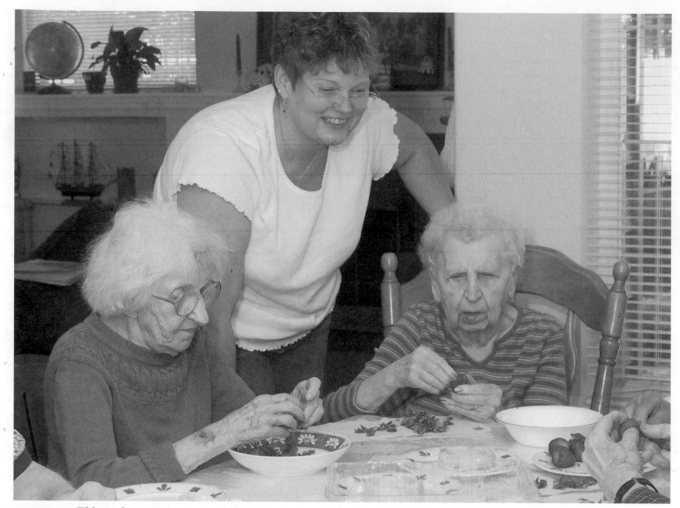

FIGURE 8-5   Elders play an important role in selecting activities that they enjoy and want to engage in.

sure that when an elder didn't want to participate in group activities, she would offer alternative one-on-one activities (Fig. 8-6).

Not all the activities were confined to the foster home. Danny and Elizabeth had a van and would occasionally take the elders to eat at local restaurants because they enjoyed getting out and eating their favorite foods. On those occasions when Arianna accompanied them, she sat close to Florence and Anthony, both legally blind, and suggested that they orient the food on their plate like a clock. Elizabeth took note and followed through with this suggestion at home with the elders. She reported that both Florence and Anthony were much happier with not needing someone to hover over them during meals. Arianna also suggested a weighted cup for Herbert and provided the phone number of a local vendor. As Arianna became more familiar with the residents, she suggested other community outings such as a trip to a lilac garden, a drive to see Christmas lights, a picnic in the park, and attending local music events at the senior center.

After working at the foster home for 3 months, Arianna expanded her services to other local adult foster homes. Danny and Elizabeth were happy with her services and passed along Arianna's business card to other adult foster home owners. She now provides group activities to five foster homes and hopes to find another COTA at the reunion who is interested in this work to expand the business.

Skilled Nursing Facility

After graduating 1 year ago, Drew moved to a rural city of 30,000 people and now works full-time at a **skilled nursing facility.** At the reunion, he shared that although he is frustrated with not being able to treat to his heart's content, he enjoys working with family members to help elders return home as soon as possible. He shared, "It's tough working toward discharge right away but then you realize most people's priorities are to get home as soon as they can." Drew primarily sees elders with CVA, as well as those with hip fractures and recent surgeries. Many have secondary complications, such as dementia, diabetes, and pneumonia.

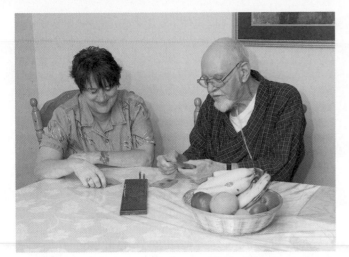

FIGURE 8-6 It is important for certified occupational therapy assistants to offer individual activities to meet each elder's needs.

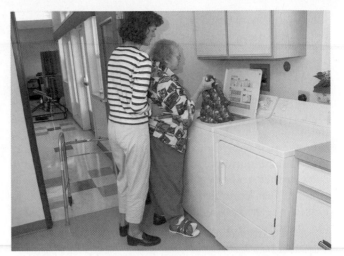

FIGURE 8-7 Certified occupational therapy assistants address the occupational roles, such as homemaker, of concern to each elder.

Drew particularly enjoys working with elders and their families to figure out the best way to manage *personal ADL* at home, including the need for adaptive equipment. One of the most problematic issues for elders leaving the SNF is toileting and bathing at home. Drew particularly prides himself on his ability to analyze each elder's performance of *personal ADL*. When observing an elder on the ward, Drew recognizes that the elder's home environment may be very different from the accessible and well-equipped rooms at the SNF. For example, he recently worked with Clarence, an elder who was admitted with a severe case of pneumonia and long-standing arthritis. Clarence and his wife were concerned about Clarence still being able to get in and out of his bathtub and soak in the warm water to relieve his arthritic pain. As best he could in the OT bathroom, Drew re-created the layout of Clarence's bathroom at home. He then observed Clarence's wife assisting Clarence to get in and out of the tub. After they tried out different methods, Drew identified the safest and least painful transfer method, and then had them practice until they felt confident. He also identified which specific equipment would best meet their needs at home. This was particularly important because many elders may not start home health immediately after discharge from the SNF and all necessary equipment needs to be in place before their departure.

Although a main focus of the SNF is promoting independence with ADL, Drew also addresses other *occupational roles* that are important to the elder (Fig. 8-7). As Clarence was a retired veterinary technician, he was also concerned that he could not take care of his many birds at home. Drew worked with Clarence and his wife to figure how Clarence could safely stand and easily reach while feeding and watering the birds and cleaning the cages. Drew also arranged with the staff for Clarence to play with the

resident dog and cat as often as possible when he was not in therapy. As Clarence also sang in the church choir, Drew worked with Clarence and his wife to develop a plan so that Clarence could conserve enough energy to attend church twice a week.

In addition to his direct work with the elders, Drew has additional responsibilities. He participates in the weekly team meetings, sharing the reporting responsibilities with Sheryl. Drew and Sheryl also collaborate to leave clear instructions for Brooke, the COTA who works on the weekend. Drew spends part of his time working with restorative aides, ensuring that they can follow through with intervention plans. Drew and Sheryl agree that he would assume primary responsibility to be aware of current regulatory and reimbursement issues related to SNF (see Chapter 6) and share the information with Sheryl.

Assisted Living Facility

Jean has been a COTA for 17 years. After graduating, she took a job at a local rehabilitation hospital and worked mainly with adults who had neurologic disorders. She enjoyed the work, but because of budgetary problems, her position was eliminated. She then worked at a long-term care facility where her level of responsibilities increased over time. Having established service competency with the OT evaluation and intervention methods used at the facility, she worked fairly autonomously with occasional OTR supervision. Four years ago, Jean returned to school on a part-time basis to complete her Bachelor's degree in health care administration. As Jean was learning management skills, she decided to apply for a position as the director of the OT department. Given her competency as a COTA and her current interest and skills in management, she was offered the position. Jean was now responsible for running the department, including scheduling therapy, coordinating the training and supervision of the employees, and maintaining communication between OT and the other services offered at the facility.

After graduation and the completion of her business degree, she began to seriously consider her future. She surveyed her life's interests and found that she enjoyed the interactions with elders and their families. She also enjoyed the management skills that she had learned and developed over the past few years as OT director. She was not sure that remaining in her current position would allow her to grow further so she began looking at other possibilities.

First, Jean compiled a list of her strengths and weaknesses. She tried to be as realistic as possible and asked for assistance from her husband, her parents, and her friends who knew her professionally. She felt that she had good supervisory, interpersonal, verbal, and written communication skills. Finally, she was familiar with health care and rehabilitation in particular. However, some of her weaknesses were that she had limited experience in marketing, operations management beyond the occupational therapy department, and budgeting.

At first, Jean looked for jobs related to OT, rehabilitation, and health care delivery and was discouraged by what she had found. Then, she expanded her search after talking with her neighbor about her mother, who was living in an assisted living complex. Jean searched the Internet for information about **assisted living** and contacted one assisted living community's corporate office and inquired about the positions that were available in her area. She learned that there were three categories of positions: activities coordinator, executive administrator, and resident services coordinator. She requested that job descriptions for each category be mailed to her.

When the three job descriptions arrived, Jean was ready to compare them with her personal analysis of her skills. The first job description that Jean reviewed was for Activities Coordinator (Table 8-3). Jean believed that this job was not challenging enough. She also knew that

according to state regulations, if there was a perception that she was providing direct OT services, she would need to have an OTR provide supervision. Besides, she felt that this was not the type of job that interested her enough to leave her current position at the long-term care facility.

The next position that she reviewed was for Executive Administrator (Table 8-4). Jean compared the job expectations with her strengths and weaknesses and realized that she was lacking in several categories. Although she has had experience at managing a small department, she lacked the marketing, budgeting, and operational management background required for this position.

The final job description Jean reviewed was for a Services Coordinator (Table 8-5). Jean studied the job description and compared it with her strengths and weaknesses. Because she believed that this was the right position, Jean contacted the assisted living organization and requested an application. She applied and was contacted for an interview. Before the interview, Jean wanted to clarify that the services she provided in this position were not those of a COTA requiring OTR supervision. She contacted her state's OT licensure board and asked them to review the job description. On careful review, the Board determined the following: (1) her status as a COTA in this position did not violate state laws and regulations; (2) although the position oversaw the coordination of programs, including OT, it did not require Jean to perform hands-on OT; and (3) Jean could use her COTA initials after her name as long as it was understood that she could not provide any OT services without the supervision of an OTR.

Meanwhile, Jean prepared for the interview by identifying the major points she wanted to emphasize. First, she wanted to stress the importance of addressing the elders' needs, including physical, social, emotional, cognitive, and spiritual, and how this belief would guide staff recruitment and development. Second, she wanted to demonstrate how she would coordinate the services

TABLE 8-3

Activities Coordinator Job Description	
Job position:	Activities Coordinator
Primary purpose:	This person is responsible for the development and coordination of individual activity programming for each resident. Responsibilities include planning and coordinating appropriate resident activities, day-to-day operations, supervising staff, and ensuring program quality.
Qualifications/skills needed:	Prefer an individual with a minimum of 2 years geriatric experience. Experience working with people with Alzheimer's disease/dementia is essential. Experience in staffing and managing the day-to-day operations is preferred. Must demonstrate good interpersonal skills and excellent written and verbal communication. Reports to resident services coordinator.

TABLE 8-4

Executive Administrator Job Description

Job position:	Executive Administrator
Primary purpose:	This person is responsible for the creation of resident-focused work teams that support the philosophy of partnering with families. Responsibilities include staffing, training, program implementation, budgeting, sales, marketing, and community relations.
Qualifications/skills needed:	Prior experience managing senior resident services is required along with a Bachelor's degree. Experience in marketing, operations management, and budgeting is essential. Strong leadership skills, including organization and interpersonal skills, are a must. Excellent verbal and written communication skills required, as well as computer experience. Occasional travel required.

in a manner that supported the assisted living organization's philosophy of partnering with families. Third, she wanted to show that her background as a COTA brought a unique perspective on quality of life for elders. She located information from the OT literature that identified that life satisfaction is multifaceted for elders (McPhee & Johnson, 2000) and that the manner in which elders occupy their time contributes to their health, well-being, and quality of life.

During the interview, Jean did well and was offered the position. Since then, she has been working with the new executive administrator, assisting her to recruit and develop resident service teams. One of the first tasks she undertook was to develop a screening tool to identify the physical, social, emotional, cognitive, and spiritual needs of the residents. Her goal was to match the services with the identified needs and eventually demonstrate how the residents' overall needs were being met.

Home Health Agency

Manisha recently changed jobs after working 9 years in an acute care hospital when she obtained a job at a **home health agency** within a major metropolitan city.

Because Manisha only used public transportation before this job, she needed to purchase her first car, one that was spacious enough to carry needed equipment and supplies. Furthermore, Manisha needed to brush up on her map reading skills because her new supervisor emphasized that she would be traveling extensively, often up to 80 miles a day. Because this agency recently converted to a computer-based documentation system, Manisha signed up for a computer course at a local community college. An important issue emphasized during her interview was client confidentiality. Although Manisha was aware of this issue from her work in acute care, Manisha would be visiting many elders during the day, carrying the required documentation from house to house, and would need to take extra care to ensure that that information was kept confidential during her visits.

During her first few weeks on the job she traveled with different team members, including nurses, physical therapists and physical therapist assistants, social workers, nutritionists, and home health aides. During these visits, Manisha was surprised by how different things were in the elder's home environment than what she "imagined" when she worked in acute care. Sometimes, solutions

TABLE 8-5

Resident Services Coordinator Job Description

Job position:	Resident Services Coordinator
Primary purpose:	This person is responsible for overseeing the delivery of resident services and supervising the resident assistant staff. As a member of the management team, responsibilities include supervising unit teams, staff development, monitoring quality of resident service and staff recruitment. Reports to executive administrator.
Qualifications/skills needed:	Person should possess a Bachelor's degree in a health-related field. Five years experience in senior resident services, including staff supervision, is required. Excellent organizational and interpersonal skills are a must. Strong verbal and written communication skills are essential. Computer proficiency is strongly preferred.

that were proposed in the hospital (similar to those proposed by Manisha when she worked there) turned out to be impractical or the elders just did not want to do them. Recognizing this, Manisha was excited to be working with elders in their own homes where she could assist them to achieve their goals within their familiar home environment, focusing on practical solutions in *context* (Fig. 8-8). Manisha looked forward to working with elders and their caregivers to achieve their goals, such as getting out in the back garden on their own, emptying the trash, getting the mail, operating the radio, or using the telephone to reorder prescription medications.

One elder, Irene, had lived by herself in a one-room apartment and was getting along fairly well despite her legal blindness. Irene recently broke her foot while getting off a high stool in her kitchen. After receiving the doctor's referral, Antonio, the OTR with whom Manisha worked, completed the initial evaluation. Antonio shared the initial evaluation results with Manisha and developed the intervention plan with Manisha, stressing that Manisha's input was important to monitor the effectiveness of the plan. Manisha then assumed primary responsibility for implementing the intervention plan and monitoring the achievement of outcomes. Although Manisha would be

visiting Irene on her own over the next month, Manisha would consult as needed with Antonio when they were both in the office in the morning. Furthermore, she frequently communicated with him, as well as with Irene's social worker and physical therapist, via cell phone calls throughout the day.

One of Irene's first priorities was to prepare her own meals rather than rely on the Meals on Wheels initially organized by the social worker. Although it was important to Irene that she prepare her own meals, she did not want to spend a lot of time doing so. After Manisha's first visit, Irene searched for recipes that would be easy to prepare and nutritious and arranged for her neighbor to purchase the necessary ingredients. During the next visit, Manisha and Irene problem solved how to safely prepare simple meals that would not compromise her fractured foot, such as safely using a low chair and safely maneuvering within the kitchen. To make it easier to transport items, Manisha also arranged for Irene to purchase a basket for her walker and to practice safely carrying her recycling items and trash down the hallway.

Because Irene was a volunteer at the blind commission, it was important for her to be able to use public transportation as soon as possible to return to her monthly meetings. Although Irene's home visits would end as soon as she became more mobile, she and Manisha problem solved how best to manage her walker while using the bus. They practiced skills such as managing doors, stepping up and down different levels while using the walker, and folding up her walker once she was seated. Another priority of Irene's was to plan and be able to execute an emergency exit from her third-floor apartment. She and Manisha developed a plan with Irene's neighbors to deal with different types of emergencies. For some situations, a buddy system would be used; for other situations, Irene could make the necessary arrangements through the telephone.

Because Irene's broken foot presented additional challenges to safely maneuver within her apartment, Manisha and she worked together to rearrange her living and dining room to make it easier and safer for her to listen to the radio and books on tape, as well as use her computer. Although Manisha works most of the time with individual elders, such as Irene, on occasion she is called in to an adult foster home to provide environmental recommendations. For example, she has recommended suitable bath and toilet equipment and more appropriate furniture arrangement to prevent falls.

Manisha enjoys working in home health because it provides a lot of variety. She visits four to five people a day, the majority of whom are elders. Because she visits elders in their own home, Manisha is particularly sensitive to being a guest, respecting the elders' privacy and following their lead to establish intervention priorities. This includes collaborating with elders and their families/caregivers as to the best approach to achieve their

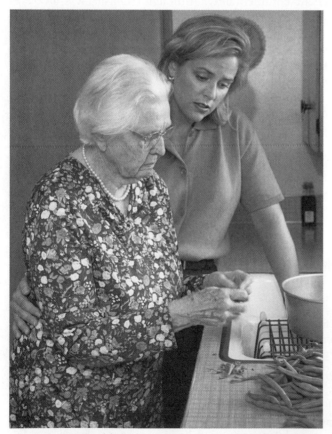

FIGURE 8-8   An elder's home provides many opportunities to work on practical solutions.

priorities. Many times this involves working closely with family members to provide education and training, emphasizing safety for not only the elders but also for the caregiver (see Chapter 11). Because Manisha is skilled with body mechanics and safety concerns/issues, she is responsible for home health aide staff training, providing them with information and skills to safely assist elders (e.g., while toileting, dressing, and bathing).

One of the most important skills that Manisha brings to this particular job is that of observation. Because the discharge summary is completed by the OTR, Manisha must provide accurate information because she has been the primary OT practitioner working with the elder. Often, detailed information is required per regulatory and facility guidelines. In Irene's case, to complete the discharge summary, Manisha needed to provide information to Antonio, not only on Irene's ADL status, but also on such factors as Irene's ability to accurately express herself, if any sanitation hazards were present in the home, which social supports she consistently relied on, and if she was capable of making safe decisions.

Community Center

Amanda graduated from the sixth OTA class at Blue Lake Community College. Her children, who were toddlers when she was in school, are now teenagers. After practicing in a variety of settings, she found it difficult to find a job that allowed her to be at home when her teenage children returned from school. Amanda found a job working for a small airline that offered her benefits and hours that fit her schedule. She enjoys watching her children play sports and volunteers once a week in her daughter's classroom.

Although she did not practice as a COTA for a number of years, to maintain her license Amanda attended continuing education courses, one of which focused on leading movement groups for persons with Parkinson's disease. This course opened up a whole new career for her. She now leads movement groups for persons with Parkinson's disease at the local **community center**. These classes are based on the premise that to deal with difficulties that stem from the loss of automatic movements, individuals need to learn to move and speak consciously (Argue, 2000). "The goal of the program is to develop a mental ability through actions and exercises that individuals do *with* their body while they are also training their minds" (p. 16). The participants develop coping strategies to speak in an artful way, one that is *mindful, graceful,* and *complete* (Argue, 2000). During group, participants repeat their mistakes in slow motion, which then helps them to figure out the right way to move. This helps them to be more *graceful* in their movements. Self-awareness and self-control are also emphasized, teaching the participants to become *mindful* of what they are doing at the time that they are doing it. To be *complete,* the participants are taught that each movement

has a beginning, middle, and end, and they should finish one action before moving on to the next (Argue, 2000).

During the class, the elders start out with warm-up stretching exercises and then move into exercises for strength and balance incorporating some Tai Chi T–stance movements. A tennis ball is used for hand exercises, and Amanda uses her creative abilities and ideas to keep the program diverse and interesting. Many symptoms associated with Parkinson's disease are addressed through exercise, including stiffness, slow movement, tremors, balance problems, difficulty walking, and speaking (Argue, 2000). During the cool-down time, speech and voice exercises are emphasized. After participating in the program, many elders report positive benefits. Irene is pleased that she now can get in and out of the church pew without pulling it over. Arthur is back on the golf course. Francisco, who could only do five 4-point push-ups, is up to 10 regular "guy" push-ups on his toes. Leanore is quick to point out that she no longer uses her cane when she walks on flat surfaces, and Edwardo, who previously fell at least once a month, has not fallen in the past 4 months.

Amanda has met other group facilitators, including a nurse practitioner, physical therapist, aerobics instructor, and personal trainer. They get together once a month for dinner and share new activities that they are incorporating into their exercise programs. They recently discussed how this program fits in with *Healthy People 2010: Understanding and Improving Health* (U.S. Department of Health and Human Services, 2000). This program emphasizes the importance of health promotion, disease prevention, and the rights of all individuals to have access to services, including those with disabilities. Although Amanda does not use the initials COTA after her name, she uses her COTA skills on a regular basis. Amanda uses her knowledge of human movement and performance of activities to help the elders to move in an *artful* manner and carry this ability into their daily activities, such as brushing their hair, washing dishes, and moving about in the community. She is able to safely transfer the elders to and from the floor using proper body mechanics. While observing the elders, her knowledge of fine and gross motor movements and upper body tension enable her to adjust the program to meet their individual needs. She is able to challenge the elders to reach their movement potential and adjust the *activity demands* for each individual elder. Amanda stated, "I am still making a positive difference in people's lives. I previously did not feel I had a lot to offer persons with Parkinson's disease beyond providing adaptive equipment and a home exercise program." The elders look forward to attending and enjoy the socialization aspect of belonging to a group. At times it is like a support group; the elders encourage each other and discuss problems they are having with their ADL. Amanda stated, "This is a perfect time for me to suggest they ask their physician for a referral to occupational therapy or to see a physical therapist."

117

Adult Day Care

Carlos works at an **adult day care** center in an urban setting. This particular setting not only has a day care center but has a continuum of care that includes assisted living, independent apartment living, and adult foster homes. The elders attend day care 5 days a week from 9:00 AM until 3:00 PM, receiving lunch, health services, and activities in which to participate. Carlos has a dual role within this setting. His primary role is similar to that of an activities director in that he identifies and plans individual and group activities for participants throughout the week. In his other role, he works with Sydney, an OTR, in providing OT services.

Carlos, who graduated 4 years ago, starts off his day by attending a team meeting. At this center, the bus drivers, the chaplain, the custodial staff representative, and home health aides attend, as well as the more typical team members, such as nurses, social workers, physicians, and physical therapy and OT practitioners. Everyone contributes during the team meetings. Recently, the bus driver reported that Mrs. Chang experiences shortness of breath while getting on the bus, and a home health aide shared the progress that Millie has made with feeding her cat by herself.

After the team meeting, Carlos works one-on-one with elders throughout most of the day. Because his primary responsibility is that of activity programming, Carlos discusses with each elder, and if possible, the family, to determine which *activities* and *occupations* would be most appropriate for the elder to engage in while at the center. For example, Carlos met with Mr. Kirov, a new participant, who identified that he enjoyed using his hands to make things and that he liked to talk with people. From this, Carlos recommended that he participate in the many craft activities offered at the center and those activities that included discussion, such as current events and reminiscence. To address *occupational problems* and initiate OT intervention, Sydney meets with each elder to identify his or her specific occupational needs. In Mr. Kirov's case, Sydney conducted an initial evaluation because he had recently fractured his humerus and was having difficulty performing activities with only one arm and hand. As a result, specific OT intervention was initiated to address his problems with performing activities.

Throughout the week Carlos divides his time; he provides one-on-one occupational therapy intervention under the supervision of the OTR, and designs and implements group activities for the participants. Because social participation is a key area of *occupation* that is integral to an elder's *health* and *well-being* (Fig. 8-9), Carlos uses his COTA background to plan and implement groups to ensure that the elders engage in social activities that they enjoy and find meaningful. One of the most popular groups is the "Helping Hands" group. The theme of this group is to provide the elders with a sense of contribution to the community. In the past, they have put together gift baskets for migrant workers, solicited personal samples for military personnel, read to preschool children, and stuffed envelopes for a local school board election. Carlos enjoys this group because he knows that elders enjoy engaging in altruistic activities in which they help other people. Other groups that Carlos plans and implements throughout the week are gardening, music, reminiscence, movement, and crafts. In addition, Carlos makes an extra effort to contact family members to discuss options for activities at home in which the elders can successfully participate and enjoy.

During one-on-one OT intervention, Carlos addresses specific concerns with performance of daily living *activities* and *occupations*. Recently, Carlos worked with Mrs. Chang after she began experiencing increased breathlessness caused by her chronic bronchitis. Mrs. Chang's family reported that during the weekends she wanted to help her daughter and son-in-law with household chores and would push herself too far and become breathless. Because Mrs. Chang valued her *occupational* role as a family member, Carlos worked with her and her family to identify which activities she considered important and which activities her family felt comfortable allowing her to do. Carlos then worked with Mrs. Chang and her family to develop a routine, incorporating energy conservation techniques that would allow her to complete activities without becoming breathless and tired. Within a month, Mrs. Chang's family reported that she was helping with household chores without getting tired and breathless. More importantly, she was extremely happy to be able to make a valuable contribution to the family and felt that her *health*, *well-being*, and *life satisfaction* was better than before.

CONCLUSION

Over the next three to four decades, the population of elders will increase significantly and the number of those

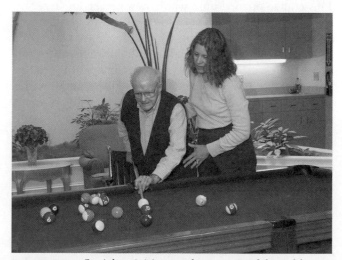

FIGURE 8-9 Social activities can be meaningful to elders and facilitate their health and well-being.

with disabilities will increase sharply (Administration on Aging, 2003). Although it is impossible to predict future health conditions of elders and the degree to which those conditions will affect their ability to engage in self-care and productive and leisure activities, current trends suggest that COTAs will have the opportunity to work with elders in both typical and emerging practice settings. Focusing on *occupations* and *daily life activities* that are meaningful to elders, COTAs provide a valuable contribution during the delivery of OT services.

After the series of presentations at Blue Lake Community College, the OTA students were excited and enthused about the variety of opportunities waiting for them after graduation. Their instructor, Chris Henson, emphasized that their unique COTA skills and knowledge prepared them to work with elders in typical settings such as SNFs, rehabilitation centers, geropsychiatric units, and home health. She went on to say that the job opportunities did not stop there. As Arianna, Jean, and Amanda had demonstrated, they used their COTA background to create new job opportunities in **emerging practice** areas. Chris Henson concluded that Carlos, who worked in adult day care, was a good example of a COTA who works in collaboration with an OTR to provide OT services but also can use his COTA background to assist elders in engaging in meaningful activities that do not require the direct supervision of an OTR. In all cases, whether in typical or emerging practice settings, the Blue Lake Community College graduates were engaged in opportunities that brought satisfaction to themselves and quality services for elders.

■ CHAPTER REVIEW QUESTIONS

1 Discuss service competency and continued competency for COTAs and ways to establish each.
2 A COTA and OTR work together in a rehabilitation setting and have different ideas regarding intervention for elders. Suggest three ways they can learn from each other and form a collaborative partnership.
3 A COTA who is a new graduate and an OTR who recently moved from another state are working to develop a supervision plan. Locate three resources to assist them, develop this plan, and explain what information they would seek from each resource.
4 Identify three activities that you consider meaningful (an occupation) and identify three that you consider "merely" an activity. Explain the differences.
5 Explain why it is important to focus on both occupations and activities to enhance an elder's health, well-being, and life satisfaction.
6 Why should COTAs consider the caregiver/significant other/spouse when collaborating to develop an intervention plan for an elder?

7 Three COTAs have been hired to work in an SNF. One is a new graduate, one has 5 years of experience working in a rehabilitation setting, and one previously worked in an outpatient adolescent psychiatric unit. Develop a continued competency for each COTA.
8 Identify five skills COTAs receive in their education that would be helpful to secure a position in an emerging practice setting.

REFERENCES

Administration on Aging (AoA). (2002). *A profile of older Americans: 2002* [WWW page]. URL www.aoa.gov

Allen, C., Earhart, C., & Blue, T. (1992). *Occupational therapy treatment goals for the physically and cognitively disabled.* Rockville, MD: American Occupational Therapy Association.

American Occupational Therapy Association (AOTA). (1999). Guide for the supervision of occupational therapy personnel in the delivery of occupational therapy services. *American Journal of Occupational Therapy, 53*, 592-594.

American Occupational Therapy Association (AOTA). (2002a). Occupational therapy practice framework: Domain and process. *American Journal of Occupational Therapy, 56*(6), 609-639.

American Occupational Therapy Association (AOTA). (2002b). Roles and responsibilities of the occupational therapist and the occupational therapy assistant during the delivery of occupational therapy services. *OT Practice, 7*(15), 9-10.

American Occupational Therapy Association Commission on Practice (AOTA COP). (1998). *Standards of practice for occupational therapy.* Bethesda, MD: The Association.

Argue, J. (2000). *Parkinson's disease and the art of moving.* Oakland, CA: New Harbor Publications.

Arthritis Foundation. (2003). People with arthritis can exercise (PACE) [WWW page]. URL http://www.arthritis.org/communities/chapters/grtrchicago/programlists/pace.asp

Black, T. (1996). COTAs and OTRs as partners and teams. *OT Practice, 1*(3), 42-47.

Howe, M. C., & Schwartzberg, S. L. (2001). *A functional approach to group work in occupational therapy* (3rd ed.). Baltimore, MD: Lippincott Williams & Wilkins.

Law, M., Baptiste, S., Carswell, A., McColl, M., Polatajko, H., & Pollock, N. (1998). *Canadian occupational performance measure* (3rd ed.). Toronto, Ontario, Canada: Canadian Association of Occupational Therapists.

McPhee, S. D., & Johnson, T. (2000). Program planning for an assisted living community. *Occupational Therapy and Health Care, 12*(2/3), 1-18.

National Board for Certification in Occupational Therapy (NBCOT). (2002). *Certification renewal handbook.* Gaithersburg, MD: Author.

Stancliff, B. L. (1996). Demonstrating continued competency. *OT Practice, 1*(9), 49-52.

Thomson, L., Lieberman, D., Murphy, R., Wendt, E., Poole, J., & Hertfelder, S. (1995). *Developing, maintaining, and updating competency in occupational therapy: A guide to self-appraisal.* Bethesda, MD: American Occupational Therapy Association.

U.S. Department of Health and Human Services (US DHHS). (2000). *Healthy People 2010: Understanding and improving health* [WWW page]. Washington, DC: US Government Printing Office. URL www.health.gov/healthypeople

World Health Organization. (2001). *International classification of functioning, disability and health* (ICF). Geneva, Switzerland: Author.

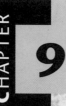

Cultural Diversity of the Aging Population

RENÉ PADILLA AND LINDA A. WALKER

KEY TERMS

diversity, culture, values, beliefs, race, sex, age, ethnicity, sexual orientation, religion, ethnocentrism, assimilation, performance context, melting pot, conformity, bias, prejudice, discrimination, minority, homosexual, cognitive style, associative, abstractive, truth, equality

CHAPTER OBJECTIVES

1. Explain the meaning of "diversity" and related terms.
2. Explore personal experiences, beliefs, values, and attitudes regarding diversity.
3. Discuss the need to accept the uniqueness of each individual and the importance of being sensitive to

issues of diversity in the practice of occupational therapy with elders.
4. Present strategies to facilitate interaction with elders of diverse backgrounds.

Today is Susan's first day at her first job as a certified occupational therapy assistant (COTA). She has been hired to work as a member of the rehabilitation team in a small nursing home in the town where she grew up. Susan is excited because this job will permit her to stay close to her family and work with elders. When she arrives at the nursing home she and the occupational therapist (OTR) discuss the elders who are participating in the rehabilitation program. Susan is told about Mr. Chu, a Chinese gentleman who experienced a stroke and often refuses to get out of bed, and Mrs. Pardo, a Filipino woman who is constantly surrounded by family

and consequently cannot get anything accomplished. The OTR also tells Susan about Mr. Cooper, an elderly man dying of acquired immunodeficiency disorder (AIDS); Mrs. Blanche, a retired university professor who is a quadriplegic; and Mr. Perez, who was a migrant farm worker until the accidental amputation of his left arm 4 weeks previously. Susan notes the distinct qualities of each of these elders.

OVERVIEW OF CULTURAL DIVERSITY

The cultural **diversity** of clients adds an exciting and challenging element to the practice of occupational therapy (OT). Each client comes from a **culture** with a unique blend of **values** and **beliefs.** This uniqueness affects all aspects of the client's life, including the occupational dimension. The ways in which a person chooses to do a task, interacts with family members, moves about in a community, looks to the future, and views health are in many ways the result of past experiences and the expectations of the people with whom that person comes in contact. Consequently, COTAs have to deal with many issues that arise from interactions with persons unlike themselves in terms of **race, sex, age, ethnicity, physical ability, sexual orientation,** family composition, place of birth, **religion,** level of education, and work experience (including retirement status) or professional status, among other factors (Johnson, 2001; Loden & Rosener, 1991) (Fig. 9-1).

Culture, **ethnocentrism, assimilation,** and diversity are discussed to provide a framework for working with elders in a sensitive manner. This chapter includes general guidelines for assessment and treatment. The challenge for COTAs is to contribute to the creation of a therapeutic environment in which diversity and difference are valued and in which elders can work to reach their goals.

WHAT IS CULTURE?

The concept of culture has long been considered important in the practice of OT. For example, the official definition of OT for licensure states, "Occupational therapy is the use of purposeful activity with individuals who are limited by physical injury or illness, psychosocial dysfunction, developmental or learning disabilities, poverty and **cultural differences**, or the aging process in order to maximize independence, prevent disability and maintain health" (American Occupational Therapy Association [AOTA], 1981, p 789). Likewise, the Standards for an

Accredited Education Program for the Occupational Therapists (AOTA, 1998), the Code of Ethics (AOTA, 2000), and the Occupational Therapy Practice Framework: Domain and Process (AOTA, 2002) all support the consideration of culture in treatment. However, the term *culture* has not been clearly defined or described in OT professional literature and has not been consistently considered in the assessment and treatment process (Bonder, Martin, & Miracle, 2002; Hasselkus & Rosa, 1997; Krefting & Krefting, 1991; Loveland, 2001). Part of the reason for this lapse may be the breadth of complex concepts encompassed by this one term. The Occupational Therapy Practice Framework (AOTA, 2002) identifies culture among the **contexts** that influence performance skills and performance patterns (observable behaviors of occupations). Culture is listed with physical, social, personal, spiritual, temporal, and virtual factors that also influence occupation. The Occupational Therapy Practice Framework describes culture as "Customs, beliefs, activity patterns, behavior standards, and expectations accepted by the society of which the individual is a member. Includes political aspects, such as laws that affect access to resources and affirm personal rights. Also includes opportunities for education, employment, and economic support" (AOTA, 2002, p. 1054). The Occupational Therapy Practice Framework describes culture as existing "outside of the person but is internalized by the person, also sets expectations, beliefs, and customs that can affect how and when services may be delivered" (AOTA, 2002). Kielhofner (2002) also offered a broad perspective when he defined culture as the beliefs and perceptions, values and norms, customs and behaviors that are shared by a group or society and are passed from one generation to the next through both formal and informal education (Fig. 9-2).

This broad and consequently vague definition of culture is not unique to the OT profession. Entire books in other fields are devoted to describing culture, and authors have been unable to agree on a single definition. Most include concepts relating to observable patterns of behavior and rules that govern that behavior. They also emphasize the conscious and subconscious nature of culture in the way it is dynamically shared among people. Some of the commonalties in those definitions, including that culture is learned and shared with others, may be used as a basis for an understanding of culture (Benedict, 1989; Hasselkus & Rosa, 1997).

Culture is learned or acquired through socialization (Fig. 9-3). Culture is not carried in a person's genetic make-up; rather, it is learned over the course of a lifetime. Obviously, then, the environment in which each person lives is central to his or her culture. A person's environment may demand or offer opportunities for some types of behaviors and restrict opportunities for other types. For example, individuals in the United States are offered

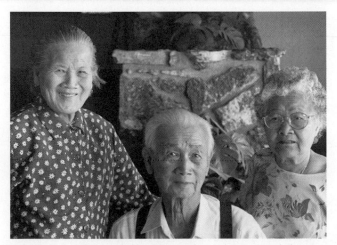

FIGURE **9-1** Cultural diversity makes occupational therapy practice exciting and challenging.

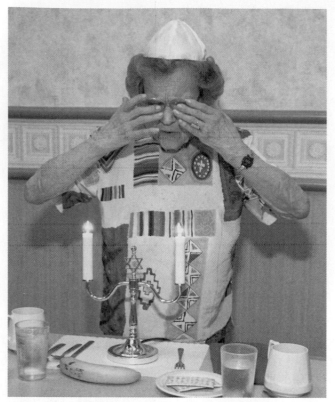

FIGURE 9-2 This Jewish elder practices a religious observance passed down from generation to generation.

the opportunity to choose the color of their clothing, but generally wearing dresses is culturally restricted to females. In the United States, persons are generally expected to drive on the right side of the street, pay taxes, and arrive at work according to schedule. Through interaction with the environment, individuals learn a variety

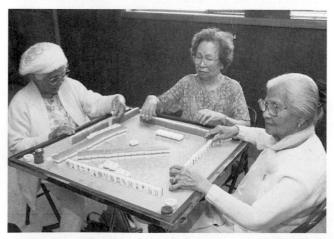

FIGURE 9-3 This group of elders enjoys a culturally shared game.

of values and beliefs and eventually internalize them. Internalized values direct the interactions among people and with the environment. As a result, people assume that others have internalized the same values and beliefs and consequently behave in the same ways (Bohannan & van der Elst, 1998; Hall, 1981). However, culture is the result of each person's unique experiences with his or her environment, and thus is an ongoing learning process.

Another commonality in the various definitions of culture is that because it is learned from others, it is also shared. What is shared as culture, however, is very dynamic. Because culture is learned throughout one's lifetime, each person learns it at a different point. On the basis of each person's status in learning culture, the person expects something from others and contributes to others' cultural education. In this way, each person learns and teaches something about culture that is unique. Over time, shared beliefs and values change. These changes in cultural beliefs and values may not be easily observed because the actual behaviors that express them seem to remain the same. However, over time, a periodic recommitment to the dynamic transmittal of beliefs and values has occurred (Baumeister, 1991). For example, the attire of women in some regions of the Arabian Peninsula has changed very little in the past 200 years. Originally the black gowns, robes, and veils were probably intended to guard the woman's modesty. Many women who wear these garments today, in addition to guarding modesty, do so as a symbol of resistance to westernization, a concern that was probably not common 200 years ago (Harris, 1989; Ross, 1993).

Finally, culture is often subconscious (Harris, 1998; Lemet, 2002; Peacock, 2002). Because learning of culture occurs formally and informally, a person is not usually aware, particularly at a young age, of learning it. Instead the person simply complies with the demands and restrictions of behavior set in particular environments and chooses behaviors from among those that are allowed. For example, when a child is not permitted to touch a frog found by a pond during a family outing, that child is being formally taught that frogs are dirty and therefore should not be touched, a value the child might internalize and then generalize to other animals. This value is informally reinforced when the child sees other people wince and make gestures of repulsion when they see certain types of animals. When the child sees a younger sibling attempting to touch a frog, the child might tell the sibling not to do so because touching it is "bad." In effect, the child internalized a value received from the culture of his or her family and passed it on to a sibling with the slight reinterpretation that it is "bad" to do the particular behavior. In a similar way all persons continue to learn culture from each physical and social environment in which they participate. When elders enter a nursing home for a short-term or long-term stay, for example, some of the facility's rules of behavior are formally explained whereas others are implied, including meal times (and consequently when elders *must* eat), visiting hours (and consequently when elders *must* and *must not* socialize), visiting room regulations (and consequently *where* and *how* elders may socialize), and "lights out" time (and consequently when elders *must* sleep). Elders also informally learn an entirely different set of rules. As they experience the daily routine in the nursing home they also learn whether it is acceptable to question the professionals who work there, to decline participation in scheduled group activities, and even to express their thoughts, feelings, desires, and concerns. Staff members have likely not formally stated, "You are not permitted to state your feelings here." However, this value may be communicated informally by staff members if they cut off conversation when an elder begins to explain feelings or simply never take time to invite an expression of the elder's feelings. In this way values and beliefs become sets of unspoken, implicit, and underlying assumptions that guide interactions with others and the environment.

Culture is a set of beliefs and values that a particular group of people share and re-create constantly through interaction with each other and their environments. These beliefs and values may be conscious or unconscious, and they direct the opportunities, demands, and behavior restrictions that exist for members of a particular group. Essentially every belief and value that humans acquire as members of society can be included in their culture, thus explaining the broadness of the concept of culture. Therefore, the beliefs and values on which we form our own understanding of elders' behaviors and the rules for these behaviors have also been socially constructed and form part of our own culture.

LEVELS OF CULTURE

Various levels exist at which values and beliefs are shared. Hasselkus and Rosa (1997) proposed that a multidimensional view of culture be adopted. In this view, culture can be defined in terms of the individual, the family, the community, and the region (Fig. 9-4). At the individual level are the relational, one-to-one interactions through which people learn and express their unique representations of culture. Examples of this level of culture are each person's use of humor, definition of personal space, coping style, and role choices. Included at the level of the family are beliefs and values that are shared within a primary social group—the group in which most of the person's early socialization takes place. This level includes issues such as gender roles, family composition, and style of worship. Each family can be seen as a variation of the culture that is shared at the level of a community or neighborhood, in which economic factors, ethnicity, housing, and other factors may be considered. Communities may be seen as variations in the culture that

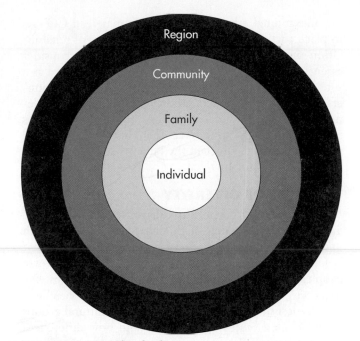

FIGURE **9-4**   Levels of culture.

is shared with a larger region, such as language, geography, and industry. Hasselkus and Rosa (1997) also noted that variation exists at each level and within each group.

Adopting a more relational framework helps overcome some of the difficulties inherent in viewing culture as synonymous with ethnicity. Ethnicity is the part of a person's identity that is derived from membership in a racial, religious, national, or linguistic group (Padilla, 2000). The viewing of culture as synonymous with ethnicity relies on generalizations about the people who belong to a particular group and can lead to mistaken assumptions about an individual's personality and beliefs. For example, the assumption that all persons of Hispanic ethnicity have brown skin and black hair is not true, because Hispanics of all racial backgrounds exist. Equally, people cannot assume that all white individuals are educated, that all Jews observe kosher practices, or that everyone who speaks English attaches the same meaning to the word "gay."

Equating ethnicity with culture can lead to many misinterpretations. In addition, this practice is often used to justify superiority of one group over another. The term *ethnocentricity* describes the belief held by members of a particular ethnic group that their expression of beliefs and values is superior to that of others, and consequently that all other groups should aspire to adopt their beliefs and values. In extreme cases of ethnocentricity, a particular ethnic group has attempted to destroy other ethnic groups, as in (Nazi) Germany, Bosnia, and the Sudan. Ethnocentrism can be and often is an underlying, subconscious belief that powerfully guides a person's behavior.

An unexamined ethnocentric attitude may lead COTAs to place particular emphasis on certain areas of rehabilitation and disregard others that elders may consider essential for their recovery. OT itself can be viewed as a subculture with beliefs and values that guide practitioners toward independence, productivity, leisure, purposeful activity, and individuality. This bias may sometimes lead practitioners to ignore the client's wishes and impose their own values in the belief that they are more important and worthwhile.

THE ISSUE OF DIVERSITY

The variety of clients that Susan, the COTA introduced at the beginning of this chapter, will work with underscores a well known fact about the United States: it is a country of immigrants, a conglomeration of diverse peoples. How is it possible that all these groups live together? The metaphor of the "melting pot" has been used to describe the way in which distinct cultural groups in the United States "melt down" and how differences between groups that were once separate entities disappear. This process is the result of the continuous exposure of groups to one another (Barresi, 1990; Bucher, 2000). Fry (1990) describes a process of **conformity** in which an individual or a cultural group forsakes values, beliefs, and customs to eliminate differences with another culture. In the United States, conformity may be demonstrated by people who Americanize their names, speak only English, abandon religious practices or social rituals, shed their ethnic dress, attend night school, and work hard to take part in the "American dream." Both conformity and the melting pot metaphor imply that new ethnic groups entering the United States will be judged by the degree to which their differences with the values and beliefs of the established American culture disappear. Some people accept the pressure to abandon their cultural identity as an inevitable or even desirable fact of life, whereas others avoid it at all costs (Bucher, 2000). This expectation can easily create **bias, prejudice,** and **discrimination** toward many individuals. The term **minority** is an outgrowth of these views. This term is used to designate not only smaller groups but also groups that have less power and representation within an established culture despite their size.

The realization that some differences such as age, race, sex, and sexual orientation can never be eliminated, even with effort and education, has led many people to discern that they should also value the characteristics that make them unique, such as their cultural heritage and their religious practices (Fig. 9-5). Cultural pluralism is a value system that recognizes this desire and focuses not on assimilation but on accepting and celebrating the differences that exist among people. Persons who value cultural pluralism believe that these differences add richness to a society rather than detract from it.

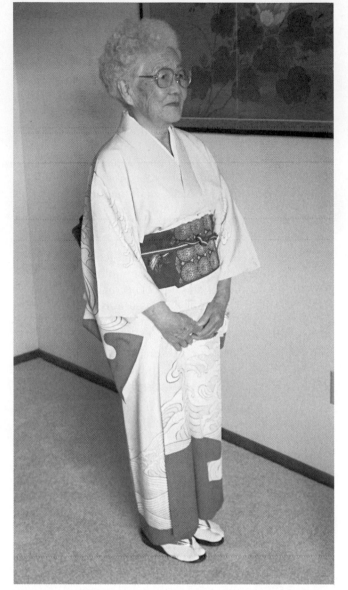

FIGURE 9-5   Maintaining one's cultural dress may be important for some elders.

Valuing Diversity

People in the United States are clearly diverse. Diversity is demonstrated through race, sex, age, ethnicity, sexual orientation, family composition, place of birth, religion, and level of education; in addition, people also differ from each other in physical ability or disability, intelligence, socioeconomic class, physical beauty, and personality type. In essence, any dimension of life can create identity groups or cohorts that may or may not be visible. Most people find that several of these dimensions have particular meaning for them.

Ironically, diversity becomes an inclusive concept when we view it as that which makes us different from each other. This view of diversity embraces everyone, because each person is in some way different from everyone else. At the same time, however, each person in some way is also similar to someone else. This viewpoint provides a framework for approaching the diversity that one encounters when working with elders: COTAs can recognize the ways in which they are both different from and similar to elders. These differences and similarities can be used during therapy to enrich the elder's life. A welcome side effect of this approach is that the COTA's life often is enriched as well.

Diversity of the Aged Population

A summary of statistical reports on the elder population is presented in Chapter 1. Each of these reports is an example of diversity. The following facts should also be taken into account when considering diversity among the rapidly growing elder population.

Persons older than 65 years represent 12.4% of the U.S. population, or about 35 million people. In 2000, 16% of elders belonged to minority populations, and this number is expected to increase to 25% by the year 2030. The number of elders in minority groups is expected to grow by 32.8% between 1990 and 2030 (American Association of Retired Persons [AARP], 1995). A growth of 81% is expected in the white non-Hispanic elder population in that same period. The growth among Hispanic elders is projected to be the largest (328%), followed by Asian and Pacific Islander elders (285%), American Indian, Eskimo, and Aleut elders (147%), and African American elders (131%) (Administration on Aging [AOA], 2002). A breakdown of the U.S. racial and ethnic population is provided in Figure 9-6. Notably, these figures represent only the numbers of elders who belong to broad categories, not cultural distinctiveness. Each of the categories listed may include numerous cultures and subcultures. These numbers are used here simply to emphasize that the population served by OT practitioners will increasingly include elders from diverse backgrounds.

No reliable figures are available regarding the sexual preference of persons in the United States who are 65 years or older. Janus and Janus (1994) estimated that 4% of men and 2% of women in the general population are exclusively **homosexual.** The figures are greater when bisexual orientation and frequency of homosexual experience are considered. Combining these figures provides the more accurate estimate that 9% of men and 5% of women may be considered homosexual (Laumann & Michael, 2000; Rosenfeld, 1999). Studies suggest that these figures are consistent for elders older than 65 years (Dorfman & Walters, 1995; Horowitz & Newcomb, 2001; Quam & Whitford, 1992). If this is true, approximately 2.3 million elders are homosexual (Fig. 9-7).

The United States is one of the most diverse countries in the world in terms of religious affiliation. Approximately 89% of people in the United States claim to have a definite

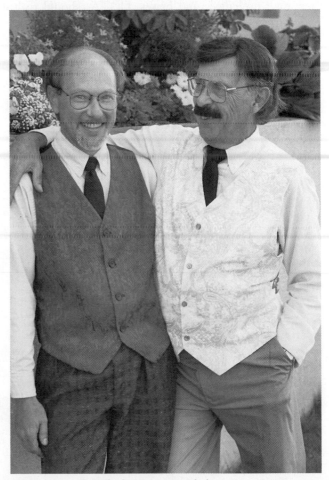

FIGURE **9-7** Certified occupational therapy assistants must be sensitive to the diversity of sex and age of life partners.

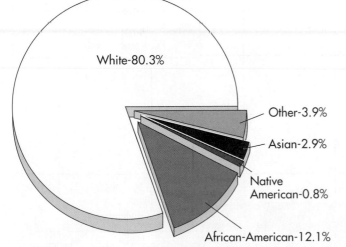

White-80.3%

Other-3.9%

Asian-2.9%

Native American-0.8%

African-American-12.1%

FIGURE **9-6** Breakdown of general population by race and ethnic origin. (Data compiled from Internet releases of the Census 2000 data by the Administration on Aging, U.S. Department of Health and Human Services.)

religious preference (Parker, 1997). The trend toward increased religious diversity is fueled both by conversion and immigration. Since 1957, the Christian population (i.e., Catholics and Protestants) in the United States has decreased from 92% to 81% of the total population, whereas the number of practitioners of other religions, including Buddhism, Hinduism, and Islam, has increased from 1% to 6%. Information on the distribution of faiths of the general U.S. population is provided in Figure 9-8.

In 2002, 10.1% of the elderly population, or 3.4 million persons, lived below the poverty line and another 6.5%, or 2.2 million elderly, were classified as "near-poor" (income between the poverty level and 125% of this level). These data are quite different when minority groups are considered individually. For example, 21.9% of elderly African Americans and 21.8% of elderly Hispanics were impoverished. More than half (50.5%, which is the highest poverty rate) of older Hispanic women who lived alone or with nonrelatives experienced poverty (AOA, 2002) (Fig. 9-9).

Sensitivity to Culture and Diversity in Treatment

To be culturally sensitive, people must acknowledge their own prejudices and biases. COTAs should realize

that prejudices are learned behaviors and can be unlearned through increased contact with and understanding of people of diverse cultural groups. Furthermore, communication always takes place between individuals, not cultures. Gropper (1996) suggests that in the clinical encounter the cultures of both the client and the clinician play important roles in successful outcomes. Groper wrote that misunderstandings and miscommunication between clients and clinicians usually result from cultural differences, and that the clinician's responsibility is to adapt to the client's culture rather than demanding that the client adapt to the clinician's culture. Kohls and Knight (1994) propose that in addition to the cultures of the client and the clinician, the culture of the institution in which the interaction takes place in many ways directs interaction between the client and clinician. In health care, institutional culture has strongly valued the biomedical approach to treatment, which places the control of health care with the physician rather than with the client. In addition, the U.S. medical system has placed little emphasis on the development of specific programs to address the needs of elders from culturally diverse groups.

Culture and diversity are extremely broad and complex concepts. Attempts to make generalizations about

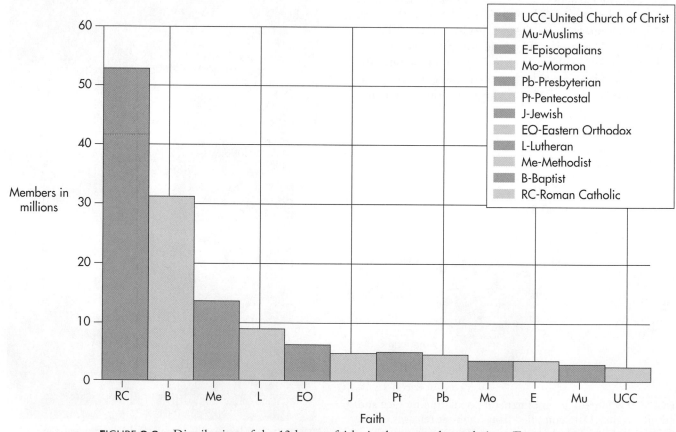

FIGURE 9-8   Distribution of the 12 largest faiths in the general population. (From *Health sciences library desk reference*. (1996). Omaha, NE: Creighton University.)

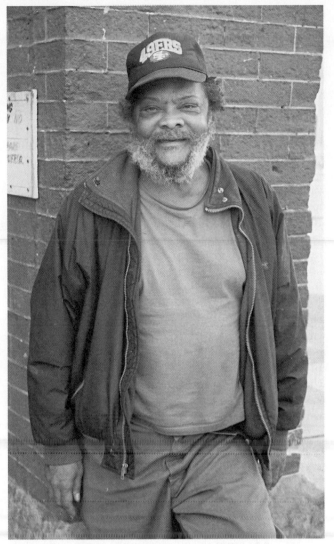

FIGURE 9-9 Approximately 10.1% of the elderly population, or 3.4 million people, live below the poverty line, and another 6.5%, or 2.2 million elderly people, are classified as "near-poor." This 72-year-old man has been in and out of homeless shelters for the past 15 years.

various groups would be useless because COTAs are certain to come across elders who do not fit into the expected behavior. Few persons are perfect representations of their culture. Generalizations may also limit the COTA's ability to see each client as a unique individual. Consequently, COTAs should be cognizant of general issues about culture that should be assessed and remembered at every step of the OT program. COTAs must realize that cultural sensitivity is an ongoing process. In addition, COTAs should not assume that by following the guidelines presented in the following sections, they have done everything necessary to provide culturally appropriate OT services. The COTA's responsibility is to develop ongoing strategies that allow the client to

maintain personal integrity and be treated with respect as an individual.

The two most important strategies COTAs can use are asking questions and observing behavior carefully. The values and beliefs that encompass "culture" direct elders in their particular way of performing activities of daily living (ADL) functions and work and leisure occupations. Consequently, COTAs must be oriented to the elder's culture to provide relevant and meaningful treatment. This cultural orientation should include an understanding of the following: (1) the cognitive style of the elder, (2) what he or she accepts as evidence, and (3) the value system that forms the basis of the elder's behavior. A fourth and final area of understanding has to do with communication style. If elders are unable to answer questions regarding these areas for themselves, COTAs should attempt to obtain this information from the elder's family or friends. If this is not an option, the COTA should obtain information about the elder's culture from other sources, such as a coworker who is of the same national origin as the elder and library materials. However, COTAs should remember that the more removed the information source is from the elder, the less likely that the information will apply to that particular elder.

Let us return briefly to Susan, the COTA starting a new job who was introduced at the beginning of this chapter. One of the elders with whom Susan would be working was Mr. Chu, a Chinese gentleman who refused to get out of bed. The OTR informed Susan that soon after Mr. Chu's admission several of the elders who had Alzheimer's disease and were disoriented had become agitated in Mr. Chu's presence because they associated him with World War II experiences. The nursing home staff did not want Mr. Chu to be offended by this behavior, so they moved him to a private room. When Susan entered Mr. Chu's room she said, "Hello! I'm from occupational therapy and I'm here to help you get out of bed and do your ADL." As anticipated, he signaled his refusal to cooperate by turning his head and closing his eyes. He remained silent whenever Susan spoke to him. When she attempted to put her hand behind his shoulder to help him sit up, he grabbed her wrist and pushed her arm away. Susan was perplexed. She called Jon, a therapist of Japanese descent whom she had met at an orientation session a week earlier, and asked him to provide any insight into Mr. Chu's behavior. Jon told Susan that in general Asians are very circumspect, preferring to be with members of their own group, and that Mr. Chu was probably reacting to Susan not being Asian. Jon suggested that a family member be called in to enlist Mr. Chu's cooperation. Susan contacted Mr. Chu's son, Edwin, who met her later that afternoon at Mr. Chu's bedside. After some discussion with his father, Edwin informed Susan that Mr. Chu refused to get out of bed because he believed he had been placed in a private room to isolate him because he was Chinese. He viewed being informed about OT intervention plans as further evidence that he was being treated differently. Susan explained the staff's concern that Mr. Chu would be offended by the comments and behavior of the other elders. Mr. Chu said he understood that such behavior was part of an illness. Susan facilitated Mr. Chu's move to a room with three other elders, and he began to participate daily in the OT program. Susan was careful to ask Mr. Chu what he wanted to accomplish in each session. Jon's report about Asians wanting to be with members of their own group was only partially true. Mr. Chu wished to be with other elders, not specifically other Chinese people. Susan was able to discover this only with the help of someone very familiar with Mr. Chu.

Cognitive Style

COTAs need to understand how elders organize information. This process does not refer to an assessment of cognitive functions that indicate the presence or absence of brain dysfunction (Allen, 1985; Allen, Earhart, & Blue, 1992). Rather, cognitive style refers to the types of information a person ignores and accepts in everyday life. Because cognitive style is the result of habits, it tends to be automatic or subconscious. Studies of cognitive style suggest that people vary along a continuum of open-mindedness or closed-mindedness, and that cultural patterns are reflected in these styles (Hofstede, 2003). Depending on the situation, people may vary along this continuum, and no one is likely to always operate from one of the poles. Open-minded persons seek out additional information before making decisions and tend to admit that they do not have all the answers and need to learn more before reaching proper conclusions. Open-minded persons usually ask many questions, want to hear about alternatives, and often ask COTAs to make personal recommendations regarding alternatives. Closed-minded individuals, however, see only a narrow range of data and ignore additional information. These persons usually take this approach because they function under strict sets of rules about behavior. For example, a devout Hindu elder would likely be appalled at being served beef at a meal and would not be willing to consider the potential nutritional benefits of this meal. Similarly, the dietitian who offers this meal to a Hindu elder may do so on the basis of a closed-minded cognitive style, assuming that beef is the ideal and only source of the particular nutrients the elder needs. Both persons are functioning under rules of behavior, with the Hindu elder's rules dictated by religious practice and the dietitian's rules dictated by professional training. Other examples of a closed-minded cognitive style include the female elder who refuses to work with a male COTA during dressing training because she believes this is not proper, and the explosive retired executive who bellows that he does not wish

to walk with a cane despite safety concerns. Both these people have attended to only part of the data available—that is, the data contrary to the rules of behavior under which they function. Their cognitive styles have limited their abilities to consider the benefits of the alternatives. Studies show that most cultures produce closed-minded citizens (Hofstede, 2003).

Another aspect of cognitive style is the way in which people process information, which can be divided into **associative** and **abstractive** processing styles. As with open-mindedness and closed-mindedness, people may vary along this continuum, and no one is likely to always operate from one of the styles. People who think associatively filter new data through the screen of personal experience—that is, these people tend to understand new information only in terms of similar past experiences. Conversely, abstractive thinkers deal with new information through imagination or by considering hypothetical situations. An example of an associative thinker is an elder who has had a stroke and wants the COTA to provide him with a set of weights because using weights was how he increased upper extremity strength when he was younger. An example of an abstractive thinker is an elderly woman who asks the COTA to write down the principles of joint protection and is able to apply that information to all situations in which she may find herself. When approaching an associative thinker with a new task, COTAs should point out the ways in which it is similar to other tasks the elder has accomplished. Often elders who are associative thinkers need one or more demonstrations of the task and do best with small incremental increases in task complexity. Alternately, when approaching an abstractive thinker with a new task, COTAs should emphasize the desired outcome and permit the elder to think of ways in which to reach the goal. For example, when teaching an elder who thinks associatively to transfer to the toilet, COTAs should point out the ways in which this transfer is similar to the transfer of getting to the wheelchair from the bed. When teaching the elder who thinks abstractly to transfer to the toilet, COTAs should point out that the goal is to maintain alignment when standing, pivot on both legs, and sit by bending the knees.

What Is Accepted as Truth

When COTAs engage people in therapy, they assume the individuals will act in their own best interest. On the basis of this assumption, COTAs can ask the question: How do clients decide if it is in their best interest to learn the task presented to them? Or, in a broader sense, what is the truth? People from different cultures arrive at truth in different ways. These methods of arriving at truth can be separated into faith, fact, and feeling. The process of evaluating truth tends to be more conscious, in contrast to the automatic cognitive style discussed previously. Furthermore, most people use combinations of methods, but for reasons of clarity, these methods are explained separately in this chapter.

The person who acts on the basis of faith uses a belief system such as that derived from a religion or political ideology to determine what is good or bad. For example, many people believe in self-sufficiency and may decline to use a wheelchair or other adaptive equipment that would clearly help them reduce fatigue. Their belief in self-sufficiency operates independently of the fact that they are too fatigued to stay awake for more than an hour. Other examples of people who act on the basis of faith include the elder who refuses a blood transfusion because this procedure is explicitly prohibited by his or her religion, and the elder who calls on a priest, rabbi, pastor, or other spiritual advisor before making a decision about care. Before OT treatment is initiated, COTAs should always ask if the elder wishes to observe any particular rules and should consider the elder's response when selecting therapeutic occupations.

Obviously, people who act on the basis of fact want to see evidence to support the COTA's recommendation or prioritization of a certain intervention. These people often want to know the benefits a certain intervention has proven to give in the past. To make plans for their future, these people often wish to know the length and cost of required OT services. People who act on the basis of fact may stop participating in a particular activity if they do not see the exact results they anticipated. COTAs may find it helpful to have these elders participate in some form of group treatment that allows them to directly observe results of OT intervention with other elders. In addition, written information about their conditions and about resources can be useful for these elders.

The most common group is people who arrive at truth on the basis of feelings (Hofstede, 2003). Such people are those who "go with their gut instincts." When faced with a difficult decision they often choose the option that "feels right" over the one that seems most logical if this option makes them too uncomfortable. People who function on the basis of feelings often need to establish a comfortable rapport with the COTA before committing themselves wholeheartedly to working with the COTA. Building a relationship with these individuals may take a long time. However, once the relationship is established it is very strong. People who function on the basis of feeling will probably want the COTA to continue treating them after they are discharged from a facility if further services are needed; they place less importance on cost considerations than on continuing the relationship. As with any client, COTAs should consistently and periodically ask elders how they are feeling about their situations and permit them time to process these feelings as needed.

Value Systems

Each culture has a system for separating right from wrong or good from evil. A person's cognitive style and the way in which the person evaluates truth provide general clues about the values of that person's culture. However, more specific value systems exist that form the basis for behavior. Althen (2002) identified eight values and assumptions that characterize dominant American culture, including the importance of individualism and privacy, the belief in the **equality** of all people, and informality in interactions with others. In addition, Althen described emphasis on the future, change, progress, punctuality, materialism, and achievement as salient American values. In this chapter, the locus of decision making, sources of anxiety reduction, issues of equality and inequality, and use of time are discussed. Numerous other value systems also direct behavior, but these four systems are discussed here because they are more related than other systems to the concerns of OT.

Locus of decision making

Locus of decision making is related to the extent to which a culture prizes individualism as opposed to collectivism. Individualism refers to the degree to which a person considers only himself or herself when making a decision. Collectivism refers to the degree to which a person must abide with the consensus of the collective group. Pure individualism and collectivism are rare. In most countries, people consider others when making a decision, but they are not bound by the desires of the group. Returning to the concept of "levels of culture" discussed previously in this chapter may be helpful in understanding individualism versus collectivism. Locus of decision making may be considered as a series of concentric circles (see Fig. 9-4). In the center is the smallest circle: the individual. At this level the individual considers mainly himself or herself when making a decision. The next circle represents a slightly larger group: usually the family. Many cultures expect the individual to consider what is best for the family when making a decision. The next circle represents a larger group: the community. This community could be an ethnic group, a religion, or even the individual's country. Some cultures expect people to consider the best interests of the entire, expansive group.

Examples of the ways people use these different levels of consideration when making a decision are easy to find in OT practice. An individualistic elder is one who makes decisions about when and how he will be discharged home without consulting his or her spouse or family. These elders might believe that their spouse or family has a responsibility to care for them—a value that may not necessarily be shared. Another elder who considers his or her family when making a decision may refuse to be discharged home out of consideration to his or her grown children because they would have to adjust their lifestyles to accommodate the elder's needs. Another elder may decide to attempt to continue living independently to defy society's stereotype of dependence of elders.

Another way of thinking about individualism versus collectivism is to consider the degree of privacy a person seeks. Elders from cultures that highly value privacy may be quite perplexed by the number of health care professionals who seem to know about their issues. Conversely, elders from other cultures that do not have rigid standards of privacy may feel isolated if they are not permitted to have constant contact with family or friends. The OT culture values independence, privacy, and individualism, but these values may be in conflict with an elder's needs if not carefully considered. One of the paradoxes of medical care in the United States is that, at the same time that we defend privacy rights in documentation, we assume that the individual will be completely comfortable undressing or toileting in our presence, and we do not give thought to the possibility that the elder may feel embarrassed by these experiences.

Sources of anxiety reduction

Every human being is subject to stress. How do individuals handle stress and reduce anxiety? Most people turn to four basic sources of security and stability: interpersonal relationships, religion, technology, and the law (Hall, 1981; Harris, 1981; Hofstede, 2003; Morrison, Conaway, & Borden, 1995). A person who must make a decision about an important health-related issue or adapt to a traumatic event is under stress. COTAs will find it helpful to know where or to whom elders turn for help and advice. If an elder is going to ask his or her spouse or family for advice, the COTA should include that spouse or family in therapy from the beginning of intervention so they clearly understand the issues involved.

Elders who rely on religion as a source of anxiety reduction often need COTAs to help them obtain special considerations regarding religious practices. Understanding every nuance in the elder's religion is not as important as acknowledging the importance and appreciating the comfort that the elder finds in religious observances.

Reliance on technology as a source of anxiety reduction can be manifested when elders seek yet another medical test to confirm or refute a diagnosis. These clients may rely on medication as the solution to their problems or may collect a myriad of adaptive equipment or "gadgets." OT practitioners often have a bias toward relieving anxiety by prescribing the use of adaptive equipment without considering fully the extent to which the elder truly needs it.

Issues of equality/inequality

An important characteristic of all cultures is the division of power. Who controls the financial resources, and who controls decision making within the family? A sacred tenet in the United States is that "All men are created equal." Despite this tenet, prejudice against many groups still exists. All cultures have disadvantaged groups. Unequal status may be defined by economic situation, race, age, sex, or other factors. Members of socially and economically advantaged classes may project a sense of entitlement to health care services and may treat COTAs and other health care workers as servants. Conversely, members of a poverty-stricken underclass may eye COTAs with suspicion or defer to any recommendation out of fear of retaliation through withdrawal of needed services.

COTAs also should analyze issues of male and female equality. Female COTAs, in particular, may find it useful to know the way women are regarded in the elder's culture. In most cultures, men are more likely to be obeyed and trusted when they occupy positions of authority, but this is not always true for women (Bateson, 2001). COTAs must understand who will be best suited to act as a caregiver on the basis of the elder's cultural values regarding gender roles. A COTA who is of the opposite sex of the elder may decide to initiate OT treatment around issues less likely to bring up conflicts regarding privacy or authority until more rapport is built and the elder is able to appreciate the COTA's genuine concern for his or her welfare.

Another factor to be considered is status awarded people because of age. *Ageism* refers to the belief that one age group is superior to another. Often the younger generation is more valued. The physical appearance of age is frequently avoided through the use of cosmetics to conceal and surgery to reverse manifestations of age. Some people attempt to delay the natural developmental process through adopting more "healthy" lifestyles of exercise, diet, rest, and so on. The avoidance of the appearance of age can contribute to the undervaluing of elders. Stereotypic descriptors such as "senile," "dependent," or "diseased" are used to describe the aging population as needy people. Because of these views of age it can be easy for the COTA to assume a position of power over elders and place them in a position of inferiority and need of services to justify the existence of the profession (Hasselkus, 2002). McKnight (1995) described how "ageism" has resulted in the view that age is a problem to be avoided. He argued that our assumptions and stereotypical myths surrounding the results of normal development contribute to ageism. These stereotypes of elders cast them as "less" in terms of sight, hearing, memory, mobility, health, learners, and even productive members of society. In contrast, McKnight (1995) described how his mother-in-law, whom he refers to as "Old Grandma," views "old":

> …finally knowing what is important…when you are, rather than when you are becoming… knowing about pain rather than fearing it…being able to gain more pleasure from memory than prospect…when doctors become impotent and powerless…when satisfaction depends less and less on consumption…using the strength that a good life has stored for you…enjoying deference…worrying about irrelevance. (p. 27)

COTAs must be prepared to overcome and critically reflect on their own bias related to growing old to provide culturally sensitive care to the elders they serve.

Use of time

Time is consciously and unconsciously formulated and used in each culture. Time is often treated as a language, a way of handling priorities, and a way of revealing how people feel about each other. Cultures can be divided into those that prefer a monochronic use of time and those that prefer a polychronic use of time (Hall, 1984). Elders from monochronic cultures will probably prefer to organize their life with a "one thing at a time" and "time is money" mentality. For these elders, adherence to schedules is highly important. They are likely to be offended if they are kept waiting for an appointment or if they perceive that the COTA is attending to too many issues at once. People from a monochronic culture prefer having the COTA's undivided attention and expect time to be used efficiently. These people are not necessarily unfriendly but prefer social "chit-chat" to be kept to a minimum if they are paying for a particular technical service. In contrast, elders from a polychronic culture organize their lives around social relationships. For them the time spent with someone is directly correlated to their personal value. Often these elders feel rushed by schedules. They may be late for an appointment because they encountered an acquaintance who they did not want to offend by rushing off to a therapy appointment. With these elders, COTAs may find that sessions are most effective when a lot of conversation takes place. People from polychronic cultures may also wish to know many details about the COTA's life as a way of showing that they value the professional. When elders of a polychronic culture arrive late for an appointment, they may be offended if the COTA refuses to squeeze them into the schedule.

Communication Style

The meaning people give to the information they obtain through interaction with others largely depends on the way that information is transmitted. Cultures differ in the amount of information that is transmitted through verbal and nonverbal language. Cultures also differ in regard to the amount of information that is transmitted through the context of the situation (Lynch, 1992). Context includes the relationship to the individual with whom one is communicating. For example, after living together for more than 50 years, an elder couple does not always have to spell things out for each to know the other's feelings. Each partner may know the other's feelings simply by the way they move and the tone of their voices. Their shared experiences over 50 years have given them high context; therefore meaning is not lost when words are not spoken.

Hall (1984) has noted that high-context cultures rely less on verbal communication than on understanding through shared experience and history. In high-context cultures, fewer words are spoken and more emphasis is placed on nonverbal cues and messages. High-context cultures tend to be formal, reliant on hierarchy, and rooted in the past; thus, they change more slowly and tend to provide more stability for their members (Hecht, Anderson, & Ribeau, 1989). When words are used in high-context cultures, communication is more indirect. People in these cultures usually express themselves through stories that imply their opinions (Bateson, 2001).

In contrast, persons from low-context cultures typically focus on precise, direct, and logical verbal communication. These persons may not process the gestures, environmental clues, and unarticulated moods that are central to communication in high-context cultures. Low-context cultures may be more responsive to and comfortable with change but often lack a sense of continuity and connection with the past (Hecht, Anderson, & Ribeau, 1989).

Misunderstanding may easily arise when COTAs and elders, family members, or caregivers use a different level of context in their communication. Persons from high-context cultures may consider detailed verbal instructions insensitive and mechanistic; they may feel they are being "talked down to." Persons from low-context cultures may be uncomfortable with long pauses and may also feel impatient with indirect communication such as storytelling. It is the responsibility of the COTA to become aware of the style of communication of the elder, family member, or caregiver and adapt to that style. COTAs must note that nonverbal communication such as facial expressions, eye contact, and touching may have completely different meanings in different cultures. COTAs can learn these things by listening carefully, observing how the family interacts, and adapting OT practice style as new discoveries are made about the elder's culture.

CASE STUDY

Mrs. Pardo is a 70-year-old Filipino woman who was admitted to a skilled nursing facility after an infection developed in her right hip. She had a total hip replacement 3 weeks before being transferred to the skilled nursing facility. Because of the infection, Mrs. Pardo had received little therapy. A week ago the OTR was finally able to complete an OT evaluation. Melissa, a newly hired COTA, is continuing the OT program. When discussing the case with Melissa, the OTR stated that although Mrs. Pardo has been trained in getting from a supine position to a sitting position at the edge of the bed and in dressing, her family routinely provides this care. The OTR has not discussed with Mrs. Pardo or her family the need for these activities to be done independently. Part of Melissa's responsibility, according to the OTR, is to "convince them to not fuss over her so much."

Melissa reviewed Mrs. Pardo's medical record before meeting her. It appeared that Mrs. Pardo's condition was stable and the infection was under control. Several professionals had documented that she was quite weak and deconditioned, presumably because of prolonged bed rest. Melissa reviewed the OT evaluation results and treatment goals, which seemed quite straightforward. The general objective was for Mrs. Pardo to become independent in ADL functions and transfers while observing specific hip precautions for at least 6 more weeks. These precautions included touch-toe weight bearing on the right leg, as well as avoiding right leg internal rotation and right hip flexion greater than 60 degrees. Melissa also noted that Mrs. Pardo was a widow who lived with one of her five adult daughters.

One of Mrs. Pardo's daughters and two of her adolescent grandchildren were present when Melissa met Mrs. Pardo. When Melissa introduced herself, Mrs. Pardo smiled and introduced her relatives. She also told Melissa she reminded her of someone she had met years ago while working as a sales representative for an American firm. Once Mrs. Pardo found out where Melissa was from she asked if Melissa knew the relatives of an acquaintance of hers, who was from Melissa's town. Finally, Melissa stated she was there to work on transfers and dressing. Because Melissa wanted to see how Mrs. Pardo performed these activities independently, she asked the relatives to leave the room for a few minutes. Once they left, Melissa sensed a change in Mrs. Pardo. Although she followed all of Melissa's directions quickly, she seemed to be avoiding eye contact. When Melissa asked her if everything was all right, Mrs. Pardo responded affirmatively. Melissa observed that Mrs. Pardo required minimal assistance to get out of the hospital bed, sit in a commode chair, and dress herself with a gown while observing all hip precautions. Noting that Mrs. Pardo appeared fatigued, Melissa said she would return at 3:00 PM to work on Mrs. Pardo's self-bathing ability. Melissa asked if Mrs. Pardo was aware of any scheduling conflicts, to which Mrs. Pardo responded, "No." When Melissa left the room, she asked Mrs. Pardo's daughter if she would be available to observe the bath that afternoon. The daughter said she would be there without fail.

Later that afternoon Melissa entered Mrs. Pardo's room at the same moment a different daughter was helping Mrs. Pardo get into bed. Alarmed that hip precautions were not being followed, Melissa immediately asked the daughter to let her take over and demonstrate the appropriate method of transferring to the bed. The daughter angrily stated that Mrs. Pardo was too tired for therapy and proceeded to complete the task without Melissa's assistance. Melissa was taken aback and told Mrs. Pardo she would return in the morning for the bath.

That evening Melissa could not stop thinking about the afternoon's events. She was aware that she had somehow offended Mrs. Pardo's daughter, and she wondered why Mrs. Pardo had gone back to bed knowing that Melissa would be coming to work with her at 3:00 PM. Melissa decided to carefully analyze what had happened. She remembered how friendly and talkative Mrs. Pardo had been at the beginning of the session, which was perhaps a sign that she valued relationships highly and wanted Melissa to know she was appreciated. Then Melissa thought about the change in Mrs. Pardo when her family left and wondered if she felt alone without family to support her. Why had Mrs. Pardo said that everything was all right but then avoided eye contact? Was this her way of letting Melissa know that she did not want to do the task without directly opposing the plan for the session? Melissa thought about the tasks they had accomplished and wondered if Mrs. Pardo had ever before been required to get out of a hospital bed, sit on a commode in front of another person, and dress in a hospital gown. Did these tasks have anything to do with her real life? Finally, Susan remembered how she had entered the room while Mrs. Pardo's daughter was helping her get into bed. Melissa realized that she had

blurted out orders without even introducing herself. Had she caused the daughter to feel embarrassed and incompetent? Was the daughter's anger a way of regaining control?

After evaluating the situation, Melissa concluded that Mrs. Pardo probably could not relate to the artificial ADL tasks presented to her. She also suspected that Mrs. Pardo relied on family members for support in making decisions and reducing anxiety. Mrs. Pardo also seemed to value the feelings of other people and avoided direct confrontation. The daughter might have been angry because Melissa confronted her directly. Melissa decided that the next day she would approach the treatment session with Mrs. Pardo differently. First, she would schedule the session when a family member could be present. She also planned to spend some time simply conversing with Mrs. Pardo and her family members, and she planned to spend more time chit-chatting during the session. Melissa decided to take Mrs. Pardo to the simulated apartment in the rehabilitation department, where they could work in a more realistic home setting with a real bed and chair, and Mrs. Pardo could also work on dressing with her own clothes.

The next day, Melissa carried out her plan with great success. Melissa had realized that Mrs. Pardo was an associative thinker who needed new tasks to be associated with more familiar routines. Melissa had also realized that Mrs. Pardo valued family ties and social relationships greatly and consequently would not risk offending others with a direct refusal. In addition, Melissa realized that Mrs. Pardo relied on family as a source of anxiety reduction. Finally, Melissa had recognized that Mrs. Pardo was from a polychronic culture that valued a more social than prescriptive approach to rehabilitation.

CONCLUSION

This chapter provides a framework that COTAs can use to approach elders from diverse backgrounds. Concepts of culture and diversity have been discussed, with special attention given to the ways these differences can contribute to the elder's ability to obtain meaning in therapy. Emphasis also was placed on the fact that both culture and diversity are very broad and complex terms. Consequently, a cultural model was presented to aid COTAs in designing individualized OT services for each elder. COTAs may use this information as a guide for culturally sensitive practice and remain open to new experiences they encounter with each elder. Before attempting to treat elders from other backgrounds, COTAs must become aware of and analyze their own prejudices and biases about the dimensions of life that create diversity (Box 9-1).

▌ CHAPTER REVIEW QUESTIONS

1 Explain why it is difficult to define the term *culture*.
2 Give examples of ways in which you have learned and shared a particular value.
3 Give examples of values and beliefs that connect individuals with the various other levels of culture, including family, community, and country.

BOX 9-1

Attitude Self-analysis

Do I believe it is important to consider culture when treating elders?

Am I willing to lower my defenses and take risks?

Am I willing to practice behaviors that may feel unfamiliar and uncomfortable to benefit the elder with whom I am working?

Am I willing to set aside some of my own cherished beliefs to make room for others whose values are unknown?

Am I willing to change the ways I think and behave?

Am I sufficiently familiar with my own heritage, including place of family origin, time of, and reasons for immigration, and language(s) spoken?

What values, beliefs, and customs are identified with my own cultural heritage?

In what ways do my beliefs, values, and customs interfere with my ability to understand those of others?

Do I view elders as a resource in understanding their cultural beliefs, family dynamics, and views of health?

Do I encourage elders to use resources from within their cultures that they see as important?

4 Explain how appreciating diversity can affect occupational therapy (OT) intervention with elders.

5 Describe your own cognitive style and explain how you base your actions on faith, fact, or feelings. Also describe how you arrive at decisions about your own health behaviors and what you rely on to reduce anxiety in difficult times.

6 Describe at least three ways in which issues of equality and inequality may affect OT intervention with elders.

7 Explain ways in which you tend to behave on a monochronic and polychronic basis. Describe how this tendency may interfere with your ability to provide treatment to elders.

8 Describe at least three other strategies Melissa could use with Mrs. Pardo that would take into consideration Mrs. Pardo's cultural context.

REFERENCES

Administration on Aging (AOA). (2002). *A profile of older Americans.* Washington, DC: U.S. Department of Health and Human Services.

Allen, C. (1985). *Occupational therapy for psychiatric diseases: Measurement and management of cognitive disabilities.* Boston, MA: Little, Brown & Company.

Allen, C., Earhart, C., Blue, T. (1992). *Occupational therapy goals for the physically and cognitively disabled.* Rockville, MD: American Occupational Therapy Association.

Althen, G. (2002). *American ways.* Yarmouth, ME: Intercultural Press.

American Association of Retired Persons. (1995). *A profile of older Americans.* Washington, DC: The Association.

American Occupational Therapy Association. (2002). Occupational therapy practice framework: Domain and process. *American Journal of Occupational Therapy, 48*(11), 1047.

American Occupational Therapy Association Representative Assembly. (1981). Official definition for licensure. *American Journal of Occupational Therapy, 35*(6), 789.

American Occupational Therapy Association. (1998). Standards of Practice in Occupational Therapy. *American Journal of Occupational Therapy, 54,* 614-616.

Barresi, C. (1990). Ethnogerontology: Social aging in national, racial, and cultural groups. In K. Ferraro (Ed.), *Gerontology: Perspectives and issues.* New York, NY: Springer.

Bateson, M. C., (2001). *Full circles, overlapping lives: Culture and generation in transition.* New York, NY: Ballantine Books.

Baumeister, R. F. (1991). *Meanings of life.* New York, NY: Guilford.

Benedict, R. (1989). *Patterns of culture.* Boston, MA: Houghton Mifflin.

Bonder, B., Martin, L., & Miracle, A. (2002). *Culture in clinical care.* Thorofare, NJ: Slack International.

Bonhannan, P., & van der Elst, D. (1998). *Asking and listening. Ethnography and personal adaptation.* Prospect Heights, IL: Waveland.

Bucher, R. (2000). *Diversity consciousness: Opening our minds to people, cultures, and opportunities.* Englewood Cliffs, NJ: Prentice Hall.

Dorfman, R., & Walters, K. (1995). Old, sad, and alone: the myth of the aging homosexual. *Gerontological Social Work, 24,* 29.

Fry, C. (1990). Cross-cultural comparisons of aging. In K. Ferraro (Ed.), *Gerontology: Perspectives and issues.* New York, NY: Springer.

Gropper, R. (1996). *Culture and the clinical encounter: An intercultural sensitizer for the health professions.* Yarmouth, ME: Intercultural Press.

Hall, E. (1981). *Beyond culture.* New York, NY: Anchor Books.

Hall, E. (1984). *The dance of life: The other dimensions of time.* New York, NY: Anchor Books.

Harris, M. (1989). *Cows, pigs, wars, and witches: The riddles of culture.* New York, NY: Vintage Books.

Harris, M. (1998). *Theories of culture in postmodern times.* Pueblo, CO: AltaMira Press.

Hasselkus, B.R. (2002). *The meaning of everyday occupation.* Thorofare, NJ: SLACK, Inc.

Hasselkus, B., & Rosa, S. (1997). Meaning and occupation. In C. Christiansen & C. Baum (Eds.), *Enabling function and well-being* (2nd ed.). Thorofare, NJ: Slack International.

Hecht, M., Andersen, P., & Ribeau, S. (1989). The cultural dimensions of nonverbal communication. In M. Asante & E. Gudykunst (Eds.), *Handbook for international and intercultural communication.* Newbury Park, CA: Sage.

Hofstede, G. (2003). *Culture's consequences: Comparing values, behaviors, institutions and organizations across nations.* Thousand Oaks, CA: Sage.

Horowitz, J., & Newcomb, M. (2001). A multidimensional approach to homosexual identity. *Journal of Homosexuality 42*(2), 1-20.

Janus, S., & Janus, C. (1994). *The Janus report on sexual behavior.* New York, NY: John Wiley & Sons.

Johnson, A. (2001). *Privilege, power and difference.* New York, NY: McGraw-Hill.

Kielhofner, G. (2002). *A model of human occupation: Theory and application* (3rd ed.). Baltimore, MD: Lippincott Williams & Wilkins.

Kohls, R., & Knight, J. (1994). *Developing intercultural awareness: A cross-cultural training handbook* (2nd ed.). Yarmouth, ME: Intercultural Press.

Krefting, L., & Krefting, D. (1991). Cultural influences on perform-ance. In C. Christiansen, & C. Baum (Eds.), *Occupational therapy: Overcoming human performance deficits.* Thorofare, NJ: SLACK International.

Laumann, E., & Michael, R. (2000). *Sex, love and health in America: Private choices and public policies.* Chicago, IL: University of Chicago Press.

Lemet, C. (2002). *Social things* (2nd ed.). Lanham, MD: Rowman & Littlefield.

Loden, M., & Rosener, J. (1991). *Workforce America: Managing employee diversity as a vital resource.* New York, NY: McGraw-Hill.

Loveland, C. (2001). The concept of culture. In R. Leavitt (Ed.), *Cross-cultural rehabilitation: An international perspective* (2nd ed., pp. 15-24). Philadelphia, PA: WB Saunders.

Lynch, E. (1992). Developing cross-cultural competence. In E. Lynch & M. Hanson (Eds.), *Developing cross-cultural competence: A guide for working with young children and their families.* Baltimore, MD: Paul H. Brookes.

McKnight, J. (1995). *The careless society: Community and its counterfeits.* New York, NY: Basic Books.

Morrison, T., Conaway, W., & Borden, G. (1995). *Kiss, bow, or shake hands: How to do business in sixty countries.* Holbrook, MA: Bob Adams.

Padilla, R. (2000). Cultural diversity and health behavior. In S. Kumar (Ed.), *Multidisciplinary approach to rehabilitation.* Woburn, MA: Butterworth-Heinemann.

Parker, P. (1997). *Religious cultures of the world: A statistical reference.* Westport, CT: Greenwood Press.

Peacock, J. (2002). *The anthropological lens: Harsh light, soft focus* (2nd ed.). London: Cambridge University Press.

Quam, J., & Whitford, G. (1992). Adaptation and age-related expectations of older gay and lesbian adults. *Gerontologist, 32,* 367.

Rosenfeld, D. (1999). Identity work among lesbian and gay elderly. *Journal of Aging Studies, 13,* 121-145.

Ross, H. C. (1993). *The art of Arabian costume: A Saudi Arabian profile.* San Francisco, CA: Players Press.

CHAPTER 10

Ethical Aspects in the Work with Elders

KATHERINE H. BROWN AND CAROL J. SCHWOPE

KEY TERMS

client autonomy, informed consent, ethical dilemma, ethical distress, distributive justice, least restrictive environment, benefits, burdens, Institutional Ethics Committee, confidentiality, empathetic relationships, whistle-blowing, American Occupational Therapy Association (AOTA) Standards and Ethics Commission (SEC), National Board for Certification in Occupational Therapy (NBCOT), State Regulatory Boards

---

CHAPTER OBJECTIVES

1. Discuss steps for ethical consideration.
2. Become familiar with the language of ethics.

3. Refine and explain personal and professional ethical commitments.

Sheila, Maryann, and Chris are three friends who graduated from the same occupational therapy assistant (OTA) program a few years ago. They have gathered to discuss a problem Sheila has been having at the psychiatric hospital where she works. Maryann works in a long-term care facility, and Chris is employed with a rehabilitation clinic. Recently, his employer expanded to home care, so Chris has begun seeing clients in their homes, as well as in the clinic.

In this chapter, the three certified occupational therapy assistants (COTAs) mentioned above discuss a variety of ethical questions arising from the complexities of their job demands. These discussions include a series of steps for ethical consideration that students and clinicians can use in responding to ethical challenges in their practices. Some of the language of ethics is reflected in the American Occupational Therapy Association Code of Ethics (American Occupational Therapy Association [AOTA], 2000). Other ethics commentaries that guide professional practice also are introduced in this chapter. The authors hope that COTAs will take the opportunity to refine and explain the ethical commitments that shape their personal integrity when working with elders.

AN OVERVIEW: ETHICS AND ELDER CARE

The health care environment is in the midst of great change. In recent years, occupational therapy (OT) practice has been especially influenced by the pressures of new technologies and cost controls. In one way, these pressures have contributed positively to OT practice. For example, technologies such as hip replacements, pacemakers, and organ transplants have increased the practitioner's capacity to respond more effectively to clients' needs.

Increased attention to the way health care dollars are spent also has made us focus on which treatments to use and why. Conversely, some technologies—especially those capable of sustaining life—sometimes pose complex questions that clients, clinicians, and society are ill prepared to answer. The ethics of continuing to artificially feed a person in a permanent vegetative state is one example. Another question concerns the ethics involved with providing access for all persons to expensive new technologies.

Cost-control strategies also can create ethical challenges for practitioners. Traditionally, health care professionals have served their clients' best interests before their own. Increasingly, however, financial constraints force practitioners to decide the best way to uphold this commitment. For instance, cost controls on health care expenditures are sometimes linked to salary incentives in managed care organizations, which can tempt practitioners away from their professional responsibilities. Other ethically problematic cost-driven practices include "creative" documentation for reimbursement and accepting referrals for marginally necessary or needless treatments. Creative documentation refers to the practice of exaggerating a problem, altering a diagnosis, or implying better prognosis so that more client visits can be approved. When actual fraud exists, such practices are liable to legal and ethical inquiry and punishment.

Frequently, cost controls can translate into fewer staff for more clients. When these staffing changes contribute to inadequate supervision or require COTAs to use modalities for which they are not sufficiently trained, COTAs are placed in another ethically questionable position in terms of their professional standards of practice.

Regardless of the clinical and financial environment of practice, special ethical concerns are raised for COTAs working with elders. Elders have a wide range of health care needs, their occupational goals are diverse, and they require personalized treatment plans, which may require the practitioner to develop particular ethical sensitivities.

Consider the example of ethical decision making in health care. Generally in the United States, most people believe that adults should be the primary decision makers about their own health care because **client autonomy** is important. Client autonomy refers to the idea that adults have the right to determine what happens to them in a health care setting.

The value of client autonomy is expressed in many ways. For instance, because of client autonomy, health care providers are careful to get **informed consent** from clients before doing a procedure, especially if the procedure has negative risks. Before consenting, clients need to know the risks and benefits of the procedure, whether there are alternatives, and the way their health will be affected if intervention is refused. Once clients have this information, client autonomy necessitates that they be allowed to accept or refuse the treatment.

How is client autonomy translated into care for elders? Elders vary in their capacities for independent function and thought, and thus their capacities for autonomous decision making. Some elders are no longer able to make decisions on their own behalf. But often the extent of this inability and its consequences for decision making are unclear. Of course, physical dependency is not always accompanied by mental dependency. COTAs must remember that clients who have lost most of their physical independence may still retain the ability to make independent decisions.

In addition, caregivers need to appreciate that an elder's capacity for independent decision making may fluctuate because of his or her physical or mental conditions. For instance, patients with Alzheimer's disease, Parkinson's disease, or stroke may be more fully alert at certain times of the day than at other times.

Elders also vary in their capacities to respond to different kinds of decision-making tasks. In a nursing home, for example, a resident who is able to walk to a dining hall without assistance at the appropriate time may be unable to choose a balanced diet. Another resident may be mentally competent to decide what to eat but is unable to keep reliable bank records. The task, the circumstance, and clients' mental and emotional states will determine their decision-making capacities.

Client decision making is just one area of ethical concern for COTAs. This chapter, through exploration of the situations presented by the three COTAs, Chris, Sheila, and Maryann, presents a number of other issues (Fig. 10-1). The chapter is organized around a four-step method for working through an ethical problem (Box 10-1). Each step is illustrated with specific cases experienced by the three friends.

AWARENESS: WHAT IS GOING ON?

The first step in approaching an ethical problem is to figure out what is going on. This may seem obvious at

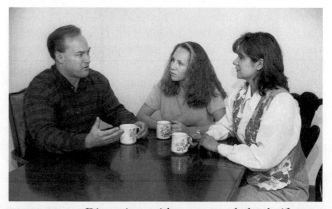

FIGURE 10-1   Discussions with peers may help clarify ethical dilemmas.

BOX **10-1**

Steps for Ethical Consideration

Awareness: What is going on?
Reflection: What do I think should happen?
Support: With whom do I need to talk?
Action: What will I do?

first, but actually the situation can be quite complicated, and before COTAs take action, they must consider a number of factors.

What Kind of Ethical Problem Is It?

COTAs may find it helpful to start by figuring out the kind of problem they are facing. Ethicists differentiate three kinds of problems: an ethical dilemma, ethical distress, and distributive justice (Purtilo, 1999). An **ethical dilemma** refers to a situation in which there are two or more ethically correct options for action. However, with each choice, the COTA compromises something of value. **Ethical distress** refers to a situation in which the COTA knows which course of action to take for the client's benefit but is unable to do so without some personal risk. The barrier often is established by someone who has more institutional authority than the COTA. **Distributive justice** problems arise when there is not enough of something that is valued. The COTA must distribute the item or service in a fair way, or in the language of ethics, a "just" way (Box 10-2).

Who Is Involved?

The question of individuals involved must be considered when approaching an ethical problem. Usually the COTA is involved, and most likely the COTA's client is involved. But who else has a stake in the ethical problem the COTA faces? It is not enough to know only who is involved; COTAs must also investigate their beliefs and values to anticipate areas of agreement and disagreement about the proposed course of action. The client's family often needs to be involved in medical decision making, but involvement may result in an ethical dilemma for the COTA.

For example, the family of one of Chris's home care clients asks him for help in placing a relative in a nursing home. The client has begun to wander from his home and has gotten lost several times. Chris knows that his client values his independence and will resist the move to a facility; however, Chris recognizes that the client might endanger himself. He respects the wishes of both the client and the client's family. What other value, besides the client's autonomy, should Chris consider? In addition to Chris, the family, and the client, who else is likely to be involved?

BOX **10-2**

Examples of Ethical Problems

Ethical dilemma
Maryann works in a long-term care facility. A client who has had a stroke asks Maryann whether she will regain fine motor control of her hand. If Maryann tells her she probably will not regain all of her fine motor control, the client is likely to fall into a deep depression. If Maryann does not tell her the full extent of her prognosis, she probably will find out anyway, and then her trust in Maryann might diminish.
 What are two of the actions Maryann could take?
 What values are compromised if either action is taken?

Ethical distress
Sheila works at a psychiatric hospital. She has just learned that her client is to be discharged tomorrow. She knows he lives alone and will most likely not be able to regulate his medications appropriately. Sheila voices her concerns, but her supervisor tells her that the client's insurance coverage has run out, so they have no choice but to discharge him.
 Is it ethically wrong to discharge this client? Why?
 What barrier(s) does Sheila confront when questioning the discharge plan?

Distributive justice
Chris works at a rehabilitation clinic but has begun seeing clients in their homes as well. One of Chris's clients has been admitted to the rehabilitation program with clear payment guidelines from his insurance company: there will be no reimbursement for equipment of any type. The client needs a wrist support splint, but this item is considered equipment by the insurance company.
 Should Chris ignore the need for a splint because of restricted payment guidelines?
 Can you name at least three other scarcities in health care that are likely to raise issues of distributive justice for you as a COTA?

Which Laws and Institutional Rules Apply?

Sometimes laws and institutional rules help clarify the role of COTAs in a given ethics problem. Some laws are federal, meaning that they apply in every state, but other laws apply only within a particular state's jurisdiction. COTAs are responsible for knowing which laws apply to their practice. Many institutions have legal counselors who can answer questions about specific legal issues. Supervisors also can help to clarify the legal and institutional responsibilities of COTAs. Each institution has established guidelines and rules that specify the expectations they have for staff, clients, and administrators.

The influence of law in defining ethical practice is illustrated in a case regarding the use of restraints that Sheila was asked to help resolve at the psychiatric hospital where she works. Sheila's client is a 68-year-old woman who was admitted to the acute care psychiatry department because of agitation and uncontrollable behavior. The client's charted diagnosis read, "Axis I schizoaffective bipolar type, axis III hypertension, degenerative joint disease, chronic obstructive pulmonary disease, chronic constipation, head trauma (grade 9; no further details)." Staff members do not particularly like this client; they often construe her behavior as violent. She calls other clients, residents, and staff derogatory names; she also tells lies about them and accuses them of mistreating her. At times, she claims she is unable to walk and demands use of a wheelchair. She often stages a fall by throwing herself from the wheelchair onto the floor. The staff recommends she be restrained in a chair for her own safety.

When Sheila brought this case to her friends for discussion, Maryann pointed out that given the client's age her case was most likely covered by Medicare. This means that legally, like the staff in her nursing home, the staff in the psychiatric hospital should follow the guidelines for restraints defined by the Omnibus Budget Reconciliation Act of 1987. Maryann explained that this federal legislation requires health care providers to ensure client safety in the **least restrictive environment.** When Chris pointed out that no one wanted to be around this client, Sheila voiced her suspicion that maybe the restraints were being used as punishment, not client safety. If this was the case, she didn't think this was an ethical use of restraints, and the others agreed. The three friends began thinking of ways that OT could help in designing the least restrictive environment for this client. "After all," said Chris, "even unpleasant clients deserve the right to make choices and have some liberty, as long as they are not hurting themselves or others."

What Guidance Does the American Occupational Therapy Association Code of Ethics Provide?

"Ethics are the human effort to catch hold of those human events and occasions that are liable to go badly and then turn them to our good as best we can" (Jonsen, 1992, p. 3). This quote is a good starting point from which to begin exploring the reasons why the AOTA Code of Ethics (AOTA, 2000) serves as a guide for OT personnel in the issues they encounter daily. The Code of Ethics has six principles. These principles are similar to a list of desired behaviors for OT personnel. OT personnel must demonstrate concern for the well-being of their clients and respect their clients' rights. OT personnel must be competent, comply with laws and rules that apply to OT personnel, and provide accurate information

about services they provide. And finally, OT personnel must be fair and discreet and demonstrate integrity with colleagues and other professionals.

Not only is the Occupational Therapy Code of Ethics a guide for behavior, it is also a regulatory code in that guidelines for conduct are stated and sanctions are provided for failure to follow the code. These sanctions are stated in the enforcement procedures for the Code of Ethics (AOTA, 2002a). Often the principles stated in the Code of Ethics are also found in local, state, and federal laws.

What Are My Options?

OT practitioners need to be aware of the range of options before deciding what action should be taken in a given ethics case. As noted, sometimes the options for a COTA are defined by law. Ethical options also may be limited by personal religious prohibitions and beliefs. Often, however, personal and professional duties are not well defined. In such cases, ethicists suggest that health care providers, clients, and families try to estimate the consequences of a given option. These consequences can be weighed against the consequences of other options. The ethically preferable course of action will be that which carries the greatest chance of a good outcome **(benefits)** and the least amount of damage **(burdens).**

This calculation of consequences is illustrated with a case Chris discussed with Maryann and Sheila. At the rehabilitation hospital where Chris works, the burn unit was considering the best way to treat a comatose 85-year-old man. The team was trying to decide whether to treat the client's severe burns or to provide him with palliative care until he died. To decide which course to take, the burn unit team was considering whether the burdens of treatment, including excruciating pain from grafts and range of motion exercises, were ethically warranted given his questionable survival. They also wondered about the quality of his life if he did survive. It was clear he would never return to his home and would need nursing facility care for the rest of his life. The client's family felt that this prospect of the future would be demoralizing for their relative because he had always cherished his independence. But some members of the staff argued that with rehabilitation the client might learn to adapt to and even enjoy a more social environment. Questions that arose for Chris out of this example include the following: What burdens are created by aggressive treatment in this case? What benefits are created by such treatment? What burdens are created by palliative care? What benefits are created by palliative care?

In accordance with professional values, COTAs should calculate these ratios of benefits and burdens in light of the client's well-being, not in terms of the staff's convenience or the client's estate. This kind of assurance is necessary for maintaining a bond of trust between health professionals and their clients, who expect professionals to work on behalf of their best interests.

Reflection: What Do I Think Should Happen?

After COTAs are aware of all the facts and options in a given case, they must decide what they want to happen and must be able to explain their position. First, COTAs must determine what actions seem most wrong or right. This process may begin as a gut feeling that persists. Sensitivity to such feelings is an important component for reflective ethical practice. In addition, the legally defined roles of COTAs or their religious tenets may affect their ethical inclinations. Ethical reflection involves careful and critical examination of feelings, a rational estimate of benefits and burdens, and a sense of professional duty.

Often this stage of ethical consideration requires some emotional and even physical detachment as COTAs step back from the problem to reflect on their ethical commitments and reasoning. Sometimes the urgency of a situation requires rapid reflection; nonetheless, ethicists recommend a conscious period be taken for serious consideration of preferences and motivations for choosing a given course of action. Each person should find personal methods of reflection that best fit his or her reasoning style.

Some health professionals find it useful to talk through a problem with a group of trusted advisors, including the occupational therapist (OTR) team partner. Such a group can be informal, like the group of COTAs highlighted in this chapter, or more formal, such as an **Institutional Ethics Committee.** Typically, Institutional Ethics Committees (sometimes referred to as Hospital Ethics Committees) are composed of staff, administrators, legal counsel, and a community representative. These committees often provide interdisciplinary consideration for a particular problem. Just as with an informal group of peers, these committees can only recommend a resolution; legally or ethically, COTAs are not usually bound to comply with the committee's advice.

When choosing to talk over an ethics problem with someone else, COTAs must respect the **confidentiality** of those involved. COTAs should make every effort to see that information about clients, colleagues, or institutions is shared in a way that does not reveal anyone's identity. The client's name should not be used, especially with persons not involved directly with the client's care. Similar care needs to be taken when the behavior of an institution or a peer is discussed.

Free writing (Goldberg, 2001) is another method used for ethical reflection. Free writing involves writing whatever comes to mind without worrying about language, spelling, and grammar. Usually the exercise is limited to 10 minutes, during which the writer does not stop writing. The key is to suspend the usual breaks in writing and let uncensored thoughts pour onto the page. The usefulness of this technique is in uncovering deep ethical feelings.

This technique may reveal previously unrealized opinions or persuasive reasons for a stance. The free writing technique requires only that COTAs trust themselves to be revealed.

Two weeks ago, Maryann was placed in a difficult position with one of her favorite clients, Mrs. Henry. Three months earlier, Mrs. Henry had come to the facility after experiencing a stroke. Despite Maryann's best efforts to help Mrs. Henry regain endurance and sitting balance, Maryann's supervising OTR concluded that Mrs. Henry was not likely to improve any further and recommended discontinuing her therapy. However, Mrs. Henry's family asked Maryann to continue the treatments. They could tell how much their mother enjoyed the attention. They were worried that Mrs. Henry would lose hope and her health would deteriorate further. Maryann explained that without demonstrable improvement, Medicare was not likely to reimburse the facility for this therapy. In response, the family appealed to Maryann's sense of loyalty to their mother, asking her to be creative about how she documented the effect of the therapy.

Maryann faced an ethical dilemma between loyalty to someone she cared for and the obligation to truthfully document OT intervention. She decided to free write for 10 minutes to better determine a response (Box 10-3). To her surprise, she found her response guided by her ethical preference.

Caring professionals are often confronted with the limits of their **empathetic relationships** with clients. Especially in long-term care environments, professionals may find that relating to their clients through the rigid shield of professional distance is unrealistic and uncomfortable. Conversely, clients must be protected from a caregiver's over-involvement, as in the extreme case of sexual liaisons, and also from a caregiver's subjective biases, as in the case of discrimination. Finding a balance between genuine caring for clients and realistic boundaries for professional involvement is a lifelong goal for all health care professionals that requires ongoing ethical introspection.

Useful tools for ethical reflection include prayer, meditation, nature walks, and reading a poem or short story, even if the content of the work seems unrelated to the current problem. Possibly, the astronomer's wisdom in finding a faint star works equally well for ethics: you can better see the star if you look just to the side of it. These and the aforementioned methods for reflective ethical practice suggest that before responding to an ethical issue, COTAs must step away from the urgency of the problem to gain perspective about their responsibilities.

BOX 10-3

Maryann's Free Writing

Let's see. It's 1:48, so that gives me until 1:58. I can't believe I'm writing this. This feels really stupid. OK. OK. The thing is, I don't know what to do for Mrs. H. She's such a sweet old lady. Even though she can't speak, she communicates with her eyes. They shine so gratefully when we are together. I can tell she appreciates my work. But it really bugs me that her family has pressured me to document progress when there isn't any. I can see their point, and in fact I want to do anything at all to help her because I really care about her. I feel really close, maybe because she can't speak, so I have to be with her when we work together. Be there for her eye to eye. That's the trouble though, it would be a lie to say she is improving from the therapy. But I don't want to give up hope. This isn't any more clear than when I started writing. What time is it? Don't stop to look. Keep writing. OK. So. What am I supposed to do? The Code says #1, we are supposed to work for each patient's well-being. But it also says we are supposed to tell the truth. So what help is that? I could get my OTR to fudge a bit on the chart, at least for a couple of weeks. But that's fraud. What is the bottom line? Why is it that caring for Mrs. H seems incompatible with telling the truth? Why not keep seeing Mrs. H., stopping by her room to cheer her up, even though insurance doesn't cover that. I wouldn't be doing therapy. I'd be there as her friend. I think that's what I'll do. I'll just have to tell the family that the therapy will end, but I won't desert their mother. And maybe I can help teach them how they can work with her so she feels like she is getting attention. I can't believe it, but I actually feel lighter. And in exactly 10 minutes to the second!

Support: With Whom Do I Need to Talk?

Although ethical issues admittedly involve conscious reflection, they should not be considered in isolation from others. Ethical commitments are shaped by social influences including upbringing, professional codes, and the circumstances of a given event. Likewise, the outcomes of most ethical decisions have social effects. Before acting according to ethical convictions, COTAs should solicit the support of others who will be affected by the issue. In many instances of ethics in health care, this means communicating with the client, the client's family, and other staff members. Sometimes the Institutional Ethics Committee also can provide institutional support for a COTA's position. Others who are more directly involved in a given issue may have more influence than the COTA when voicing their ethical positions. In addition, others may have more moral authority given the particular circumstances under

consideration. The usual practice in the United States is to prioritize the wishes of adult clients above those of others, even when the adult's wishes run counter to expert opinion. Other professionals on the health care team, by virtue of status, training, and tradition, also may claim decision-making authority.

When COTAs have limited influence, they must express their position and the reasons that support it so that others have the benefit of these insights. Also, by expressing their positions, COTAs can sometimes avoid the experience of ethical distress when asked to participate in an intervention that conflicts with their ethical views. The more rational the COTAs' arguments in support of their position, the more persuasive COTAs will be in defending their objections, even if the course of events cannot be changed.

In cases in which COTAs are asked to do something that is ethically questionable, they have the responsibility to involve those with supervisory jurisdiction over them. COTAs should document such communications, especially if there are legal ramifications or if job security is at risk. Following is an example of this kind of dilemma.

In the last year, since his rehabilitation clinic changed to a managed care model, Chris has observed that he is increasingly asked to do treatments that OTRs previously did. Most of the time Chris appreciates the opportunity for more responsibility and feels comfortable doing what is asked of him. However, recently he was asked by the referring physician to work with a client who needed paraffin baths for her arthritic fingers. After he explained the situation, Chris and his friends discussed the issue.

"Absolutely not! You haven't had any training for this modality, and you might burn the client or something," said Sheila.

"I think it's really unfair that they asked you to do this, Chris. This puts you in a tough position about something that isn't your problem. They are just trying to save money by asking you to do this instead of asking an OTR," added Maryann.

"That may well be," replied Chris, "but I still have to deal with it one way or another."

"What you have here is a perfect example of ethical distress, I'd say. And I don't envy you at all," stated Sheila.

"So what are you going to do?" asked Maryann.

"Well, I like my job and I don't think this is worth quitting over, at least not without first communicating my distress to my supervisor. Like you, Maryann, I worry that I might hurt someone inadvertently, and this goes against my sense of professional duty to do no harm. You know how strongly this is reinforced by the AOTA code. I think there may also be legal liability issues involved, so maybe I need to talk with the risk manager of the clinic. But first I will talk with my supervisor and ask her what she thinks. I will also ask her to negotiate on behalf of the patient to get someone more qualified to do the paraffin baths."

"We're behind you on this one, buddy. The other COTAs at the clinic will be, too. I bet if you called the AOTA national office, their ethics consultant would back you up," suggested Sheila.

"But whatever you do, I think you better carefully document everything that is said and done so there is a clear record of your reasons for refusing and your efforts to negotiate a change in your assignment," cautioned Maryann.

Action: What Will I Do?

Inevitably, even in the most complex ethics cases, COTAs need to take some action. Doing nothing can also be perceived ethically as an action. If the previous steps have been considered in good conscience and the client's best interests have been prioritized, COTAs usually have an ethical basis for action. COTAs may retain a sense of uncertainty, but at least they will have the comfort of knowing that they have given deep thought to their position to articulate the basis for their action. Generally speaking, COTAs will most likely not have to act alone because of the input received from others.

Reporting the unethical behavior of a professional colleague or an institution is one of the most difficult actions to take. Nevertheless, if unethical conduct has been observed, COTAs have an ethical obligation to report this behavior to the authorities. In some states, this obligation is underscored by law. Thus, if COTAs know of a wrongdoing and do not report it, the law considers them guilty also.

Reporting another's unethical behavior is sometimes referred to as **whistle-blowing.** Especially when the COTA's job may be threatened, it can take courage to follow through with such a report. If possible, COTAs should work with the support of others, especially those in a supervisory position. Obviously this is difficult when a supervisor is the person being reported. Regardless of the circumstance, COTAs should make sure to document their actions so that their systematic efforts to address the problem are well established, especially if the COTA is in a less powerful position than the person being reported. Sometimes in a twist of logic, the whistle-blower becomes a scapegoat, or is blamed for another's unethical behavior. If COTAs have kept good records of their attempts to correct or resolve the situation, they will be more easily cleared of such an accusation.

Often, coworkers also will have observed unethical behavior and may feel similarly vulnerable. COTAs can sometimes increase the effectiveness of their responses if they work with others. When sharing information with others to gain support for their actions, COTAs must respect the confidentiality of persons and institutions by providing information fairly and appropriately.

If warranted, the authorities will dispense an appropriate punishment for wrongdoing after an investigation.

Who are the relevant authorities? The **AOTA Standards and Ethics Commission (SEC)** prepared a detailed discussion of where to go to seek guidance about reporting unethical conduct. It names three major bodies with jurisdiction over professional behavior (AOTA, 2002a).

COTAs may call or write the AOTA SEC. After discussing the possible violation of the Code of Ethics, COTAs can decide whether to file a formal complaint with the SEC. The SEC is responsible for writing the Code of Ethics and for imposing sanctions against AOTA members who do not follow it. Depending on the seriousness of the unethical behavior, the SEC will suggest public censure, temporary suspension of membership, or revocation or permanent loss of membership (AOTA, 2002a).

The **National Board for Certification in Occupational Therapy (NBCOT)** is responsible for certifying OTRs and COTAs. Depending on the significance of the unethical behavior that is reported, and after a thorough and confidential investigation, the NBCOT may take action against the practitioner in question. The most severe punishment available through the NBCOT is permanent denial or revocation of certification. (The NBCOT maintains a web page with up-to-date information at http://www.nbcot.org)

State Regulatory Boards, created by state legislatures, also may be helpful. These boards have the power to intervene if they determine the public to be at risk because of a practitioner's incompetence, lack of qualifications, or unlawful behavior. State boards can publicly reprimand a practitioner or, if warranted, may even prohibit someone from practicing in that state.

Finally, COTAs should gather copies of their state's licensure laws, the AOTA Code of Ethics (AOTA, 2000), and other documents from the AOTA that can help clarify ethical issues. Documents such as "Standards of Practice for Occupational Therapy" (AOTA, 1998), "Guide for Supervision of Occupational Therapy Personnel" (AOTA, 1999), and "Roles and Responsibilities of the Occupational Therapist and Occupational Therapy Assistant During the Delivery of Occupational Therapy Services" (AOTA, 2002b) also can give COTAs a basis for their ethical arguments.

CONCLUSION

Working with elders carries special rewards and responsibilities. Clinical and ethical competency is necessary to maximize clients' functional capacities and contribute to the dignity and self-worth required for autonomous decision making. COTAs bring comfort to their clients through skillful treatment and by acting as the client's agent in ensuring ethical care. A healing bond of trust is reinforced each time clients witness COTAs responding with a sense of ethical commitment in the fulfillment of their clients' best interests.

This chapter reviewed ethical challenges in geriatric care settings and presented a step-by-step method for responding in a conscientious, informed manner. The authors hope that readers will follow the strategies described when responding to events in their practices.

■ CHAPTER REVIEW QUESTIONS

1 Recall the discussion Sheila, Maryann, and Chris had about one of Sheila's clients at the psychiatric center who was being placed in restraints. At the end of that conversation, Chris stated, "After all, even unpleasant clients deserve the right to make choices and have some liberty, as long as they are not hurting themselves or others." What ethical term did you learn earlier in the chapter that summarizes Chris's statement?

2 Reread the case of Chris, the COTA expected to use paraffin baths with a client.
   a Identify the benefits and burdens to the client if Chris were to administer the paraffin bath.
   b Based on your calculations, is it ethical for Chris to do the procedure?
   c Who, if anyone, would you involve in supporting your decision if you were asked to use a modality for which you had not been trained?

3 Imagine that you are sitting with the three COTAs discussing the case that is described below. Suggest how you would guide their response to the ethical challenges facing Chris.

   Chris is concerned about recent changes in his supervision at the rehabilitation clinic, especially in the new home care work he is doing. He never sees his supervising OTR anymore. She does her evaluations in the evenings or on weekends, when he is not at work. She wants him to mail his notes for her to cosign, but he worries about client confidentiality, especially if the notes got lost in the mail. However, Chris is most concerned about some of the treatment being ordered for his older home care clients. He often feels pushed to

provide three or four units (15 minutes) of treatment when his older clients seem able to tolerate only one or two units per session. He suspects that the extra treatments are motivated by financial reasons and not by the well-being of his clients.
   a Awareness
      1 What kind of ethical problem(s) is Chris facing?
      2 Who is involved?
      3 What laws and institutional rules apply?
      4 What guidance does the AOTA Code of Ethics give?
      5 What are Chris' options?
   b Reflection
      1 Suggest strategies Chris can use for reflection.
      2 Provide reasons for your preferred response(s) to the problem(s) he faces.
   c Support
      1 Suggest strategies Chris might use for building support.
   d Action
      1 What should Chris do?

REFERENCES

American Occupational Therapy Association. (1998). Standards of practice for occupational therapy. *American Journal of Occupational Therapy, 52,* 866-869.

American Occupational Therapy Association. (1999). Guide for supervision of occupational therapy personnel. *American Journal of Occupational Therapy, 53,* 592-594.

American Occupational Therapy Association. (2000). Code of ethics. *American Journal of Occupational Therapy, 54,* 614-616.

American Occupational Therapy Association. (2002a). Enforcement procedure for the occupational therapy code of ethics. [WWW page]. URL http://www.aota.org/members/area2/links/link07.asp?PLACE=/members/area2/links/link07.asp

American Occupational Therapy Association. (2002b). Roles and responsibilities of the occupational therapist and occupational therapy assistant during the delivery of occupational therapy services. *OT Practice, 7*(15), 9-10.

Goldberg, N. (2001). *Thunder and lightning: Cracking open the writer's craft.* New York: Doubleday.

Jonsen, A. R. (1992). *The new medicine and the old ethics.* Cambridge, MA: Harvard University Press.

Purtilo, R. (1999). *Ethical dimensions in the health professions* (3rd ed.). Philadelphia, PA: WB Saunders.

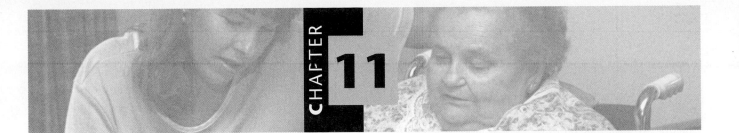

CHAPTER 11

Working with Families and Caregivers of Elders

ADA BOONE HOERL AND BARBARA JO RODRIGUES

KEY TERMS

social support system, family, caregivers, education, role changes, stress, community resources, abuse, neglect

CHAPTER OBJECTIVES

1. Define the role of the certified occupational therapy assistant in family and caregiver training.
2. Understand role changes within family systems at the onset of debilitating conditions in elders.
3. Discuss communication strategies that maximize comprehension during elder, family, and caregiver education.
4. Identify stressors that affect quality of care, ability to cope, and emotional responses in the elder/caregiver relationship.
5. Identify techniques to minimize caregiver stress.
6. Define and identify signs of elder abuse and neglect and discuss reporting requirements.

To provide optimal care, certified occupational therapy assistants (COTAs) must consider the many factors that influence an elder's functional abilities. When planning treatment, the occupational therapist (OTR) and COTA team consider not only physical and cognitive skills but also psychosocial factors that affect occupational performance potential. **Social support systems** such as spouse and **family** can significantly affect the outcome of occupational therapy (OT) intervention (Walens, 1996). COTAs must be able to interact with elders and their social support systems, especially the family, and treat elders and their families as units of care. This chapter addresses interaction between family members and **caregivers**.

ROLES FOR CERTIFIED OCCUPATIONAL THERAPY ASSISTANTS

For COTAs to define their roles in facilitating family interaction, they must first understand the family caregiver's role. Family members are not necessarily inherently skilled at caregiving. Frequently this role is unfamiliar and possibly unwanted. Caregivers must keep elders safe and clean and ensure that their daily physical needs are met. They must help elders maintain socialization and a sense of dignity. These tasks can be overwhelming for a family member who has little or no experience with debilitating and chronic illness. Ensuring that caregivers and elders work together effectively is crucial (Park, 1996).

COTAs should act as facilitators, educators, and resource personnel.

Development of elders' and caregivers' skills is achieved through selected activities with graded successes facilitated by COTAs. Activities that include family members and caregivers should be introduced as early as possible in the OT program to minimize dependence on COTAs. Facilitating interdependence between elders and their families and caregivers will ease the transition from one level of care to the next.

Effective elder, family, and caregiver **education** is a central component of care. Knowledge is empowering and encourages elders, family members, and caregivers to be responsible. Activities selected during the early stages of intervention need not be complex. They may include directions on positioning, simple passive range of motion exercises, and communication strategies. More training can follow as discharge planning progresses and the role of the caregiver becomes more clearly defined. Elder, family, and caregiver education is often required for activities of daily living, mobility, upper extremity management, behavioral management, and cognitive intervention strategies (Fig. 11-1). COTAs may help elders, family members, and caregivers understand the physician's diagnosis and prognosis of the medical condition and the functional implications of the condition. Insight regarding the specific physical, cognitive, and psychosocial impairments will aid caregivers in providing safe and appropriate assistance. Sometimes understanding the reasons for doing

a certain task is more important than demonstrating proficiency in its performance (Snow, 1988). For example, understanding principles of wrist protection that can be applied to every situation is more important for caregivers than correctly supervising the elder's use of radial wrist deviation to open a door each time. To maximize the effectiveness of the education, COTAs need to develop communication strategies (Box 11-1).

COTAs also act as resources for elders, family members, and caregivers. Depending on facility role delineation, COTAs may provide information about community and support services, as well as medical equipment vendors, paid caregivers, and respite programs. In collaboration with OTRs, COTAs may also serve as liaisons with other services. (Some resources are listed in the Appendix.)

COTAs can learn much about elders', family members', and caregivers' values, desires, and insights through frequent and close interaction. Elders may be unable to

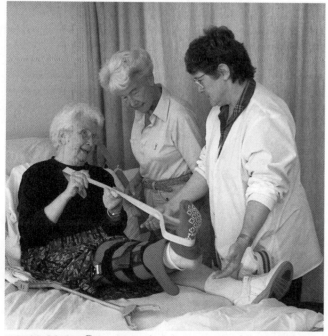

FIGURE 11-1 Caregiver education is a central component of the care that certified occupational therapy assistants provide.

BOX 11-1

Considerations for Effective Communication

1. Initially, make frequent, brief contacts to develop the relationship. This will familiarize the elder, family members, and caregivers with COTAs and their purpose.
2. Manage the environment in which communication occurs. Minimize distractions and interruptions.
3. Use responsive listening techniques. Maintain good eye contact, intermittently acknowledge statements made, and use body language that allows all parties to listen and respond. Be an active listener.
4. Use common terminology that nonmedical individuals understand. If a common term is available, use it. For example, use *shoulder blade* for *scapula*. Otherwise, define and explain concepts in simple terms.
5. Always respect client confidentiality. If able, secure permission from clients before discussing details with others.
6. Use open-ended questions to encourage self-expression. Be comfortable with brief silences.
7. Organize your ideas and avoid skipping between subjects. Focus on one topic at a time and clarify what you don't understand.
8. Provide education that will enable elders and their families to make informed choices. Do not offer advice or your personal opinion. Always acknowledge the right of choice.
9. Communicate with respect and warmth. Be supportive. Respond to feedback when given.
10. Do not promise if you cannot deliver.

express themselves for many reasons. Some limitations may be premorbid, whereas others, such as aphasia, may result from illness. COTAs may act as advocates for elders, helping meet needs that might otherwise go unacknowledged. COTAs may also act as advocates for family members and caregivers.

Like elders, families and caregivers may have needs that become evident only after close and frequent interaction. Because each individual's ability to provide caregiving differs, the OTR and COTA team must consider everyone's abilities when planning for facility discharge and family training.

All members of the treatment team, including COTAs, must educate elders, family members, and caregivers about the team's treatment recommendations. Recommendations may include plans for discharge, supervision, follow-up treatment, and home programs, and they must be clearly documented. When elders, families, and caregivers choose not to follow the team's recommendation, it is crucial to document all responses and actions to serve as a legal record if anyone is harmed. The more elders, family members, and caregivers are included in the formulation of plans, the more likely they are to comply with home programs and other discharge recommendations (Nolan, Davies, & Grant, 2001).

ROLE CHANGES IN THE FAMILY

Greater therapeutic outcomes are achieved when intervention does not focus solely on elders but also includes families and caregivers (Laver, 1996; Park, 1996). In addition to developing the elder's performance skills, "in the family-centered approach, the emphasis is on enabling the family to maximize function and social interaction of the dependent family member" (Humphrey, Gonzalez, & Taylor, 1993). This is especially important when lifestyle changes are required because of functional impairments.

Ideally, elders will consult family members when caregiving needs become evident. However, many variables affect a family system's abilities to meet the elder's needs. Some of these variables may include the treatment setting itself, cognitive deficits, psychological issues, the prior quality of family relationships, cultural and social influences, geographic distance, scheduling conflicts, financial resources, and advanced directives. COTAs must take all these factors into consideration during collaborative planning.

COTAs must consider role changes that occur for both elders and family during the course of an illness. OT should be designed around elders' and family members' skill levels. From that foundation, COTAs can facilitate adjustment to disability. With the onset of illness or disability, elders may feel a loss of independence, which can mean a major change in their sense of control and their role within the family.

Role changes also occur within the family unit during an elder's illnesses. Spouses may feel a deep sense of loss of a partner and may resent being solely responsible for previously shared tasks. In addition to a sense of loss, children must deal with the role reversal of being a parent to their own parent. Elders' disabilities and needs for caregiving may come at a time in children's lives when, for the first time, they find themselves free of family responsibilities and are planning for their own retirement. Family members are usually unprepared for the sudden changes that may occur with acute illnesses.

Roles within the family unit tend to be adjusted and adapted to gradually when elders have chronic or degenerative diseases. However, as the functional impairments accumulate into a major disability with significant activity limitations, modifications in roles are required (Rogers, 1996). Not knowing the length of the illness is often a source of added frustration. In addition, chronic conditions may involve long-term adaptations that demand a greater degree of self-care and responsibility on the part of elders and caregivers (Rogers, 1996).

Caregiver Stresses

An entire generation is moving into the caregiving role for their aging parents. These caregivers are changing their lives to assist their parents through the illness process. In addition to grieving for their parent, these caregivers may also be experiencing a loss of their own independence, privacy, financial security, safety, and comfort within their own homes. These losses may leave caregivers ultimately feeling guilty about their inadequacies or angry toward the debilitated elder.

Life changes for caregivers and their families. This changing process may be gradual, beginning with the elder experiencing mild confusion and only requiring assistance with bills. The change also may be sudden and immediate, with the elder surviving a stroke and needing total physical care. The care required may be temporary or permanent with no hope for rehabilitation. No matter what the situation, this change of life is stressful for everyone involved.

Approximately 12 million people in the United States assist 5 million ill family members or friends who need help to remain at home. Statistics indicate that 75% of caregivers are women, 25% of whom are caring for their own children and their elder parent. Half of all caregivers also work outside the home (U.S. Department of Health and Human Services, 2000). An estimated 16% to 23% of families across the United States are caring for adults with cognitive impairments, and 70% of the 4 million Americans with Alzheimer's disease are cared for at home (Family Caregiver Alliance, 1996). Financial concerns and home and life management add **stress** to caregivers' lives (Fig. 11-2).

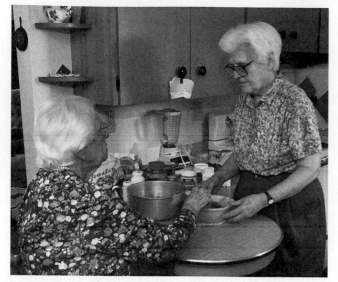

FIGURE 11-2   About 75% of caregivers are women, 25% of whom are caring for their own children and their elder parent.

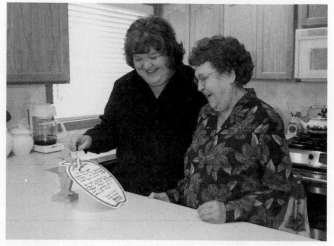

FIGURE 11-3   Caregiving may require various levels of assistance. This 90-year-old elder only needs a reminder to function in her environment while her daughter is at work.

Advice from physicians, nurses, and therapists and attempts at self-education about an unfamiliar illness also can add stress. The need to learn the language of health care workers can be stressful, especially for caregivers for whom English is a second language or caregivers who are functionally illiterate.

Stress also may be increased by family members who offer suggestions for caring for elders. When decisions are made by several relatives but one family member or caregiver is responsible for following through with the group's decisions, the caregiver can easily become overwhelmed and feel resentful.

Elders who need caregiving may require various levels of assistance, and their conditions may change frequently. At times little assistance may be needed, but there may be long periods when much more assistance is required (Fig. 11-3). Other family members may not understand the fluctuating assistance levels, and their perceptions of the work required to maintain the elder at home may not be accurate.

Family members may not understand their own emotions or those of the primary caregiver. Family members may deny feelings of guilt, frustration, anger, or grief. They also may be in denial about the level of care required and may not be ready to assist. Family members who are unable to understand their own emotions or the illness and needs of the elder may become angry with the caregiver for not allowing the elder more independence. They may be resentful and suspicious of the caregiver's motives or intentions, which can devastate caregivers and reduce the level of care they are willing to provide.

The demands and constraints of caregiving can become overwhelming. Caregivers may feel isolated and believe that they must be the sole providers of care. They may think they have no time for friends or support systems. Responsibilities can quickly become burdens, and caregivers may feel that they are not providing the needed assistance and are failing in their responsibilities to the elder. Caregivers may refuse assistance from others because they feel the home is not clean enough for others to visit, or they believe they are the only ones who can properly care for the elder. Caregivers may forget that the level of care they now provide is the result of months of practice and learning through trial and error. COTAs must become adept at identifying signs of caregiver stress to ensure that the elder's needs are being met (Box 11-2).

Family Resources

COTAs should continually assess the family's needs and resources and offer the best referrals possible, keeping in mind that family members may feel isolated and disconnected or may be reluctant to ask for assistance. It may first be necessary to assist family members in identifying their needs and willingness to accept assistance. The suggestion that they read a book about caregivers or attend a caregiver support group may be met with resistance. However, COTAs must provide support and guidance while family members go through the process of realizing their own needs. When family members are ready to ask for assistance, COTAs must be ready with reliable resources and referrals. Successful experiences encourage families to use available **community resources.** COTAs must help

BOX 11-2

Signs of Caregiver Stress

Too much stress can be damaging to both the caregiver and the elder. The following stress indicators, experienced frequently or simultaneously, can lead to more serious health problems.

1. The caregiver may deny the disease and its effect on the person who's been diagnosed. "I know Mom's going to get better."
2. The caregiver may express anger that no effective treatments or cures currently exist for chronic conditions such as Alzheimer's disease* and that people don't understand what's going on. "If he asks me that question one more time, I'll scream."
3. The caregiver may withdraw socially from friends and activities that once brought pleasure. "I don't care about getting together with the neighbors anymore."
4. The caregiver may express anxiety about facing another day and what the future holds. "What happens when he needs more care than I can provide?"
5. The caregiver may experience depression, which eventually breaks the spirit and affects coping ability. "I don't care anymore."
6. The caregiver may be exhausted, which makes it nearly impossible to complete necessary tasks. "I'm too tired for this."
7. The caregiver may experience sleeplessness caused by worrying. "What if she wanders out of the house or falls and hurts herself?"
8. The caregiver may express irritability, which may lead to moodiness and trigger negative responses and reactions. "Leave me alone!"
9. Lack of concentration on the part of the caregiver makes it difficult to perform familiar tasks. "I was so busy, I forgot we had an appointment."
10. The caregiver experiences mental and physical health problems. "I can't remember the last time I felt good."

Adapted from the Alzheimer's Association. (1995). *Ten signs of caregiver stress.* Chicago: The Association.
*For more information on Alzheimer's disease and services provided by the Alzheimer's Association, call 1-800-272-3900.

family members and caregivers understand that caring for themselves and accepting help will ultimately help them care for the elder. Caring for themselves and accepting help may also make it possible to offer care at home for a longer period (Box 11-3; Fig. 11-4).

Many community and national resources are available for families and caregivers. Support groups, publications, videos, and resources can be found in virtually every large community. In rural areas, organizations may be contacted by phone, in writing, or through computer technology. (An extensive resource and referral list is included in the Appendix.)

RECOGNIZING SIGNS AND REPORTING ELDER ABUSE OR NEGLECT

Unfortunately, **abuse** and **neglect** of elders do occur. All professionals working with elders must be informed of their responsibilities and prepare themselves to act on the elder's behalf should suspicion of abuse or neglect arise. Federal definitions of elder abuse have been included in the Older Americans Act since 1987. Each state also has its own definition of elder abuse through legislation on adult protective services. COTAs should contact their state's ombudsman or Adult Protective Services Office for more detailed and specific guidelines. Only general definitions and guidelines are presented in this chapter. Elders have a right to direct their own care, refuse care, and receive protection from being taken advantage of or hurt by others.

The National Aging Resource Center on Elder Abuse has identified and defined six types of elder abuse (Tatara & Kuzmeskus, 1999). Physical abuse is identified as nonaccidental use of physical force that results in bodily injury, pain, or impairment. Sexual abuse is defined as nonconsensual sexual contact of any kind with an elder. Emotional or psychological abuse is willful infliction of mental or emotional anguish by threat, humiliation, or other verbal or nonverbal abusive conduct. Neglect is the willful or nonwillful failure by the caregiver to his or her obligations or duties as a caretaker. Financial or material exploitation is an unauthorized use of an elder's funds, property, or resources. Self-abuse and neglect are abusive or neglectful methods of conduct of elders directed at themselves that threaten their health or safety.

Abuse may occur in the home or community setting, as well as in residential care, skilled nursing facilities (SNFs), or day health programs. In an effort to protect elders, every health care provider must be aware of signs and indicators of abuse. Indicators of abuse have been outlined in many documents available through agencies on aging (Disk, 1992). Physical abuse indicators include the presence of unexplained, inconsistent, and incompatible injuries. These may be bruises or welts, particularly if bilateral, clustered, or in patterns, or if in various stages of healing. Other signs are burns, particularly those that appear to be caused by cigarettes, caustic materials, and friction from ties; fractures or sprains; and lacerations or abrasions. Evidence of confinement, such as food dishes or remnants, excretory vessels, and ties on furniture should be evaluated. Behavioral signs of physical abuse include extremes in behavior, fearfulness, nonresponsiveness,

BOX 11-3

Ways to Reduce Caregiver Stress

1. Get a diagnosis as early as possible.

Symptoms may appear gradually, and if a person seems physically healthy, it's easy to ignore unusual behavior or attribute it to something else. See a physician when warning signs are present. Some dementia symptoms are treatable. Once you know what you're dealing with, you'll be able to better manage the present and plan for the future.

2. Know what resources are available.

For your own well-being and that of the person for whom you are caring, become familiar with care resources available in your community. Adult day care, in-home assistance, visiting nurses, and Meals on Wheels are just some of the community services that can help.

3. Become an educated caregiver.

As the disease progresses, different caregiving skills and capabilities are necessary. Care techniques and suggestions can help you better understand and cope with many of the challenging behavior and personality changes.

4. Get help.

Trying to do everything by yourself will leave you exhausted. The support of family, friends, and community resources can be an enormous help. If assistance is not offered, ask for it. If you have difficulty asking for assistance, have someone close to you advocate for you. If stress becomes overwhelming, don't be afraid to seek professional help. Support group meetings and help lines are also good sources of comfort and reassurance.

5. Take care of yourself.

Caregivers frequently devote themselves totally to those they care for and, in the process, neglect their own needs. Pay attention to yourself. Watch your diet, exercise, and get plenty of rest. Use respite services to take time off for shopping, a movie, or an uninterrupted visit with a friend. Those close to you, including the one for whom you are caring, want you to take care of yourself.

6. Manage your level of stress.

Stress can cause physical problems (blurred vision, stomach irritation, high blood pressure) and changes in behavior (irritability, lack of concentration, loss of appetite). Note your symptoms. Use relaxation techniques that work for you and consult a physician.

7. Accept changes as they occur.

Elders change and so do their needs. They often require care beyond what you can provide at home. A thorough investigation of available care options should make transitions easier, as will support and assistance from those who care about you and your loved one.

8. Do legal and financial planning.

Consult an attorney and discuss issues related to durable power of attorney, living wills and trusts, future medical care, housing, and other key considerations. Planning now will alleviate stress later. If possible and appropriate, involve the elder and other family members in planning activities and decisions.

9. Be realistic.

The care you provide does make a difference. Neither you nor the elder can control many of the circumstances and behaviors that will occur. Give yourself permission to grieve for the losses you experience, but also focus on the positive moments as they occur and enjoy your good memories.

10. Give yourself credit, not guilt.

You're only human. Occasionally, you may lose patience and at times be unable to provide all of the care the way you'd like. Remember, you're doing the best you can, so give yourself credit. Being a devoted caregiver is not something to feel guilty about. Your loved one needs you, and you are there. That's something to be proud of.

Adapted from the Alzheimer's Association. (1995). *Ten signs of caregiver stress.* Chicago: The Association.
For more information on Alzheimer's disease and services provided by the Alzheimer's Association, call 1-800-272-3900.

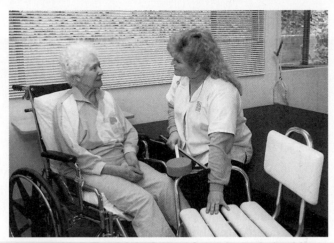

FIGURE 11-4 Careful discharge planning can help elders and caregivers feel less overwhelmed with changes.

agitation, trembling, hesitation to talk openly, implausible stories, anger, depression, withdrawal, contradictory statements not caused by mental dysfunction, and confusion (Disk, 1992). Because many of these indicators are also common symptoms of dementia and other forms of mental illness, careful observation skills are required to confirm or rule out causes of behaviors.

Indicators of neglect include unattended physical or mental problems such as neglected bedsores, untreated injuries, skin disorders and rashes, poor hygiene, and torn or unwashed clothing. Hunger, malnutrition, dehydration not caused by illness, and pallor, sunken eyes, and sunken cheeks may be potential signs of neglect. Unsanitary conditions in the home, fire hazards, inadequate heating or cooling, and insufficient food and water supply are associated with elder neglect. Neglect also may be indicated by the elder's helplessness, nonresponsiveness, and dependent behavior. Refusal to be helped, desire for social isolation, aggressiveness, agitation, detachment, hopelessness, and low self-esteem also may indicate other types of abuse, such as mental suffering or abandonment (Disk, 1992).

Sexual abuse may go unreported because of the elder's fear, embarrassment, shame, communication difficulties, or concern for the abuser. Sexual abuse may be identified by the presence of sexually transmitted diseases, genital discharge or infection, physical trauma to the anal or genital area, difficulty walking or sitting because of genital or anal pain, and painful urination or defecation. Behavioral indicators of sexual abuse may include changes in customary behavior, eating or sleeping disturbances, fears, phobias, overly compulsive behavior, inability to make eye contact, weeping, and fear of being left alone (Disk, 1992).

Fiduciary abuse indicators include inappropriate activity in bank accounts such as withdrawals from the automatic teller machine when the client is unable to leave home,

elder's lack of understanding of having given power of attorney to a care custodian, and another person's unusual interest in the amount of money being spent on care. Refusal to spend money on care, unpaid or overdue bills, and change of title of the elder's home suggest the possibility of fiduciary abuse. Other possible indicators include a recently redrawn will of an elder who is confused, lack of amenities for elders when their estate can afford them, and missing personal belongings. Isolating elders from friends and family, promising lifelong care in return for property, and requesting signatures on checks of incapacitated elders are additional signs of abuse (Disk, 1992).

Many states have enacted mandatory reporting laws that require professionals who regularly work with elders, including health workers such as COTAs, law enforcement personnel, and human service personnel, to report abuse. State and local agencies designated to receive and investigate reports and provide referral services to victims, families, and elders at risk for abuse include the Adult Protective Services Agency, long-term care ombudsman programs, law enforcement or local social service agencies, area agencies on aging, aging service providers, and aging advocacy groups. If elder abuse is suspected, these agencies can assist COTAs.

COTAs must report physical abuse if they witness an incident that reasonably appears to be physical abuse; find a physical injury of a suspicious nature, location, or repetition; or listen to an incident related by an elder or dependent adult. An immediate telephone call followed by a written report is often required. This report should include identifying information about the person filing the report, the victim, and the caregiver. In addition, the incident and condition of the victim and any other information leading the reporter to suspect abuse must be included. Although many facilities have designated personnel to carry out reporting, it is each individual's duty to report suspected abuse. Failure to report is a legally punishable misdemeanor in states with mandatory reporting laws.

CASE STUDY

Edward is an 85-year-old man who was referred for OT after triple bypass heart surgery. During the operation, he had a cerebrovascular accident (CVA) resulting in left side hemiplegia and neglect. Other symptoms were severe dysphagia and aspiration pneumonia requiring the use of a nasogastric feeding tube. Chronic urinary tract infections and incontinence required the use of a Foley catheter, supplemental oxygen was required at all times, and intravenous antibiotics were being administered daily.

Before being admitted to the hospital, Edward had been living with his wife, Valerie, and was functioning independently with an active social life. His daughter, Elaine, lived in the same small town and provided assistance when necessary. The plan was for Edward to stay in an SNF near his home until he stabilized medically and then to transfer to a rehabilitation hospital in a larger city. He would then return home when he was ready to live independently again.

During the OT evaluation and initial treatments, Valerie asked for thorough explanations of every aspect of therapy. She questioned how more activity could help her husband regain his strength. Edward quickly began to regain some usage of his left side and became involved in his own care. Valerie was pleased with Edward's recovery and enthusiastic about the care he was receiving. Edward seemed to look forward to the therapy sessions and saw them as important to his recovery. Valerie and Edward decided that he would stay at the SNF and continue rehabilitation services until he was independent enough to return home.

Over the next few weeks Edward showed improvement in activities of daily living, using adaptive equipment for dressing, and shaving with an electric razor. He gained strength and mobility in his left arm. Although he demonstrated increased independence during therapy or while alone, he began to show more dependence when Valerie was present. When dining alone or with the speech therapist, Edward ate independently with set-up, whereas when Valerie was present, he insisted that she feed him each bite of food and wipe his chin.

Edward's daughter approached the therapists about Edward's inconsistent behavior. She reported that although he could do things for himself, he saw it as her mother's responsibility to take care of him. Elaine suggested that all therapists involved in Edward's care make a list of things that Edward was capable of doing for himself. This list could be used as a reminder of what he could do safely. Elaine also asked that Edward be taught how to empty his catheter bag, as he had done before his surgery. She expressed concerns that her mother would try to do too much for her father and eventually would be unable to cope herself.

A meeting was arranged between Edward, Valerie, Elaine, and all therapists. Edward joked that he was "born lazy," and Valerie concurred that she tended to "baby" him. Elaine reminded Edward that if he wanted to return home he would need to be more independent. Edward again stated that his goal was to go home, although he admitted that it was easier and faster to let other people do things for him. The COTA invited Valerie to attend Edward's therapy sessions to simulate home activities with him. Although outwardly Edward showed no signs of depression, everyone involved in his care agreed that he seemed to have lost some of his motivation to return home. The meeting ended with setting up a home visit to assess any barriers for functional activities.

After the home evaluation, Edward appeared more motivated and stated that therapy seemed more relevant because he realized that it was preparing him for returning home. The final OT sessions included training for Edward and Valerie with transfers on a bath bench and using adaptive equipment, providing a home exercise program for Edward to follow, and suggesting that Valerie continue to encourage Edward to perform activities independently. Home health services were coordinated, and after tearfully thanking everyone, Edward was discharged.

Several weeks later, the home health agency contacted OT, inquiring about Edward's level of function at discharge, because during therapy visits it appeared that he was almost totally dependent on Valerie for all tasks and that she seemed overwhelmed caring for him.

CASE STUDY QUESTIONS

1 What communication strategies could the treatment team use to integrate the different viewpoints of Edward and his family?
2 How can the treatment team ensure that the gains in independence that Edward made in therapy will be self-sustaining?

CHAPTER REVIEW QUESTIONS

1 While working at a skilled nursing facility you approach a new elder who says, "My husband just left me here all alone. Oh, please help me, I want to go home." How should you respond?
2 You work in a rehabilitation unit. You recommend a tub transfer bench for an elder with hemiplegia. Medicare will not cover the expense of this bench. The family says, "We'll just rig something up when we get home." How should you respond?
3 You are working on an Alzheimer's disease special unit. An elder comes up to you, grabs your arm and says, "Momma, where have you been? I've been so afraid." As the elder continues to cling to your arm, you notice the elder's family members are watching. The elder's behavior escalates whenever a family member approaches. How should you respond?
4 The grown daughter of an elder approaches you and states, "My father has been an alcoholic all my life. He has been so mean to my mother. His being in the hospital is the first peace she's had in years. Please don't let my father come home." How should you respond?
5 You have worked closely with an elder for 2 weeks. After a week-long vacation you return to learn that the elder has refused treatment most of the week you were absent. The elder had stated, "I don't want anyone new! My family doesn't know how to help me." What steps should you have taken to minimize the elder's dependence on you?
6 On admission of their 87-year-old widowed father to an acute-care hospital, three adult children state that it is their desire to take him home and share the caregiving responsibilities when he is ready for discharge. During the 3-week hospitalization, staff members have seen the children visit only once. They also have not returned repeated phone calls by the social worker. What input should the certified occupational therapy assistant give to the treatment team in preparation for discharge?

REFERENCES

Administration on Aging. (2002). *Elder action: Action ideas for older persons and their families.* Washington, DC: Department of Health and Human Services.

Disk, K. (1992). *The elderly and dependent adults as crime victims: Abuse and neglect of California's elderly.* Sacramento, CA: State Department of Health.

Family Caregiver Alliance. (1996). *About brain impairments: Quick facts about common brain impairments.* San Francisco, CA: The Alliance.

Humphrey, R., Gonzalez, S., & Taylor, E. (1993). Family involvement in practice: issues and attitudes. *American Journal of Occupational Therapy, 47*(7), 587.

Laver, A. (1996). The Occupational Therapist Intervention Process. In K. Larson, R. Stevens-Ratchford, L. Pedretti, & J. Crabtree (Eds.), *The role of occupational therapy with the elderly.* Rockville, MD: American Occupational Therapy Association.

Nolan, M., Davies, S., & Grant, G. (2001). *Working with older people and their families.* Philadelphia, PA: Open University Press.

Park, S. (1996). Restoring occupational performance: Rehabilitation services for older adults. In K. Larson, R. Stevens-Ratchford, L. Pedretti, & J. Crabtree (Eds.), *The role of occupational therapy with the elderly.* Rockville, MD: American Occupational Therapy Association.

Rogers, J. (1996). Ability and disability: The performance areas. In K. Larson, R. Stevens-Ratchford, L. Pedretti, & J. Crabtree (Eds.), *The role of occupational therapy with the elderly.* Rockville, MD: American Occupational Therapy Association.

Snow, T. (1988). Working with the family. In L. Davis & M. Kirkland (Eds.), *The role of occupational therapy with the elderly.* Rockville, MD: American Occupational Therapy Association.

Tatara, T., & Kuzmeskus, L. (1999). *Types of elder abuse in domestic settings.* Washington, DC: National Center on Elder Abuse.

Walens, D. (1996). Collaboration as an effective approach to treatment. In K. Larson, R. Stevens-Ratchford, L. Pedretti, & J. Crabtree (Eds.), *The role of occupational therapy with the elderly.* Rockville, MD: American Occupational Therapy Association.

CHAPTER **12**

Addressing Sexuality of Elders

HELENE **L**OHMAN

KEY **T**ERMS

sexuality, values, myths, homosexuality, physiologic changes, nursing facilities,
permission, limited information, specific suggestions, and intensive therapy model

CHAPTER **O**BJECTIVES

1. Discuss the ways values can influence attitudes about elder
   sexuality.
2. Identify primary myths about elder sexuality.
3. Discuss how elder homosexuals have been ignored by
   society.
4. Describe normal, age-related, sexual, physiological changes.
5. Discuss the treatment team members' roles in addressing
   elders' sexual concerns.
6. Discuss the ways elders' sexuality is commonly dealt with
   in nursing facilities.

7. List the components of the permission, limited information, specific suggestions, and intensive therapy model and
   discuss ways the certified occupational therapy assistant
   can apply this model.
8. Identify strategies for elder sexual education.
9. List treatment ideas for addressing sexual concerns
   of elders who experience strokes, heart disease, and
   arthritis.
10. Increase personal comfort to discuss elder sexual
    concerns.

Jennifer is a certified occupational therapy assistant
(COTA) employed at an acute care hospital. A large part
of her caseload is elders who have sustained total hip
replacements. Treatment approaches are routine because
they are based on clinical pathways. Transfers, home situation, and safety precautions are typically reviewed
with people who have total hip repairs. One day a circumstance happened that resulted in Jennifer changing
her treatment approach. Jennifer was working with Sam,

an elder who had sustained a right total hip replacement.
After Jennifer went through the protocol for total hip
replacements she asked him if he had any questions.
"Yes," he responded, "my wife and I want to know when
we can have intimate relations." Jennifer felt a variety of
emotions. She felt perplexed, because she did not know
how to respond. She recalled blushing with embarrassment, stammering through a sentence stating that she
would get back with Sam, and abruptly leaving the room.

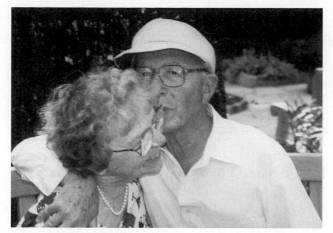

FIGURE **12-1**   Sexual expression is an important part of a person's life at any age. (Courtesy Helene Lohman, Creighton University, Omaha, NE.)

Afterwards Jennifer reflected about the situation. She wondered why she felt so embarrassed and what she could have done differently. She questioned whether she harbored feelings that elders should not be sexually active. After further reflection Jennifer took the initiative to learn more about sexuality and elders and to incorporate this knowledge into treatment.

COTAs who provide thorough treatment get to know elders as human beings first and develop an understanding of the person's daily life routines. Part of the daily life routines of many elders may involve sexual functioning. Sexual expression can be an important part of a person's life at any age and is related to a person's "self concept, self esteem and body image" (Pangman & Sequire, 2000). However, despite sexuality being so integral to human sexual expression, it may be ignored in clinical treatment for many reasons, including discomfort with one's own sexuality or with an elder or disabled person remaining sexually active. Other reasons may include a lack of understanding of normal sexual changes with aging and a lack of knowledge about sexual function with regard to age and disability. Dealing with the elder's concerns about sexual function should be part of clinical treatment. This chapter helps the COTA learn about this important but often ignored area of activities of daily living (ADL) intervention. Furthermore, the chapter helps to clarify myths and misconceptions (Fig. 12-1).

VALUES ABOUT SEXUALITY

Each generation has certain values reflective of society. In addition, all individuals have their own value systems. The current elder population is from a generation that did not often discuss sexuality (Goodwin & Scott, 1987). For some it was a necessity for procreation and

not a source of enjoyment. These are deeply held values that can influence the elder's comfort level when discussing sexual feelings during clinical treatment. In addition, the COTA may feel uncomfortable discussing sexual concerns with the elder, because sexuality is not usually an open topic. But generational values change, and it is predicted that the Baby Boomer generation, especially the women from that generation, may embrace more openness about sexuality (Jacoby, 1999). Exercises 12-1 and 12-2 should be completed before further reading to explore values regarding elders and sexuality.

Exercise 12-1: Generational Sexual Attitudes/ Values Inventory

Answer the following questions while considering your generation and the current elder generation (that is, 65 years and older). Fill in "yes" or "no" for each question, then discuss or contemplate your findings.

Yes = Acceptable
No = Unacceptable

1. It is appropriate to openly discuss sexual needs and concerns.
   Your generation _____
   Current elder generation _____
2. Sexual activity is acceptable in a non-marriage situation.
   Your generation _____
   Current elder generation _____
3. Sexual activity is appropriate if the purpose is physical pleasure.
   Your generation _____
   Current elder generation _____
4. Sexual activity is only for procreation.
   Your generation _____
   Current elder generation _____
5. The naked body is very private. Nudity is unacceptable.
   Your generation _____
   Current elder generation _____
6. Women should discuss their sexual needs with their partners.
   Your generation _____
   Current elder generation _____
7. It is appropriate for women to initiate sex.
   Your generation _____
   Current elder generation _____
8. Masturbation is a normal sexual act.
   Your generation _____
   Current elder generation _____
9. Sexual activity between people of the same sex is acceptable.
   Your generation _____
   Current elder generation _____

10. Sexual activity between adults of different generations is unacceptable.
    Your generation _____
    Current elder generation _____

These questions were adapted from a module by Goldstein & Runyon (1993).

■ Exercise 12-2: Personal Values Assessment

This exercise helps identify personal values and attitudes. Answer the following questions. On completion of this exercise, any uncomfortable feelings may be handled by using this chapter as an educational tool to help dispel myths and misconceptions and to clarify normal physiologic changes resulting from aging. After reading the chapter, the COTA can retake this personal value assessment to determine whether uncomfortable feelings have decreased.

1. Elders in nursing facilities should not be sexually active.
   Agree _____ Disagree _____
2. My grandparents (or parents) should not be sexually active.
   Agree _____ Disagree _____
3. It is acceptable for elder men to remain sexually active.
   Agree _____ Disagree _____
4. It is acceptable for elder women to remain sexually active.
   Agree _____ Disagree _____
5. It is immoral for elders to engage in recreational sex.
   Agree _____ Disagree _____
6. Sexual education is not necessary for elders.
   Agree _____ Disagree _____
7. Sexual education is not necessary for nursing facility staff.
   Agree _____ Disagree _____
8. Nursing facilities should provide large enough beds for couples to sleep together.
   Agree _____ Disagree _____
9. Nursing facilities should provide privacy for residents who desire sexual activity.
   Agree _____ Disagree _____

These questions are adapted from a scale developed by White (1982).

MYTHS ABOUT ELDERS AND SEXUAL FUNCTIONING

The media have provided people with misinformation and myths about elder sexual functioning. Television and magazine advertisements encourage people to ignore or to cover up the aging process. Greeting cards make fun of aging and suggest that lying about age is acceptable. Some media sources encourage myths about sexuality such as "the dirty old man syndrome." In addition, myths can be perpetuated by family members, peers, or elders themselves. With this inundation of misinformation, many people believe myths instead of truths about the sexual functioning of elders. Exercise 12-3 helps determine personal myths about elders and sexuality.

■ Exercise 12-3: Myths About Geriatric Sexuality

For each question below, answer T if the statement reflects a myth or F if the statement does not reflect a myth (the answers appear at the end of the chapter directly before the References).

1. T F   Elders are no longer interested in sexuality.
2. T F   Elders no longer engage in sexual activity.
3. T F   Elders engage in a wide variety of sexual activity, including intercourse, cuddling, caressing, mutual stimulation, and oral sex.
4. T F   Elders in nursing facilities should be segregated according to sex; sexual functioning should be prohibited.
5. T F   Elder women are unattractive.
6. T F   More elder men remain sexually active than elder women.
7. T F   Elders are too frail to engage in sexual activity.
8. T F   Inability to maintain an erection (erectile dysfunction) is *not* a natural consequence of aging.
9. T F   All elders are heterosexual.

These questions were adapted from Comfort & Dial (1991), Goodwin & Scott (1987), Hammond (1989), Morrison-Beedy & Robbins L (1989), and Pfeiffer, Verwoerdt, & Wang (1968).

Discussion of Myths

Findings from a recent survey study by the American Association of Retired Persons (AARP; n = 1384) (AARP, 1999) provide perspective about some of these myths about geriatric sexuality. A key finding was that elders of both sexes considered sexuality and the accompanying relationships as contributing to their quality of life (Fig. 12-2). However, a greater percentage of elder men than women valued sexual activity as contributing to their quality of life. Nevertheless, sexuality was perceived as an integral part of these elders' lives, not something they avoided. Furthermore, many elder men found their partner to be attractive, with the greatest percentage (63%) having this viewpoint being male respondents older than 75 years. This same finding occurred in more than 57% of the elder women older than 75 years. In addition, women older than 75 years were more likely to describe their partners as romantic as compared with their younger

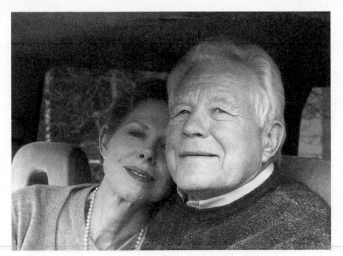

FIGURE **12-2**   Elders consider sexuality and satisfying relationships as contributors to their quality of life.

counterparts (53% older than 75 years compared with 29% younger than 60 years) (Jacoby, 1999). Thus, these findings contradict the societal myths that equate age with unattractiveness and lack of romance. Health decline and lack of partners were major contributing factor to decreased sexual activity (AARP, 1999). However, partners who were strongly connected emotionally continued having sexual relationships even with health problems (Jacoby, 1999).

The AARP study (AARP, 1999) together with other literature (Meston, 1997) suggests that for women sexual activity often stops because of lack of a partner. Approximately half of older women are widows and there are almost four times as many widows as widowers (U.S. Department of Health and Human Services [DHHS], 2001). In addition, some elder women believe the myth that they are unattractive and therefore should remain abstinent from sexual relationships. Furthermore, the current elder generation's values are strongly against women being sexually active without a husband. A finding from the AARP study (AARP, 1999) verified this concept. Values against sexual relationships outside of marriage were strongest among elder women older than 75 years, but were not strong among elder male subjects of any age (Jacoby, 1999).

Both older men and older women may experience pressure from their children to remain abstinent. Some adult children may find it difficult to think of their parents as having normal sexual desires, especially if the parent is in a nursing facility (Gibson, Bol, Woodbury, Beaton, & Janke, 1999).

Most men experience occasional impotence or erectile dysfunction by the time they are elder (Starr, 2001) because of fatigue, stress, illness, or alcohol (Lerner, 2000).

However, erectile dysfunction is not considered to be a normal part of aging (Meston, 1997). In the AARP study (1999), approximately one in four men admitted to some degree of erectile dysfunction. Men can continue to have normal sexual activity throughout their lives. Minor physiologic changes may have some effect on sexual functioning. For example, a benefit from physiologic aging can be delayed ejaculation, which can increase sexual pleasure for the partner (Laflin, 2002).

For elder men who have erectile dysfunction, new medications can help, such as Viagra (Pfizer U.S. Pharmaceutical Group, New York), which increases the vascular flow to the genitals. However, caution must be taken in prescribing Viagra because erectile dysfunction is complex, involving physical and psychological factors. In addition, Viagra, like any medication, has side effects and interactions with other medications (Starr, 2001). Media coverage about Viagra may have a positive impact in opening up discussions about erectile dysfunction, a subject not commonly discussed (Jacoby, 1999).

Most elders, especially the young old (that is, those 65 to 75 years of age), have active lives in which sexuality can remain an important component. Most likely, if a couple has always been sexually active, they will continue to be so as they grow older. As with any age group, communication is important for a positive sexual relationship. Frailty and disability do not automatically necessitate cause for an elder to be abstinent, although as findings from the AARP study suggest, having a disability or health problem does contribute to decreased sexual activity (AARP, 1999) (Fig. 12-3).

ELDER HOMOSEXUALS

Society has often ignored homosexuality in elders. Overall, society has embraced a "heteronormativity"

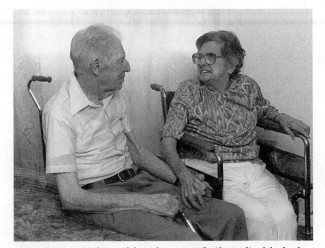

FIGURE **12-3**   When elders become frail or disabled, they do not necessarily become asexual.

viewpoint, or "a general perspective which sees heterosexual experiences as the only, or central view of the world" (Harrison, 2001, p. 143). Obviously, the elder cohort is diverse in terms of income, race, health status, and sexual orientation. Within this cohort the elder homosexual population also has a diverse background (Kimmel, 2001). The invisibility of the homosexual population is reflected in the paucity of research about homosexual elders (Wojciechowski, 1998). In occupational therapy literature, only a few articles have considered the homosexual experience (Birkholtz & Blair, 1999; Jackson, 1995, 2000; Walsh & Crepeau, 1998), and even fewer have considered elder homosexuals (Harrison, 2001).

Many elder homosexuals may be uncomfortable sharing about their sexuality, having grown up in a time when overt prejudice was expressed toward homosexuals (Wojciechowski, 1998). Homosexuality was defined as a mental illness in the *Diagnostics and Statistical Manual of Mental Disorders* until 1986 (Wojciechowski, 1998). Discrimination continues to exist with examples of lesbian couples who want to live together in long-term care facilities being denied rooms (Wojciechowski, 1998). Social Security does not recognize a life-long companion for benefits, and many medical and other legal decisions are made by family members rather than a person's partner (Kimmel, 2001).

COTAs can help dispel myths by simple actions such as the use of more inclusive language. As Harrison (2001) suggests, asking who are significant others in a person's life rather than who is a person's spouse can help create a more open conversation. Times are changing and there are now organizations that advocate for elder homosexuals, such as the National Association of Lesbian and Gay Gerontology, Lesbian and Aging Issues Network, and a Lesbian and Gay Aging Network with the American Society on Aging (Harrison, 2001; Kimmel, 2001).

Normal Age-related Physiological Changes in Men and Women

With normal aging, physiological changes might affect sexual functioning. Knowledge of these changes may help the COTA counsel the elder (Box 12-1). Not all these changes happen to every elder, and the degree varies among individuals (Glass & Dalton, 1988). In addition, COTAs should be aware of the concept "use it or lose it." Elders who remain sexually active may not experience some of these physiological changes or not to the same degree as elders who do not remain sexually active.

BOX 12-1

Age-related Physiologic Changes and Sexual Responses

Women
1. Decrease in rate and amount of vaginal lubrication may possibly lead to painful intercourse (Meston, 1997; Zeiss & Kasl-Godley, 2001).
2. Orgasmic phase decrease may occur in elder women (Laflin, 2002).
3. Structural changes or atrophy may occur in the labia or uterus, in addition to a reduction in the expansion of the vagina width (Laflin, 2002; Meston, 1997; Zeiss & Kasl-Godley, 2001).
4. Thinning of the lining of the vagina can result in irritation and painful intercourse (Meston, 1997).

Men
1. Erection is slower, less full, and disappears quickly after orgasm. Erection has a longer refractory period. A man in his 80s may need to wait several days as compared with a man in his 20s, in whom refractory period is a few minutes (Schiavi & Rehman, 1995).
2. Elder men may experience a decrease in penile rigidity (Schiavi & Rehman, 1995).
3. A decreased volume of sperm occurs; although fertility level is decreased, men do not become sterile (Laflin, 2002).
4. Decreased penile sensitivity results in increased need for direct penile stimulation over other forms of stimulation such as visual or psychological (Schiavi & Rehman, 1995).
5. Ejaculatory control increases, and ejaculation may occur every third sexual episode as a result of less preoccupation with orgasm (Laflin, 2002).
6. Ejaculation is less strong, and orgasm is often less intense (Laflin, 2002; Meston, 1997).
7. Decrease in ejaculatory testosterone occurs, although most elder men have the minimal level for sexual functioning (Meston, 1997).
8. Reduced size of testicles and increased size of prostate gland (Schiavi & Rehman, 1995).

Adapted from Goldstein & Runyon (1993).

Furthermore, these physiologic changes are just one aspect of sexuality. Sexuality is complex and involves psychological, spiritual, social, and cultural dimensions of a human being (Pangman & Sequire, 2000). The ways a person reacts to and perceives these physiologic changes ultimately affect sexual functioning. COTAs can apply this knowledge to educate elders. For example, a commercially available lubricant can supplement decreased vaginal secretion and can help reduce abrasion from thinning of the vaginal lining. Lubrication may also prevent dyspareunia, or painful intercourse (Lohman & Runyon, 1995). Kegel exercises help preserve vaginal tone and reduce symptoms of incontinence (Mueller, 1997).

ROLE OF TREATMENT IN SEXUAL EDUCATION

COTAs, occupational therapists (OTRs), and elders should collaborate to address concerns about sexuality. In addition, COTAs should be aware of other team members' areas of expertise. Sexual dysfunction such as erectile problems, ejaculatory disturbances, anorgasmia (lack of orgasm), and pain during intercourse may be caused by side effects of medication and other physiologic reasons. The physician and pharmacist must be notified about these concerns. Sexual dysfunction has a psychological component. Therefore, the client should be referred for counseling with a social worker or psychologist who has expertise with elders who have disabilities and sexual dysfunction. In addition to the OTR/COTA team, some physical therapists and nurses may educate the client about sexual positioning. Speech therapists may assist elders who have difficulties with communication (Lohman & Runyon, 1995).

ADDRESSING ELDER SEXUALITY IN A NURSING FACILITY

Trends in public policy and in professional literature suggest a more accepting attitude of sexual activity in nursing facilities (Fig. 12-4). Federal laws regulate privacy for institutionalized patients (Omnibus Budget Reconciliation Act, 1987). Professional literature since the 1990s has generally encouraged a more accepting attitude of sexuality in nursing home settings (Gibson, Bol, Woodbury, Beaton, & Janke, 1999). However, despite these positive trends, challenges still exist in nursing home facilities. These challenges include availability of privacy (Gibson, Bol, Woodbury, Beaton, & Janke , 1999), dealing with sexual behavior of residents who have cognitive impairments (Doyle, Bisson, Janes, Lynch & Martin, 1999), and addressing sexual concerns of residents with chronic conditions (Ghusn, 1995). In addition, negative attitudes and viewpoints against sexual activity of elders are expressed by some staff (Doyle, Bisson, Janes, Lynch, & Martin, 1999), spouses, and residents (Gibson, Bol, Woodbury, Beaton, & Janke, 1999). Staff may express

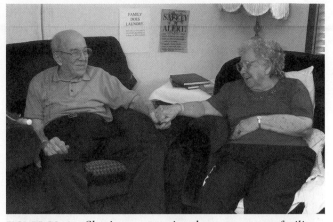

FIGURE 12-4 Sharing a room in a long-term care facility, these elders are able to enjoy the companionship of their lifelong spouse.

their disapproval in many ways. One subtle way is by joking about sexual activity, which may serve as a means to make elders conform to the expectation of asexuality in some nursing facilities.

In some institutional settings, envisioning elders being interested in sex is difficult and the elders themselves may be intolerant of peer engagement in sexual behavior (Gibson, Bol, Woodbury, Beaton, & Janke, 1999). Generational beliefs or societal expectations may influence these attitudes (Ghusn, 1995). Mulligan and Palguta (1991) found that male elders in nursing home facilities displayed continued interest in sex and were sexually active if a partner was available.

Sexuality does not only include sexual intercourse. It also involves touching, hugging, masturbation, and expressing the self as a sexual being (Lyder, 1991). COTAs participating in program planning can suggest dances and other social events that encourage romance and human touch. They can encourage elders to be well dressed and well groomed. In addition, COTAs should always be aware of respecting client privacy. Shutting a curtain between beds or going to another room for treatment with personal ADL functions helps to preserve privacy rights (Figs. 12-5 and 12-6).

Elders should reside in a supportive environment that encourages involvement in sexual activity (Ghusn, 1995). Residents should be involved in setting standards for sexual behavior within the community (Gibson, Bol, Woodbury, Beaton, & Janke, 1999) because most nursing home residents and staff support sexual rights (Ghusn, 1995).

Finally, education can help dispel myths and misconceptions about sexuality and elders (Lohman & Aitken, 1995). COTAs who have positive attitudes and are educated about sexuality and elders can help to dispel the ageist attitudes sometimes held by nursing home staff, family members, or the elders themselves.

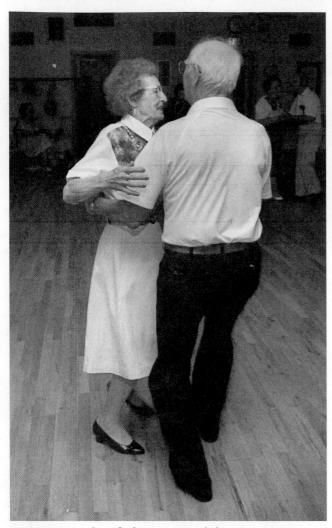

FIGURE 12-5   Certified occupational therapy assistants may suggest dances and other social events that encourage romance and affectionate touch.

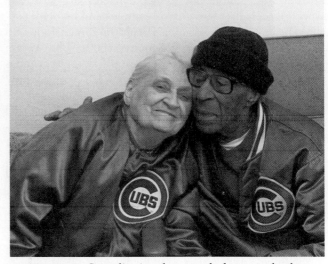

FIGURE 12-6   Sexuality involves touch, hugs, and other forms of expression.

EDUCATING AND COUNSELING THE ELDER CLIENT
The Permission, Limited Information, Specific Suggestions, and Intensive Therapy Model

Treatment models may help to provide sexual education to elders. The permission, limited information, specific suggestions, and intensive therapy (PLISSIT) model developed by Annon (1974, 1976) is a useful format for presenting sexual education information (Box 12-2).

COTAs can use the first, second, and third stages of this model during treatment. The elder must be assured of confidentiality throughout the educational process. In the first stage of the PLISSIT model, permission, the COTA applies therapeutic listening skills. The verbal and nonverbal body language of the COTA must show comfort with the topic. COTAs can ask questions in a

nonthreatening manner to encourage communication about sexual functioning during the ADL assessment (Goldstein & Runyon, 1993). In addition, the COTA can convey that sexuality is a normal part of every human's needs throughout a lifetime (Kessel, 2001). Elders who are interested in discussing sexuality may have general questions about normal sexual changes with aging or common myths. The spouse or partner should be encouraged to join the discussion.

In the second stage of the model, the COTA can apply limited information by relating knowledge of sexuality gleaned from this chapter and other relevant sources. The COTA can provide specific suggestions in the third stage. Many suggestions to help elders who have disabling conditions and their partners maintain sexual function are discussed in this chapter. The COTA should refer the elder who needs psychological support at any point of the education process to the appropriate counselor. The fourth stage of the model, intensive therapy, involves the skills of a trained counselor and is especially important for those elders experiencing sexual dysfunction.

Role of the Certified Occupational Therapy Assistant in Sexual Education

To provide elders with adequate sex education, COTAs must have a general knowledge about medical conditions, awareness of psychological issues, and an understanding of the importance of good communication. Understanding the effects of a disease or disabling condition on sexual performance is necessary. COTAs must remember that the manifestations of a disease or condition differ with each person, and often sexual functioning has to do with how a person adapts to life changes

BOX 12-2

The PLISSIT Model

P = Permission
This stage involves listening in a nonjudgmental, knowledgeable, and relaxed manner as the client discusses sexual concerns. General questions can be asked in an intake or screening evaluation (for example, "Do you have any concerns about the effects of your disease on sexual function?").

LI = Limited information
At this level, the elder can be educated about normal physiologic changes with aging, myths and stereotypes about the elder population, and sexuality and psychosocial factors that may inhibit or stress the elder.

SS = Specific suggestions
At this level, COTAs may make appropriate suggestions for improved sexual functioning. Elders also may need to be referred to specialists such as social workers, psychologists, and physical or occupational therapists.

IT = Intensive therapy
This level of counseling involves the expertise of a skilled social worker, psychologist, or psychiatrist.

Adapted from Lohman & Runyon (1995).

(Lerner, 2000). The following are some general education suggestions:

1. Encourage elders to maintain good communication with their partners in all aspects of their lives, not just about sexuality (Laflin, 2002).
2. Encourage elders to experiment with different sexual positions for comfort (Laflin, 2002).
3. Provide instruction on energy conservation techniques. Suggest resting before sexual activity (Goldstein & Runyon, 1993).
4. Encourage elders with decreased energy to explore other forms of sexual expression such as caressing, masturbation, and oral sex (Laflin, 2002).
5. Reassure elders that once they are medically stable and their physician has assessed them they can reassume sexual activity (Mueller, 1997).
6. Talk with elders about any fears they may have about resuming sexual functioning (Goldstein & Runyon, 1993).

The specific sexual concerns of elders who have experienced cerebrovascular accidents (CVAs), heart disease, and arthritis are discussed in the following sections.

EFFECTS OF HEALTH CONDITIONS ON ELDER SEXUALITY
Cerebrovascular Accident

COTAs commonly work with elders who have sustained CVAs or strokes. Dealing with sexual concerns after a stroke is often ignored (Miracle & Miracle, 2001). Addressing sexuality should be one of many aspects of a thorough evaluation. Just as the outcomes after a stroke are complex and different for each person, so are the impacts of a stroke on sexuality. It is not unusual for someone after a stroke to experience a decreased desire for sexual activity and decreased satisfaction with sexual activity (Edmans, 1998; Korpelainen, Nieminen & Myllyla, 1999). Changes after a CVA have been linked to a person's attitude about sexual activity and to fears about having erectile dysfunction, experiencing rejection, or having another stroke (Korpelainen, Niemulen & Myllyla, 1999; Monga & Ostermann, 1995). Changes in one's body image and one's coping skills can be psychological manifestations (Monga & Ostermann, 1995). Being aphasic, having functional changes, displaying difficulties in arousal, and taking certain medications that have side effects on sexual performance also can influence sexual activity (Monga & Ostermann, 1995). Many of these changes may indicate a need for intervention about sexuality, and COTAs can play a strong role because of their background in working with people who have had CVAs. However, in considering any intervention, COTAs should keep in mind the concept that sexual dysfunctions after a CVA will likely result from multilateral causes (Monga & Ostermann, 1995); therefore, use of clinical reasoning skills (Mattingly & Fleming, 1994) will be important.

COTAs should observe for motor abnormalities and other symptoms that can affect sexual function, including hemiplegia; perceptual, cognitive, and visual spatial disturbances; speech problems; emotional manifestations; and sensory deficits. For example, if elders are depressed, they may have no interest in sex. Anxiety may cause sexual performance problems such as male impotence and decreased female lubrication leading to painful intercourse. If elders have unilateral neglect, they may ignore one side of the body during sexual performance. Expressive aphasia may result in difficulty stating sexual needs. Sensory deficits such as esthesia or hyperesthesia on the affected side may affect sexual pleasure (Zukas, Ross-Robinson, 1991). Motor disturbances such as muscle weakness or hypertonia can make sexual performance awkward (Zukas, Ross-Robinson, 1991). (See Chapter 19 for a detailed discussion about CVA.)

After identifying the symptoms that affect sexual performance, the OTR and the COTA should collaborate with the elder to develop specific treatment suggestions. For example, clients with hemiplegia are sometimes advised to lie on the affected side so that the unaffected arm is free to caress the partner (Burgener & Logan, 1989), or to just find a comfortable position (Laflin, 2002). Simple adaptations such as using pillows under the affected side, raising the headboard, and adding a bed trapeze can help with motor manifestations of the CVA (Zukas & Ross-Robinson, 1991). Touch and other forms of nonverbal communication are useful with elders who have expressive aphasia (Laflin, 2002). The partners of elders with visual field deficits should be encouraged to approach from the impaired side and use touch on both sides. Minimizing environmental distractions during sexual activity may help elders with cognitive deficits involving concentration (Neistadt & Freda, 1987).

Beyond the physical effects of a CVA, some elders may experience low self-esteem and depression. These symptoms can affect sexual desire and performance (Monga & Ostermann, 1995). Elders who are in some way dependent on a partner may feel ambivalent about resuming a sexual relationship because of role changes (Mooradian, 1991). In addition, elders may worry about sustaining another CVA (Monga & Ostermann, 1995). Elders with these psychological manifestations may require counseling.

Heart Disease

Heart disease is one of the most common chronic ailments affecting the elder population (DHHS, 2001). Elders can have acute cardiac conditions, such as myocardial infarctions (MI), or chronic cardiac conditions, such as hypertension. With either type of cardiac condition the possible impact on sexuality should not be ignored. Elders should consult their physician for recommendations about sexual activity and cardiac conditions. DeBusk et al. (2000) developed a classification system to use as a guideline for physician's recommendations to manage sexual activity in patients with cardiac disease. With this classification system patients are divided into low, medium, or high cardiac risk. Patients with low risk, such as having controlled hypertension or mild stable angina, are recommended to safely resume sex. Patients with moderate risk, such as sustaining a recent MI or displaying moderate angina, require further cardiac evaluation. Patients in the high-risk category, such as having unstable angina or hypertension, are recommended to be stabilized before reassuming sexual activity. Table 12-1 summarizes this classification system.

Once stabilized, some elders with cardiac conditions may be instructed to resume sexual activity in a gradual manner (Steinke, 2000). For elders who gradually reassume sexual activity alternative forms of sexuality other than intercourse can be suggested. However, before reassuming sexual activity, elders should be instructed by the medical team about precautions and when to notify their physician.

Examples of precautions for sexual activity are chest pain, shortness of breath, excessive fatigue, and continuous increase in blood pressure after sex or heart palpitations lasting longer than 15 minutes after sex (Mueller, 1997; Steinke, 2000). The medical team also should be aware of negative side effects of common cardiac medications, herbal supplements, or illicit drugs that can influence libido or result in sexual dysfunction (Mueller, 1997; Steinke, 2000).

Sustaining a cardiac condition can impact a person psychologically, resulting in fears about resuming sexuality. The resumption of sexual activity after a heart attack is believed by some people to cause future cardiac incidents and even death (Steinke, 2000). Findings from a study (n = 1774) published in the *Journal of the American Medical Association* helps to clarify anecdotal information. Sexual activity was found to contribute to MIs in a small number of the subjects (0.9%), and regular exercise was related to a decreased risk (Muller, Mittleman, Maclure, Sherwood, & Tofler, 1996). Elders need to be educated that the physical demands of sexual activity are equal to mild to moderate exercise ("heart rate rarely increases to greater than 130 beats per minute and systolic blood pressure is rarely greater than 170 mm Hg"; DeBusk et al., 2000, p. 176).

Relaxation is important because fears and anxieties are common after cardiac incidents, especially about reassuming sexual relationships (Westlake, Dracup, Walden, & Fonarow, 1999). In addition, it is not uncommon to be depressed (American Heart Association, 2002). Sexual dysfunctions can develop because of these anxieties (Laflin, 2002). Sexual dysfunctions such as erectile problems also can result from physical reasons such as arteriosclerosis (hardening of the arteries) (Miracle & Miracle, 2001). Furthermore, one must consider the sexual activity of the person before the cardiac incident (Lerner, 2000). Using positions that require less energy expenditure and encouraging relaxation with sexual activity are helpful suggestions (American Heart Association, 2002). COTAs can teach elders stress reduction techniques. Energy conservation

TABLE **12-1**

Management Recommendations Based on Graded Cardiovascular (CV) Risk Assessment

Grade of risk	Categories of CVD	Management recommendations
Low risk	■ Asymptomatic, <3 major risk factors for CAD ■ Controlled hypertension ■ Mild, stable angina ■ Post-successful coronary revascularization ■ Uncomplicated past MI (>6-8 wk) ■ Mild valvular disease ■ LVD/CHF (NYHA class 1)	■ Primary-care management ■ Consider all first-line therapies ■ Reassess at regular intervals (6-12 mo)
Intermediate risk	■ ≥3 major risk factors for CAD, excluding gender ■ Moderate, stable angina ■ Recent MI (>2, <6 wk) ■ LVD/CHF (NYHA class II) ■ Noncardiac sequelae of atherosclerotic disease (e.g., CVA, peripheral vascular disease)	■ Specialized CV testing (e.g., ETT, Echo) ■ Restratification into high risk or low risk based on the results of CV assessment
High risk	■ Unstable or refractory angina ■ Uncontrolled hypertension ■ LVD/CHF (NYHA class III/IV) ■ Recent MI (<2 wk), CVA ■ High-risk arrhythmias ■ Hypertrophic obstructive and other cardiomyopathies ■ Moderate/severe valvular disease	■ Priority referral for specialized CV management ■ Treatment for sexual dysfunction to be deferred until cardiac condition stabilized and dependent on specialist recommendations

From DeBusk et al. (2000), with permission of Excerpta Medica, Inc.
CAD, coronary artery disease; CHF, congestive heart failure; CVA, cerebrovascular accident (stroke); CVD, cardiovascular disease; Echo, echocardiogram; ETT, exercise tolerance test; LVD, left ventricular dysfunction; NYHA, New York Heart Association.

techniques also may be helpful for those who are gradually building up their endurance. It is also beneficial to wait 1 to 3 hours after meals to allow the heart to pump blood to assist with the digestive process (Steinke, 2000). Per the PLISSIT model (Annon 1974, 1976), COTAs may need to refer the elder to an expert to address any sexual dysfunction. (See Chapter 23 for a more detailed discussion about cardiac concerns and the elderly.)

Arthritis

Arthritis is another common chronic condition among elders. All types of arthritis, including osteoarthritis and rheumatoid arthritis, can influence sexual function with physical and psychological effects. Physical concerns can be pain, functional limitations, fatigue, medication side effects, and genital lesions with some types of arthritis. Psychological problems include but are not limited to depression, anxiety, and loss of self-esteem (Lim, 1995). In addition, less opportunity to meet potential partners because of isolation and physical separation from one's partner because of repeated hospitalizations are other psychological concerns (Lim, 1995).

Elders with joint inflammation and pain may be particularly prone to sexual performance problems. A common treatment goal for people with rheumatoid arthritis is to maintain or increase functional abilities in all areas of life (Yasuda, 2002), including sexual function. COTAs can make specific suggestions to help elders reduce joint pain and discomfort and preserve energy. Exercises to increase and maintain muscle strength affect the motor aspect of sexual performance. Elders should be encouraged to use a heating pad or tub bath before sexual activity to help decrease joint pain and inflammation. Elders and their partners also may experiment with various sexual positions that decrease joint pressure. Rest and energy conservation techniques may help make sexual performance less fatiguing (Goldstein & Runyon, 1993). Finding the best time of day for sexual activity when the elder is less fatigued helps sexual performance (Whittington, Mansour & Sloan, 1995).

Joint Replacements

Elders with a history of arthritis commonly sustain joint replacements. Elders after total hip replacements are counseled to follow certain precautions in all areas of their lives, including sexuality. For an elder who has had a total hip replacement (posterolateral approach), it is important to review that with any sexual activity, or life activity, the elder should not flex the affected hip more than 90 degrees (Whittington, Mansour, & Sloan, 2001) and that the affected hip should not be adducted or externally rotated (Coleman, 2002). Once past the customary healing period of approximately 6 weeks and with physician approval, these elders can resume sexual activity as long as they follow precautions.

For intercourse, it is preferable with either sex that the elder with the total hip replacement be positioned supine (on back) with hips abducted (apart), knees in extension (straight), and legs in neutral (toes pointed up), and not in external rotation (toes pointed out) (Whittington, Mansour, & Sloan, 2001). Intercourse in a side lying position for the involved elder woman is accomplished by lying on her unaffected side with a minimum of two pillows between her legs to keep them abducted. The involved man using a side lying position should also lie on his unaffected side and should "use his partner's legs to support his affected leg." Thus, the man's affected leg is on top of his partner's leg during sexual intercourse. The elder man's partner should have a minimum of two pillows between her legs for support and to help her partner follow precautions (Whittington, Mansour, & Sloan, 2001, p. 7). Other suggestions are pillows between the knees to help maintain the hip joints in abduction, and pillows under the knees while in a supine position can prevent extreme external rotation (Coleman, 2002).

After a total knee replacement, elders should be instructed to find the most comfortable position for intercourse. When the involved person is in a supine position, pillows can be placed under the knee and the person can bend the knee within a comfortable range (Whittington, Mansour, & Sloan, 2001). A side lying position is often most comfortable after surgery, and pillow support under the knee is beneficial (Whittington, Mansour, & Sloan, 2001).

■ Exercise 12-4: Role Play

Addressing sexual concerns in treatment will become more comfortable for COTAs with practice. The purpose of this role play exercise is to increase comfort levels when discussing sexual issues. It also serves as a review of chapter material. To begin the exercise, choose four people to be part of a radio talk show panel made up of knowledgeable professionals who are experts on the sexuality of elders. Then choose people who will read the scenarios listed below. Members of the radio talk show panel are allowed to consult notes and have

a commercial break if they want to discuss a situation before responding.

■ *Situations for Role Play: Radio Talk Show*

- I am 78 years of age and have rheumatoid arthritis. Over the years, I have developed increasingly painful joints, particularly in my hips. I am currently a widow but will soon marry a wonderful man. I would like to enjoy my new sexual relationship. Do you have any suggestions?

- I am a 65-year-old man who had a heart attack 8 weeks ago. My doctor says that it is safe to begin sex again. Still, I have tremendous fears. Are these fears normal and what can I do about them?

- I am a nurse's aide who works in a nursing facility. I have recently noticed male and female patients taking an interest in each other. They are constantly holding hands and have been observed kissing. The other aides make fun of them and have told them to stop, but they continue openly expressing their affection. I feel that they have a right to express their romantic side. Who is right?

- I am an 82-year-old man. My wife and I continue to have a satisfying sexual relationship. However, I have noticed in recent years that my first erection is slower and it takes me even longer to achieve an erection the second time. I am afraid to ask my physician about this. Am I normal?

- I am a 64-year-old man who had a heart attack 2 years ago. I have been impotent since getting out of the hospital. What should I do?

- I have a two-part question. I am 65 years old and have recently had a minor stroke. I am uncomfortable asking my physician about this. I have noticed over the years that sexual activity with my lover has become painful because of less vaginal lubrication. Is this normal, and is there anything I can do about it? Concerning the stroke, my left side is impaired and weakened. Do you have any suggestions for sexual positioning?

- I am an 87-year-old lesbian. I can now more openly state that fact because times are changing. However, in most of my lifetime I have had to hide my sexuality. Because of having arthritis and high blood pressure I have found it more difficult to get around and am now looking into relocating to an assisted living facility with my partner. With interviews at the facilities we have been open about our sexual relationship. Although none of the directors has directly stated that they do not want us to move into their facility, it has been obvious from their body language that we are less than welcome. We realize that we will likely experience some prejudice from other residents wherever we move. Do you have any suggestions on how to approach finding a place? Also, as long as you are consulting do you have suggestions about my arthritis and maintaining sexual relations with my partner?

▉ CHAPTER REVIEW QUESTIONS

1 Discuss common myths related to elder sexuality.

2 Discuss the viewpoint held by society about elder homosexuals.

3 Identify some of the normal age-related physiological changes for women and some simple treatment suggestions for them.

4 Identify some of the normal age-related physiological changes for men.

5 List the members of the treatment team and discuss ways the team can work together to address elders' sexual concerns.

6 Discuss the ways attitudes of health care workers in nursing home facilities affect elder sexuality.

7 Describe ways COTAs help facilitate elder sexual expression in a nursing home setting.

8 List and describe the parts of the PLISSIT model.

9 Describe ways COTAs may apply the PLISSIT model in treatment.

Answers to Exercise 12-3 questions: 1. T; 2. T; 3. F; 4. T; 5. T; 6. F; 7. T; 8. F; 9. F.

REFERENCES

American Heart Association. (2002). Sexual activity and heart disease or stroke [WWW page]. URL http://www.americanheart.org/pre-senter.jhtml?identifier=4714

American Association of Retired Persons (AARP). (1999). AARP modern maturity sexuality survey-summary of findings [WWW page]. URL http://www.research.aarp.org/health/mmsexsurvey_l.html

Annon, J. S. (1974). *The behavioral treatment of sexual problems: brief therapy* [brochure]. Honolulu, HI: Kapiolani Health Services.

Annon, J. S. (1976). *The behavioral treatment of sexual problems: brief therapy*. New York: Harper and Row.

Birkholtz, M., & Blair, S. (1999). "Coming out" and its impact on women's occupational behaviour—a discussion paper. *Journal of Occupational Science, 62,* 68-74.

Burgener, S., & Logan, G. (1989). Sexuality concerns of the post-style patient. *Rehabilitation Nursing, 14*(4), 178-195.

Coleman, S. (2002). Hip fractures and lower extremity joint replacement. In L. W. Pedretti & M. B. Early (Eds.), *Occupational therapy: Practice skills for physical dysfunction* (5th ed.). St. Louis, MO: Mosby.

Comfort, A., & Dial, L. (1991). Sexuality and aging: An overview. *Clinics in Geriatric Medicine, 7*(1):1-7.

DeBusk, R., Drory, Y., Goldstein, I., Jackson, G., Kaul, S., Kimmel, S., Kostis, J., Kloner, R.A., Lakin, M., Meston, C. M., Mittleman, M., Muller, J. E., Padma-Nathan, H., Rosen, R. C., Stein, R. A., & Zusman, R. (2000). Management of sexual dysfunction in patients with cardiovascular disease: Recommendations of the Princeton consensus panel. *The American Journal of Cardiology, 86,* 175-181.

Doyle, D., Bisson, D., Janes, N., Lynch, H., & Martin, C. (1999). Human sexuality in long-term care. *Canadian Nurse, 95*(1), 25-29.

Edmans, J. (1998). An investigation of stroke patients resuming sexual activity. *British Journal of Occupational Therapy, 61*(1), 36-38.

Ghusn, H. (1995). *Sexuality in institutionalized patients. Physical medicine and rehabilitation: State of the art reviews, 9, 2.* Philadelphia, PA: Hanley & Belfus.

Gibson, M. C., Bol, N., Woodbury, M. G., Beaton, C., & Janke, C. (1999). Comparison of caregivers', residents' and community-dwelling spouses' opinions about expressing sexuality in an institutional setting. *Journal of Gerontological Nursing, 25*(4), 30-39.

Glass, C., & Dalton, A. (1988). Sexuality in older adults: a continuing education concern. *Journal of Continuing Education in Nursing, 19,* 61-64.

Goldstein, H., & Runyon, C. (1993). An occupational therapy module to increase sensitivity about geriatric sexuality. *Physical and Occupational Therapy in Geriatrics, 11*(2), 57-75.

Goodwin, A. J., & Scott, L. (1987). Sexuality in the second half of life. In P. B. Doress, & D. L. Siegal (Ed.), *The midlife and older women book project: Ourselves growing older.* New York: Touchstone, pp. 79-99.

Hammond, D. (1989). Love, sex, and marriage in later years. In E. S. Deichman, & R. Kociechki (Eds.), *Working with the elderly: An introduction.* Buffalo, NY: Prometheus Books;

Harrison, J. (2001). "It's none of my business": Gay and lesbian invisibility in aged care. *Australian Occupational Therapy Journal, 48,* 142-145.

Jackson, J. (1995). Sexual orientation: Its relevance to occupational science and the practice of occupational therapy. *American Journal of Occupational Therapy, 54,* 26-35.

Jackson, J. (2000).Understanding the experience of non-inclusive occupational therapy clinics: Lesbians' perspectives. *American Journal of Occupational Therapy, 54,* 26-35.

Jacoby, S. (1999). Great sex. 'What's age got to do with it?' *Modern Maturity,* 1-8 [WWW page]. URL http://www.aarp.org/mmaturity/sept_oct99/greatsex.html

Kessel, B. (2001). Sexuality in the older person. *Age and Aging, 30,* 121-124.

Kimmel, D. C. (2001). Homosexuality. In R. C. Atchley (Ed.), *The Encyclopedia of aging: A comprehensive resource in gerontology and geriatrics: Vol. 1* (3rd ed.). New York: Springer.

Korpelainen, J. T., Nieminen, P., & Myllyla, V. V. (1999). Sexual functioning among stroke patients and their spouses. *Stroke, 30,* 715-719.

Laflin, M. (2002). Sexuality and the elderly individuals. In C. B. Lewis (Ed.), *Aging: The health-care challenge* (4th ed.). Philadelphia, PA: FA Davis.

Lerner, S. (2000). Sexuality and myths: A study of aging factors. *Focus on Geriatric Care and Rehabilitation, 13*(10), 3-12.

Lim, P.A.C. (1995). Sexuality in patients with musculoskeletal diseases. *Physical Medicine and Rehabilitation: State of the Art Review, 9*(2), 401-415.

Lohman, H., & Aitken, M. (1995). Influence of education on knowledge and attitude toward older adult sexuality. *Physical and Occupational Therapy in Geriatrics, 13,* 51.

Lohman, H. & Runyon, C. (1993). An occupational therapy module to increase sensitivity about geriatric sexuality. *Physical and Occupational Therapy in Geriatrics 11*(2), 57.

Lohman, H., & Runyon, C. (1995). *Counseling the geriatric client about sexuality issues in counseling and therapy: Lesson 5.* New York: Hatherleigh Company.

Lyder, C. H. (1991). Examining sexuality in long term care. *Journal of Practical Nursing 41*(4), 25-27.

Mattingly, C., & Fleming, M. H. (1994). *Clinical reasoning: Forms of inquiry in a therapeutic practice.* Philadelphia, PA: FA Davis.

Meston, C. M. (1997). Successful aging: Aging and Sexuality. *Western Journal of Medicine, 167*(4), 285-290.

Miracle, A., & Miracle, T. S. (2001). Sexuality in late adulthood. In B. R. Bonder & M. B. Wagner (Eds.), *Functional performance in older adults* (2nd ed.). Philadelphia: FA Davis.

Monga, T. N., & Ostermann, H. J. (1995). Sexuality and sexual adjustment in stroke patients. *Physical Medicine and Rehabilitation State of the Art Reviews, 9*(2), 345-359.

Mooradian, A. D. (1991). Geriatric sexuality and chronic diseases. *Clinics in Geriatric Medicine, 7*(1), 113-131.

Morrison-Beedy, D., & Robbins, L. (1989). Sexual assessment and the aging female. *Nurse Practitioner 14*, 36.

Mueller, L. W. (1997). Common questions about sex and sexuality in elders. *American Journal of Nursing, 97*(7), 61-64.

Muller, J. E., Mittleman, M. A., Maclure, M., Sherwood, J. B., & Tofler, G. H. (1996). Triggering myocardial infarction by sexual activity: Low absolute risk and prevention by regular physical exertion. *Journal of the American Medical Association, 275*(18), 1405-1409.

Mulligan, T., & Palguta, R. F. (1991). Sexual interest, activity, and satisfaction among male nursing home residents. *Archives of Sexual Behavior, 20*(2), 199-204.

Neistadt, M. E., & Freda, M. (1987). *Choices: A guide to sexual counseling with physically disabled adults.* Malabar, FL: Robert E. Krieger.

Omnibus Budget Reconciliation Act (OBRA). (1987). *Health Care Financing Administration.* Baltimore, MD: Health Care Administration.

Pangman, V. C., & Sequire, M. (2000). Sexuality and the chronically ill older adult: A social justice issue. *Sexuality and Disability, 18*(1), 49-50.

Pfeiffer, E., Verwoerdt, A., & Wang, H. S. (1968). Sexual behavior in aged men and women, *Archives in General Psychiatry, 19*, 753-758.

Schiavi, R. C., & Rehman, J. (1995). Sexuality and aging. *Urologic Clinics of North America, 22* (4), 711-726.

Steinke, E. E. (2000). Sexual counseling after myocardial infarction. *American Journal of Nursing, 100*(12), 38-44.

Starr, B. D. (2001). Sexuality. In R. C. Atchley, *The Encyclopedia of aging: A comprehensive source in gerontology and geriatrics: Vol. 2* (3rd ed.). New York: Springer.

U.S. Department of Health and Human Services (DHHS). (2001). *A profile of older Americans.* Washington, DC: Author.

Walsh, A., & Crepeau, E. (1998). "My secret life": The emergence of one gay man's authentic identity. *American Journal of Occupational Therapy, 52*, 563-569.

Westlake, C., Dracup, K., Walden, J. A., & Fonarow, G. (1999). Sexuality of patients with advanced heart failure and their spouses or partners. *The Journal of Heart and Lung Transplantation, 18*, 1133-1138.

White, C. B. (1982). The aging sexuality attitudes and knowledge scale (ASKAS): A scale for the assessment of attitudes and knowledge regarding sexuality in the aged. *Archives of Sexual Behavior 11*(6), 491-502.

Whittington, C., Mansour, S., & Sloan, S. L. (2001). *Sex after total joint replacement: A guide for you and your partner.* Atlanta, GA: Media Partners.

Wojciechowski, C. (1998). Issues in caring for older lesbians. *Journal of Gerontological Nursing, 24*, 28-33.

Yasuda, Y. L. (2002). Rheumatoid arthritis and osteoarthritis. In C. A. Trombly (Ed.), *Occupational therapy for physical dysfunction* (5th edition). Baltimore, MD: Williams & Wilkins.

Zeiss, A. M., & Kasl-Godley, J. (2001). Sexuality in older adults' relationships. *Generations, 25*, 18-25.

Zukas, R. R., & Ross-Robinson,L. (1991). Sexuality and the disabled woman. *Occupational Therapy Practice, 2*, 1.

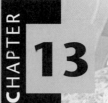

CHAPTER 13

Use of Medications by Elders

BARBARA L. FLYNN AND BRENDA M. COPPARD

KEY TERMS

self-medication programs, over-the-counter, as needed (prn), polypharmacy, delirium, adverse drug reactions, drug interactions, storage pill box, medication diary

---

CHAPTER OBJECTIVES

1. Define polypharmacy and identify recommended interventions to diminish drug-related problems of polypharmacy in elders.
2. Identify factors that predispose elders to adverse drug events and discuss strategies to detect medication problems.
3. Identify classes of medications commonly associated with adverse drug reactions in elders.
4. Identify common symptoms of adverse drug reactions in elders.
5. Identify and describe skills needed for safe self-medication.
6. Explain the ways that adaptive devices help compensate for skills needed for safe self-medication.
7. Describe elder and caregiver education needs regarding self-medication.

"He arose at the crack of dawn when he began to take his secret medicines: potassium bromide to raise his spirits, salicylates for the ache in his bones when it rained, ergosterol drops for vertigo, and belladonna for sound sleep. He took something every hour, always in secret, because in his long life as a doctor and teacher he had always opposed prescribing palliatives for old age: it was easier for him to bear other people's pains than his own. In his pocket he always carried a little pad of camphor that he inhaled deeply when no one was watching to calm his fear of so many medicines mixed together."

From Gabriel Garcia Marquez, *Love in the Time of Cholera* [p. 8]

Omar, a certified occupational therapy assistant (COTA) working in a long-term care facility, asked the facility's consulting pharmacist to review one of the resident's medications. The resident, Ellie, had been falling frequently and seemed tired and confused. Omar wondered if any of her medications might be causing problems.

The pharmacist reviewed Ellie's chart and found that the medications were contributing to her falls and changes in mental status. Omar was wise to be concerned about Ellie's medications, especially because one of her falls resulted in a hip fracture. Elders tend to be very sensitive to drug effects. If Ellie's medications had not been adjusted, her progress in occupational therapy (OT) may have been hindered.

COTAs often work with elders on a daily basis in a variety of treatment settings. Because COTAs spend a considerable amount of time with the elder population, they are a valuable asset in addressing medication routines. COTAs also may convey vital information regarding medications and side effects to the health care team. Common medications and medication-related problems encountered by elders are discussed in this chapter. Skills for **self-medication** and intervention programs for elders and caregivers are also discussed. More specific medication information is available from textbooks such as *Physician's Desk Reference* (PDR) and *Physician's GenRx*.

Some elders have many chronic and debilitating illnesses. Therefore, they use many medications to manage these conditions. It is estimated that elders consume more than 40% of all **over-the-counter** (OTC) medications (Lucas, Noyes, & Stratton, 1995). Elders living in long-term care facilities tend to take more medications than those residing in the community. For example, elder women residing in the community have been estimated to use five routinely administered and three as needed **(prn)** medications daily (Lucas, Noyes, & Stratton, 1995). Elders in long-term care facilities may take seven to eight routinely administered medications and several as needed (prn) medications daily (Avorn & Gurwitz, 1995).

MEDICATIONS COMMONLY PRESCRIBED FOR ELDERS

COTAs should always check the medication sections of elders' medical records to determine which medications are being used. This information helps COTAs to be aware of possible side effects and drug interactions that might be observed in clinical treatment. COTAs should contact the elders' physicians and pharmacies with any medication-related concerns or questions. (Common drug-related abbreviations and definitions are listed in Table 13-1.)

Medications commonly prescribed for elders include those used to manage chronic diseases such as high blood pressure, diabetes, arthritis, and depression. Cardiovascular drugs (digoxin, diuretics, high blood pressure medications, medications for chest pain, and blood thinners), hypoglycemic agents (insulin and oral agents), gastrointestinal agents (antacids, laxatives, and antiulcer medications), and analgesics and antiinflammatory agents are commonly prescribed (Hussar, 1991). Antianxiety and antipsychotic medications are frequently used to manage behavioral disturbances such as psychosis, anxiety, and dementia caused by Alzheimer's disease (AD) and other diseases. Psychosis is thought to affect up to 38% of elders who live in long-term care facilities. In addition, 20% to 50% of these elders are estimated to receive an antipsychotic medication (Frederickson & Boult, 1995).

MEDICATION-RELATED PROBLEMS

Medication-related problems for elders include multiple drug usage, adverse reactions to drugs, being prescribed and using wrong or unnecessary medications,

TABLE 13-1

Common Drug-Related Terminology

Abbreviation	Definition
Po	By mouth
Qd	Once daily
Bid	Twice daily
Tid	Three times daily
Qid	Four times daily
Prn	As needed
IM	Intramuscular (injection into the muscle)
IV	Intravenous (injection into the vein)

being prescribed improper drug dosages, and failure to take drugs correctly. One of the most frequently overlooked aspects of drug therapy is periodic reevaluation. Often medications intended for short-term therapy are not discontinued. With elders, drug dosages may be excessive. Some elders benefit from starting with one third to one half of the typical adult dosage. The adage "start low, go slow" certainly applies to initiating medications with elders.

Medication problems can lead to problems affecting daily function and may include confusion, depression, delirium (mental status changes), insomnia, urinary retention, incontinence, weakness, lethargy, loss of appetite, falls, and changes in speech and cognition. Elders must know the medical reason for every medication they are receiving. Surprisingly, this basic information frequently is not conveyed to elders, their families, or other members of the health care team. Some medications are prescribed for multiple diagnoses. Diuretics, for example, have multiple indications for use. Is the individual receiving a diuretic for high blood pressure or to manage heart failure? The medical reason for use of the drug is vital information to all persons involved in the elder's care.

Polypharmacy

Polypharmacy is the term describing the use of many medications by one person. It not only increases the cost of drug therapy dramatically, but also increases the incidence of adverse side effects (Cipolle, Strand, & Morley, 1998) and drug–drug interactions (DDIs). Polypharmacy may occur when several physicians are caring for one person and communication between them is limited. Another factor is elders using several different pharmacies, and one pharmacy cannot keep track of all of their medicines. An additional problem may arise when elders are given samples by a physician, and the pharmacist or other physicians involved in the care of the elder may not be aware of their use. Confused elders may not be able to give accurate medication-related information to their physicians or pharmacists. Polypharmacy may also result when elders misunderstand directions about the use of medications. For example, when a currently prescribed medication is ineffective and a new drug is initiated, elders may not understand that they are to stop taking the initial medication.

Adverse Drug Reactions

Given the complexity of drug regimens, it is not surprising that elders are prone to **adverse drug reactions (ADRs)** and DDIs or drug–nutrient interactions. Lucas, Noyes, & Stratton (1995) estimated that 39% of patients admitted to the hospital for ADRs and 51% of deaths caused by ADRs occurred in elders older than 60 years. (Medications and common side effects are listed in Table 13-2.) Some medications must not be taken with certain foods, such as fruit juices. Other medication activity and ADRs may be affected if the medicine is taken with food or on an empty stomach.

Many factors are involved in the increased incidence of drug toxicity in elders. With aging, kidney and liver functions decline. Many medications are excreted by the kidney and metabolized, or degraded, by the liver. Therefore, changes in organ function may frequently lead to increased drug accumulation in the body. This accumulation leads to ADRs, which in elders are commonly manifested by hypotension (decrease in blood pressure), constipation, urinary incontinence or the inability to void urine, confusion, memory loss, restlessness, falls, anxiety, and depression.

Movement disturbances, which are called *extrapyramidal syndromes (EPSs)*, may also occur in elders receiving antipsychotic medications. Extrapyramidal side effects (EPSEs) most commonly manifest as abnormal oral–facial movements such as obsessively putting one's tongue in cheek, sticking out the tongue, or teeth clenching or grinding. Poor dentition also should be ruled out. Gait disturbances, such as a "shuffling" gait, extreme muscle

TABLE 13-2

Disease States, Medications, and Common Side Effects

Disease state	Medication	Common side effect
Hypertension	Diuretics: Bumex, Lasix, Dyazide, Maxzide Antihypertensives: Cardizem, Levatol, Lopressor, Procardia, Vasotec, Captopril	Dizziness, low blood pressure, fall risk, changes in electrolyte levels
Arthritis	Nonsteroidal anti-inflammatory drugs: Advil, Ascriptin, Feldene, Motrin, Naprosyn, Orudis, Celebrex, Vioxx	Upset stomach, ulcers, mental confusion, fluid retention
	Narcotic analgesics: Darvocet, Darvon, Demerol, Empirin with codeine, morphine, Percocet, Tylenol with codeine, Tylox, hydrocodone	Mental confusion, constipation, stomach upset
Depression	Antidepressants: Anafranil, Asendin, Desyrel, Elavil, Norpramin, Pamelor, Prozac, Sinequan, Tofranil, Wellbutrin, Zoloft, Lexpro, Celexa, Remeron, Trazodone	Dizziness, low blood pressure with posture changes, mental confusion
Congestive heart failure	Digoxin, Bumex, Lasix, Aldactone, Dyazide, Maxzide, nitrates, hydralazine, Capoten, Vasotec, Altace	Mental confusion, weakness, slow heart rate, arrhythmias
Diabetes	Insulin Oral hypoglycemics: DiaBeta, Diabinese, Glucotrol, Humulin, Micronase, Orinase, Glucophage	Low blood sugar, dizziness
Anxiety/insomnia/ psychosis/behavioral disturbances	Antianxiety drugs: Atarax, Ativan, BuSpar, Serax, Tranxene, Valium, Vistaril, Xanax Sedatives: Dalmane, Halcion, Restoril Antipsychotics: Clozaril, Compazine, Haldol, Loxitane, Mellaril, Navane, Prolixin, Risperdal, Stelazine, Thorazine, Seroquel, Zyprexa	Falls, sedation, unsteady gait, confusion, blood pressure changes

spasms of the neck (torticollis), or upward fixation of the eyes may also occur. EPSEs are serious events that require professional assessment and treatment.

Elders are more sensitive to the effects of certain medications such as narcotic analgesics, blood thinners, and heart medications. Any medication that has central nervous system side effects may become problematic because of this increased sensitivity in elders. Any medication with any potential central nervous system side effects is greatly exacerbated, particularly in elders with a cognitive condition such as AD.

Many medications prescribed for elders may impair functional capabilities. Drug-induced **delirium**, for example, is characterized by an acute and reversible confusion state (DeMaagd, 1995). Because of the prevalence of this side effect, OT practitioners must be familiar with drugs that may cause delirium in elders. COTAs should discuss any mental changes they witness with the other members of the health care team. Medications reported to cause delirium include antihistamines, antipsychotics, antianxiety agents, antidepressants, and seizure medications. High blood pressure medications, analgesics, antibiotics, cardiac drugs, drugs used to treat or prevent ulcers, and drugs used in managing Parkinson's disease may also induce drug delirium. Delirium usually resolves with discontinuation of the involved medication.

The risk for falls is greatly increased because of medications commonly prescribed to elders. Many of these medications cause dizziness, mental confusion, sedation, and changes in blood pressure, thereby predisposing elders to falls. The clinical consequences of falls can be very serious. (Refer to Chapter 14 for further discussion of the consequences of falls.) Falls may also be the result of poor judgment (such as in patients with AD), lack of following directions to seek assistance when transferring out of bed, or from a urinary incontinence episode (the elder slips in a pool of urine on the floor). It is important not to give diuretics too late in the day, to prevent the need for frequent trips to the bathroom at night, when lighting conditions may be low. Keeping a night light on is a good idea for all elders to assist with nighttime trips to the bathroom.

Drug–Drug Interactions

DDIs may also affect functional status. Although common in elders, not all interactions are clinically significant. Drug interactions occur for several reasons. Interactions are more commonly based on the number of prescriptions, OTC medications, and herbal supplements taken by elders. Age-related changes that predispose elders to adverse outcomes from DDIs may also play a role.

Drug interactions occur by many different mechanisms. Some interactions involve cumulative effects when medications with similar side effects are used simultaneously. For example, antianxiety agents and narcotic analgesics both possess sedative properties, which may lead to excessive sedation if used together. Another drug interaction results when medications with opposing actions are used together. For example, use of an antiinflammatory medication such as Advil (ibuprofen) may cause fluid retention, thereby counteracting the diuretic effect of Lasix.* Drug interactions may also result from declining organ capabilities in elders. Decreased liver and kidney function have already been mentioned. Other drug interactions involve depletion or accumulation of electrolytes such as potassium, or are complicated by metabolic problems or disease states.

Detection of Medication Problems in Elders

Mental confusion is one of the most common medication side effects in elders. Other common side effects include dizziness, weakness, upset stomach, constipation, and difficulty with urination. Many disease states also may present with these symptoms. Clinical differentiation between disease and medication-related problems can be challenging. For example, mental confusion caused by medications can be misdiagnosed as AD.

Detailed questioning about an elder's compliance with the drug regimen is critical. This questioning can be part of the occupational therapist and COTA team's evaluation of activities of daily living (ADL) functions (American Occupational Therapy Association [AOTA], 1994). Many elders may customize their drug regimens without consulting a health care professional because of cost concerns or drug side effects. For examples, some elders cut tablets in half or take their medicine every other day in an effort to save money. The pharmacist is in an ideal role to suggest a less expensive alternative to the prescribing physician. Elders should be questioned about the exact manner in which the medication is taken because many do not follow the directions printed on labels.

COTAs should consult other health care professionals about medication-related concerns. Optimal care involves a multidisciplinary approach. Each discipline reviews the elder's status from a different perspective. For example, an elder with AD is experiencing falls. A physician may be focused on issues such as poor judgment or progression of the disease. A pharmacist will be scrutinizing medications that the elder is taking. The occupational therapist and COTA will evaluate the elder from a functional perspective. This is the optimal scenario for evaluating the elder experiencing falls in this example. Timely communication with a pharmacist is vital, and such consultation may be initiated verbally or by written consultation when a pharmacist is not directly available (Fig. 13-1).

---

*Manufactured by Mylan, Morgantown, WV.

Resident: _____   Room #: _____

Consult requested by: _____   Date: _____

Therapeutic problem: _____

Consult completed by: _____   Date: _____

Could problem be drug related?   No _____

                                 Yes _____   (See recommendations)

Recommendations:

Drug therapy interventions (dosage reduction, drug discontinuation, switch to

different drug, or other): _____

_____

Laboratory monitoring: _____

_____

Nursing monitoring: _____

_____

Other recommendations: _____

_____

Should you have any further questions, please contact the pharmacist completing
this evaluation. Thank you.

FIGURE **13-1**   Interdisciplinary drug therapy consult form.

SKILLS REQUIRED FOR INDEPENDENT SELF-MEDICATION

Medication routines of clients are often not addressed by OT (Potts, 1994). This is evident in the lack of literature on **self-medication programs** and OT interventions with medication routines. Instruction in proper use of medication should be dealt with as part of ADL routines (Lewis, 1989). A medication routine includes obtaining medication, opening and closing containers, following prescribed schedules, taking correct quantities, reporting problems and adverse effects, and administering correct quantities by using prescribed methods (AOTA, 1994).

Various skills and abilities are needed for elders to medicate themselves safely and efficiently. In addition to normal swallowing (if given orally), these skills may include manual dexterity, visual acuity, hearing, memory, problem solving, motivation, ambulation/transportation, and communication.

Manual Dexterity

Usually a great deal of fine motor coordination, finger dexterity, and some degree of strength are needed to open and close medication containers. Fine grasp patterns are required when picking up pills or tablets. Therefore, elders with conditions such as rheumatoid arthritis or Parkinson's disease may have difficulty opening childproof containers. Non-childproof tops can be provided by the pharmacist,

if requested. If nonsafety caps are dispensed by the pharmacist, it is essential that elders store their medication out of the reach of children.

Vision and Visual Perception

Visual perception skills may be required by elders who take multiple medications. Visual perception skills include color discrimination, depth perception, and figure-ground perception. Visual acuity and perception are required to distinguish between different containers of medication and to read instruction labels. If needed, glasses should be worn when elders self-medicate. Adaptations may be used to assist elders who have visual impairments (Fig. 13-2). Magnifying lenses and large type or contrasting print may be helpful. For severe visual impairments, different size, different shape, or multicolor containers can be used for medication storage. Instructions for administration can be tape recorded to relay information that cannot be read. Depth perception skills are needed to obtain pills in a multipartition container. Figure-ground perception also is needed to see white pills in a white pill box. COTAs should suggest that elders use colored pill containers for white pills.

Hearing

Approximately 33% of elders older than 65 years have hearing impairments (National Center for Health

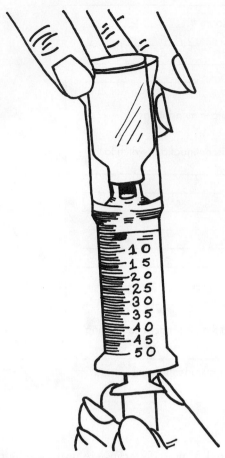

FIGURE 13-2 This magnifier device consists of a plastic cylinder in which the medication and syringe fit at each end and permits elders with visual impairments to view amounts easily.

Statistics, 2004). COTAs should remember this when educating elders, family members, and caregivers. The ability to hear is important for elders to understand medication dosages and changes. COTAs should give both verbal and written instructions when educating elders. For example, Kathy, a COTA, meets with Vladimir, who has difficulty hearing, to review his discharge program. She first checks to make sure Vladimir is wearing his hearing aid and then reviews the information in his client education packet. Kathy speaks slowly and clearly and is sitting directly at eye level with Vladimir. She also frequently asks Vladimir whether he has any questions and encourages him to repeat back to her what he understands (see Chapter 16).

Strength

Manipulating medication containers requires strength. Occasionally, a medication routine involves crushing pills or splitting them in half. Such assists as pill crushers and pill splitters can help an elder who has poor hand strength.

Elders should *never* use a razor blade to cut tablets. Many medications that are released over time (known as "extended" or "sustained release") and should not be crushed. A pharmacist is an invaluable resource person to find out whether a tablet can be crushed. Furthermore, sometimes a liquid form of the medication (if available) may be a better choice for an elder who needs to crush several medicines.

Memory

Both long-term and working memory (Andiel & Liu, 1995) are required for independent self-medication. Elders need long-term memory to understand which condition is being treated. Understanding and remembering the nature of the regimen also is required for self-medication. Elders also need long-term memory to remember where the medication is stored. Working memory, which includes simultaneous storing and processing of information, is needed to avoid undermedication or overmedication. This frequently occurs when elders do not remember whether they took a medication. Various items such as programmable alarms or auditory devices that exclaim, "time to take your pill," and pill storage boxes can aid self-medication. Home health aides and pharmacists may assist in filling self-medication boxes. A fee may be charged for this service. One advantage of involving home health or a pharmacist is that they can make sure the elder is actually taking the medicine, as prescribed, when it is time to refill the storage container.

Problem Solving

A great deal of problem solving is needed to properly self-medicate. Elders must decide whether to contact the physician when changes in a condition occur. For example, Ken goes to his physician because he wonders whether his frequent headaches indicate that his blood pressure medication is not working or whether he needs a new prescription for his glasses. Problem solving also is needed to determine when refills need to be obtained and how to safely store medication.

Motivation

Elders must be motivated to comply with their medication regimen. Depression, uncertainty, misunderstanding, financial worries, lack of confidence, side effects, and social or cultural taboos are all factors that may contribute to a lack of motivation. For example, Hazel, a 74-year-old woman with a history of angina and high blood pressure, sometimes takes her Procardia* tablets only once a day instead of three times a day as prescribed. Hazel does this when she feels "better" to save money. In addition, some elders are embarrassed by the diagnosis of depression, or other emotional disorders, and are reluctant to take

---

*Manufactured by Pfizer, New York, NY.

prescribed antidepressants or other medicines used to treat psychological problems.

Ambulation and Transportation

Elders taking medications need to have a way of getting prescriptions filled on a regular basis. Elders who do not drive or are wheelchair-bound may seek community resources to obtain rides to medical appointments and the pharmacy. Some pharmacies will deliver medications for a fee. In addition, some communities have volunteer programs that provide this service at no cost. For example, Antonio is unable to drive because of his poor vision, but he is able to renew prescriptions by using a free transportation service provided by his church. Automated systems are available at many pharmacies, which allow people to renew their prescriptions over the phone.

Communication

Elders must be able to communicate their medication regimen with health care providers and caregivers. Health care providers must reciprocate communication in an effective manner. Demonstration, verbal, and written formats can be used for communication. Elders may find it helpful to keep names, phone numbers, and addresses of health care providers and agencies in a regular place so they are available for emergencies. Posting this information on the refrigerator may also be helpful. For example, Greta has been deaf since birth but is able to communicate by using a notebook that contains information regarding her past and present medical condition. She stores this notebook in a drawer in the nightstand by her bed. She also has notified family members where the notebook is located in case of an emergency.

ASSISTIVE AIDS FOR SELF-MEDICATION

Many commercial or homemade aids can assist individuals with self-medication (Meyer, 1993). Each aid has advantages and disadvantages.

Commercial Aids

Calendars

Calendars are helpful for tracking medication schedules. A pocket calendar or a calendar hung near the place where medication is taken can be used to mark each time medication is taken. At the end of the day, marks are counted to make sure that the medication schedule was followed. The advantage of using calendars is that the medications are stored in their original containers and remain properly labeled. Calendars are also inexpensive and readily available. The disadvantage of using a calendar is that it requires some basic reading, comprehension, and memory skills to mark the calendar each time medications are taken (Meyer, 1993).

Pill storage boxes

Storage boxes are containers with compartments in which to put medications (Fig. 13-3.) **Storage pill boxes**

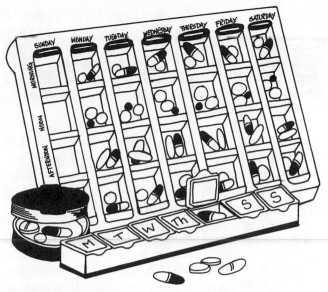

FIGURE 13-3 Various pill boxes are available with compartments for single or multiple daily and weekly doses.

are available to organize medications for one day, one week, or one month. Pill boxes require manual dexterity skills to open and close and to manipulate pills. Visual discrimination also is required to identify desired pills. Pill boxes usually do not provide tight storage for medications that require tight containers, such as nitroglycerin. In addition, the pills are no longer in labeled, childproof containers.

There are advantages and disadvantages for using daily and 7-day pill boxes (Meyer, 1993). An advantage of a daily pill box is a better chance of taking all daily doses. Any errors made in setting up this pill box would be experienced for only one day. A disadvantage of a daily pill box is that each compartment could contain several unlabeled pills. The elder would have to identify the medication(s) by physical appearance. This is a serious safety concern if pills are similar in size, shape, or color, especially if the elder has impaired vision or is easily confused.

Weekly pill boxes store medication for 7 days. The design of some pill boxes allows separation of multiple daily doses. These boxes often consist of four rows and seven columns. The four rows are marked with times of the day (morning, noon, evening, bedtime), and the seven columns are marked with the day of the week. The advantage of using a 7-day pill box is that setup is required only once a week. The disadvantage is that setup requires more accuracy (Meyer, 1993). If there is a mistake, it may occur seven times.

A pill box with an alarm is an option for elders who must take their medication at specific times. The advantage of this type of pill box is that it alerts elders of the medication schedule. A disadvantage is that elders must be able to read, understand, and follow in-depth instructions. These devices often need to be programmed and may require very fine manipulation to set the clock or the alarm. If the device breaks, repairs may be difficult and expensive. Another disadvantage is the risk of not hearing the alarm when it sounds.

Insulin holders

Insulin holders are intended for one-handed use. The device holds an insulin bottle so that a person can manipulate a syringe to obtain the proper amount of fluid. Often the device has suction cups or a nonskid surface to prevent the device from sliding on a table top.

Pill splitters

Pill splitters are useful devices when a pill must be split for proper dosage or to reduce the pill size for easier swallowing (when appropriate). Pill splitters are often lightweight and use a leverage design to reduce the amount of strength needed to use it. As previously stated, a razor blade should never be used to cut a tablet.

Pill crushers

A pill crusher is a device used to pulverize tablets into a fine powder. Similar to the design of pill splitters, pill crushers use a leverage system so that an abundance of strength is not required. Pill crushers can be beneficial when individuals have difficulty swallowing whole tablets. (Remember that not all tablets can be crushed or split.)

Talking and shaking alarms, watches, and prescription bottles

For elders who experience difficulty remembering to take their medications or what their medication routine is, several devices such as talking or shaking alarms and talking prescription bottles may be beneficial. Talking alarms are devices that are programmed to send a "beep," voice message, or visual cue when it is time to take a medication. Shaking alarms can be clipped to the bedding to wake elders when it is time to take their medication. The device can be put in one's pocket when in public and it will provide a quiet vibration to indicate the medication time. A talking prescription bottle is a device attached to a prescription bottle. A pharmacist or physician records the prescription information into the device. To operate, one pushes a button on the device to play a recorded message about the contents; how many pills to take, when, and what for; and any warnings. The talking prescription bottle is intended for those who have low vision or hearing impairments. It is also beneficial for elders for whom English is a second language or for elders who have difficulty reading.

Homemade Aids

Medication diary

A medication diary is another aid for tracking medication use (Table 13-3). COTAs may assist elders in making a diary, which can be kept in a notebook. This information can then be shared with other health care professionals, as needed.

Storage cups

Storage cups can be made at home by using small plastic or paper cups that are stacked and ordered according to the number of times the medication must be taken throughout the day. The cups should be marked in relation to when medications are taken (for example, morning, noon, dinner, and bedtime) (Fig. 13-4). After the morning medication is taken, the "morning" cup is moved to the bottom of the stack. This allows the next medication dose to be on the top. This system requires that elders have good manual dexterity, visual-perceptual, and memory skills. A similar system can be made using egg cartons. For liquid or powder medications, a system can be set up using small, labeled, airtight containers. Using a homemade system is simple and inexpensive. However, using a homemade system may cause medication to be exposed to improper storage conditions (Meyer, 1993). Also, pills in open view may tempt small children who live in or visit the elder's home. This risk can be reduced by storing the medication out of view and reach.

SELF-MEDICATION PROGRAM

A formal self-medication program may help to prevent problems with polypharmacy (Potts, 1994). The program is designed to: (1) use an interdisciplinary team approach, (2) educate elders about their medications, (3) develop elders' motor skills for proper administration, (4) offer practice opportunities to elders, (5) assess elders for any adaptive devices that may be useful, and (6) evaluate elders' skills in medication administration before discharge.

The elder's treatment plan should include interventions to maximize independence with self-medication. Depending on elders' limitations and deficits, COTAs

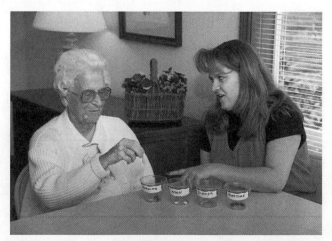

FIGURE 13-4   Storage pill cups can be made at home by simply using small plastic or paper cups.

TABLE 13-3

Contents of a Medication Diary

Section	Information
1: Demographics	Name Date Address Phone number Date of birth Medication allergies: date of occurrence and type of reaction Vaccinations (year, date) Flu shots (year, date)
2: Health care providers	List names and phone numbers of all health care providers (tape their business cards here).
3: Past medications	List all medical conditions that required treatment with medication over the years. List all medical conditions that currently require treatment with medication.
4: Special equipment	List all adaptive or special equipment required (such as a nebulizer, ostomy products, and incontinence products). Include the brand, size, and model, and the supplier's name and phone number.
5: Recent medications	Enter the name of new medications used, the date, the reason the medication is being used, the strength of the medication, and how often the medication is taken each day. Keep track of any dosage changes, discontinuation, the date, and the reason for the change or discontinuation.
6: Over-the-counter medications	List any over-the-counter medications used for the eyes, ears, skin, and other organs and tissues. Enter how often the medications are used.
7: Questions for health care providers	List any questions to ask the doctor or pharmacist.

should engage them in simulated medication tasks. An example of such a task is using small colored candy pieces to practice color discrimination and fine prehensile patterns. Reading and comprehending general labels can aid in reading medication labels. Opening and closing medication containers should be practiced. In addition, elders should master any adaptive aids before being discharged from OT (Fig. 13-5).

Relatives, friends, and home care personnel who assist in the delivery of medications often have not been included in discussions of medications (Wieder & Wolf-Klein, 1994). Family and caregivers should be able to name the elder's medications, describe the purpose of each medication, and describe any precautions associated with each medication (Box 13-1).

CASE STUDY

Olivia is an 83-year-old woman living at home with her 85-year-old husband. Olivia is currently under the care of two physicians: her primary medical physician and a psychiatrist. A few weeks ago Olivia fell and fractured her hip. Her mental status fluctuates. Her husband is in charge

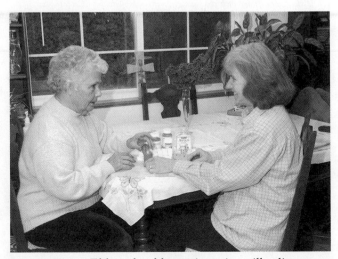

FIGURE 13-5 Elders should practice using pill splitters and filling and removing medications from pill boxes.

BOX 13-1

Guidelines for Caregivers Who Administer Medications

Elders most at risk to experience problems with medications are those who are:
- Seeing many physicians
- Taking many medications
- Using many pharmacies

Keep track of the following information on the elder(s) you are caring for:
- *All* the prescription drugs the elder is taking
- *All* the nonprescription (OTC) drugs the elder is taking
- *All* other medicinal items the elder uses from a health food store or supermarket
- When and how much medicine to give
- What results to expect from the medicine
- Any physical or mental change in the elder (report to physician)
- What to do if a dose is missed

Prescriptions

The need for the medications should be reevaluated at least every 3 to 6 months.

Do not save unused medication for future use without the physician's approval.

Flush unused medication down the toilet. Do not share medications with anyone. Closely check expiration dates and dispose of expired medicine.

Do *not* be satisfied with directions such as:
- Take as directed
- Take before meals
- Take as needed
- Take four times a day

Ask the pharmacist to put the specific directions on the label and to tell you exactly how to follow them.
- What does four times a day really mean?
- Does it mean every 6 hours? Does it mean with meals and at bedtime?
- Can this medicine be taken with other medications?

To reduce the risk for aspiration and swallowing problems, *never* give tablets or capsules while the elder is lying down. *Always* give medications with plenty of fluids to reduce stomach upset unless directed otherwise.

Medication storage

Store medications properly. If you count or measure medications, keep them in a cool, dry place, away from the sunlight and away from children. Keep the label on the medication container until all medicine is used or destroyed. If traveling, take the original medicine container with you in case of an emergency.

Take precautions with the following:
- *Chewable tablets: Elders often do not like chewable tablets because they can interfere with dentures. One option is to have the elder suck on the tablet to dissolve it. Chewable tablets should not be swallowed whole.*
- *Crushing tablets or opening capsules: Many pills should not be crushed because they are designed to be long-acting. Other pills should not be crushed because the contents may cause stomach upset or inflammation.*

Always check with the pharmacist. Occasionally a liquid substitute is available.
- Liquid medications: Because liquid medications are difficult to measure accurately, ask the pharmacist for a measuring device to ensure the correct dose.
- Applying ointments: Because medications applied to the elder's skin will have an effect on your skin, wash hands after each application. Use gauze or gloves to apply.
- Applying patches: Always remove old patches. Know how often and where to apply the patch on the body. Remove old patches *gently*, because elders have delicate skin. Notify the pharmacist if the skin becomes irritated or the patch does not stick.
- Giving injections: Practice administration techniques with a nurse or pharmacist.

(Continued)

BOX 13-1

Guidelines for Caregivers Who Administer Medications—cont'd

- Tube feedings: Tube feedings with medication require special instructions. Liquid medications, if available, work best when medicine needs to be given down a feeding tube. Some medications, such as Dilantin,* may actually directly interact with the enteral supplement (such as Osmolite). Contact the pharmacist for instructions on exactly how to give the medication.

Discharge plans from the hospital or nursing home
This can be a very confusing time! Medications often change while the elder is in the hospital. Everyone must know which medications to take and which *not* to take.
- Know about any generic drugs. Tablets or capsules may look different and have a different name, but the medications contain the same ingredient in the same amount. Know exactly what each generic medication is. Keep an accurate list or bring all the medications when visiting every doctor. Shop at one pharmacy to avoid medication duplication. If moving to another area, ask the pharmacist to forward your prescription records to your new pharmacist.
- Monitor the elder's nutrition, diet, and fluids. Pay attention to the elder's appetite and notify the physician if there are any concerns such as weight gain or loss. Know whether the elder requires a special diet, including foods/liquids to avoid and to encourage. Administer medication by offering plenty of liquids, unless otherwise instructed.

*Manufactured by Parke-Davis Pharmaceuticals, Ltd., Vega Baja, PR.
Data from Simon & Silverman (1986) and Parke-Davis Center for the Elderly (1995).

of administering medications. Her problems and medications are listed as follows:

Disease state	Medication
High blood pressure	Lasix (diuretic, or water pill)
Insomnia and anxiety	Ativan* (antianxiety)
Rheumatoid arthritis	Aspirin (pain reliever)
Depression	Prozac (antidepressant)
Insomnia	Benadryl (nonprescription sleep aid)

■ CASE STUDY QUESTIONS

1 Which medication-related problems might be of concern to COTAs?
2 Could any of Olivia's current medical problems be caused by her medications? If so, which medications cause which side effects?
3 What other factors may place Olivia at risk for polypharmacy and medication-related problems?
4 The COTA is concerned about the frequency of Olivia's falls and the risk for another hip fracture but is unsure whether any medications are contributing to the falls. What is a reasonable course of action to address this plausible medication-related concern?
5 What skills for safe self-medication are affected in Olivia's case?
6 What assistive devices may help with her medication routine and why?
7 Who should be involved in a self-medication program to help Olivia with her medications?

■ CHAPTER REVIEW QUESTIONS

1 Considering the information in this chapter, explain why the certified occupational therapy assistant

*Manufactured by Wyeth-Ayerst, Philadelphia, PA.

(COTA) is an important player in the health care team to address medication issues with elders.
2 What are some reasons for polypharmacy among elders?
3 What is one side effect of each of the following: diuretics, nonsteroidal antiinflammatory drugs, narcotic analgesics, antidepressants, digoxin, insulin, antipsychotics?
4 What is a common symptom of elders having adverse medication reactions?
5 What resources and personnel are available to address the concerns or questions of COTAs regarding medications?
6 Explain eight skills needed for safe self-medication.
7 What aids are available to elders with poor vision, memory, or hearing, or lack of transportation?
8 What should be included in a medication diary?
9 What are some essential components to a self-medication program?
10 What information should COTAs provide to educate caregivers?

REFERENCES

American Occupational Therapy Association. (1994). Uniform terminology for occupational. *American Journal of Occupational Therapy, 48*, 1047.
Andiel, C., & Liu, L. (1995). Working memory and older adults: Implications for occupational therapy. *American Journal of Occupational Therapy, 49*, 681-686.
Avorn, J., & Gurwitz, J. H. (1995). Drug use in the nursing home. *Annals of Internal Medicine, 123*, 195.
Cipolle, R. J., Strand, L. M., & Morley, P. C. (1998). *Pharmaceutical care practice.* New York: McGraw Hill.
DeMaagd, G. A. (1995). Review of the pharmacologic causes of delirium in the elderly. *Consultant Pharmacists, 10*, 461.

Frederickson, T. W., & Boult, C. (1995). Federal regulation and the use of antipsychotic medications in nursing homes. *Nursing Home Medicine, 3,* 41.

Hussar, D. A. (1991). *Drug interactions in the elderly.* East Hanover, NJ: Sandoz Pharmaceutical Corp.

Lewis, S. C. (1989). *Elder care in occupational therapy.* Thorofare, NJ: Slack.

Lucas, D. S., Noyes, M. A., & Stratton, M. A. (1995). Principles of geriatric pharmacotherapy. *Clinical Consultant, 14.*

Márquez, G. G. (1988). *Love in the time of cholera.* New York: Penguin Books.

Meyer, M. E. (1993). *Coping with medications.* San Diego, CA: Singular Publishing Group.

National Center for Health Statistics. Data Warehouse on Trends in Health and Aging, http://www.cdc.gov/nchs/agingact.htm. January 13, 2004.

Parke-Davis Center for the Elderly. (1995). *The caregiver's medication guidelines.* Morris Plains, NJ: Parke-Davis Elder Care Program.

Potts, J. M. (1994). Developing a patient self-medication program for the rehabilitation setting. *Rehabilitation Nursing, 19,* 344.

Simon, G. I., & Silverman, H. M. (1986). *The pill book* (3rd ed.). New York: Bantam Books.

Wieder, A. J., & Wolf-Klein, G. P. (1994). When medications change, tell the caregiver, too. *Geriatrics, 49,* 48.

CHAPTER 14

Considerations of Mobility

KEY TERMS

restraints, restraint reduction, environmental adaptations, psychosocial approaches, activity alternatives, fall prevention, aging in place, environmental hazards, mobility, transit, driving, pedestrian, paratransit

CHAPTER OBJECTIVES

1. Discuss Omnibus Budget Reconciliation Act regulations pertaining to the use of physical restraints.
2. Describe steps in the establishment of a restraint reduction program.
3. Describe the role of the certified occupational therapy assistant in restraint reduction.
4. Identify three reasons why elder adults are at a greater risk for falls than the general population.
5. Identify environmental, biological, psychosocial, and functional causes of falls.
6. Describe the process of obtaining a fall history using the acronym "SLIPPED" to collect information.
7. Describe recommended interventions to prevent falls.
8. Discuss ways elders may gain access to public transportation.
9. Describe ways elders may become safer pedestrians.
10. Describe a driving evaluation and identify criteria for this assessment.
11. Describe visual and physical changes in elders that may affect their ability to drive.
12. Outline the basic steps in evaluating the fit of a wheelchair.
13. Describe the major precautions to consider when elders should use wheelchairs.

KAI GALYEN

PART 1 Restraint Reduction*

HISTORY

Physical **restraints** have been used in this country since the 1700s to manage psychotic behavior. More recently,

*Updated by Candice Mullendore and Ivelisse Lazzarini.

restraint use has been associated with cognitive impairment (Atkins, 1996; Castle & Mor, 1998). Until the late 1980s, use of restraints was almost universal in nursing homes (Eigsti &Vrooman, 1992). This practice was based on institutional tradition rather than on nstrated benefit (Donius & Rader, 1994; Kane, 01).

The literature indicates that restraints are essentially ineffective in eliminating serious injury secondary to falls and that they cause agitation, behavioral difficulties, and a myriad of problems associated with immobility (Rader, 1995; Stolley, 1995) (Box 14-1). Concern among health care professionals, consumers, and advocates for elders about these detrimental effects and the right of elders to self-determination, mobility, and dignity led to a movement for **restraint reduction** that contributed to the historical Nursing Home Reform Act, part of the Omnibus Budget Reconciliation Act (OBRA) of 1987 (Sullivan-Marx, 1995).

Omnibus Budget Reconciliation Act Regulations

OBRA was drafted to protect elders from abuse and to promote choice and dignity. The ultimate goal is that each person reach his or her highest practical level of

BOX 14-1

Negative Effects of Restraints	
Psychosocial	**Physical**
Depression	Hazards of immobility
Lethargy	Incontinence
Withdrawal	Constipation
Anxiety	Disturbed spell pattern
Distress	Loss of balance
Fear	Falls
Panic	Pressure ulcers
Anger	Bone demineralization
Agitation	Loss of muscle tone and mass
Increased aggression	Respiratory difficulties
Reduced opportunity	Pneumonia
for social contact	Infection
Threat to identity	Thrombophlebitis
Embarrassment	Dehydration
Humiliation	Impaired circulation
Demoralization	Respiratory problems
Decreased feelings	Orthostatic hypotension
of dignity	Decreased appetite
Decreased sense of	Decreased ability to care
self-esteem	for self
Decreased autonomy	Abrasions
Helplessness	Cuts
Dependence	Bruises
Regression	Decreased functional status
Increased confusion	Loss of freedom
Increased disorientation	Death caused by suffocation
Increased disorganized	or strangulation
behavior	
Broken human spirit	

well-being. A reduction in the use of restraints is only a small part of this intent. OBRA requires caregivers to develop an individualized plan of care that supports each elder in the least restrictive environment possible (Health Care Financing Administration [HCFA], 1995, 2001). COTAs should become familiar with OBRA guidelines regarding restraints.

Two types of restraints are used: chemical and physical. Chemical restraints are drugs prescribed to control mood, mental status, and behavior for purposes of discipline or convenience rather than management of a medical condition. Physical restraints are any method, device, material, or equipment that is difficult to self-remove and restricts freedom of movement or normal access to one's body. Restraints are permitted only when they enable greater functional independence, restrict the elder from interfering with the provision of life-saving treatment, or are necessary because less restrictive devices have failed. A documented medical need and physician's order for restraints must exist. Clients must be released at least every 2 hours, and the restraints can be used only as a temporary intervention (HCFA, 2001).

Despite these guidelines, improper use of restraints continues in the United States. COTAs have an ethical and legal obligation to report elder abuse, which includes using restraints as punishment for clients or as a convenience to staff. COTAs also should participate in educating others about restraints and may wish to initiate a restraint reduction program in their own facility.

ESTABLISHING A RESTRAINT REDUCTION PROGRAM

The move toward eliminating the use of restraints must be done in a gradual, planned, systematic way. Factors to consider include gaining administrative support, training staff, and developing strategies to assure that restraints become an unacceptable option in the facility.

Philosophy

A fundamental philosophical concept in the care of elders is the empowerment of both elders and staff. This empowerment is expressed in collaborative solutions to problems. The ability to contribute to solutions allows elders dignity and adds meaning and quality to their lives (Kari & Michels, 1991; Knowlton, 2002). Making choices, including the choice to take a risk, is an essential part of life and contributes to maintaining self-respect. Caregivers must recognize that decisions concerning risk must include input from even cognitively impaired elders (Rader, 1995; Capezuti, et al., 1999). Caregivers have been indoctrinated with the concept that safety automatically includes the use of restraints (Mason, O'Connor, & Kemble, 1995; Guttman, Altman, & Karlan, 1999). After years of viewing restraints only as safety devices, caregivers find it difficult to accept that these measures are often unsafe. Caregivers may also have trouble accepting that freedom and choice precede safety in importance. We need to become elder centered rather than system or task centered (Kapp, 1994; Neufeld, et al., 1999).

Policy

Administrative stability, involvement, and demonstration of support by the clear articulation of policy are essential to the success of any restraint elimination program (Mahoney, 1995; Guttman, Altman, & Karlan, 1999). Research indicates that reducing restraints is cost effective, especially because of decreased medical complications from immobility and fewer serious falls (Bradley, Siddique, & Dufton, 1995; Capezuti, Talerico, Cochran, Becker, Strumpf, & Evans, 1999). Studies also indicate that reduction of restraints is usually accomplished with no additional staff (Bloom & Braun, 1991; Castle & Mor, 1998). Because restraints have been shown to be potentially harmful, litigation is more likely to occur from applying restraints than from withholding them. In addition, Medicare and Medicaid sanctions (such as decertification and even delicensure of the facility) are more likely to result from imposing restraints than from removing them (Kapp, 1994).

Education

Practitioners must teach these new concepts not only because they have been mandated by federal regulation but because, as Brungardt (1994) indicates, elders' function cannot improve "if they are tied down or drugged up." We should recognize that even those of us without dementia would not react positively to being restrained, even for our own good (Rader, 1995). Sullivan-Marx (1995) has likened the symptoms resulting from the trauma of restraint to posttraumatic stress disorder, learned helplessness, or battered-woman syndrome. Including the teaching of such concepts in a restraint reduction training program creates disequilibrium, which is necessary to change belief systems. Another teaching strategy is to provide practical and applicable information (Strumpf, Evans, Wagner, & Patterson, 1992; Strump, Evans, & Bourbonniere, 2001). Including an experiential component, such as applying a variety of restraints to participants, also adds to the effectiveness of the training. Few individuals can imagine choosing restraints as an appropriate intervention for themselves. Feeling the helplessness and degradation of being restrained sensitizes staff to the use of restraints on elders. Education should use and affirm participants' life experiences. Including board members, volunteers, and all facility employees (kitchen workers, bookkeepers, administration, chaplains, and maintenance workers) in this educational program has been identified as a factor leading to decreased reliance on restraints (Janelli, Kanski, & Neary, 1994; Strump, Evans, & Bourbonniere, 2001). Kapp (1994) and Capezuti, Strumpf, Evans, & Maislin (1999) recommend mandatory training sessions provided on a continuing basis and introduction to this subject in orientation material.

Steps for Success

All members of the team, including families, staff from each shift, consultants, contract personnel, ombudsmen, state surveyors, physicians, and elders themselves, should be included in all stages of the program. Dialogue between these participants from the beginning makes the transition to restraint-free care much smoother. All team members play an important role. Family members can, for example, describe the elder's previous routines and preferences. Kari and Michels (1991) assert that Certified Nursing Assistants (CNAs) have essential knowledge of elders and that their usual lack of influence in decision making negatively affects the quality of care. CNAs may be the team members who first notice behavioral changes and the need for removal of restraints in elders (Janelli, Kanski, & Neary, 1994). Strumpf, Evans, Wagner, & Patterson (1992) indicate that respect for the dignity of their work is vital for any significant reduction in the use of restraints. An interdisciplinary team assessment of the need for restraint is helpful in reducing reliance on restraints (Mion & Mercurio, 1992; Strump, Evans, & Bourbonniere, 2001).

A procedure outlining steps for implementing use of any restraint in a variety of situations should be developed. A committee should be formed to review existing and new requests for restraints (Atkins, 1996; Guttman, Altman, & Karlan, 1999). In addition, restraints should be removed from the unit so that they are unavailable without consultation (Rader, 1995).

Most successful restraint-free programs have adopted permanent staffing (J. Rader, personal communication, 1996). This model assigns daily a "primary" CNA (and registered nurse, housekeeper, therapist, among others) to each elder. When these staff members are not working, they should have regular replacements. Permanence in staffing fosters relationships between elders, families, and staff that contribute to feelings of safety and connectedness and are particularly important to elders with cognitive impairment.

Interventions to eliminate restraint use should be individualized to produce a safer and more comfortable environment for elders. Individualized interventions are paramount to the quality and success of restraint elimination programs (Burgener, Shiver, & Murrell, 1993). Mion and Mercurio (1992) suggest starting with an elder who has been identified as a good candidate for removal of restraints. Initial success will help staff members feel confident about continuing restraint reduction. Finally, each individualized intervention should be reassessed on a regular basis (Janelli, Kanski, & Neary, 1994).

Rader (1995) has found that the biggest obstacles to eliminating restraints are our fears, biases, and unwillingness to change. She proposes that caregivers, clients, advocates, and regulators work together to create new interventions on the basis of the elder's perspectives and wishes. Reducing restraints should be only the beginning of providing safe care in a dignified and less restrictive environment that promotes the elder's abilities (Werner, Koroknay, Braun, & Cohen-Mansfield, 1994; Neufeld, et al., 1999).

ROLE OF THE CERTIFIED OCCUPATIONAL THERAPY ASSISTANT

In collaboration with an occupational therapist (OTR), COTAs may assess the need for restraints, consult with staff about alternatives to restraint, and provide intervention to eliminate restraint use. Before restraints are used, supportive documentation is required regardless of the reason for restraint or the person who identified the need.

Assessment

Once need for intervention is documented and an occupational therapy (OT) order has been received, the OTR/COTA team performs an evaluation. Specific assessments of posture, alignment, balance, strength, and visual acuity are necessary. Assessments of head control, trunk stability, upper extremity support, and ability to self-propel are added to evaluate seating needs (Ericson, 1991; Tideiksaar, 2001). Perceptual and cognitive assessments should be included only as appropriate. Practitioners should not embarrass or agitate cognitively impaired elders by assessing areas already documented as deficient.

Consultation

The assessment may reveal minimal intervention needs, perhaps only consultation. Patterson, Strumpf, & Evans (1995) include the roles of advocate, observer, teacher, information specialist, team problem solver, and identifier of resources and alternatives in their definition of *consultant*. They also report that the combination of consultation with formal restraint reduction training significantly reduces the use of restraints. COTAs are uniquely qualified to function as consultants in developing alternatives to restraints, especially if they are familiar with restraint reduction principles, OBRA regulations, and the basic principles of positioning. For example, an elbow air splint may be all that is necessary for an elder who continually scratches at sutures on a healing incision. Although an air splint certainly is restrictive, it allows more movement than wrist restraints, thereby meeting the criterion for "least restrictive environment." Because wound healing is temporary, the air splint is a temporary measure. A protocol for use of the air splint should be provided. The care plan should document the reason why the splint is being used, the way it will be used, and the way it will be reassessed by nursing staff.

COTAs may recommend other environmental, psychosocial, and activity-related alternatives (Box 14-2). The alternatives outlined are not a complete list. Options are limitless, depending on the COTA's creativity. Each measure considered should provide as much free choice and control as possible for elders. Eigsti & Vrooman (1992) claim that the basic ingredient in reducing restraint use is teaching staff to understand and believe that alternatives exist.

Environmental Adaptations

Environmental adaptations are an important source of restraint alternatives. For example, many different styles of chairs are found in nursing homes. The one selected must be comfortable both physically and emotionally for the elder. However, replacing a belt or vest restraint with a reclined chair from which the elder is unable to rise is not an acceptable alternative. An inexpensive and less restrictive alternative for the confused elder who rises unsafely from a chair might be a personal alarm. Several such alarms are on the market. They do not prevent the elder from rising, but they do alert staff. An elder's attempt to rise usually occurs for a reason and warrants attention from the caregiver. However, a personal alarm may frighten or agitate the elder or surrounding residents. Therefore, the use of the alarm should be with caution and take into account the environment, elder, and other residents.

A wrap-around walker with a seat is an alternative device that allows independent ambulation for some elders who would otherwise require assistance (Kerr, 1994) (Fig. 14-1). It can provide a means for safe and comfortable ambulation, allowing an elder who previously sat alone all day the opportunity to engage in social interaction and exercise. With supporting documentation, this walker should be interpreted as a beneficial orthotic device. If it makes the elder feel confined or agitated, however, it is considered a restraint. A wrap-around walker with wheels can be used for independent ambulation with more mobile elders.

Many facilities have discovered that nursery intercoms are an inexpensive and effective way to monitor safe ambulators who wander. Directional signs may help these elders locate their rooms and deter them from entering someone else's room. An alternative to direction signs are signs with familiar pictures instead of words. Families should be encouraged to help elders decorate their rooms with familiar objects, pictures, and even furniture, which help elders feel more connected to their surroundings and reduce the likelihood of wandering.

Psychosocial Approaches

Psychosocial approaches to reduce restraint use are important. Rader, Doan, & Schwab (1985) define *agenda behavior* as the plans and actions of cognitively impaired elders that result from an effort to fulfill physical, emotional,

BOX 14-2

Alternatives to Restraints

Environmental adaptations
Chairs
  Deep seats
  Tilted
  Recliners
  Rockers
  Gliders
  Bean bag
  Adirondack type
  Customized

Monitoring systems
  Television monitoring
  Enclosed courtyards
  Alarms
  Exit alarms
  Door buzzers
  Nursery intercom
  Personal alarms
  Pressure-sensitive pads
  Positional alarms
  Limb bracelet alarms

Signs
  Directional
  Stop or Keep Out
  Identifying (elder's name)

Environmental adaptations
Safety adaptations
  Nonskid surfaces
  Low bed
  Mattress or sleep mat on floor

¾- to ½-length bed rails
  (instead of full length)
Lowered or no bed rail
Accessible call lights
Safe furniture arrangement
Accessible light switches
Safe walking routes
Encouraged use of handrail
Bedside commode or urinal
Items within reach
Shoes or nonskid socks worn in bed

Personalized room
  Familiar furniture
  Familiar objects to hold
  Meaningful pictures and photographs

Other adaptations
  Bean bags (different sizes)
  Pillows
  Foam
  Nonslip mats
  Firm wheelchair seats
  Air-splints
  "Wrap-around" walkers with seats

Psychosocial Approaches
Behavioral strategies
  Remotivation
  Reality orientation (if helpful)
  Frequent reminders
  Active listening
  Responding to agenda behavior

Decrease or increase
  Interactions
  Visiting
  Sensory stimulation (especially noise
    such as that from overhead paging,
    television, radio, among others)
  Identification of antecedent to the
    unwanted behavior and appropriate
    measures to address

Activities
  Structured daily routines
  Self-care
  Permit or encourage wandering and
    pacing
  Exercise
  Bowling
  Nature walks
  Wheelchair aerobics, dances, ball
    games
  Ambulation programs
  Toileting every 2 hours
  Nighttime activities
  Volunteer and family assistance
  Buddy system
  Activity kits
  Diversional opportunities
  Relaxation techniques
  Massage
  Therapeutic touch
  Warm bath
  Music specific to elder tastes

or social needs. The authors indicate that such behavior often follows feelings of loneliness or separation. Wandering or attempts to get up from a chair may be part of an elder's agenda behavior and may lead to agitation if the elder is restrained. Evans, Forceia, Yurkow, and Sochalski (1999) indicate that the keys to responding successfully to agenda behavior are to allow elders to act on their plans, identify a point at which they may accept a suggestion or guidance, and allow them to keep their dignity throughout an incident. The important difference in the result of this approach compared with others is that allowing the elder to play out the behavior provides a sense of identity and promotes feelings of belonging, safety, and connectedness, diminishing the elder's need to seek those feelings elsewhere. Further incidences of wandering are subsequently decreased or eliminated (Gallo, et al., 1999). Brungardt (1994) adds that this method works well if the elder's welfare is considered before the needs or routines of the facility.

Activity Alternatives

Providing meaningful activity alternatives can decrease behavior such as restlessness that has traditionally led to the use of restraints. An activity kit, perhaps in the form of a sewing basket, briefcase, fanny pack, or tackle box, may be helpful. The kit may be assembled by family members who are familiar with the elder's interests. (Rader, 1995; Plautz & Camp, 2001). The idea is to provide something familiar, comfortable, and safe that engages the elder's attention.

Treatment

Although not all referrals require intervention beyond consultation, the assessment may identify a need for

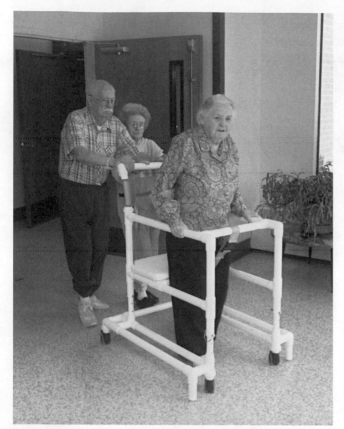

FIGURE **14-1**   A wrap-around walker allows independent ambulation for this elder who would otherwise need assistance.

ongoing treatment. Examples of treatment to eliminate the need for restraint include development of self-care techniques, upper body positioning, and seating adaptations.

Because restraint use is associated with the inability to perform self-care, elders and their caregivers should be taught strategies for accomplishing this goal. Determining the routines the elder followed in the past to maintain a sense of continuity and predictability is particularly important. Because part of the objective is to reduce anxiety and agitation, self-care must be done according to the elder's agenda and routine rather than those of the COTA or facility.

Elders with hemiplegia are often provided with lapboards to assist with upper body positioning. Because these elders need the best support possible for their upper extremities, this is one of the few cases in which it may be advantageous to begin with the most restrictive device, a full lapboard, and adapt if necessary. If a full lapboard causes agitation or seems too restrictive (perhaps the elder is unable to use a urinal independently), a swing-away half lap tray may be used. Another solution is a foam wedge or cylindrical bean bag, which can extend the width of the armrest for safe positioning without

a lapboard. As with any restrictive device, however, less than perfect positioning may be necessary to accommodate the elder's choice.

Another specific OT intervention aimed at reducing the need for restraints is a positioning assessment for elders who are wheelchair bound. Ill-fitting wheelchairs contribute to restraint use, which can lead to abnormal sitting posture and eventual loss of function (Greenburg, 1996). For example, wheelchairs usually found in nursing homes were not designed for independent mobility or long-term sitting. Necessary adaptations for comfort and function include dropping the seat so that elders can reach the floor with their feet, replacing the sling seat with a firm seat and cushion, and replacing the sling back with a firm back. A narrower chair may help elders propel themselves more comfortably (Jones, 1995). Knowledge of the principles of positioning is essential. (Basic alignment principles applicable to any elder are outlined in Chapter 19.) Once adaptations have been designed and implemented, the elder's verbal, behavioral, and postural response must be observed. The system should be reassessed and adapted as necessary until the positioning goals have been met. Documentation should accompany every step of this process, especially if the elder declines the intervention. With very difficult cases, consultation with a seating expert may be helpful. However, even the nonexpert can make many "low-tech" foam supports. More detailed information on wheelchair positioning is included in Part 4 of this chapter.

Relatively inexpensive foam is available in large sizes at the local building or craft store and can easily be cut and shaped with an electric knife. This type of foam works well for the addition of width to an armrest, fabrication of forearm wedges to elevate edematous upper extremities, or provision of lightweight lateral trunk support. Egg crate foam is another inexpensive material suitable for limited purposes. Neither of these low-density foams is adequate to support entire body weight while sitting or during episodes of spasticity. For long-term positioning, manufactured cushions of mixed density foam, gel, or air cushions are more durable and are recommended for both comfort and maintained skin integrity. The therapeutic role of orthotic devices in achieving proper body position, balance, and alignment and improving overall functional capacity without the potential negative effects of restraint use is recognized by HCFA (1995, 2001). This recognition does not provide license to use wedges, reclining chairs, or seat belts as restraints, even for cognitively intact elders. However, it does allow the legitimate use of positioning devices to increase function, given a demonstrated necessity. Any adaptation should maintain the dignity of elders and augment their quality of life.

CONCLUSION

COTAs have a responsibility to clearly state their professional opinion and recommendations. Clients must choose whether to act on that advice. True restraint reduction requires an examination of our attitudes about the rights of elders, especially those with cognitive impairment, to make choices and take risks. We must be willing to become advocates for elders. An understanding of OBRA regulations and positioning principles and the ability to

be flexible and creative within a team framework permit COTAs to contribute effectively to restraint elimination programs. If we have honestly attempted to increase function and honor the dignity of the elders we serve, we will have followed not only the letter of the law but the intent and spirit as well.

CANDICE MULLENDORE

PART 2 Wheelchair Seating and Positioning
Considerations for Elders

In 1997, approximately 19% of individuals aged 65 years and older relied on a wheelchair for their mobility within the household and community (Russell, Hendershot, LeClere, Howie, & Adler, 1997). As the population in this age range continues to grow, this percentage is expected to rapidly increase. The use of assistive devices such as wheelchairs for mobility has increased with the population growth, technologic advances, and initiatives in public policies (Russell, Hendershot, LeClere, Howie, & Adler, 1997). Public policies such as the Technology Related Assistance for Individuals with Disabilities Act (1998) and the Rehabilitation Act Amendments of 1986 have contributed to the increased access to wheelchairs by elders. The use of a wheelchair for mobility in the home or community, or both, is important in improving individuals' level of independence and their ability to participate in chosen occupations.

Health professionals frequently have a "one size fits all" approach to wheelchair seating and positioning. This is often true with elders because Medicare has strict guidelines regarding wheelchair rental and purchase. However, elders have numerous conditions associated with aging that increase the likelihood of complications from improper wheelchair seating and positioning. Such conditions include joint replacements, osteoarthritis, osteoporosis, musculoskeletal changes including kyphosis and scoliosis, cerebrovascular accident, Alzheimer's disease, amyotrophic lateral sclerosis, Parkinson's disease, dementia, chronic obstructive pulmonary disease, diabetes, congestive heart failure, and hypertension (Krasilovsky, 1993).

A wheelchair should be selected with the unique needs of the individual person in mind. The overall outcomes for a person in a proper position in his or her wheelchair include increased independence, prevention of skin breakdown, decreased need for caregiver(s), and a general overall improvement in quality of life (Rader, Jones, &

Miller, 2000). The result of an elder seated improperly in his or her wheelchair can be fixed or flexible deformities, as well as a decrease in overall function (Perr, 1998).

A proper wheelchair seating and positioning assessment should be conducted by an OTR. The COTA may collaborate in this process. Areas considered in such an assessment include diagnosis, prognosis, age, cognition, perception, level of independence with activities of daily living (ADL) and occupations, functional mobility, body weight distribution, posture, sensory status, presence of edema, skin integrity, and time spent in the wheelchair. It is important that the elder be involved in the decision about a wheelchair. Wheelchair abandonment is more likely to occur when the individual's needs are not addressed (Cook, 1982; Zola, 1982). Once a proper wheelchair has been determined, the COTA must help monitor the patient in any of the areas assessed as listed earlier.

Certain aspects of wheelchair seating and positioning are of particular importance to elders. Because of musculoskeletal changes, the elder's posture needs to be monitored continuously. In addition, elders are more at risk for skin breakdown. Therefore, the COTA should help monitor this and educate the elder about the need for pressure relief on a regular schedule. The COTA may also be responsible for making sure the components of a wheelchair are working properly. If a needed repair is identified, the COTA can help facilitate a follow-up visit with the wheelchair vendor.

Skin breakdown can occur quickly with elders. There are several types of skin breakdown related to improper seating, including abrasion, pressure, and shearing. Abrasion occurs when the skin rubs against a surface and causes damage to the tissue (Perr, 1998). An example of this may be if an overweight individual sits in a standard size wheelchair and his or her hips rub against the armrest. In addition, rubbing against any sharp areas can cause an abrasion. Elders generally have fragile skin and an abrasion can occur with very little rubbing (Perr, 1998). A COTA should be aware of this risk and evaluate if any abrasions occur.

Pressure occurs when the forces of two surfaces act against each other. In an optimal wheelchair seating system, pressure will be equally distributed between the person and the seating system. Unfortunately, this equal distribution can be difficult to achieve and maintain, and therefore pressure sores may develop. A pressure sore occurs when the blood circulation to an area is decreased. Subsequently, oxygen does not flow to those cells and death of the cells may occur. After death of the cells occurs, necrosis takes place and a pressure sore results. Pressure sores develop from the inside out, generally in areas with bony prominences. The ischial tuberosities and sacrum are areas in which pressure sores commonly occur because of improper seating. A COTA should be aware of this risk and continually monitor if an elder is at risk for pressure sores. Elders who are particularly slender may be at more risk for a pressure sore. All elders should be seated on some type of wheelchair cushion after a proper OT evaluation.

Shearing is another cause of skin breakdown. Shearing also occurs when two surfaces rub against one another. It is not uncommon for shearing to happen with elders seated improperly in sling wheelchairs. The sling does not support the pelvis adequately and elders may slump in their chair, causing shearing at the ischial tuberosities and sacral areas. In addition, the risk for shearing in those same areas and in the spinous processes increases with a chair that reclines (Perr, 1998).

The COTA can help elders learn how to monitor their skin for potential breakdown. Any areas of redness, particularly over bony prominences, can quickly turn into an abrasion or pressure ulcer. The COTA can advise the elders and their caregivers about how to complete a skin inspection. The COTA also can help to adapt or modify mirrors to help elders view their skin.

It is important for the COTA to be aware of the optimal seating position. The most important element of proper seating is the position of the pelvis. The pelvis is the base of support when one is sitting. The pelvis should be in a neutral position with weight equally distributed between the left and right ischial tuberosities. The trunk should have slight lordosis in the lumbar area, slight kyphosis in the thoracic region, and a small amount of cervical extension (Perr, 1998). The elder's femurs should be in neutral position, with slight abduction of the hips and 90 degrees of flexion at the hip, knee, and ankle. The arms should be supported by the armrests with the elbows slightly forward of the shoulders (Perr, 1998). The armrests should be an adequate height to support the arms, but not to elevate the shoulders (Fig. 14-2).

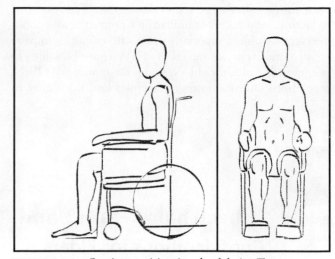

FIGURE 14-2   Seating position in wheelchair. (From Perr, A. [1998]. Elements of seating and wheeled mobility intervention. *Occupational Therapy Practice*, *3*(9), 16-24.)

Improved posture in a wheelchair can help physiologic functions such as breathing, swallowing, and digestion (Rader, Jones, & Miller, 2000). In addition, adjusting posture can improve socialization by simply changing the elder's eye gaze to allow for more interactions in the environment. Comfort is often improved with proper seating, which may also impact elders' tolerance and endurance to sit in their wheelchair for longer periods.

The COTA can observe the posture of elders in their wheelchair and make note of any abnormalities such as posterior tilt of the pelvis, sliding forward in the wheelchair, leaning to one side, inadequate arm support, and inability to propel self in the wheelchair. Should a COTA identify problems in an elder's current wheelchair system, a referral to an OTR would be indicated for reevaluation of the seating system. The negative impact of poor seating on frail elders is summarized in Table 14-1 (Rader, Jones, & Miller, 2000).

Because of insurance restrictions, elders often find themselves in rental wheelchairs with sling upholstery. Sling-upholstered wheelchairs were not designed to be primary or long-term seating systems; they were designed to transport people short distances (Rader, Jones, & Miller, 2000). People seated for long periods in sling-upholstered wheelchairs often develop poor posture including posterior pelvic tilt and kyphosis in the thoracic and lumbar regions. This type of posture increases the possibility of skin breakdown and limits elders' ability to engage in their occupations. Simple remedies such as inserting a solid seat or back, or both, can significantly improve the situation for elders. COTAs can help to identify problems associated with poor wheelchair seating

TABLE 14-1

Negative Impact of Poor Seating on Frail Elders		
Seating problem	**Result on body**	**Potential negative impact**
Wheelchair too tall	Feet do not touch the floor Inability to move self Migration of pelvis out of chair	Agitation Circulatory problems Edema in legs Decreased activity Poor sitting posture Increased restraint use Pain
Poor back support	Compression of trunk, chest, abdomen Sliding out of chair Increased posterior pelvic tilt	Skin breakdown on back and sacrum Impaired digestion, elimination, chewing, swallowing, breathing, and coughing
Wheelchair too heavy	Inability to move chair Requires more energy to move chair	Decreased activity, socialization Fatigue
Wheelchair too wide	Shifting pelvis from side to side Leaning out of chair Inability to access hand rims	Sheering of skin Poor posture, circulation Increased restraint use Pain Agitation
Hammocking effect of sling seat	Pelvic obliquity Scoliosis Sliding out of chair Requires more energy to stay in chair	Poor posture and circulation Increased restraint use Decreased wheelchair tolerance Pain Sheering of skin Fatigue Agitation
Foot rests too high	Lack of femoral support Unequal pressure distribution Increased ischial tuberosity pressure	Poor posture Pain Skin Breakdown

From Rader, J., Jones, D., & Miller, L. (2000). The importance of individualized wheelchair seating for frail older adults. *Journal of Gerontological Nursing, 26,* 24–32.

and positioning and help recommend changes to improve independence.

Pain and agitation also have been associated with improper positioning of elders in wheelchairs (Feldt, Warne, & Ryden, 1998). As a result, elders with these symptoms may find themselves with restraints in their wheelchairs. Unfortunately, this usage of restraints can cause further agitation and can decrease the elder's level of alertness and ability to participate in occupations. Other elders may find themselves sliding or leaning in the wheelchair. Caregivers often use seating restraint to help with posture (Rader, Jones, & Miller, 2000). The use of a restraint to correct posture does not address the cause for the misalignment, which is poor seating and positioning. Therefore, the COTA should be careful when monitoring the elder's posture in a wheelchair. See Part 1 of this chapter for a review of proper usage of

restraints, and see Box 14-3 for common seating observations (Rader, Jones, & Miller).

COTAs also can help to determine an elder's functional levels in their current seating system. Because of insurance restrictions from Medicare noted earlier, elders often are set up with heavy, standard-sized wheelchairs that can impede their ability to participate in activities. A study of nursing home residents by Simmons et al. (1995) indicated a positive correlation between hand-grip strength and wheelchair endurance. This study revealed that simple modifications such as extending brake handles, modifying seat to floor height, and prescribing lightweight wheelchairs when appropriate would increase the elder's participation within the nursing home.

If a COTA notices a decrease in an elder's functional activity, it would be important to determine whether the seating system is impairing the elder's ability to participate

BOX 14-3

Observations That Should Trigger a Seating Assessment

Leaning or sliding in chair
Use of a tie-on restraint
Use of gerichair or recliner as restraint
Crying and yelling behaviors in wheelchair-bound elders
Agitation and restlessness in wheelchair-bound elders
Seatbelts that go over or above the abdomen
Tray tables, lap pillows, wedges, or bolsters used for positioning

From Rader, Jones, & Miller (2000). The importance of individualized wheelchair seating for frail older adults. *Journal of Gerontological Nursing*, 26, 24-32.

in certain activities. Of particular importance would be to determine if the elder's strength has decreased. A decrease in any level of strength may also mean a decrease in elder's ability to transfer to and from a wheelchair and/or propel themselves to activities. The COTA can discuss with elders what factors are impeding their participation in activities. It may be that a simple solution such as extending the hand brakes or oiling the flip-up footplates can facilitate increased participation in an activity.

A good wheelchair seating system can support improvements in posture, comfort, independence, and endurance, while preventing skin breakdown. Furthermore, a good system can help elders increase their tolerance for being in the wheelchair, increase socialization, and decrease the burden on caregivers (Rader, Jones, & Miller, 2000). The COTA should work closely with elders, caregivers, the OTR, and the interdisciplinary team to ensure an optimal wheelchair seating system for each elder.

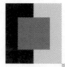

SANDRA HATTORI OKADA

PART 3   Fall Prevention*

COTAs must be aware of the high risk of falls among the elderly and the importance of **fall prevention.** Falls can be a major cause of immobility, premature nursing home placement, and even death. Some risk factors include a history of falls, neurologic illness, multiple medications, poor eyesight, deconditioning, and age-related changes such as decreased protective responses. More importantly, delicate balance exists between biological and psychosocial factors and common environmental hazards. Therefore, even a small disruption in this dynamic system can lead to a devastating fall.

Elders older than 75 years have falls more frequently than any group except infants and toddlers. However, elders face a significantly greater risk for sustaining a severe or fatal injury. Accidents are the sixth leading cause of death for those older than 65 years, and falls are the leading type of accident in the home (Tideiksaar, 2001). Once a fall occurs, 1 of 40 elders will be admitted to the hospital. Of those elders in the hospital after a fall, only about half will be alive one year later.

By the year 2030, the elder population is expected to more than double to approximately 70 million people (Kinsella & Velkoff, 2001). Over a third of persons aged

*Updated by Candice Mullendore and Ivelisse Lazzarini.

65 and older experience a fall each year (Gillespie, et al., 2002; Rubenstein, 2001; Tinetti, Speechley, & Ginter, 1988). Accidents are the sixth leading cause of death for those older than 65 years (Josephson, Fabacher, & Rubenstein, 1991; Lamb, Miller, & Herrnandez, 1987; Tideiksaar, 2001). Once a fall occurs, 1 of 40 elders will be hospitalized (Campbell, Reinken, Allan, & Martinez, 1981), and one fifth of all falls will require some level of medical attention (Gillespie, Gillespie, Robertson, Lamb, Cumming, & Rowe, 2002). Of those elders admitted to the hospital after a fall, only about half will be alive 1 year later (Gryfe, Amies, & Ashley, 1977; Rubenstein & Robbins, 1989). As the elder population increases in the next 30 years, so will the incidence of falls. Therefore, it is important to be knowledgeable about the causes of falls in elderly persons.

CAUSES OF FALLS
Environmental Causes

Accidents related to the environment are the primary cause of falls among elders (Tideiksaar, 1987, 2001; Rubenstein & Robbins, 1989). Approximately one third of falls occur in the home (Hettinger, 1996). Disease processes associated with aging are often strong determinants for falls, but environmental factors in the home may be a more common cause (Perry, 1985, as cited in Walker and Howland, 1991). About 30% of older adults are **aging in place** (growing old at home), a 32% increase from 13 years ago (Administration on Aging, 2003). A poorly kept home or yard may be an environmental sign of age-related changes. As people age, they may lose the endurance, strength, and cognitive ability to structure tasks and deal with their environment. Common **environmental hazards** in the home include poor lighting or glare, uneven stairs, lack of handrails by stairs, and uneven or unsafe surfaces (frayed rug edges, slippery floors in the shower and tub, polished floors, cracks in cement, high doorsteps, and so on). Other hazards may involve old, unstable, or low furniture (chairs, beds, or toilets); pets; young children; clutter or electric cords in walkways; inaccessible items; and limited space for ADL functions (Fig. 14-3). New, used, or improperly installed equipment and unfamiliar environments may also be hazardous.

According to Reinsch, MacRae, Lachenbruch, and Tobis (1992), approximately 51% of falls in the elderly population occur outside the home. Common areas in the community where falls occur include public buildings, streets, sidewalks, transferring to or from transportation, or another person's home. In addition, the greatest proportion of persons with repeated falls occurred in the community, specifically on the street or sidewalk. The most common activities that elderly persons were engaging in when they fell include walking on uneven ground, tripping (over curbs, rugs, or objects), and slipping on wet surfaces. Other examples of activities associated with falls include lifting heavy objects, reaching, balancing on items of unstable support (overturned box), or turning quickly. Therefore, the OTA should take into consideration the home, community, and activity during fall when determining a fall prevention plan (Reinsch, MacRae, Lachenbruch, & Tobis, 1992; Capezuti, 2000).

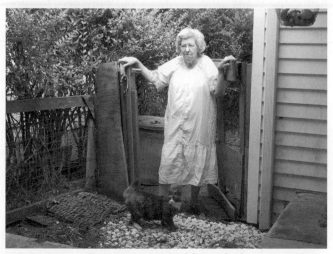

FIGURE 14-3 Common potential hazards that may cause falls include rugs and pets underfoot.

Biological Causes

Sensory

Visual changes associated with aging that may influence falls include decreases in depth perception, peripheral vision, color discrimination, acuity, and accommodation. Approximately 30% of persons aged 65 and older have visual impairments (Desai, Pratt, Lentzner, & Robinson, 2001). As the elderly population grows, so will the number of persons with visual impairments. A visual impairment can affect a person's ability to participate in functional mobility in the home and the community.

Stairs may become more difficult to maneuver. Knowing the location of the next step and judging its depth can become a big challenge. That 75% of all stair accidents occur while descending the stairs, most in the second half of the flight, is also noteworthy (Brummel-Smith, 1990; Tideiksaar, 2001). New bifocals or trifocals may require adjustment time, and looking down stairs requires constant head and eye adjustments.

Medical conditions affecting vision include macular degeneration, cataracts, diabetic retinopathy, glaucoma, and stroke (Desai, Pratt, Lentzner, & Robinson, 2001). These conditions may manifest as scotomas (blind spots), which impair safety in mobility. Objects on the floor, such as pencils and telephone cords, may not be apparent. Elders with visual impairments may also run into furniture. Decreased visual input caused by disease processes may result in a decrease in postural stability (Poole, 1991). In turn, this affects an elder's balance and may contribute to the greater incidence of falls among this population.

A disorder involving spatial organization or figure ground may cause an elder to perceive a change in rug color or flooring as a stair, and glare on the linoleum as spilled liquid. A dark stairway may be perceived as a ramp. Misinterpreting this information may cause a misjudged step and a fall. (Chapter 15 provides more detailed information on age-related changes in vision and recommended adaptations.)

Neurologic/Musculoskeletal

Conditions that affect posture and body alignment cause changes in center of gravity, gait, stride, strength, and joint stability, all of which increase the risk for falls. Age-related changes in postural control include decreased proprioception, slower righting reflexes, decreased muscle tone, and increased postural sway (Poole, 1991; Steinmetz and Hobson, 1994). Changes in gait include decreased height of stepping. Men tend to have a more flexed posture and wide-based, short-stepped gait, whereas women tend to have a more narrow-based, waddling gait (Kane, Luslander, & Abrass, 1994). Medical conditions that affect instability include degenerative joint disease, deconditioning, malnutrition, dehydration, and neurologic disorders such as neuropathy, stroke, Parkinson's disease, and dementia (Brummel-Smith, 1990; Kane, Luslander, & Abrass, 1994;

Tideiksaar, 2001). Elder women are more susceptible to brittle bones, with a greater incidence of osteoporosis after menopause. In the case of brittle bones, it may be a fractured bone that causes the fall rather than vice versa. However, falls in the elderly cause 90% of the incidence of hip fractures (Carter, Kannus, and Khan, 2001). Musculoskeletal conditions that contribute to falls in the elderly include osteoarthritis, spondylosis, and a general decrease in joint range of motion (McIntyre, 1999).

To compensate for changes in gait and decreased balance, elders may "furniture glide" by holding on to furniture for support while they walk (Fig. 14-4). They may also drag a foot or lose their balance toward their weaker side (stroke), have a shuffling gait (Alzheimer's disease), or fall forward (Parkinson's disease) during ADL training. Older adults may hold onto faucets to get into the tub or shower or lean against the shower wall for stability while bathing.

Cardiovascular

Age-related changes include orthostatic hypotension, which affects approximately 30% of the elder population (Brummel-Smith, 1990; Sullivan, 2001). Other medical conditions that cause blood pressure changes include hypertension, neuropathy, and diabetes. In addition, these changes can occur as side effects of certain medications. Arrhythmias may cause up to 50% of syncopal episodes in elders (Sullivan, 2001). Elders may experience a greater incidence of dizziness or light-headedness, with lower cardiac output, autonomic dysfunction, impaired venous return, and prolonged bed rest. Underlying cardiac

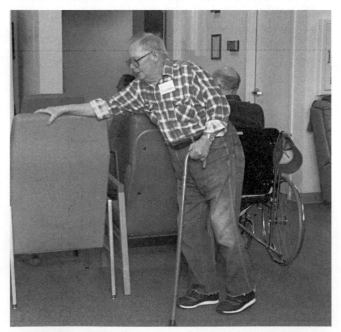

FIGURE 14-4 Elders often "furniture glide" by holding on to furniture to compensate for changes in gait and decreased balance.

disease is the most common cause of syncope that may result in a fall (Rubenstein & Josephson, 2002). Together with extrinsic, or environmental, factors, these biological, or intrinsic, factors are the primary causes of falls among elders (Tideiksaar, 1987, 2001; Rubenstein & Robbins, 1989).

Cognitive/Psychosocial Causes

Psychosocial and cognitive risk factors that may influence falls include poor judgment, insight, and problem-solving skills; confusion; and inattention resulting from fatigue, depression, and dementia. Other factors may include reactions to psychotropic medications, fear of falling, unfamiliarity with a new environment or caregiver, and a strong drive for independence. Elders and their families may not comply with recommended safety modifications because of cultural or personal preferences, aesthetic values, and limited financial or social resources. Consequently, both the caregiver and the client are at greater risk for having a fall.

Functional Causes

Performing ADL functions becomes increasingly challenging for elders. In 1997, 14% of the elder population reported difficulties with ADL and 22% reported difficulties with instrumental ADL (IADL; U.S. Bureau of Census, 2002). Functional mobility problems that may lead to falls include difficulty with performing transfers (to or from lounge chair, bed, toilet, tub or shower, wheelchair, and car), dressing and bathing (especially the lower body), reaching, sitting, standing, and walking unsupported. Other factors may include the lack of assistive aids for ambulation or an inability to use them. Elders with dementia may forget where they left a cane or walk carrying their walker rather than using it for support. Old, lost, borrowed, or smudged glasses may impair vision. Poorly fitting shoes, loose pants with dragging hems, and flimsy sandals with nylons can affect balance. Falls most commonly occur in places where elders perform most self-care activities: by the bed and in the bathroom (Tideiksaar, 1987, 2001).

FALL PREVENTION

Fall prevention is an issue for the entire health care team. Falls have multifactorial causes; therefore, the interdisciplinary team must obtain an accurate history of falls to prevent their future occurrence. Team members, including the COTA, can help to identify the frequency and location of the falls, the medical history and symptoms, medications taken and their side effects, and gait analysis (Tideiksaar, 1989, 2001). The acronym *SLIPPED* can be used to collect information (Box 14-4).

When asking about functional status, COTAs should not only ask whether the elder is able to perform ADL functions but also observe the way these are done.

BOX 14-4

Work-Up for Falls

S　Environmental hazards
L　Length of time at residence
I　Important activities to continue doing
P　Performance: how the activity was done
P　Personal assistance, time left alone
E　Environmental hazards
D　Devices used or not used

For example, when the COTA asked Mr. Owen if he could get off the toilet by himself, he responded that he was independent with toileting. When the COTA asked him to demonstrate this transfer, Mr. Owen hooked his cane on a towel rack to pull himself off the toilet. The COTA was able to determine a high risk for falling only because the transfer was observed. If the COTA had simply accepted Mr. Owen's report of independence, she would not have been able to recommend a raised toilet seat and toilet rails or replacement of the towel racks with sturdy grab bars.

COTAs should encourage elders to wear sturdy, comfortable, rubber-sole footwear (for example, tennis shoes) to help obtain a more secure footing. Some elders may wear slip-on shoes because tying or fastening shoes is difficult. Assistive devices such as elastic laces or Velcro closures may help address this difficulty and provide the elder with more stable footwear to help prevent falls. When dressing, elders should pull pant legs above their ankles before standing. Pants should be pulled down *after* transferring from the wheelchair to the toilet to avoid tripping.

Fogel (1992) observed that elders with a reach of less than 6 to 7 inches also were limited in their mobility skills and were the most restricted in ADL activities. Older adults who have difficulty reaching and carrying objects may require reachers, extended handles on bath brushes or shoe horns, carts, walker trays or bags, and sock aids. COTAs also can help problem solve—for example, they can determine the best way to attach the reacher to the walker or rearrange items around the living space so they are within reach. Higher electrical outlets also could be recommended to limit the need to reach and bend. Redesigning or rearranging an elder's environment is often an inexpensive and effective fall prevention technique. However, it is important to consider that rearranging furniture may disorient an elder, which could increase the possibility of a fall. Environment redesign should only occur with the consent of the elder, and follow-up visits are recommended to assess the transition.

Difficulty with transfers and **mobility** during ADL functions may require safety training with the cane, walker, or wheelchair. This is particularly important because many falls occur in transit during transfers. Elders with nocturia, a normal age change involving increased frequency of urination at night, have a particular need for night lights and a clear passage to the toilet. Before rearranging furniture to provide wider walkways, COTAs must first make sure elders do not need the furniture for stability when ambulating. A consultation with a physical therapist may help clarify the most appropriate and safe assistive device for ambulation.

Bathroom modifications may include a tub or shower bench with armrests and back, a handheld shower hose, grab bars, or a raised toilet seat. Throw rugs should be removed, or nonskid backing should be applied under them. Nonskid stripping or rubber mats can be placed on tub or shower floors. Sliding glass doors should be removed to allow for wider access into the tub. A shower curtain may be hung from a pressure mounted bar to provide privacy if the glass doors are removed. Heat-sensitive safety valves also can be installed to prevent scalding. If the elder uses a wheelchair and the door to the bathroom is too narrow, a rolling shower bench or commode chair with wheels may help. Placing a commode chair by the bed may eliminate unsafe night transfers to the bathroom toilet. A three-in-one commode chair is an inexpensive solution. This type of commode is light and can be used at bedside, over the toilet, or in the tub or shower. Caregivers should remember, however, that emptying the commode bucket and lifting and relocating the commode can be difficult for elders. They should be discouraged from using soap dispensers, towel racks, and toilet paper holders for support. Hygiene items should be placed within reach. Mirrors may be tilted or lowered for better viewing during ADL functions. Doors under the sink should be removed to give the elder more leg room while sitting in front of the sink.

Similar precautions should be taken in the kitchen. Step stools should be avoided, and frequently used utensils and dishes should be rearranged so they are within safe reach. Use of energy conservation techniques during meal preparation may decrease the risk for falling because of fatigue or orthostatic hypotension. Simple meal preparation packages are widely available in grocery stores. Use of a microwave can help decrease the amount of time an elder spends standing at a stove to prepare a meal.

About 30% of all falls in the elderly occur in the home (Reinsch, MacRae, Lachenbruch, and Tobis, 1992). Of those elders who fell during ADL, 22% had falls that occurred when they tried to get out of bed or up from a chair (Reinsch, MacRae, Lachenbruch, and Tobis, 1992). The height of seats (beds, sofas, chairs) can be increased with firm cushions. Worn mattresses or cushions should be rotated. Chairs with armrests are recommended to facilitate

189

rising from the chair. Chairs with wheels should be avoided, and the brakes of wheelchairs and commodes must be secured before transfers are attempted. Elders should lean forward in the wheelchair only when both feet are flat on the floor (not on the footrests). Electronic lift chairs are typically available in furniture stores.

Caregivers must ensure that stairs are well lit, with no glare, and equipped with railings running along the entire length of the stairwell on both sides. Stripping of various colors can be used at the edge of each step to distinguish them from each other. Safety grip strips may be placed on each step as well. Light switches should be within reach at both the top and bottom of the stairway. COTAs should discuss with elders safe ways to change a light bulb. User-friendly, touch-sensitive, and motion-sensor light switches also are available. Transition areas such as doorways, garages, and patios are common sites for falls. COTAs should look at the outdoor environment, transition areas, and the indoor environment to help prevent falls.

Interventions to compensate for visual loss include increased lighting with limited glare, improved contrast for steps and furniture, decreased clutter in walkways, and well maintained flooring. COTAs should anticipate elders' performance at different times of the day, with varied natural lighting and indoor lighting. Referrals to vision specialists may be appropriate to ensure elders are wearing the appropriate eyewear.

Elders who report dizziness with a change in position may be experiencing a decrease in blood pressure that could result in a fall with or without syncope. Blood pressure should be monitored, and elders should be allowed to make slow transitions from supine to sitting or sitting to standing positions. A few minutes may be necessary to allow the blood pressure to accommodate to the change in head position. By teaching elders different techniques for dressing and bathing and instructing them in the use of long handle devices, COTAs can help elders limit and modify their bending. A typical recommendation is that the elder get dressed while seated to help accommodate for orthostatic hypotension. The rest of the health care team should be informed of reports of dizziness and unstable changes in blood pressure.

Gradual increases in activity are recommended for people with conditions that affect endurance (such as cardiac conditions and deconditioning). Strategically located sturdy chairs may be useful for elders who require rest periods when going from one room to another. Sitting while bathing and avoiding long hot baths also are recommended. A commode chair by the bed may save energy. Activities that involve straining and holding one's breath (such as during toileting, strenuous transfers, or exercise) can cause light-headedness and should be monitored.

General strengthening programs incorporated in the elder's daily routine can help to decrease deconditioning, especially that caused by a sedentary lifestyle. Exercise programs have been proven as an effective measure in fall prevention. COTAs may refer elders to physical therapy for general lower extremity strengthening and balance exercises (Steinmetz and Hobson, 1994). Community exercise programs such as dancing, water aerobics, swimming, and walking clubs also are appropriate recommendations. A study by Gillespie, Gillespie, Roberston, Lamb, Cumming, and Rowe (2002) reviewed the literature to determine effective fall prevention programs in the United States. The study revealed that the most effective measures included muscle strengthening, balance retraining, Tai Chi group exercise, home assessment and modification, and decreasing psychotropic medications. Cuming (2002) reported similar findings.

COTAs, elders, family members, and caregivers should work together to identify activities important to elders that can be modified to prevent falls. Family members should be included because elders may depend on them to help with preparation and assistance. Elders may prefer to perform toileting activities independently but may not mind assistance with feeding. COTAs should identify personal and shared spaces in the elder's living environment. If family members do not want to modify the only bathroom in the home with a raised toilet seat and grab bars, a commode chair by the elder's bed may be appropriate. COTAs should help elders and their family members address safety concerns and practice giving assistance in a safe environment.

Additional areas to consider are the frequency and occurrence of falls. If elders experience repeated falls, their confidence levels may decrease, which could result in a decrease in participation in ADL and IADL (Walker & Howland, 1991). The time of day that a fall occurs also is important information to obtain. About 64% of elders in a study reported falls in the afternoon to late afternoon period (Walker & Howland, 1991). The afternoon is generally a time of increased activity for elders, and assessment of ADL and IADL should address the time factor.

COTAs should make sure that strategies exist for emergency situations. Typical questions include the following: If a curtain is not drawn, will the neighbor know that this may be an indication of trouble? If an elder falls, will he or she know the proper way to get up from the floor if no injuries are apparent? Is a telephone within reach? Is a list of emergency phone numbers placed by the phone? If the elder is at home alone, are there emergency alert systems available to signal for help? Is a telephone reassurance program available in which a volunteer calls daily? Is it safer to soil clothes than risk an unassisted transfer to the toilet? All these questions should be addressed to ensure the elder's safety before discharge from OT.

PENNI JEAN LAVOOT

PART 4 Community Mobility*

Most elders prefer the freedom of traveling by automobile (Fig. 14-5). Driving is an important factor in their independence and mental health (Malfetti & Winter, 1986; Ekelman, Mitchel, & O'Dell-Rossi, 2001). By the year 2030, 1 in 5 American drivers will be 65 years of age or older (Savoye, 2001). In 2000, elders represented 9% of the general population, but accounted for 13% of all traffic fatalities (U.S. Department of Transportation, 2003). In the past decade, highway traffic fatalities decreased by 10% in the general population, but increased by 33% in the elderly population (U.S. Department of Transportation, 2003).

Elders are becoming increasingly more reliant on automotive transportation. This could be because the majority of elders live in rural or suburban communities. Often in these communities there are limited or no resources available for transportation options for seniors. COTAs can help elders assess the resources within the elders' local community.

Elders may experience age-related changes that can negatively affect their ability to drive, including decreased visual acuity, color discrimination, and peripheral vision, and increased sensitivity to glare (Okada, 1990). Other factors that may influence driving and mobility include unrecognized disease processes, deconditioning, psychosocial issues, medications, dementia, and environmental issues such as small print on signs. Physical changes contributing to driving abilities of elders also include a decrease in reaction time and in decision-making abilities.

Age-related changes affect the mobility of elders, whether they are pedestrians, drivers, or users of public transportation. For example, pedestrians may have difficulty stepping up or down from curbs or crossing streets within the time allotted by crossing signals (Fig. 14-6). Drivers may have difficulties merging, yielding the right of way, negotiating intersections, backing up, handling quick maneuvers, reading traffic signs, and making left turns (Okada, 1990). Physical barriers may make public transportation inaccessible. All these challenges may rob elders of the freedom and independence they may have enjoyed throughout their lives.

A common goal of OT is to assist elders in being as independent as possible in their homes and communities. As with most adults, elders regularly go to the doctor's office, grocery store, and pharmacy. These places may be around

*Updated by Candice Mullendore and Ivelisse Lazzarini.

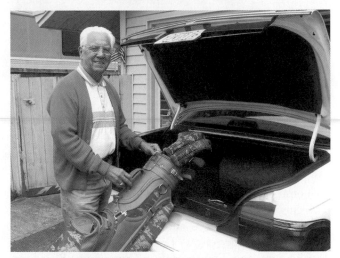

FIGURE **14-5** Most elders prefer to travel by automobile.

the corner or many miles from the elder's home. The role of the COTA in helping to identify realistic goals and treatment plans for elders often includes increasing their ability to move in the community. To do this effectively, COTAs must explore as many options for community mobility as possible (Box 14-5). Community transportation options vary greatly among rural areas and cities.

PEDESTRIAN SAFTEY

Walking safely is an important factor in community mobility. Elders account for 17% of all pedestrian fatalities (U.S. Department of Transportation, 2003). COTAs should evaluate the ability of elders to walk outdoors. Box 14-6 lists precautions for safe walking in an elder's community.

Elders who use wheelchairs, walkers, and scooters usually have more difficulty and require more time conquering crosswalks, curbs, and uneven sidewalks. These elders need training to negotiate cut-out curbs because electric scooters or wheelchairs may overturn when descending. Electric scooters with three wheels tend to tip more often than those with four wheels. A mobility expert should conduct an evaluation to determine the type of equipment needed. This evaluation should take into consideration the elder's cognition, physical impairments, home environment, and seating and positioning needs, and the progression of disease. Whenever possible, COTAs should provide safety training with the exact type of mobility equipment that elders will be using in

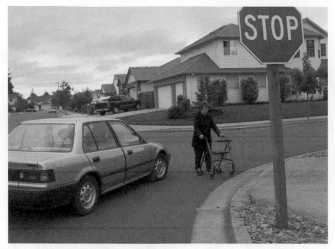

FIGURE 14-6   Elder pedestrians may need more time to cross streets than other people.

the community. COTAs also can help elders advocate for curb cuts or longer crossing times at various intersections to ensure independence and safety in the community. To this end, the city's Traffic Commission or the Architectural and Transportation Compliance Board can be of assistance.

Elders who fatigue easily or are unable to walk long distances may consider using an electric scooter or wheelchair

(Fig. 14-7). Golf carts can be especially helpful for elders who live in a planned retirement community and stay within the closed community area. An obstacle course can be set up to determine the elder's ability to maneuver before this expensive device is purchased. An evaluation by

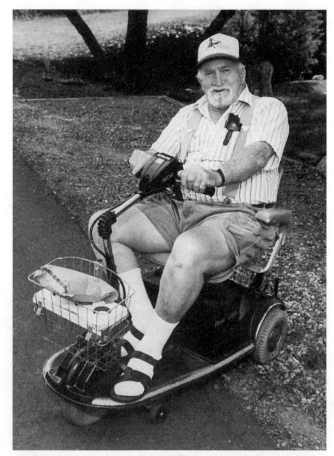

FIGURE 14-7   Elders may use electric scooters to move around freely in the community.

a specialist in wheelchair and scooter prescriptions also is recommended before purchase.

If elders need to transport a wheelchair or scooter in their personal vehicle, community mobility becomes much more complicated. Electric wheelchairs should only be transported in a van fitted with an electric lift of the appropriate size and weight. A driver rehabilitation professional should evaluate each case before a van or lift is purchased to prevent expensive mistakes such as incompatible equipment. A driver rehabilitation professional takes into account many factors, including the type of wheelchair or scooter that must be transported, whether the person needing this equipment will be a driver or passenger, and the length of time this equipment will be needed. The diagnosis of the elder also is important. An elder with a progressive illness has different needs than an elder without a progressive illness. A driver rehabilitation professional can be found by contacting the Association of Driver Rehabilitation Specialists (ADED) or using the American Automobile Association (AAA) Mobility Guide (AAA, 1995). (Refer to the Appendix for these and other resources.)

The driver rehabilitation professional also can provide resources for vendors who install adaptive equipment for vehicles in a particular geographic area. Before an electric lift or scooter carrier is purchased, the prospective user should demonstrate an ability to perform the entire loading process using the recommended equipment. COTAs can assist elders by providing information on driver rehabilitation specialists in the area.

In contrast to electric wheelchairs, electric scooters can be transported in a variety of ways. They can be stored in the trunk of some cars or on the back of the vehicle. The elder and caregivers must practice *every* step of this process before the equipment is purchased. The mobility device and personal vehicle must be compatible for safety reasons. Checking with the manufacturer of the vehicle to see whether it can handle the extra weight of a scooter carrier is necessary.

COTAs can assist the elder driver in applying for a disabled parking placard, usually issued by the Department of Motor Vehicles (DMV) of each state. This entitles the driver of the car to park close to buildings and may also include assistance at the gas station. Some elder drivers do not apply for this placard because they do not understand the application procedure. Other elders may not apply because of a perceived social stigma. It is important for the COTA to help the elder determine the requirements for a disabled parking placard. In many states, the form must be filled out and signed by a licensed physician.

ALTERNATIVE TRANSPORTATION

When planning OT intervention, COTAs must take into consideration the individual's lifestyle and needs. This is especially true for elders who have never driven,

are now unable to drive because of impairments, voluntarily decide not to drive, or want the option of using community transportation in addition to their personal vehicle. Elders who relied on others for transportation may need to learn to drive, especially if those people are no longer available. COTAs should help the elder investigate community transportation resources available where the elder currently resides or is planning to live. Information on alternative transportation can be obtained by calling city hall, a local senior citizens' center, the local DMV, local transportation agencies, the area's Office on Aging, and the local American Association of Retired Persons (AARP) offices. Independent living centers in the community may also be good sources of information. When calling these agencies, COTAs should help the elder obtain information about application procedures, cost, distance traveled, eligibility requirements, and the type of additional equipment available on the vehicles.

Title II of the Americans with Disabilities Act (ADA) addresses many needs of elders with disabilities. This act states that no qualified individual with a disability shall, by reason of that disability, be excluded from participating in or be denied the benefits of the services, programs, or activities of a public entity. According to the ADA, a *qualified individual* is defined as a person with a disability who meets the essential eligibility requirements for receiving services or participating in programs or activities provided by a public entity. The individual may meet these qualifications with or without reasonable modifications to rules, policies, or practices. They may also qualify with or without the removal of architectural barriers or the provision of auxiliary aids and services. *Public entity* refers to any state or local government or instrumentality of a state or local government. The **paratransit** and other special transportation services provided by public entities are designed to be usable by individuals with disabilities, be they physical or mental, who need the assistance of another individual to board, ride, or disembark from any vehicle on the system. Individuals for whom no fixed and accessible route transit (usually public bus) is available are also eligible for paratransit and special transportation services. However, fixed, accessible route transit should be used if available (West, 1991; Ekelman, Mitchel, & O'Dell-Rossi, 2001) (Fig. 14-8).

Elders who have impairments that prevent them from traveling to or from a boarding location for fixed transportation may also be eligible for special services. Under the law, any individual accompanying the person with the disability may be eligible for paratransit services provided that space is available and other people with disabilities are not displaced (West, 1991) (Fig. 14-9). This means that if elders with a disability cannot use the available bus system, another transportation system that can pick them up directly from their home must be provided. COTAs working with

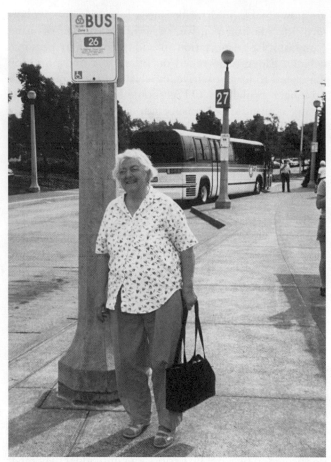

FIGURE 14-8 Elders may need to learn to use community transportation in addition to their personal vehicle.

elders who have a disability must know the ADA as it relates to transportation and accessibility. COTAs also should become knowledgeable about the paratransit services in the local community.

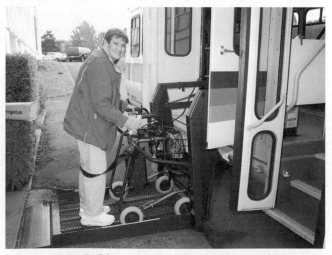

FIGURE 14-9 Public transportation may be a viable option for elders who may no longer be able to drive.

As good as paratransit services may be, they almost never help elders in leaving their homes. Regardless of whether elders are using a bus, paratransit service, or personal vehicle, their ability to exit their homes safely is of critical importance and must be evaluated to determine whether available services should be used. Information regarding this issue can be found in Part 2 of this chapter. The elder may be unable to climb stairs or even unlock or lock the door. COTAs should consider these factors and include them when training in the use of transportation services.

Some elders find the process of applying for special transportation services overly complicated and confusing. COTAs should have applications available and know the eligibility requirements for these services. If possible, COTAs should schedule an outing with elders to use particular services and help them resolve any difficulties that arise. Elders may need encouragement to be assertive when they require assistance. If the outing is successful, elders are more likely to use the service independently or with a friend or family member.

SAFE DRIVING

Aging is a highly complex process that varies tremendously among individuals. Chronologic age alone is not a good predictor of driving performance. The physical effects of aging in combination with a disability make driving safety an important issue. Although driving may seem simple because so many people do it, it is an extremely complex occupation that requires constant attention and concentration (Malfetti & Winter, 1991; Ekelman, Mitchel, O'Dell-Rossi, 2001). Driving involves a number of abilities. The abilities of sensing, deciding, and acting are critical in operating a vehicle. Drivers must perform a series of coordinated activities with their hands and feet while using input from their eyes and ears. Drivers must make many decisions on the basis of what they see and hear in relation to other vehicles on the road, other drivers, traffic signs, signals, and road conditions. These decisions result in the actions of braking, steering, and accelerating, or a combination of all three to maintain or adjust the position of the vehicle in traffic. Because fluctuations in traffic occur quickly, the coordination between decisions and actions must be smooth. Drivers make about 20 decisions for each mile traveled, demonstrating that the occupation of driving is complex and fast paced (Malfetti & Winter, 1991). Age- or disability-related decreases in sensorimotor skills may compromise driving safety by reducing the speed with which an elder can sense, decide, and act in traffic.

The sense dimension of driving includes visual acuity, visual accommodation, field of vision, dark adaptation, color vision, visual searching, and hearing. Glare and illumination, as well as certain diseases of the eye, may also affect the way the driver senses environmental changes.

Integrity of muscles and joints and reaction time also are intimately related to driving. Elders may not perceive, interpret, and react to sensory stimulation as acutely or quickly as younger people. Approximately 30% of all persons aged 65 years and older have a visual impairment (Desai, Pratt, Lentzner, & Robinson, 2001). As the size of our elder population increases, the number of people with visual impairments will increase significantly. Visual impairments are a primary consideration in safe driving and should be assessed accordingly.

Vision is usually defined as visual acuity or the ability to see fine details. Static acuity (such as looking at an eye chart) is tested in driver licensing examinations. Dynamic acuity (subject or target moving) is more closely related to traffic accidents but is seldom tested. Up to ages 40 or 50 years, little change in visual acuity occurs, but visual acuity declines markedly in individuals older than 50 (Malfetti & Winter, 1991; Ekelman, Mitchel, & O'Dell-Rossi, 2001). By age 70 years, most elders have poor acuity without correction. The implications of this decline for driving are that drivers find distinguishing between objects increasingly difficult and need to be closer to objects to clearly perceive them. To compensate for this, elders may drive slowly to distinguish hazards on the road in time to avoid them. Some diseases of the eye, such as macular degeneration, can be improved with devices such as bioptic lenses. However, in some states driving with these lenses is illegal.

Accommodation is defined as the ability to focus the eyes on nearby objects. With aging, changes in the lenses of the eyes and in the muscles that adjust them decrease their capacity for accommodation. For this reason, many elders need bifocal or trifocal eyewear, which affects driving because more time is required to change focus from near to distant objects, such as when looking from the instrument panel to the road and vice versa. A younger person can change focus in about 2 seconds, whereas adults older than 40 years take 3 seconds or more. This delay is potentially hazardous.

The retina of the normal eye receives about one half as much light at age 50 as at age 20 years, and about one third as much at age 60 as at age 20 years (Fordyce, 1999; Maddox, 2001). This change is primarily because of a decrease in the size of the pupil. Elders who complain of night blindness have good reason not to drive at night, because less light is available. Choosing well-lighted highways and instrument panels and keeping headlights, windows, and eyeglasses clean are helpful measures.

Field of vision decreases with age, and this decrease can contribute to the possibility of collisions. For example, people who can see only directly ahead confront a greater risk for accidents at intersections because they cannot see vehicles approaching from the sides. Compensations for a decreased field of vision can include the use of special panoramic mirrors and the habit of turning the head more often to check for traffic. Many elders may also not be aware of their blind spot on the side of the vehicle. Reminders to look over the shoulder before all lane changes may be necessary.

Glare occurs when too much light or light from the wrong direction or source is present. If excessive light shines on a highway sign, the elder may not see it. Quick recovery from oncoming headlights is necessary for safe driving. In the elder driver, eye recovery is slower and sensitivity to glare increases.

Dark adaptation is the process whereby eyes adjust for better vision in low light. Elders not only see less clearly in darkness but also require more time to accommodate to it. This can be a particular problem when driving in and out of tunnels. Many elders decide on their own not to drive at night for this reason.

Elders may not identify the color of traffic signs or signals as well as younger people, especially when the light is dim or glare is present. This can be a problem because elders require additional time to read road signs, which diverts their attention from the road and traffic (Ekelman, Mitchel, & O'Dell-Rossi, 2001). According to the AARP (2001), elders may be able to compensate for some visual limitations. They should have their vision checked at least yearly and avoid eyeglass frames that obstruct peripheral vision. Learning the general meaning of traffic signs by their shapes and colors and avoiding driving at night whenever possible are useful precautions.

Approximately 37% of people older than 65 years experience some hearing loss (Desai, Pratt, Lentzner, & Robinson, 2001). This loss can cause problems during driving because horns, sirens, and train whistles may be difficult to hear. It may also prevent elders from realizing that the turn signal indicator is on when no turns are being made. Elders should have their hearing tested by a qualified professional. When adjusting to any hearing assistive device, elders should keep the volume of the car radio as low as possible, leave the air conditioning or heating units on the lowest possible setting, and visually check turn signals. (Resources for drivers with hearing difficulties are listed in the Appendix).

The aging process also affects muscles and joints in ways that may affect driving. Elders may experience back pain, making it difficult to sit for long periods. Special cushions may be helpful. Arthritis may cause stiffness in the neck, which makes turning to check for traffic painful. Fatigue and discomfort are also problems that may distract elders and lessen their awareness of traffic conditions. Power steering and power brakes can help tremendously. A wide variety of mirrors are available to compensate for stiffness in the neck. Using tilt steering and arm rests may also help.

Reaction time is extremely important in safe driving. Reaction time is the time required by the eyes to see and the brain to process, decide what to do, and transmit the information to the proper body parts. For example, after seeing that the traffic ahead has stopped, a driver extends the right leg and pushes on the brake pedal. The ability to respond quickly may decrease with age, but specific safety measures can be used to compensate for the loss. One strategy is to maintain a safe distance from the car ahead. When stopping, the driver should be able to see the tires of the car in front. Other strategies are to avoid rush hour traffic and to take someone else along, especially when traveling to a new destination. If elders are upset or ill, they will probably have a slower reaction time. Education on compensatory techniques can help elders to change unsafe habits. The AARP and the AAA offer various programs and courses for elder drivers (Fig. 14-10). The driver safety course offered by the AARP covers many issues, including decreased reaction time, visual and hearing losses, the effects of certain medications, and hazardous situations (AARP, 2003). The fee for these courses is nominal, and many insurance companies will offer a rebate on automobile insurance after successful completion of a driver safety course. However, these classes do not include behind-the-wheel testing. COTAs should discuss concern about the elder's ability to drive safely with the supervising OTR and physician whenever possible.

A behind-the-wheel evaluation is the best method for determining driver safety. A driving evaluation program that specializes in working with persons with disabilities can determine safety and equipment needs. The Handicapped Driver's Mobility Guide (AAA, 1995) and the Association of Driver Educators for the Disabled can assist COTAs in locating driver evaluation programs. These programs also can instruct COTAs in the proper procedures for reporting unsafe or questionable drivers to the DMV of each state.

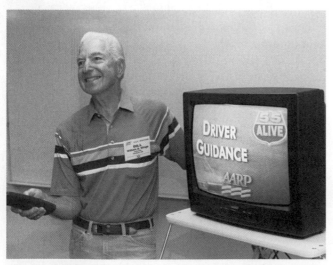

FIGURE 14-10   There are various programs and courses in the community to assist elder drivers.

COTAs should clearly document all recommendations to elders. For example, if the COTA recommends that an elder's driving ability be evaluated after a stroke, this recommendation must be clearly stated in the medical chart. To demonstrate thorough care, COTAs are advised to document the names of at least three resources given to the client.

A wide variety of equipment is available to help elders continue driving. This equipment is available from a variety of sources, including equipment catalogs, vendors, and automobile manufacturers (Table 14-2). (Refer to the Appendix for addresses of organizations to contact for additional resources.)

CASE STUDY

Mr. Thomas is 62 years old. One year ago he had a right cerebrovascular accident and has a nonfunctional left upper extremity. For long distances, he uses a manual wheelchair, which he pushes with his right lower extremity. For short distances, he slowly ambulates using a quad cane. Other medical conditions include a seizure disorder controlled by medication and a left hip joint replacement that causes pain and discomfort with prolonged sitting. A former physical education teacher, Mr. Thomas enjoys working with students at the high school level and is anxious to return to work in some capacity. His wife works full time and he receives occasional assistance in transportation from friends. Mr. Thomas believes he is ready to drive, but his wife is very concerned for his safety.

Mr. Thomas received a driving evaluation, during which he exhibited difficulties such as weaving out of the lane and forgetting to turn off his turn signal. After driving for 20 minutes, he drifted across two lanes and lost concentration. The driving instructor had to take over the steering wheel to pull the car over to the side of the road. Mr. Thomas stated that his "leg hurt."

After the evaluation, the deficits observed during driving were discussed. Mr. Thomas demonstrated insight into his difficulties and expressed the desire to begin training to improve his driving skills. Equipment needs included a spinner knob to allow him to steer with one hand and a right crossover directional device that enabled him to use his right hand for directional use. Training strategies included asking Mr. Thomas to tell the driving instructor when he was starting to have pain in his leg and to pull over when it was safe. He was reminded to turn off his directional signal after use and to look ahead while driving. After three training sessions, Mr. Thomas was able to demonstrate safe driving skills. He received a driving test from the DMV and passed. He is now able to return to part-time work and independent living.

■ CASE STUDY QUESTIONS

1   Considering the case of Mr. Thomas, identify some relevant recommendations for driving if he had experienced a spinal cord injury rather than a cerebrovascular accident.
2   Identify alternatives for transportation appropriate for Mr. Thomas if he had failed the driving evaluation.

TABLE **14-2**

Adaptive Equipment Ideas

Difficulty	Effect on driving	Resources to assist elder drivers
Decreased neck ROM or pain when turning head	Limited scope of view of traffic around car	Install panoramic mirrors (Brookstone) or convex mirrors (can be installed by vendors); refer to driving program for evaluation; instruct client in use of head support
Decreased shoulder ROM or pain in shoulders	Difficulty steering, reaching for seat belt, and adjusting rearview mirror	Use arm supports already in vehicle; automobile upholsterer can build up existing arm supports to support elbows, which usually decreases client's shoulder pain; client may need effort of steering reduced, which can be determined by driving evaluation (driving program can refer to appropriate vendor for this modification); instruct elder in use of stick to adjust rearview mirror and tilt steering wheel
Decreased ROM or pain in fingers and hands	Difficulty turning key, opening door, adjusting radio, air conditioning, and so on; possible difficulty holding onto steering wheel safely	A wide variety of key holders and door openers are available from medical supply catalogs; knob extensions can be made by car vendors; refer client for driving evaluation to determine need for steering device or built-up steering wheel
Back pain	Decreased concentration caused by pain; difficulty turning to check traffic	A wide variety of cushions and lumbar supports are available from medical supply companies and vendors; these should be tried before purchase; driving programs also can evaluate and provide resources
Impairment or loss of both lower extremities	Inability to operate gas and brake pedals	Refer to driving program for evaluation of ability to use hand controls
Impairment or loss of right lower extremity	Difficulty using gas and brake pedals	Refer to driving program for evaluation of ability to use left foot accelerator
Impairment or loss of left upper extremity	Difficulty using turn signal and turning	Refer to driving program for evaluation of ability to use right crossover directional and spinner knob
Impairment or loss of right upper extremity	Difficulty steering, shifting gears in automatic or manual cars	Refer to driving program for evaluation of ability to use spinner knob
Hearing impairment	Inability to hear emergency sirens; failure to turn off turn signal	Elder drivers can purchase equipment to amplify sound of blinker; hearing aids can help clients hear sirens better
Cognitive impairment	Decreased judgment and decision making; slow reaction time; unsafe driving	Refer to driving program for detailed evaluation; discuss concerns with occupational therapist; document recommendations clearly
Visual impairment	Compromised ability to read signs; overly slow driving; generally unsafe driving skills	Refer to optometrist for vision check-up; if elder has low vision, refer to ophthalmologist who specializes in low vision

Adapted from Lillie, S. (1993). Evaluation for driving. In T. T. Yoshikawa & E. Lipton (Eds.), *Ambulatory geriatric care*. St. Louis, MO: Mosby.
ROM, range of motion.

CHAPTER REVIEW QUESTIONS

1 Explain the reason that Omnibus Budget Reconciliation Act regulations involving use of restraints were drafted and discuss related requirements for health providers.

2 Explain the steps to be taken in establishing a restraint reduction program.

3 Explain the role of the certified occupational therapy assistant (COTA) in consultations regarding use of restraints.

4 Describe at least three environmental adaptations that may help to reduce the use of restraints.

5 Identify psychosocial approaches to reducing the use of restraints with an elder who wanders.

6 Explain the ways activity aids in the reduction of restraints.

7 Describe the ideal position in which an elder should sit in a wheelchair.

8 List five precautions to consider when monitoring the appropriate fit of a wheelchair for an elder.

9 Identify three reasons that many falls go unreported.

10 Explain the reason that some elders and their family members are reluctant to change the environment when personal safety and prevention of falls are a concern.

11 Explain the need for assessment of an elder's nighttime toileting skills.

12 Describe ways the home can be modified to prevent falls if elders have vision impairments and poor standing balance.

13 Identify three emergency strategies for an elder who lives alone and has a history of falls.

14 List the issues that must be considered when recommending community transportation.

15 Describe strategies to alleviate the elder's fear of using transportation.

16 Describe the actions of the COTA when the client's ability to be a safe driver is in question.

REFERENCES

Administration on Aging. (2003). *A profile of older Americans: 2002.* Washington, DC: U.S. Department of Health and Human Services.

American Association of Retired Persons. (2001). *Older driver skill assessment and resource guide.* Washington, DC: The Association.

American Association of Retired Persons. (2003). Driving safely while aging gracefully [WWW page]. URL http://www.nhtsa.dot.gov/people/injury/olddrive/Driving%20Safely%20Aging%20Web/index.html

American Automobile Association. (1995). *The disabled driver's mobility guide.* Heathrow, FL: Traffic Safety and Engineering Department.

American Automobile Association. (1993). *Walking through the years.* Heathrow, FL: Traffic Safety and Engineering Department.

Atkins, C. (1996). Teamwork is the real key to reduced use of restraints. *Advance for Occupationl Therapists 12*(1), 5.

Bloom, C., & Braun, J. (1991). Restraints in the 90's: Success with wanderers. *Geriatric Nursing 12*(1), 20.

Bradley, L., Siddique, C. M., & Dufton, B. (1995). Reducing the use of physical restraints in long-term care facilities. *Journal of Gerontologic Nursing 21*(9), 21.

Brummel-Smith, K. (1990). Falls and instability in the older person. In B. Kemp, K. Brummel-Smith, & J. W. Ramsdell (Eds.), *Geriatric rehabilitation.* Boston, MA: College Hill Press.

Brungardt, G. (1994). Patient restraints: New guidelines for a less restrictive approach. *Geriatrics, 49*(6), 43.

Burgener, S. C., Shiver, R., & Murrell, L. (1993). Expressions of individuality in cognitively impaired elders. *Journal of Gerontological Nursing 19*(14), 13.

Campbell, A. J., Reinken, J., Allan, B. C., & Martinez, G. S. (1981). Falls in old age: A study of frequency and other related factors. *Age and Ageing, 10,* 264.

Capezuti, E. (2000). Preventing falls and injuries while reducing siderail use. *Annals of Long-Term Care, 8,* 57-63.

Capezuti, E., Strumpf, N., Evans, L., & Maislin, G. (1999a). Outcomes of nighttime physical restraint removal for severely impaired nursing home residents. *American Journal of Alzheimer's Disease, 14*(13), 1-8.

Capezuti, E., Talerico, K. A., Cochran, E., Becker, H., Strumpf, N., & Evans, L. (1999b). Individualized interventions to prevent bed-related falls and reduce siderail use. *Journal of Gerontological Nursing, 25*(11), 26-34.

Carter, N. D., Kannus, P., & Khan, K. M. (2001). Exercise in the prevention of falls in older people: A systematic literature review examining the rationale and the evidence. *Sports Medicine, 31,* 427-438.

Castle, N. G., & Mor, V. (1998). Physical restraints in nursing homes: A review of the literature since the Nursing Home Reform Act of 1987. *Medical Care Research and Review, 55*(2), 139-170.

Cuming, R. G. (2002). Intervention strategies and risk-factor modification for falls prevention: A review of recent intervention studies. *Clinics in Geriatric Medicine, 18,* 175-189.

Desai, M., Pratt, L. A., Lentzner, H., & Robinson, K. N. (2001). Trends in vision and hearing among older Americans. *Aging Trends, 2,* 1-8.

Donius, M., & Rader, J. (1994). Use of siderails: Rethinking a standard of practice. *J Gerontological Nursing 20*(11), 23.

Eigsti, D. G., & Vrooman, N. (1992). Releasing restraints in the nursing home: It can be done. *J Gerontological Nursing 18*(1), 21.

Ekelman, B., Mitchel, S., & O'Dell-Rossi, P. (2001). Driving and older adults. In B. Bonder & M. Wagner (Eds.), *Functional performance in older adults* (2nd ed.). Philadelphia, PA: FA Davis.

Ericson, L. L. (1991). Restraints in the nursing home environment. *Occupational Therapy Forum, 6*(4), 1.

Evans, L. K., Forceia, M. A., Yurkow, J., & Sochalski, J. A. (1999). The geriatric day hospital. In P. Katz, M. Mezey, & R. Kane (Eds.), *Emerging systems in long-term care* (pp. 67-87). New York: Springer Publishing Company.

Feldt, K. S., Warne, M. A., & Ryden, M. B. (1998). Examining pain and agitation in aggressive cognitively impaired older adults. *Journal of Gerontological Nursing, 24*(11), 14-22.

Fogel, B. S. (1992). Simple balance measure proven effective (measure frailty). *Brown University Long Term Care Quality Letter, Winter 2*(2), 2-4.

Fordyce, M. (1999). *Geriatric pearls.* Philadelphia, PA: FA Davis.

Gallo, J. J., Busby-Whitehead, J., Rabins, P. V., Silliman, R. A., Murphy, J. B., & Reichel, W. (Eds.) (1999). *Reichel's care of the elderly: Clinical aspects of aging* (5th ed.). Philadelphia, PA: Lippincott Williams & Wilkins.

Gillespie, L. D., Gillespie, W. J., Roberston, M. C., Lamb, S. E., Cumming, R. G., & Rowe, B. H. (2002). Interventions for preventing falls in elderly people. *The Cochrane Library* (CD000340).

Greenberg, D. (1996). Geriatric seating and positioning: Definitely a therapy task. *Gerontology Special Interest Section Newsletter, 19*(3), 1.

Gryfe, C. I., Amies, A., & Ashley, M. J. (1977). A longitudinal study of falls in an elderly population: Incidence and morbidity. *Age and Ageing, 6,* 201.

Guttman, R., Altman, R. D., Karlan, M. S. (1999). Use of restraints for patients in nursing homes. *Archives of Family Medicine, 8*(2), 101-105.

Health Care Financing Administration. (1995). *Interpretive guidelines Rev. 250: Part II guidance to surveyors for long-term care facilities tag #s f221-241.* Washington, DC: U.S. Department of Health and Human Services. (pp 44-53).

Health Care Financing Administration. (2001). *42 Code of Federal Regulations, Part 483 Subpart B, Requirements for long term care facilities.* Washington, DC: U.S. Department of Health and Human Services.

Hettinger, J. (1996). Encouraging activity in older adults. *OT Week, 15.*

Janelli, L. M., Kanski, G. W., & Neary, M. A. (1994). Physical restraints: Has OBRA made a difference? *Journal of Gerontological Nursing, 20*(6) 17.

Jones, D. A. (1995). Seating problems in long-term care. In E. M. Tornquist (Ed.), *Individualized dementia care: Creative compassionate approaches.* New York: Springer.

Josephson, K. B., Fabacher, D. A., & Rubenstein, L. Z. (1991). Home safety and fall prevention. *Geriatric Home Care, 7,* 707-731.

Kane, R. (2001). Regulation in long term care. In G. Maddox (Ed.), *The encyclopedia of aging: A comprehensive resource in gerontology and geriatrics* (3rd ed.). New York: Springer.

Kane, R. L., Luslander, J. G., & Abrass, I. B. (1994). Instability and falls. In J. D. Jeffers & M. Navrozov (Eds.), *Essentials of clinical geriatrics.* New York: McGraw-Hill.

Kapp, M. B. (1994). Reduce legal risks through restraint reduction plan. *Provider, 17*(8), 48.

Kari, N., & Michels, P. (1991). The Lazarus project: The politics of empowerment. *American Journal of Occupational Therapy, 45*(8), 719.

Kerr, T. (1994). Making "merry walkers" of once-restrained residents. *Advances in Occupational Therapy, 10*(6), 42.

Kinsella, K., &Velkoff, V. (2001). *An aging world: 2001* (U.S. Census Bureau, Series P95/01-1). Washington, DC: U.S. Government Printing Office. Retrieved October 7, 2003 from http://www.census.gov/pod/2001pubs/p95-01-1).

Knowlton, L. (2002). Ethical issues in the care of the elderly. *Geriatric Times, 3*(2). Retrieved December 22, 2003 from http:/www.geriatrictimes.com/g020301.html

Krasilovsky, G. (1993). Seating assessment and management in a nursing home population. *Physical and Occupational Therapy in Geriatrics, 11,* 25-38.

Lamb, K., Miller, J., & Hernandez, M. (1987). Falls in the elderly: Causes and prevention. *Orthopedic Nursing, 6,* 45-49.

Lillie, S. (1993). Evaluation for driving. In T. T. Yoshikawa & E. L. Cobbsl (Eds.), *Ambulatory geriatric care.* St. Louis, MO: Mosby.

Maddox, G. (2001). *The encyclopedia of aging: A comprehensive resource in gerontology and geriatrics* (3rd edition). New York: Springer.

Mahoney, D. F. (1995). Analysis of restraint-free nursing homes. *Image: The Journal of Nursing Scholarship 27*(2), 155.

Malfetti, J., & Winter, D. J. (1986). *Drivers 55 plus: Test your own performance: A self rating form of questions, factors and suggestions for safe driving* [brochure]. Falls Church, VA: American Automobile Association Foundation for Traffic Safety.

Malfetti, J., & Winter, D. J. (1991). *Concerned about an older driver? A guide for families and friends* [brochure]. Washington, DC: Safety Research and Education Project and AAA Foundation for Traffic Safety.

Mason, R., O'Connor, M., & Kemble, S. (1995). Untying the elderly: Response to quality of life issues. *Geriatric Nursing, 16*(2), 68.

McIntyre, A. (1999). Elderly fallers: A baseline audit of admissions to a day hospital for elderly people. *The British Journal of Occupational Therapy, 62,* 244-248.

Mion, L. C., & Mercurio, A. (1992). Methods to reduce restraints: Process, outcomes, and future directions. *Journal of Gerontological Nursing, 18*(11), 5.

Neufeld, R. R., Libow, L. S., Foley, W. J., Dunbar, J. M., Cohen, C., & Breuer, B. (1999). Restraint reduction reduces serious injuries among nursing home residents. *Journal of the American Geriatrics Society, 47*(10), 1202-1207.

Okada, S. (1990). Should Miss Daisy drive? *Geriatric Rehabilitation, 2*(3), 1.

Patterson, J. E., Strumpf, N. E., & Evans, L. K. (1995). Nursing consultation to reduce restraints in a nursing home. *Clinical Nurse Specialist, 9*(4), 231.

Perr, A. (1998). Elements of seating and wheeled mobility intervention. *Occupational Therapy Practice, 3*(9), 16-24.

Plautz, R., & Camp, C. (2001). Activities as agents for intervention and rehabilitation in long-term care. In B. Bonder, & M. Wagner (Eds.), *Functional performance in older adults* (2nd ed.). Philadelphia, PA: FA Davis.

Poole, J. L. (1991). Age related changes in sensory system dynamics related to balance. *Physical and Occupational Therapy in Geriatrics, 10,* 55-65.

Rader, J. (1995). In E. Tornquist (Ed.), *Individualized dementia care: Creative, compassionate approaches.* New York: Springer Publishing.

Rader, J., Doan, J., & Schwab, Sr. M. (1985). How to decrease wandering, a form of agenda behavior. *Geriatric Nursing 6*(4), 196.

Rader, J., Jones, D., & Miller, L. (2000). The importance of individualized wheelchair seating for frail older adults. *Journal of Gerontological Nursing, 26,* 24-32.

Reinsch, S., MacRae, P., Lachenbruch, P. A., & Tobis, J. S. (1992). Why do healthy older adults fall? Behavioral and environmental risks. *Physical and Occupational Therapy in Geriatrics, 11,* 1-15.

Rubenstein, L. Z. (2001). Falls and balance problems. The *AGS Foundation for Health in Aging.* URL http://www.healthinaging.org/public_education/pef/falls_and_balance_problems.php

Rubenstein, L. Z., & Josephson, K. R. (2002). The epidemiology of falls and syncope. *Clinics in Geriatric Medicine, 18,* 141-158.

Rubenstein, L. Z., & Robbins, A. S. (1989). Falling syndromes in elderly persons. *Comprehensive Therapy, 15,* 6.

Russell, J. N., Hendershot, G. E., LeClere, F., Howie, L. J., & Adler, M. (1997). Trends and differential use of assistive technology devices: United States, 1994. *Advance Data, 292,* 1-10.

Savoye, C. (2001). States to try to help elderly stay behind the wheel. *Christian Science Monitor, 93,* 3.

Simmons, S., Schnelle, J., MacRae, P., & Ouslander, J. (1995). Wheelchairs as mobility restraints: predictors of wheelchair activity in non-ambulatory nursing home residents. *Journal of American Geriatrics Society, 43,* 384-388.

Steinmetz, H. M., & Hobson, S. J. (1994). Prevention of falls among the community dwelling elderly: An overview. *Physical and Occupational Therapy in Geriatrics, 12,* 13-29.

Stolley, J. M. (1995). Freeing your patients from restraints. *American Journal of Nursing, 12*(3) 27.

Strumpf, N. E., Evans, L. K., Wagner, J., & Patterson, J. (1992). Reducing physical restraint: Developing an educational program. *Journal of Gerontological Nursing 18*(11), 21.

Strumpf, N., Evans, L., & Bourbonniere, M. (2001). Restraints. In M. Mezey (Ed.), *The encyclopedia of elder care* (pp. 567–569). New York: Springer.

Sullivan, R. J. (2001). Cardiovascular system overview. In G. Maddox (Ed.), *The encyclopedia of aging* (3rd ed.). New York: Springer.

Sullivan-Marx, E. M. (1995). Psychological responses to physical restraint use in older adults. *Journal of Psychosocial Nursing and Mental Health Services, 33*(6), 20.

Tideiksaar, R. (1987). Fall prevention in the home. *Topics in Geriatric Rehabilitation, 3,* 1.

Tideiksaar, R. (1989). Geriatric falls: Assessing the cause, preventing recurrence. *Geriatrics, 44*(7), 57.

Tideiksaar, R. (2001). Falls. In B. Bonder, & M. Wagner (Eds.), *Functional performance in older adults* (2nd ed.). Philadelphia, PA: FA Davis.

Tinetti, M. E., Speechley, M., & Ginter, S. (1988). Risk factors for falls among elderly persons living in the community. *New England Journal of Medicine, 319,* 1701-1707.

U.S. Department of Transportation (2003).*Traffic Safety Facts: 2000 National Center for Statistics and Analysis.*

Washington, DC: National Highway Traffic Safety Administration.

Walker, J. E., & Howland, J. (1991). Falls and fear of falling among elderly persons living in the community: Occupational therapy interventions. *The American Journal of Occupational Therapy, 45,* 119-122.

Werner, P., Koroknay, V., Braun, J., & Cohen-Mansfield, J. (1994). Individualized care alternatives used in the process of removing restraints in the nursing home. *Journal of the American Geriatrics Society, 42* (3), 321.

West, J. (1991). *The Americans with Disabilities Act.* New York: Milbank Memorial Fund.

CHAPTER

15

SECTION TWO
PSYCHOLOG
VISION I
OCCUPATI
OCCUPATIO

Working with Elders Who Have Vision Impairments

REBECCA BOTHWELL

KEY TERMS

cataracts, glaucoma, retina, lens, macular degeneration, diabetic retinopathy, visual acuity, contrast sensitivity, visual cognition, visual memory, pattern recognition, scanning, visual attention, oculomotor control, visual fields, eccentric viewing, scotoma, hemi-inattention, diplopia, strabismus

CHAPTER OBJECTIVES

1. Describe the typical physiologic changes affecting vision that occur with aging.
2. Name and describe the major ocular diseases affecting vision in elders.
3. Describe the common vision deficits resulting from neurological insult in elders.
4. Provide a framework for addressing visual impairments.
5. Identify general principles to enhance vision and to increase independence in elders with low vision.
6. Identify general principles in the treatment of vision dysfunction after brain insult.

Visual impairments are common in the elderly population. One in six adults aged 65 or older has a visual impairment and this number is expected to double by the year 2030 (American Foundation for the Blind, 2002). The odds of development of a visual impairment worsen with age, as one in four adults aged 75 years or older experiences either a moderate or severe visual impairment (Lighthouse, Inc. 1995). In addition to vision loss from ocular disease, many adults are disabled by visual impairments resulting from head trauma, stroke, or neurological insult. Between 40% and 75% of individuals with head trauma or stroke are estimated to experience visual impairments requiring rehabilitation (Warren, 1998). These statistics demonstrate the need for certified occupational therapy assistants (COTAs) to possess a thorough understanding of the causes of vision loss and appropriate treatment techniques. Regardless of the particular setting, any COTA working with elders is likely to encounter many clients with visual impairments.

...GICAL IMPLICATIONS OF
...MPAIRMENTS

Almost 25% of adults with visual impairment report symptoms of depression compared with 10% of those without visual impairment (Center on an Aging Society, 2002). The thought of losing one's vision is one of the most devastating disabilities imaginable. Without vision, the ability to perform many of the daily activities normally taken for granted is lost. Without vision, a means of social connectedness is lost because it is no longer possible to make eye contact or to read subtle facial expressions. The thought of vision loss conjures up a terrifying world of blackness. However, although most people think of vision loss as total blindness, most individuals with visual impairments are not totally blind. In fact, in one report, 80% of those who reported being legally blind actually had some degree of "useful vision" (American Foundation for the Blind, 1999d). It is often difficult for family members and friends of those with partial sight to understand what their limitations and capabilities are (Friedman, 2000). It is not uncommon for partially sighted individuals to be labeled as "fakes" when others observe that they are capable of one task that requires some degree of vision but are incapable of another task (Friedman, 2000). This confusion about the abilities of those with partial sight may produce more psychological distress than does total blindness (Friedman, 2000; Rolland, 1994).

In addition to the ambiguity associated with being partially sighted, individuals often find it difficult to adjust to their vision loss because of the uncertainty of their condition. For many, it is difficult to know whether their vision will improve, stay the same, or get worse. There is often an internal struggle with a desire to be independent and a desire to be cared for. In some situations, they may want assistance but feel unable to ask for it. Mood swings and erratic behavior are common (Friedman, 2000). Friedman (2000) describes the stages of coping that individuals with vision loss experience as closely paralleling those that Kubler-Ross (1969) describes in her study on death and dying, which include initial shock and denial, then guilt, bargaining, anger, depression, and, finally, adaptation.

EFFECTS OF THE NORMAL AGING PROCESS ON VISION

Although elders are more likely to experience visual impairments because of some specific ocular and neurological pathologies, they also experience many age-related changes that affect visual functioning. These normal changes must be taken into consideration when working with this population.

The **retina** is a multilayered lining of neural tissue on the innermost part of the eye (Fig. 15-1). It receives visual messages and transmits them through the optic

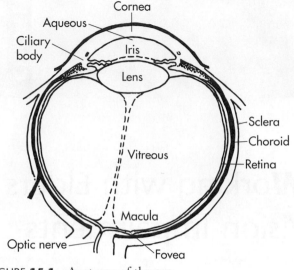

FIGURE **15-1**   Anatomy of the eye.

nerve to the brain (Mogk, 2000). The central area of the retina, or macula, has a concentration of cone cells that enable color vision and fine-detail discrimination. Rod cells are extremely sensitive to light and provide peripheral vision and night vision (Mogk, 2000). As the retina ages, it gradually loses neurons. Central or peripheral vision may be affected, depending on which retinal neurons die. The rate of retinal deterioration and the resultant visual field loss varies among individuals, but generally, elders experience shrinkage of the peripheral field, experience difficulty with light and dark adaptation, and require an increased time to recover from glare. Because the pupils also decrease in size with age, elders require more illumination for fine-detail tasks (Bennett, 1992).

Changes may also occur in the **lens** of the eye with age (see Fig. 15-1). The lens is responsible for properly focusing the image on the retina. It does this by changing shape according to the distance of the object being viewed (Scheiman, 2002b). As the lens ages, it loses some of its elasticity, making shape change or accommodation more difficult. This condition, called *presbyopia*, affects focal ability at near distances, making it difficult to read print or perform close-vision tasks (Scheiman, 2002a). The greatest change occurs between the ages of 40 and 45 years (Scheiman, 2002a). Reading glasses or bifocals are often prescribed at this time. In addition to this loss of elasticity, the lens also becomes more yellow with age. This deeper yellow can affect the ability to differentiate between colors and discriminate objects with low contrast (Lighthouse International [n.d.]).

SPECIFIC OCULAR PATHOLOGIES

In addition to the natural aging process, several specific pathologic conditions have a more profound effect

TABLE 15-1

Functional Outcomes of Ocular Conditions

Condition	Cause	Functional outcome
Cataract	A protein degeneration in the lens results in opacification	Hazy, blurred vision Increased sensitivity to glare Difficulty with night driving Difficulty finding appropriate lighting
Glaucoma	An increase in pressure inside the eye results in damage to the tissues, especially the optic nerve	Decreased peripheral vision, initially Can potentially lead to total blindness Difficulty adjusting to changes in lighting Shadow like halos around lights Increased sensitivity to glare
Diabetic retinopathy	Hemorrhaging of blood vessels and/or formation of microaneurysms results in damage to the retina	Fluctuating, blurred vision Change in focal ability Loss in visual field, peripheral or central
Macular degeneration	The central portion of the retina undergoes a deterioration, in some cases brought on by hemorrhaging blood vessels	Central field loss Decreased acuity

on functional abilities. Four major conditions that affect an elder's vision are **macular degeneration, cataracts, glaucoma**, and **diabetic retinopathy.** These conditions can occur in isolation, but they commonly coexist in elders, creating greater challenges for elders to remain independent (Table 15-1).

Macular Degeneration

Macular degeneration is the leading cause of vision loss in older Americans (American Foundation for the Blind, 1999b). The macula is the central portion of the retina where the clearest vision is found. Macular degeneration, therefore, leads to a "blind spot" in the center of the field of view (Fig. 15-2). Macular degeneration does not result in total blindness (American Foundation for the Blind, 1999b). However, because the macula is responsible for fine-detail vision, activities such as reading, doing needlework, recognizing faces, and writing can be become extremely difficult.

There are two types of macular degeneration: the "dry" type and the "wet," or hemorrhagic, type. Dry age-related macular degeneration (ARMD) is more common and is the result of yellowish deposits, or drusen, forming under the macula. This causes the macula to thin and dry out. The wet form of ARMD is caused by the rapid growth of small blood vessels beneath the macula. These blood vessels leak and eventually form scar tissue that creates vision loss (American Foundation for the Blind, 1999b).

The wet form of ARMD can sometimes be treated with photocoagulation, or laser surgery. This treatment can slow the rate of vision loss; however, there is no known treatment that prevents macular degeneration or that can reverse the loss of vision (American Foundation for the Blind, 1999b).

Cataracts

With aging, the lens may undergo a protein degeneration resulting in opacification, or clouding, which is known as a *cataract* (American Foundation for the Blind, 1999a). Cataracts prevent an adequate amount of light from reaching the retina. Individuals with cataracts have hazy or blurred vision, increased sensitivity to glare, difficulty with night driving, and difficulty seeing objects that have

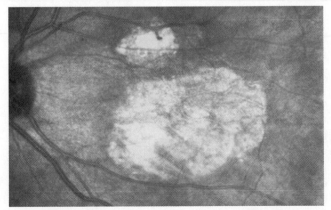

FIGURE 15-2 This photograph, which was taken with a scanning laser ophthalmoscope, shows the deterioration of a retina (white areas) in an elder client who has macular degeneration.

203

low contrast with their background (American Foundation for the Blind, 1999a).

Cataracts can now be successfully treated with surgery and are no longer considered to be a major cause of permanent visual impairment in developed countries. The most common procedure is the removal of the opacified lens followed by the insertion of an intraocular lens implant (American Foundation for the Blind, 1999a).

Glaucoma

Glaucoma is a serious ocular condition that involves excessively high pressure inside the eyeball. This increased pressure results from a buildup of excess fluid in the eye (Mogk, 2000). Increased intraocular pressure can eventually cause damage to the optic nerve or to the blood vessels that supply the optic nerve (Mogk, 2000). One of the first effects of this optic nerve damage is usually a loss of vision in the peripheral field (Fig. 15-3). This loss of peripheral vision is often not noticed by the individual initially and the disease frequently progresses substantially before it is noticed (American Foundation for the Blind, 1999c). If left undetected and untreated, this loss can lead to total blindness. Elders should be encouraged to have routine ophthalmologic visits so that glaucoma may be diagnosed at an early stage. When the diagnosis is early, individuals respond well to medication and, if necessary, surgery to improve the balance of fluid in the eye (Mogk, 2000).

There are many types of glaucoma, but open-angle glaucoma is by far the most common (Mogk, 2000); other types include closed- or narrow-angle, traumatic, and low tension glaucoma (Mogk, 2000). Open-angle glaucoma involves an eye with normal anatomy that, for unknown reasons, is not able to drain the fluid as efficiently as it produces it. This leads to a slow, gradual buildup of intraocular pressure over time (Mogk, 2000).

Closed- or narrow-angle glaucoma is less common. This type of glaucoma progresses rapidly and symptoms are immediately apparent. Nausea, headaches, severe redness of the eye, and pain may be symptoms of an acute attack of narrow-angle glaucoma (Jose, 1985) Emergency surgery often is required to reduce the intraocular pressure.

The functional implications of glaucoma vary greatly depending on the severity of the disease, which is usually related to its time of diagnosis. When diagnosis is early, glaucoma can be treated and many people may have little need to adjust their lifestyles. If the disease is allowed to progress, individuals may experience decreased peripheral vision, difficulty adjusting to changing light, fluctuating and blurred vision, shadowlike halos around lights, and an increased sensitivity to glare (Bennett, 1991, 1992). Individuals with undiagnosed glaucoma may lose all of their vision beginning with their peripheral field and eventually extending into their central vision.

Diabetic Retinopathy

Diabetic retinopathy, one of the complications of diabetes mellitus, is another leading cause of visual impairment in elders. Diabetic retinopathy occurs in two stages: background and proliferative diabetic retinopathy. In background retinopathy, microaneurysms form but are reabsorbed by the retina (Mogk, 2000). If background retinopathy progresses to proliferative retinopathy, more severe changes in visual acuity may occur and total blindness may even result (Mogk, 2000). The term *proliferative* is used to indicate the new blood vessels that grow throughout the retina during this stage of retinopathy. These vessels easily rupture and produce bleeding into the eye, often resulting in scotomas, or blind spots in the central visual field. When the new network of vessels and its accompanying fibrous tissue contract, traction retinal detachments may also occur (Mogk, 2000).

The functional implications of diabetic retinopathy, like glaucoma, vary depending on early diagnosis and severity of the disease. Some individuals may have a mild degree of retinopathy and may not need to make any adaptations in their lifestyles. Others, however, may need to make major life changes as their disease continues to progress. They may eventually need to learn blind techniques for all ADL functions. Symptoms may include fluctuating and blurred vision, decreased contrast sensitivity, difficulty with color discrimination, poor night vision, "spotty" losses in visual field, and possibly total blindness (Mogk, 2000).

Diabetic retinopathy may be treated either by photocoagulation or a procedure known as *vitrectomy* (Mogk, 2000). Photocoagulation with a laser to treat diabetic retinopathy is similar to the procedure used to treat macular degeneration. A vitrectomy may be performed to remove blood and scar tissue from the vitreous if photocoagulation does not stop the bleeding or when it is not an option (Mogk, 2000). Although two thirds of patients experience improved vision after these procedures, the benefits are relative. Individuals with diabetic retinopathy typically have significant visual impairment both before and after surgery (Mogk, 2000).

VISUAL DYSFUNCTIONAL AFTER NEUROLOGICAL INSULT

The discussion of visual impairments in elders thus far has focused on impairments as a result of ocular conditions. However, the visual system is not composed of the eyeballs alone. To perceive visual information, the data must travel through a complex nervous system and must be processed by appropriate cerebral centers. In addition, effective control of eye movements depends on proper impulses from the brain. Thus, successful adaptation to the environment through the visual sense requires the proper functioning of both ocular and neurological components.

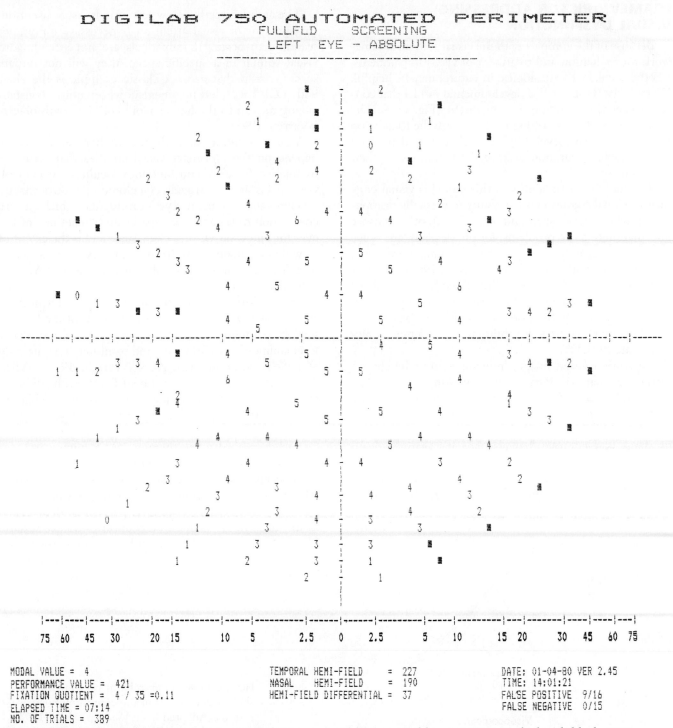

FIGURE 15-3 This printout from an automated perimeter test indicates visual loss in points marked with black squares. Note the peripheral distribution.

Causes of brain insult can include trauma, cancer, multiple sclerosis, and cerebrovascular accidents (CVAs), or strokes. The vision system is vulnerable to strokes or other types of brain insult (Warren, 1993). A host of various visual disorders can result from brain insult including visual field disorders, reduced visual acuity, reduced contrast sensitivity, problems with stereopsis (depth perception), difficulty adapting to changes in lighting conditions, visual–spatial disorders, and oculomotor dysfunction (Kerkhoff, 2000).

FRAMEWORK FOR ADDRESSING VISUAL DYSFUNCTION

Because of the complexity of the visual system, a framework for evaluation and treatment of visual impairments, whether ocular or neurological in nature, may be helpful. Warren (1993) suggests a developmental model that conceptualizes vision abilities in a hierarchy (Fig. 15-4). The abilities at the bottom of Figure 15-4 form the foundation for each successive level. Higher level abilities depend on the complete integration of lower level abilities for their development.

The highest vision ability in this model is **visual cognition.** Visual cognition is the ability to mentally manipulate visual information and integrate it with other sensory information to solve problems, formulate plans, and make decisions. This ability is required for reading, writing, and solving mathematical problems (Warren, 1993).

Visual memory is the ability directly below visual cognition in Warren's model. Visual cognition depends on visual memory because mental manipulation of a visual stimulus requires the ability to retain a mental picture (Ratcliff, 1987).

To store a visual image, individuals must be able to recognize a pattern. **Pattern recognition,** the next ability level, involves identification of the salient features of an object (Julesz, 1981, 1985). An individual must not only be able to identify the holistic aspects of an object such as its shape and contour, but also specific features of an object such as its color detail, shading, and texture.

The ability to scan the environment is necessary for effective pattern recognition. **Scanning,** therefore, is foundation ability for pattern recognition. The eye must record all the details of a scene systematically and follow an organized scan path (Warren, 1993).

The ability directly below scanning is visual attention. Engagement of visual attention is necessary for proper scanning to occur. If individuals are not attending to visual stimuli in a specific space, they will not initiate scanning into that area. A classic example is the elder with a CVA with left hemineglect who requires constant cueing to scan to the left to avoid colliding with objects (Warren, 1993).

Visual attention and all the higher level abilities depend on three primary visual abilities that form the foundation for all vision functions: oculomotor control, visual fields, and visual acuity. Oculomotor control enables efficient and conjugate eye movements, which ensure completion of accurate scan paths and "teaming" of the eyes for binocular vision. The visual field is the extent of view that a person has in front of each eye. Visual acuity describes the sharpness or clearness of vision (Warren, 1993).

Evaluation and treatment of visual dysfunction should begin with a thorough examination of the foundation abilities followed by an assessment of the next higher level abilities: visual attention and scanning. The majority of deficits occur in these areas (Warren, 1993). When deficits are observed, the treatment focus can be directed at correcting or compensating for these deficient abilities. Deficits that are apparent in higher level abilities often are alleviated by improving the deficient foundation level skills.

Earlier occupational therapy (OT) frameworks for addressing visual skills often borrowed the terminology and concepts used by other disciplines such as psychology. This results in a "top-down" approach in which therapists are able to label a high level perceptual deficit such as impaired figure ground perception or visual closure. However, this approach does not help to direct treatment.

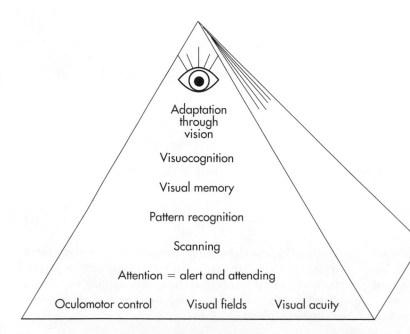

FIGURE **15-4**   Hierarchy of visual perceptual skills development in the central nervous system. (Adapted from Warren, M.L. [1993]. A hierarchical model for evaluation and treatment of visual perceptual dysfunction in adult acquired brain injury, part 1. *American Journal of Occupational Therapy, 47,* 42–54.)

Using Warren's hierarchical model often helps therapists locate deficits in foundation areas that, if improved, often impact the higher level perceptual skills. One example is to consider how deficits in visual attention and scanning could affect a skill such as figure ground perception. Someone who has difficulty carrying out a systematic scan pattern and attending to the salient features of each object would also likely have difficulty locating a key that is lying on a cluttered table, an example of the higher level skill of figure ground perception.

PRINCIPLES OF TREATMENT

When an OT visual screen reveals deficits that are affecting ADL, the client should then be referred to an ophthalmologist or optometrist to obtain a comprehensive visual examination. If available records and clinical observation indicate the client's visual impairment is caused by an ocular disease, it would be best to refer the client to a low vision specialist (see later discussion of professionals for collaboration). If, conversely, diagnostic and clinical information indicate the client's visual impairment is caused by a neurological insult such as a head injury or stroke, a consultation with a neurophthalmologist or neurooptometrist is recommended. If either of these scenarios is not possible, a consultation with a trusted ophthalmologist would be the next choice. Ideally, a good working relationship should be established with low vision specialists and neurophthalmologists in the area to facilitate the speed of referral and communication between professionals.

The information provided by an ophthalmologist or optometrist may vary depending on the condition and the professional's area of specialty, but a report from these professionals typically includes many of the following visual functions: visual acuity, visual field, contrast sensitivity function (the ability to distinguish subtle degradations in contrast between an object and its background), oculomotor control, intraocular pressure (the pressure inside the eyeball), best correction for eyeglasses prescription, and the general health of ocular structures. Low vision specialists often also make recommendations for special optical devices to access printed materials if visual acuity cannot be corrected to a functional range. This information, as well as that gathered during the OT evaluation, is invaluable in guiding treatment.

DECREASED ACUITY

The input of an eye care specialist is crucial in addressing reduced acuity. Some elders are simply in need of an updated eyeglass prescription. In the case of a head injury or stroke, acuity may be reduced initially, but often resolves spontaneously in a few months. Reduced acuity secondary to ocular diseases such as macular degeneration cannot be improved through a change in eyeglass prescription. Recommendations for special optical devices

may be made in this case. Diabetic retinopathy often not only causes reduced acuity, but also causes fluctuating acuity. It is important to follow the advice of the eye care specialist when planning treatment related to acuity.

As mentioned earlier, one method to compensate for reduced acuity is to use special optical devices to magnify or enlarge print. It is recommended that occupational therapists and assistants receive specialized training in optical devices before attempting to train individuals in their use. There are many unique concepts and techniques involved in the proper use of these devices and elders typically require very clear instructions and encouragement to become proficient in their use. Some commonly used optical devices are shown in Figures 15-5 and 15-6. Other examples of using enlargement to compensate for decreased acuity are the use of large print materials and writing larger using a felt tip pen.

When an elder has decreased acuity, there are other techniques to help maximize function such as the use of proper illumination, reduction of pattern and clutter in the environment, and the use of organizational systems. Proper lighting is usually critical for optimal performance. However, some individuals may also be photophobic or sensitive to light, which presents a challenge in finding appropriate lighting. Good room lighting is necessary for ease and safety in ambulating. A directional, focal type of light source, such as a gooseneck lamp, is recommended for fine-detail or low contrast tasks such as reading and sewing. Proper positioning of the lamp must be considered to avoid glare. Directing the light from behind the elder's shoulder so that the glare source is not in the eyes and from a position opposite the dominant hand to avoid shadows when writing usually works best.

Patterned backgrounds and clutter in the environment tend to "camouflage" objects that an elder is seeking (Fig. 15-7). This can be remedied by using solid colors for background surfaces such as bedspreads, place mats,

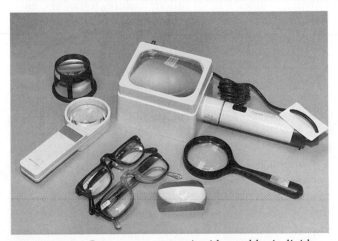

FIGURE 15-5 Some common optic aids used by individuals with low vision.

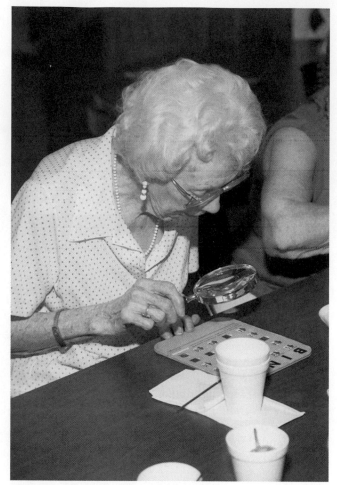

FIGURE 15-6   This elder is able to pursue a hobby by using a low-tech device.

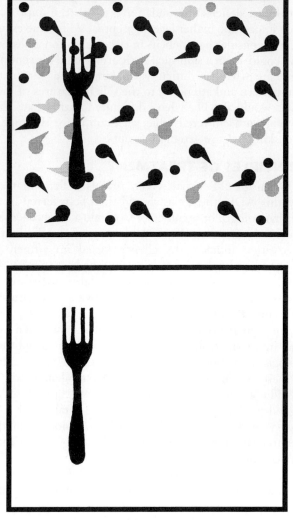

FIGURE 15-7   A patterned background can make it difficult to locate objects.

tablecloths, rugs, and furniture coverings. Care also should be taken to reduce clutter where possible by limiting the number of objects in the environment and arranging the remaining objects in an orderly fashion. Once the environment is rearranged and simplified, every effort should be made to keep it organized (Fig. 15-8).

There are many national and local services available for those with impaired visual acuity (and other visual impairment). Most of these services are free of charge. They can be found by investigating the resource section of the public library or by contacting organizations such as The American Foundation for the Blind or The Lighthouse (see Appendix for contact information for these organizations), which is an example of one such service in which books and magazines on cassette tapes are loaned and sent to individuals free of charge. There are also many catalogs that offer low-tech adaptive devices for the visually impaired such as talking clocks, large print playing cards and bingo cards, assistive devices for diabetic management, and many others (see Appendix).

VISUAL FIELD LOSS

Elders who have a visual field loss may be taught to compensate for this loss in daily activities. The first step, however, is to increase the elder's awareness of the visual field loss. Having accurate information on the extent and location of field loss is critical for teaching elders proper methods of compensation. The exact type and scope of visual field loss will vary depending on the cause of the disorder or disease and on individual presentation. In general, those with ocular conditions experience relatively "spotty types" of field loss, whereas those with neurological disorders exhibit more uniform or extensive field loss. Of course, there are definitely exceptions to this rule as some ocular conditions can lead to an extensive and even total loss of visual field. Small concentrated areas of visual field loss also have been found in those with head injuries (Williams, 1995).

208

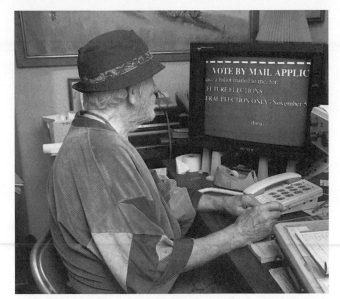

FIGURE 15-8 This elder would be able to function in his environment more effectively if the clutter were removed.

Elders who have central field loss, such as that seen with macular degeneration, must learn to compensate by directing their gaze to the side of the target rather than directly at the target. This technique, called eccentric viewing, enables the individual to place the target outside of the blind spot so it can be seen. This requires a conscious effort on the elder's part to override the natural tendency to direct the fovea, the most central area of the retina, to the target. Central field loss usually affects fine-detail vision tasks, but does not significantly interfere with mobility. Those with more peripheral field loss typically require intervention aimed at increasing safety and independence in mobility skills. Elders with a homonymous hemianopsia occurring after a stroke may be taught to compensate for this loss of half the visual field by systematically training them to turn the head and scan into the impaired field during functional activities such as reading, shopping, and mobility (Kerkhoff, Munbinger, & Meier, 1994, Warren, 1998).

OCULOMOTOR DYSFUNCTION

Treatment for oculomotor dysfunction is likely one of the most complex areas for beginning practitioners to comprehend and implement effectively. It is highly recommended that the entry level COTA attend continuing education seminars, develop a mentoring relationship, and establish service competency in this area before attempting any of the treatment strategies suggested. It is also strongly recommended that therapists and assistants work under the close supervision of an optometrist or ophthalmologist when treating oculomotor impairments. Oculomotor impairments are seen in individuals who have experienced some type of neurological insult.

Ocular conditions do not affect the muscular or neural mechanisms that control eye movements.

A strabismus, or misalignment of an eye (Scheiman, 2002a), is often seen as a result of extraocular muscle weakness after a stroke or other neurological insult. This misalignment of the eyes results in diplopia, or double vision. The primary treatment methods used to address diplopia include occlusion, eye exercises, application of prisms, and surgery (Warren, 1998).

Occlusion is essentially the "patching" of an eye to eliminate the double image (Scheiman, 2002a). Care must be taken to follow an occlusion protocol that optimizes the elder's comfort and reduces the likelihood of developing contractures in the muscles opposite the weak ones. Occlusion should not be carried out by simply patching the affected eye during all waking hours because this does nothing to encourage the use of the weak muscles. The protocol is typically directed by an ophthalmologist or optometrist.

Eye exercises can be used in conjunction with occlusion to help strengthen the affected muscles. One basic method would be to patch the unaffected eye and have the client track an object through all ranges of motion (Warren, 1998). An optometrist may suggest additional exercises to be carried out under his or her direction.

Another strategy to treat diplopia is the application of prisms (Scheiman, 2002a). Prisms are sometimes prescribed and used to create a single image in the primary direction of gaze. The prism displaces the image to one side causing the disparate images created by the strabismus to overlap and fuse into a single image. The prism can be permanently ground into the client's eyeglass lens or can be temporarily applied to the eyeglass lens using press-on prisms. If the strabismus is resolving, the elder should be gradually weaned from the prism by reducing its strength over time (Scheiman, 2002a). An ophthalmologist or optometrist determines the strength of the prism and directs the treatment.

In some specific cases, surgery to correct the strabismus may be warranted (Warren, 1998). This is further testimony to the necessity of consulting with appropriate eye care professionals to obtain optimal treatment for the individual. In most cases, the general approach to the surgery is to make the action of one or more eye muscles weaker or stronger by changing its attachment position. This is done by an ophthalmologist who is specially trained in strabismus surgery (Warren, 1998).

REDUCED CONTRAST SENSITIVITY

Contrast sensitivity may be affected by both ocular and neurological conditions. This function is different than visual acuity, which only reveals the size of high contrast black and white letters that the individual is capable of seeing. Contrast sensitivity is the capacity to discriminate between similar shades (Mogk, 2000).

In daily life, good contrast sensitivity is necessary to see a gray car on a cloudy day, to detect unmarked curbs and steps, and to distinguish subtle contours on people's faces in order to recognize them. Deficits in contrast sensitivity typically are addressed through environmental adaptation. For persons with low contrast sensitivity, the world often loses its definition. The primary technique to compensate for this deficit is to simply add contrast to the environment whenever possible. Many items used in daily activities can be changed to add more contrast and definition (Box 15-1). Proper illumination (as described earlier under "Decreased Acuity") also is helpful in enhancing contrast.

IMPAIRED VISUAL ATTENTION AND SCANNING

Deficits in attention and scanning are seen in those with neurological involvement, not in those with ocular conditions. One type of impairment in this area is hemiinattention, or hemineglect. This refers to a lack of attention to one half of a person's visual space. A neglect of the left half of visual space is more common, but right hemiinattention also is occasionally seen (Diamond, 2001). Individuals with hemiinattention are not able to take in visual information in the orderly, sequential, and comprehensive pattern needed to complete many daily activities safely such as grooming, meal preparation, and functional mobility. Initial treatment of deficits in visual attention and scanning often involves increasing the elder's awareness of the deficit followed up with appropriate compensation or remediation techniques, or both. Research has shown that individuals with left visual neglect may be trained to reorganize their scanning strategies by beginning the scan path in the impaired space (Weinberg et al., 1979). This is accomplished through treatment strategies similar to those described earlier in treating homonymous hemianopsia. Activities are used that require and encourage a systematic left-to-right scan pattern with an

anchor placed to the left (or right as appropriate) as a cue if necessary. There is some evidence that the effects of this training on patients with hemiinattention may be task-specific and may not generalize to overall ADL function (Gordon et al., 1985; Wagenaar, Van Wieringen, Netelenbos, Meijer, & Kuik, 1992). The presence of hemineglect also has been associated with poor rehabilitation outcome (Fullerton, Mackenzie, & Stout, 1988; Kalra, Perez, Gupta, & Wittink, 1997; Kaplan & Hier, 1982).

HIGHER LEVEL VISUAL–PERCEPTUAL DEFICITS

Warren's (1993) proposed treatment for higher level visual deficits includes addressing the foundation visual skills that may affect these areas, education of the patient to increase awareness of the deficit, and, last, instruction in the use of compensatory strategies for the deficit. (See Warren [1993] for a more detailed description of these techniques.)

SETTINGS IN WHICH VISUAL IMPAIRMENTS ARE ADDRESSED

Because visual impairments are a common result of neurological insult and because ocular diseases are relatively common in the elderly, COTAs working in any geriatric or neurorehabilitation setting should be well educated in visual dysfunction and treatment techniques. This may include inpatient and outpatient rehabilitation, subacute rehabilitation facilities, long-term care facilities, and home health agencies.

However, low vision rehabilitation is becoming a specialty area in the field of OT and COTAs may also find opportunities to work in a low vision rehabilitation clinic. Occupational therapists and COTAs work in conjunction with other trained professionals to provide comprehensive services to individuals with vision impairments. The majority of individuals treated in low vision clinics have impairments caused by ocular pathologies. Macular degeneration accounts for 60% of low vision cases (Scheiman, 2002a), whereas glaucoma and diabetic retinopathy are ranked second and third, respectively (Stuen, 1996). For this reason, the term "low vision" is typically associated with visual impairments caused by ocular diseases. However, individuals with visual impairments secondary to neurological insult also may seek treatment in some low vision clinics.

COTAs working in low vision rehabilitation must have specialized training in areas such as optics and use of optical devices, eccentric viewing techniques, blind techniques for ADL, and vision enhancement techniques for ADL, as well as a good working knowledge of the extensive adaptive equipment available for low vision clients. They also must possess a good understanding of available resources to direct clients to appropriate support groups and other services.

BOX 15-1

Examples of Modifications Using Contrast in the Environment

- Use a black felt tip marker for writing.
- Add strips of contrasting tape (usually orange or yellow is best) to the edge of steps.
- Use a white coffee cup so the level of coffee can be seen against the white background when pouring.
- Use a black and white reversible cutting board and slice light-colored items, such as onions, on the black side and vice versa.
- Mark light switches with contrasting fluorescent tape to increase visibility.

There are many other low vision rehabilitation professionals with whom the COTA can collaborate to provide the most comprehensive program for their clients. Orientation and mobility specialists address travel needs directly related to vision loss. They typically hold Master's degrees and have a wealth of knowledge in this area. The goal of their services is to develop independent travel skills within the client's home, neighborhood, or community. These specialists may work in many settings including public school systems, private agencies, and state-supported programs. Rehabilitation teachers are professionals who are trained at the university level to address ADL that have been affected by visual impairment. They provide instruction in using adaptive techniques or adaptive equipment to increase independence in areas such as communication, household management, self-care, and other ADL. Rehabilitation teachers may work in private agencies, itinerant state services, residential schools, and independent living centers. The areas addressed and the knowledge base of these professionals may overlap at times with OT professionals. As long as there is open communication and collaboration, each profession will likely learn valuable techniques from the other and the client will receive an optimal rehabilitation program.

Ophthalmologists and optometrists specializing in low vision also help to ensure that comprehensive low vision services are provided. They evaluate the client's visual function and prescribe optical devices and training to compensate for vision loss. They may see low vision clients in their own broader-based private practice or they may work in low vision clinics. (For more information regarding a program using ophthalmology and OT to provide low vision rehabilitation in an outpatient rehabilitation setting see Warren [1995].)

SUMMARY

Visual impairments in elders may result from either ocular or neurological pathology. Normal physiologic changes that may occur with aging include shrinkage of the peripheral field, increased time required to recover from glare, difficulty with light and dark adaptation, increased need for illumination, loss of elasticity in the lens, and yellowing of the lens. The most common ocular diseases that may occur in elders are macular degeneration, cataracts, glaucoma, and diabetic retinopathy. Elders are also at risk for CVAs, which may disrupt any of several neurological components necessary for effective visual functioning.

COTAs can play vital roles in helping elders with visual impairments learn to function as independently as possible. By providing education about a particular vision loss, COTAs may be able to offer the first sense of security these individuals have had since being diagnosed as visually impaired. COTAs also may give instruction in the techniques for compensating for vision loss in daily activities.

Finally, COTAs may make environmental adaptations to help the elder function more independently.

The loss of vision in elders is a common occurrence, whether it results from the natural aging process, ocular disease, or disruption of neurological components. Vision loss has significant functional implications and can complicate the elder's rehabilitation process with other physical impairments. This emphasizes the need for COTAs to familiarize themselves with the causes and types of vision loss and effective treatment techniques, whether they are working in low vision clinics, general rehabilitation centers, or acute care hospitals.

CASE STUDY

George is 67-year-old widower who lives alone and following an amputation below the right knee was just admitted to the rehabilitation unit where you work. He has diabetes mellitus and has had many complications of the disease including the peripheral vascular disease that led to his amputation and diabetic retinopathy. George states that he did not manage his condition well in the past, but wants to do everything he can now to keep these complications from getting any worse. He states that he finds it difficult to see the numbers and lines on his syringes when drawing his insulin. He also has some trouble seeing the blood sugar reading on his glucometer. He needs to check his blood sugar three times a day with this machine and adjust his insulin dosage accordingly. The OT visual screen reveals that George has moderately decreased visual acuity and decreased contrast sensitivity.

George has good upper body strength and uses his walker well on the unit. He will need to use the walker at discharge while waiting for his leg to heal before being fitted for a prosthesis. Fortunately, you will be able to conduct a home evaluation to make recommendations before discharge.

■ CASE STUDY QUESTIONS

1 What are some specific areas of concern/potential hazards that you would look for on George's home evaluation visit?
2 What are some recommendations you could make to address these concerns and improve safety and ease of functioning in George's home?
3 You would like to increase George's independence in his diabetic management, but do not know what techniques or adaptive equipment is available to accomplish this. Where could you turn for help?

■ CHAPTER REVIEW QUESTIONS

1 What are some natural age-related changes in the eye and what implications do they have for function?
2 What are the three primary ocular conditions that account for the majority of referrals to low vision rehabilitation clinics?
3 Which ocular conditions could potentially lead to total blindness?

4 What are some possible vision problems after a stroke or other neurological insult?

5 What are the primary vision abilities that form the foundation for all other vision abilities?

6 What type of impairment would be seen more frequently in a low vision rehabilitation setting: diplopia or decreased acuity?

7 Name some other professionals with whom the COTA could collaborate regarding a low vision client.

REFERENCES

American Foundation for the Blind. (1999a). Fact sheet: Cataracts [WWW page]. URL http://www.afb.org/info_document_view.asp?documentid=193

American Foundation for the Blind. (1999b). Fact sheet: Visual impairment and age-related macular degeneration [WWW page]. URL http://www.afb.org/info_document_view.asp?documentid=202

American Foundation for the Blind. (1999c). Fact sheet: Visual impairment and glaucoma [WWW page]. URL http://www.afb.org/info_document_view.asp?documentid=705

American Foundation for the Blind. (1999d). Statistics and sources for professionals [WWW page]. URL http://www.afb.org/info_document_view.asp?documentid=1367

American Foundation for the Blind. (2002). Facts about aging and vision [WWW page]. URL http://www.afb.org/info_documents.asp?kitid=8&collectionid=2 and http://www.afb.org/info_document_view.asp?documentid=1809

Bennett, S. H. (1991). Visual changes associated with aging: Influence on practice. *Occupational Therapy Practice, 3*(1), 12.

Bennett, S. H. (1992). Low vision: Clinical aspects and interventions. In J. Rothman & R. Levine (Eds.), *Prevention practice strategies for physical therapy and occupational therapy* (pp. 258-269). New York: WB Saunders.

Center on an Aging Society. (2002). Visual impairments data profile, no. 3. [WWW page]. URL http://ihcrp.Georgetown.edu/agingsociety/pdfs/visual.pdf

Diamond, R. (2001). Rehabilitative management of post-stroke visuospatial inattention (review). *Disability and Rehabilitation, 23*(10), 407-412.

Friedman, D. B. (2000). Psychosocial factors in vision rehabilitation. In D. M. Albert, & F. A. Jakobiec (Eds.), *Principles and practice of ophthalmology, Vol. 5* (pp. 3667-3670). Philadelphia: WB Saunders.

Fullerton, K. J., Mackenzie, G., & Stout, R. W. (1988). Prognostic indices in stroke. *Quarterly Journal of Medicine, 250*, 147-162.

Gordon, W. A., Hibbard, M. R., Egelko, S., Diller, L., Shaver, M. S., Lieberman, A., & Ragnarsson, K. (1985). Perceptual remediation in patients with right brain damage: A comprehensive program. *Archives of Physical Medicine and Rehabilitation, 66*, 353-360.

Jose, R. T. (1985). The eye and functional vision. In R.T. Jose (Ed.), *Understanding low vision* (pp. 3-42). New York: American Foundation for the Blind.

Julesz, B. (1981). Texton, the elements of texture perception and their interactions. *Nature, 290*(12), 91.

Julesz , B. (1985). Preconscious and conscious processing in vision. In C. Chagas & R. Gattass (Eds.), Pattern recognition mechanisms. *Experimental Brain Research, 11* (suppl 11), 333.

Kalra, L., Perez, L., Gupta, S., & Wittink, M. (1997). The influence of visual neglect on stroke rehabilitation. *Stroke, 28*, 1386-1391.

Kaplan, J., & Hier, D. B. (1982). Visuospatial deficits after right hemisphere stroke. *American Journal of Occupational Therapy, 36*, 314-321.

Kerkhoff, G. (2000). Neurovisual rehabilitation: Recent developments and future directions. *Journal of Neurology, Neurosurgery, and Psychiatry, 68*, 691-706.

Kerkhoff, G., Munbinger, U., & Meier, E. (1994). Neurovisual rehabilitation in cerebral blindness. *Archives of Neurology, 51*, 474-481.

Kubler-Ross, E. (1969). *Death and dying* (pp.11-138), New York, NY: Macmillan.

The Lighthouse, Inc. (1995). The Lighthouse national survey on vision loss: The experience, attitudes, and knowledge of middle-aged and older Americans. New York: The Lighthouse, Inc.

Lighthouse International. (n.d.). Normal changes in the aging eye: What we all can expect. [WWW page]. URL http://www.lighthouse.org

Mogk, L. G. (2000). Eye conditions that cause low vision in adults. In M. Warren (Ed.), *Low vision: Occupational therapy intervention with the older adult: A self-paced clinical course from AOTA.* Bethesda, MD: American Occupational Therapy Association.

Ratcliff, G. (1987). Perception and complex visual processes. In M. J. Meier, A. L. Benton, & L. Diller (Eds.), *Neuropsychological rehabilitation.* New York: Guilford.

Rolland, J. S. (1994). *Families, illness, and disability: An integrative treatment model* (pp. 127-164). New York: Basic Books.

Scheiman, M. (2002a). Management of refractive, visual efficiency, and visual information processing disorders. In M. Scheiman (Ed.), *Understanding and managing vision deficits: A guide for occupational therapists* (pp. 117-162). Thorofare, NJ: Slack Inc.

Scheiman, M. (2002b). Review of basic anatomy, physiology, and development of the visual system. In M. Scheiman (Ed.), *Understanding and managing vision deficits: A guide for occupational therapists* (pp. 9-15). Thorofare, NJ: Slack Inc.

Stuen, C. (1996). New concepts and treatments. *Vision and Aging News, 8*(1), 8.

Wagenaar, R. C., Van Wieringen, P. C. W., Netelenbos, J. B., Meijer, O. G., & Kuik, D. J. (1992). The transfer of scanning training effects in visual inattention after stroke: Five single-case studies. *Disability and Rehabilitation, 14*, 51-60.

Warren, M. L. (1993). A hierarchical model for evaluation and treatment of visual perceptual dysfunction in adult acquired brain injury, part 1. *American Journal of Occupational Therapy, 47*, 42-54.

Warren, M. L. (1995). Providing low vision rehabilitation services with occupational therapy and ophthalmology: A program description. *American Journal of Occupational Therapy, 49*, 877-884.

Warren, M. L. (1998). *The brain injury visual assessment battery for adults test manual.* Lenexa, KS: visABILITIES Rehab Services, Inc.

Weinberg, J., Diller, L., Gordon, W. A., Gerstman, L. J., Lieberman, A., & Lakin, P. (1979). Visual scanning training effect on reading-related tasks in acquired right brain damage. *Archives of Physical Medicine and Rehabilitation, 60*, 479-486.

Williams, T. A. (1995). Case report: Low vision rehabilitation for a patient with traumatic brain injury. *American Journal of Occupational Therapy, 49*(9), 923-926.

Working with Elders Who Have Hearing Impairments

SHARON STOFFEL

KEY TERMS

sensorineural hearing loss (sensory, neural, mechanical), conductive hearing loss, cochlear implants, tinnitus, hearing aid, assistive listening device, audiologist

CHAPTER OBJECTIVES

1. Describe sensorineural and conductive hearing losses.
2. Describe ways that slow, progressive changes in the auditory system interfere with occupations that require communication.
3. List environmental modifications that reduce background noise in homes and institutions.
4. Describe possible safety recommendations for home and institutional environments where hearing-impaired elders reside.

5. Describe the effect of age-related hearing loss on socialization, communication, and travel and its possible contribution to feelings of isolation for hearing-impaired elders.
6. List suggestions for improving communication with hearing-impaired elders.
7. Describe possible behaviors that may indicate hearing impairment.

The voice of a loved one, the chimes of a grandfather clock, a violin concerto—these are sounds many people not only enjoy, but take for granted. For elders who have hearing impairments, these sounds may be either misinterpreted or missed altogether. Hearing impairments may also be associated with reduced ability to hear warning signals, ambulation difficulties, balance problems, and increased incidence of falls (Garstecki & Erler, 1998; Tobis et al., 1990). Hearing impairments can contribute to social isolation. Safety related to hearing impairments

may become a concern when elders are unable to hear alarms and other warning signals.

Hearing loss is more prevalent than any other chronic condition (Garsteck & Erler, 1998; Rieske & Hostege, 1996). By the year 2050, 26 million people are expected to have a hearing impairment (Kinderknecht & Garner, 1993; Rieske & Hostege, 1996). Although persons of all ages experience hearing impairments, elders are primarily affected (Hooper, 2001). Elders between the ages of 65 and 74 years experience an estimated 25% hearing loss.

entage increases to 40% for those older than
rs, and some studies indicate that 85% to 90% of
rsing home residents have hearing impairments that
limit function (Hooper, 2001).

Even though hearing impairments are more prevalent
than vision loss, they are often more difficult to distinguish. Changes in hearing are often subtle and occur
gradually. Many elders with significant hearing losses
often wait as long as 5 years before seeking assistance
with their hearing (Lichtenstein, Bess, & Logan, 1991).
Elders, family members, and health care personnel may
not recognize hearing losses. Some may accept the loss as
an inevitable and unalterable aspect of aging.

Because elders seldom seek assistance or plan interventions to enhance their hearing, certified occupational
therapy assistants (COTAs) must be able to distinguish
the various types of hearing impairments. In addition,
COTAs should be aware of interventions, services,
devices, and activities that can enhance occupational performance for elders who are hearing impaired. This
chapter provides an overview of the most common types
of hearing losses that affect elders. The possible psychosocial effects that a hearing impairment may have on
elders, their families, and their friends also are addressed.
Rehabilitation considerations are discussed, including
communicating with an elder who has a hearing impairment, methods for modifying home, public spaces, and
institutional environments, and recommendations for
assisting elders in the use of hearing aids and assisted
listening devices (ALD).

HEARING CONDITIONS ASSOCIATED WITH AGING

Elders who have a hearing loss should see a physician to
determine cause and rule out or treat other underlying
pathological processes (Kinderknecht & Garner, 1993).
Generally, hearing losses are divided into the three following areas: sensorineural, conductive, and mixed. These
conditions may affect one or both ears.

The most common type of hearing loss in elders is the
result of sensorineural damage to the hearing organ itself
or to the peripheral or central nervous system (or both).
Although elders rarely have just one type of **sensorineural loss,** the most common type of loss is caused
by hair cell damage or loss of the sensory hair cells of the
cochlea. As individuals age, these hair cells are slowly lost,
and the ability to hear high-frequency sounds is diminished. One of the most frustrating and handicapping
aspect of this loss is the ways sounds are changed or distorted. Although the elder may hear someone speaking,
the signals that allow him or her to understand what is
being said are not clear. Such losses can have serious consequences in both social and therapeutic settings. For
example, at a party someone may say, "How are you?" and
the elder may respond, "Seventy-one." An elder in a clinic

setting who is asked to hand the COTA a "dime" may
respond with the correct "time." Such responses often
raise questions about mental status and often lead to a loss
of confidence in interacting with others (Cherney, 2002).
In such situations, the COTA should seek assistance to
rule out the presence of sensorineural loss before questioning the elder's orientation or ability to follow directions. In addition, because women's voices are usually
higher pitched than men's, female occupational therapy
(OT) practitioners must understand that their voices can
contribute to decreased comprehension by elders.

Elders living in areas with low exposure to loud or high-
pitched noise levels may experience less sensorineural
hearing loss than those living in noisy, industrial areas.
Although those with better overall health seem less likely
to experience this type of loss, some sensorineural loss
eventually affects elders regardless of environmental conditions. However, continued exposure at any age to loud
noises for long periods, such as listening to headphones
at high volumes, may cause permanent damage, resulting
in premature hearing impairments (Hooper, 2001).

Three types of sensorineural hearing loss have been
identified: **sensory, neural,** and **mechanical** (Cherney,
2002; Hooper, 2001). Sensory loss is caused by atrophy
and degeneration of the hair cells at the base of the basi-
lar membrane. It produces a loss of high-frequency
sounds but does not interfere with the discrimination of
speech. Neural loss is caused by the loss of auditory nerve
fibers. It affects the ability to distinguish speech sounds,
especially in the higher frequencies, but does not affect
the ability to hear pure tones. Mechanical loss is characterized by degeneration of the vibrating membrane
within the cochlea. This type of loss leads to gradual
impairment of hearing in all frequencies. In situations
where several sounds in various frequencies are present at
the same time, the ability to distinguish between the
sounds becomes increasingly difficult. Table 16-1 lists
common hearing conditions of elders.

A sensorineural hearing loss may be unnoticed in the
early stages because the high-frequency tones that are
initially lost are above the functional range used in most
environments. As the condition progresses, elders may
notice that they cannot hear the ringing of the telephone,
the buzz of the doorbell, the ticking of a clock, or the
water dripping from a faucet. With further progression,
the sounds of certain consonants such as *s, z, t, f,* and *g*
become increasingly difficult to distinguish. Eventually,
elders may strain to hear and understand conversations
and one-syllable words (Cherney, 2002).

A second hearing condition, **conductive hearing loss,**
results in an inability of the external ear to conduct sound
waves to the inner ear. Conductive hearing losses may be
related to the buildup of cerumen (earwax), fluid accumulation in the middle ear from eustachian tube dysfunction, or an upper respiratory infection. These conductive

TABLE 16-1

Common Hearing Conditions of Elders

Condition	Cause	Symptoms
Sensorineural losses Sensory	Atrophy and degeneration of the hair cells at the base of the basilar membrane	Loss of high frequency sounds; condition does not interfere with speech discrimination
Neural	Loss of auditory nerve fibers	Condition affects ability to distinguish speech sounds in higher frequencies; does not affect ability to hear pure tones
Mechanical	Degeneration of the vibrating membrane within the cochlea	Condition leads to gradual loss of hearing in all frequencies, ability to distinguish sounds becomes increasingly difficult
Conductive hearing loss	Inability of the external ear to conduct sound waves to the inner ear; may be related to buildup of earwax, fluid accumulation in the middle ear, or upper respiratory infection	Condition can often be corrected by cleaning the ear, medications, or surgery; hearing aids or cochlear implants may be considered
Tinnitus	May be related to conductive or sensorineural loss, Ménière's disease, otosclerosis, presbycusis, earwax buildup, lesions, or fluid in middle ear	Buzzing, ringing, whistle, roar in ears, most noticeable at night; may be necessary to rule out underlying conditions before implementing treatments designed to symptoms

problems often can be corrected by cleaning the ear, administering medications, or performing surgery. Hearing aids may be effective for persons who have untreatable or residual conductive hearing loss. A hearing aid amplifies incoming sound and requires functioning hair cells and an intact nerve to transmit the sound to the central auditory pathways. For older adults whose residual hearing is greatly limited because of an absence of hair cells, cochlear implants may be considered (Hooper, 2001). Cochlear implants are only appropriate when minimal or no benefit is possible when a conventional hearing aid is used. Cochlear implants are prosthetic replacements for the functions of the lost hair cells by converting mechanical energy (sound waves) into electrical energy capable of exciting the auditory nerve. Cochlear implants are placed within the inner ear. They bypass the hair cells of the cochlea and directly stimulate the endings of the auditory nerve. The system consists of an external microphone, processor, and transmitter and an internal receiver–stimulator and electrode. Figures 16-1 and 16-2 show the external and internal placements for a cochlear implant.

Tinnitus is a subjective auditory problem consisting of a ringing, whistling, buzzing, or roaring noise in the ears. Tinnitus may occur as part of a conductive or sensorineural hearing loss. It may also be associated with Ménière's disease, otosclerosis, sensorineural loss, an accumulation of cerumen pressing on the eardrum, tympanic membrane lesions, and fluid in the middle ear. Medications such as the doses of aspirin prescribed for arthritis or other medical conditions can be additional contributing factors (Hooper, 2001). Before planning interventions to mask the symptoms of tinnitus, possible underlying conditions such as cardiovascular disease, anemia, and hypothyroidism should be ruled out by a physician.

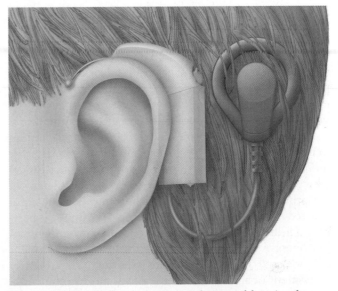

FIGURE 16-1   External placement for a cochlear implant. (From Cochlear Ltd, Engelwood, CO.)

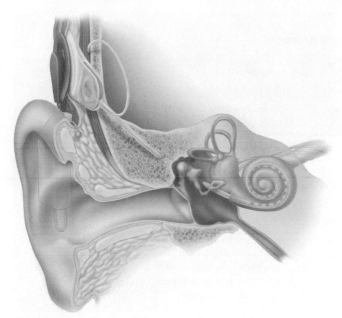

FIGURE 16-2   Internal placement for a cochlear implant. (From Cochlear Ltd, Engelwood, CO.)

Tinnitus is often most noticeable at night when other noises are reduced. A radio, tape recording, or appropriate hearing aid may mask the tinnitus so the individual can fall asleep. Other therapeutic interventions may include relaxation techniques and biofeedback (Garstecki & Erler, 1998).

PSYCHOSOCIAL ASPECTS OF HEARING IMPAIRMENTS

Even though much information about the environment is learned through the sense of hearing, the importance of hearing during travel, while working, and in personal and social situations often goes unnoticed. Some researchers suggest that when hearing loss is the only loss elders' experience, they can adjust well (Cherney, 2002). Others suggest that a hearing loss may lead to isolation and even paranoia (Garstecki & Erler, 1998). Unfortunately, many elders experience other losses or lifestyle changes at the same time hearing loss occurs. Retirement may lead to a loss of role identity, income, and social contacts. Adjusting to the death of a spouse or undergoing changes in vision or mobility may take priority over a loss of hearing. Elders who are predisposed to loneliness or have difficulty in initiating or maintaining relationships may become more isolated or avoid interpersonal relationships if they experience a hearing loss. This can result in an increased sense of loneliness or isolation, especially if the hearing impairment is associated with other losses (Cherney, 2002). Early assessment of a perceived hearing loss and recommendations for adaptations may help to reduce an elder's sense of loneliness.

The elder with a hearing loss often guesses at or misses the content of conversations, is reluctant to ask for clarification, or is embarrassed when mistakes are made because of a misunderstanding. This can occur when an elder with a hearing impairment is traveling. Studies involving elderly airline travelers have found that misunderstanding or not hearing overhead paging information has resulted in missed flights (Canadian Transportation Agency, 2002). Hearing changes also make it difficult to detect and understand speech in crowded and stressful situations. Limited hearing may decrease an elder's sense of security and increase feelings of vulnerability, making travel more difficult. As a result, some elders may either limit their travel or stop engaging in that occupation (Garstecki & Erler, 1998).

Communication can be exhausting for elders with a hearing impairment. For example, an 85-year-old man registering for OT treatments at a rehabilitation clinic will likely be embarrassed if he misinterprets the receptionist's request for his address as a request to undress. He may also experience isolation if his accompanying family member interrupts and answers all remaining questions. Repeated frustrating and embarrassing experiences can contribute to feelings of vulnerability, insecurity, and doubts related to self-esteem that can lead to withdrawal from travel, social, cultural, and family contacts.

Some elders with hearing impairments may hear well at home and only struggle to hear in other social settings. Others may be isolated not only from family and friends but also from the broader world because they cannot get information from television, radio, movies, and even telephone conversations. Elders may become increasingly frustrated as family, friends, and even health care workers begin to make decisions for them.

An age-related hearing loss may only further complicate the effects of illnesses and mental health conditions such as Alzheimer's disease. Hearing loss in elders can lead to or exacerbate paranoid ideas, suspicions, loss of contact with reality, and related tendencies (Cherney, 2002). Corso (1990) stated that a hearing loss can magnify previously existing paranoid personality attributes. Continued expression of suspicions, hostilities, and accusations of lying may result in friends and family members avoiding the hearing-impaired elder.

REHABILITATION AND THE HEARING-IMPAIRED ELDER

Rehabilitation often is an overlooked option for elders with hearing impairments and is seldom considered for those who are in the old-old age range (Commission on Education of the Deaf, 1989). The contributions of OT practitioners in the areas of occupations that have value and interest for the individual—functional communication, socialization, and environmental assessment of home, work, and public and private institutions—are an integral part of enabling elders to live independent and productive lives (Mann, 1994). Without rehabilitation, elders may be at risk for increased frequency of falls, functional dependence, loss of self-esteem, and institutionalization.

The effectiveness of rehabilitation for maximizing occupational independence is based on many factors. Those related to hearing loss may include age-related changes at the time of onset of the hearing impairment, such as vision and mobility losses, retirement, death of a spouse, and loss of clearly defined life roles. Other factors include the severity and rapidity of the loss, the degree of residual hearing, the presence of other medical conditions, and the involvement of the individual and family members in the rehabilitative process. COTA and occupational therapist (OTR) teams may work together to identify elders who have hearing impairments through observation of behaviors (Box 16-1). The Self-Rating Hearing Inventory also can be an effective tool for assessing the effects of a hearing impairment on perceived occupational performance (Janken & Cullinan, 1990). The American Academy of Otolaryngology–Head and Neck Surgery has developed a 5-minute hearing test to determine the need for referral to a hearing specialist (Fig. 16-3). For more profound hearing losses, a consultation and referral regarding use of a **hearing aid,** individual or computerized

BOX 16-1

Observable Behaviors That May Indicate Hearing Loss

- Inappropriate volume increase when speaking—for example, appearing to shout while talking to a person nearby
- Turning the television or radio volume inordinately high when there is no one else in the room and no noises in the background
- Turning in a chair or turning the head to get a better hearing position when being addressed
- Consistently asking for statements to be repeated
- Not responding to verbal questions or conversation
- Responding to verbal questions only when there is accompanying visual cueing
- Looking disoriented or confused or giving inappropriate responses to questions—for example, answering "yes" to a multiple choice question
- Answering questions addressed to another person when there are several persons conversing simultaneously in the same room
- Withdrawing from social situations
- Exhibiting short attention span, which is especially apparent when two people are talking simultaneously

Adapted from Kane, R. L., Ouslander, J. G., & Abrass, I. B. (1999). *Essentials of clinical geriatrics* (4th ed.). New York: McGraw-Hill.

training in speech reading (lip reading), and instruction regarding the use of an **ALD** may be needed. In addition, referrals for accessing both formal and informal support services through public and community agencies may be beneficial. Individuals for whom none of these interventions are effective may be candidates for cochlear implants.

COTAs may be involved in direct treatment interventions to assist individuals in engaging in the occupations of their choice. They may also assist in adapting environments for individuals, groups, or institutional facilities. The skills and experience of COTAs may be directed toward designing and implementing individual or institutional activities. These recommendations, intended to promote successful adaptation for hearing-impaired elders, also can assist families, friends, and institutional personnel.

RECOMMENDATIONS FOR IMPROVING ELDER COMMUNICATION

Psychosocial issues associated with hearing impairments often affect family members and friends, as well as the hearing-impaired elder. Information and education about the various types of age-related hearing losses and conditions may help COTAs in assisting elders to develop coping strategies (Hooper, 2001). The COTA should encourage family members and friends to be involved in the education and consultation process so that conversational and environmental adaptations that encourage inclusion of the elder can be promoted.

Hearing-impaired elders may need to gain confidence in requesting adaptations that help them adjust to their hearing losses. Having elders role play situations in which they request specific needs or adaptations may increase self-confidence for reentering social situations that they may have been avoiding.

Environmental adaptations should first center on identifying and minimizing the influence of background noises. Background noises greatly limit enjoyment of conversations and often contribute to avoidance of social gatherings (Christenson & Taira, 1990). Common sources of background noise include music, conversations on television or of persons in the room, dishes being clanked, fans in use, outside traffic, overhead intercoms in use, and ice machines in use. Personnel shifts and changes in the institutional environment may also create background noise.

COTAs can recommend environments that reduce background noise. Examples include going to restaurants during times that they are less crowded, requesting to sit in less crowded areas, or sitting away from distracting background noises such as kitchen traffic or music. When traveling, to help compensate for difficulty in hearing overhead paging systems, elders can be encouraged to frequently check overhead flight monitors, or check in frequently with airport staff, or both. Using theaters and church communities that offer ALDs that amplify specific

Five-Minute Hearing Test

	Almost always	Half of the time	Occasionally	Never
1. I have a problem hearing over the telephone.				
2. I have trouble following the conversation when two or more people are talking at the same time.				
3. People complain when I turn the TV volume too high.				
4. I have to strain to understand conversations.				
5. I miss hearing some common sounds like the phone or doorbell ringing.				
6. I have trouble hearing conversations in a noisy background such as a party.				
7. I get confused about where sounds come from.				
8. I misunderstand some words in a sentence and need to ask people to repeat themselves.				
9. I especially have trouble understanding the speech of women and children.				
10. I have worked in noisy environments (jackhammers, assembly lines, jet engines).				
11. Many people I talk to seem to mumble (or don't talk clearly).				
12. People get annoyed because I misunderstand what they say.				
13. I misunderstand what others are saying and make inappropriate responses.				
14. I avoid social activities because I cannot hear well and fear I'll reply improperly.				
To be answered by a family member or friend: 15. Do you think this person has a hearing loss?				

Scoring
To calculate your score, give yourself 3 points for every time you checked the "Almost always" column, 2 for every "Half of the time," 1 for every "Occasionally" and 0 for every "Never." If you have a blood relative who has a hearing loss, add another 3 points. Then total your points. The American Academy of Otolaryngology–Head and Neck Surgery recommends the following:
- 0 to 5: Your hearing is fine. No action is required.
- 6 to 9: Suggest you see an ear-nose-and-throat (ENT) specialist.
- 10 and above: Strongly recommend you see an ear physician.

FIGURE 16-3   5-Minute hearing test. (©1993 by the American Academy of Otolaryngology–Head and Neck Surgery, Alexandria, VA.)

sounds are other ways to reduce interference from background noises in public spaces.

Personal environmental modifications for reducing background noise include adding carpet to floors and acoustical tiles to ceilings, hanging drapes on windows, hanging banners from high ceilings, and replacing wood or metal furniture with upholstered furniture. Although these recommendations are intended to help absorb sound, they also can add aesthetic appeal to a home or institution (Christenson & Taira, 1990).

Additional interior modifications to reduce background noise within institutions include adding insulated sheetrock around noisy areas such as kitchen, maintenance, and mechanical areas, and tightening window weather seals.

COTAs can assist individuals, families, and facility administrators in weighing the benefits of certain recommendations against the expenses of purchasing them. COTAs also can point out that, in some situations, background noises may provide helpful cues to locations of activity rooms, lounges, and beauty shops.

Environmental safety issues and concerns may center on the difficulties that hearing-impaired elders may have in locating the source of sounds in their home. Inability to locate sounds may contribute to a sense of insecurity in an individual's own environment and to the possibility of auditory illusions. Fire and smoke alarms tend to have high-pitched sounds that are difficult for persons with sensorineural losses to hear (Hooper, 2001). Adding visual cues such as flashing lights is recommended for alarms. Flashing lights, lower-pitched rings, or low-toned musical chimes are also available options for telephones and doorbells. COTAs should recommend adapting telephones with volume and tone controls for persons who need these modifications. Portable telephones, although convenient for some individuals, may add to confusion and frustration for persons with hearing impairments. The ring of a portable telephone may not be heard or the telephones may be difficult to locate if needed for an emergency (Statch & Stoner, 1991).

Tobis, Block, Steinhaus-Donham, Reinsch, & Tamaru (1990) report a greater incidence of falls in hearing-impaired individuals than in those who are not hearing impaired. Studies indicate that instruction in ways to substitute visual cues for hearing cues reduces the incidence of falls. COTAs also should make family members and health care providers aware that approaching hearing-impaired elders from the back and talking to and touching them may startle them and possibly cause them to lose balance. COTAs should recommend that hearing-impaired individuals be approached from the front, where visual contact can be made before beginning a conversation or expecting a response to a question.

To enhance conversations in areas where groups gather, COTAs should recommend that hearing-impaired individuals stay away from windows and plaster walls. Standing or sitting near soft materials that absorb sound, such as draperies, bookshelves, and upholstered furniture, also is recommended. Sitting in high-backed, upholstered chairs can help shield background noise. Focusing on the speaker's lips during conversation can help to increase comprehension. If an individual has more impairment in one ear than the other, the individual can find the position that maximizes hearing with the unaffected ear (Cherney, 2002).

For family members and friends who want to improve communication with hearing-impaired elders, COTAs should recommend that they position themselves in the elder's field of vision and get the elder's attention before speaking. While conversing, they should look directly at the elder, reduce the rate of speech, and speak distinctly with a low tone. Additional recommendations include asking the elder to repeat what was said and providing written instructions to reinforce verbal directions. COTAs should stress that a hearing impairment does not reduce an individual's intelligence. Accommodations for the hearing impairment should not be overly exaggerated or simplified to the point where elders with hearing loss feel that their intelligence or judgment is in question.

Because sensorineural hearing loss and its corresponding reduction in the ability to hear high-pitched sounds is the most common hearing disorder in elders, lowering the voice is especially important for women who address hearing-impaired elders. Increasing volume only increases tone and contributes to personal and social embarrassment.

In restaurants and institutional and private dining rooms, seating no more than four persons at a table so eye contact can be easily made can enhance the social aspects derived from conversations during meals. In larger dining rooms, padded room dividers between tables can absorb sounds from surrounding tables. General recommendations regarding reduction of background noises also should be considered.

The effects of glare on the visual and nonverbal cues that enhance auditory communication should be considered when speaking with hearing-impaired elders. Sources of glare may include windows, lights, and glass surfaces either from behind the person speaking or reflected from eyeglasses. Before beginning a conversation, the COTA, family member, or friend should adjust blinds or shades, adjust lighting, and reposition seating arrangements as needed (see Chapter 15 for more information on visual adaptations with aging).

Entertainment through television, music, and radio offers opportunities for stimulation that are not dependent on other people. When elders control the times and selections for television and radio programs and music, the cognitive stimulation can be rewarding. When televisions and radios are on constantly or programs selected are not those the elder would choose, they become an additional source of background noise rather than a source of stimulation (Hooper, 2001; Statch & Stoner, 1991). Closed-captioned television is an additional option to suggest. COTAs should identify and reduce sources of glare on the screen when positioning elders for television viewing. ALDs offer a means of controlling the volume for the hearing-impaired elder without disturbing others. Adjusting the volume and sound for music for those individuals with sensorineural hearing loss requires increasing the bass and decreasing the treble. Developments in technology have made the cost of these devices quite reasonable when weighed against the potential benefits (Statch & Stoner, 1991). Table 16-2 summarizes environmental adaptations for the hearing-impaired elder. (See the Appendix for additional resources.)

TABLE 16-2

Environmental Adaptations for the Hearing-Impaired Elder

Problem	Intervention
Background noises (institutional and home)	Add carpeting to floors, acoustical tiles to ceilings, and drapes on windows, and replace wood and metal furniture with upholstered furniture.
Background noises (institutional)	Hang banners from ceilings; add insulating sheetrock around kitchens, maintenance, and mechanical areas; tighten window weather seals. In dining rooms, seat no more than four persons at a table and add padded room dividers between tables to absorb sound. On special care units, eliminate ringing telephones, televisions, and intercoms; serve meals in small groups; pass medications at times other than meal times.
Background noises (public places)	Go to restaurants at less crowded times; request to sit in areas away from music and kitchen. Seek out theaters and churches that offer listening devices to amplify specific sounds.
Safety (home)	Add flashing lights or lower-pitched rings to smoke detectors, doorbells, and telephones. Add volume controls to telephones. Learn to substitute visual cues for hearing cues to reduce incidence of falls.
Communication (conversation)	Focus on lips, get visual attention before speaking, look directly at person, speak clearly, lower voice tone, reduce glare.
Communication (television, radio, music)	Position to reduce glare, add closed captioning, use assisted listening devices. Use remote controls to select programming, and alternate between music, television, and radio.

PROVIDING ASSISTIVE HEARING DEVICES

One of the most common assistive devices for persons with a hearing impairment is a hearing aid. An **audiologist** assists in determining if a hearing aid would be appropriate. The audiologist also determines whether other factors associated with aging, lifestyle, and personality are compatible with a hearing aid. COTAs may refer elders to a physician or audiologist for assessment and evaluation.

Recent improvements in hearing aid technology have made hearing aids more acceptable. The improved devices are smaller and fit in the ear, and therefore are more cosmetically appealing (Fig. 16-4). In addition, they dampen certain frequencies. Some evidence indicates that younger individuals report more satisfaction than do elders with hearing aids (Kane, Ouslander, & Abrass, 1989; Rieske & Hostege, 1996; Stoneham, 1994). This increased satisfaction may result from several factors. The onset of age-related hearing loss is often gradual, and elders may have accommodated to their hearing loss over an extended period, eventually finding the sudden amplification of all sound to be invasive and disturbing. In addition, the fine finger and hand dexterity required to manipulate volume and frequency controls and change batteries makes the hearing aid difficult to operate. Possible cognitive changes and short-term memory loss may affect the elder's ability to remember to turn the device on and off. The cost of replacement batteries and the elder's acceptance of new technologies are other factors

to consider when determining the appropriateness of a hearing aid (Statch & Stoner, 1991; Stoneham, 1994). Goals for an elder who uses a hearing aid may include identifying alternative ways of operating it, building handles for tools used with the controls, changing or testing batteries with less difficulty, and learning the proper way to insert the device. (See the Appendix for additional information on hearing aids.)

Even with improved technology, hearing aids may not be effective for some individuals. For others, sound distortions may be louder with a hearing aid. When hearing

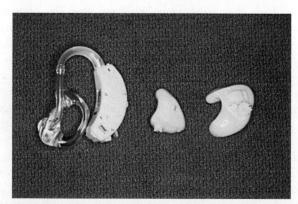

FIGURE 16-4   Hearing aids. (From Bingham, B. J. G., Hawke, M., & Kwok, P. [1991]. *Atlas of clinical otolaryngology*, St. Louis, MO: Mosby.)

aids are not effective, ALDs may be used. ALDs consist of a microphone to capture spoken sounds, an amplifier to increase sound volume, and a headset worn by the hearing-impaired person (Figs. 16-5 and 16-6). Because the amplified sound from an ALD reaches the ear directly, background noises are reduced. ALDs can augment hearing in a noisy clinic or hospital room. When an ALD is plugged into a television, the sound is amplified only for the hearing-impaired person. Use of an ALD also should be considered when visual impairment does not allow the elder to read lips or to supplement hearing loss by responding to other nonverbal cues.

CONCLUSION

As the number of elders with hearing impairments increases, the challenges and opportunities for COTAs continue to grow. The occupational performance and psychosocial and environmental issues that surround a hearing impairment demand that COTAs be informed and able to recommend appropriate interventions. COTAs can assist elders in attaining both performance and quality of life expectations by identifying limitations in hearing, referring elders for additional evaluation and treatment, and providing appropriate interventions.

CASE STUDY

Oscar is an 82-year-old man who has resided at The Garden View Nursing Home for the past 7 years. His diagnoses include dementia, congestive heart failure, and most recently an increase in hearing loss. Until recently, Oscar's social history had been active and included participation in recreational activities and daily socializing with staff and other patients. At a recent care conference the recreation director reported that his participation in activity groups had decreased from nine to four groups a week. The nurse working with Oscar stated that he was less social during meals and had started to sleep in the afternoons. The social worker shared her current assessments of Oscar and stated

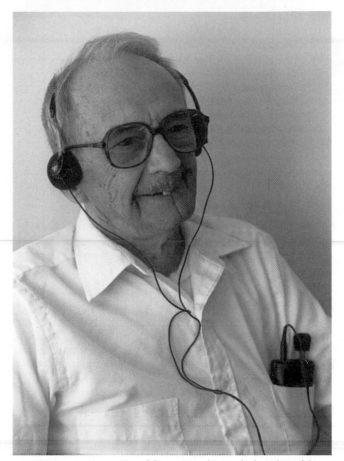

FIGURE **16-6** An assisted listening device helps this elder participate more fully in social interactions.

that he seemed to be isolating himself from others, including his roommate. When the social worker and other staff asked him how he was doing, he seemed to have difficulty understanding the question and changed the subject to talk about the weather. The staff thought his dementia could be contributing to the confusion or perhaps changes in the level of his hearing loss. The team recommended referrals for a professional hearing evaluation and an OT assessment of Oscar. The referral for OT included an evaluation of Oscar's current level of occupational functioning and suggestions for adapting his environment. In addition, staff was seeking suggestions from OT on how staff and others might interact more effectively with Oscar. The OTR is a new graduate and has only been at the Garden View Nursing Home for 2 months. She has asked the COTA who has worked at the nursing home for 5 of the 7 years that Oscar has been a resident at the home to assist her with the assessment.

■ CASE **S**TUDY **Q**UESTIONS

1 Using information from the case study and the chapter identify why staff would think that Oscar's hearing loss might have an effect on his social interaction with others.
2 Describe how Oscar's recent decrease in social interaction may be influencing his mood.

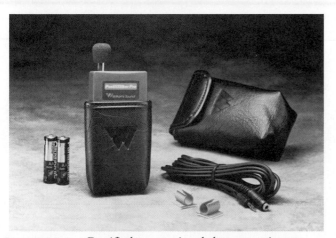

FIGURE **16-5** Certified occupational therapy assistants may need to instruct elders on maintenance of assisted listening devices such as cleaning and battery change.

3 As the long-standing COTA member of the OT department, what assistance can you provide for the OTR? For Oscar?

4 Using information from the chapter identify assessments that may be useful for Oscar.

5 What recommendations would you consider to adapt Oscar's environment to make it more purposeful and accommodating for him?

6 What types of assistive devices would be considered for Oscar?

7 You have been asked to prepare an inservice on hearing impairments and elders and provide recommendations that will assist all staff to be more effective when interacting with those who have a hearing impairment.
- How will you organize this inservice?
- What information do you think would be most helpful for staff?
- How will you engage the staff in the learning process?

CHAPTER REVIEW QUESTIONS

1 Referring to the whole chapter, what are some age-related hearing changes in elders?

2 How do age-related hearing impairments in elders affect their communication and socialization skills, as well as their safety?

3 How can certified occupational therapy assistants (COTAs) contribute to improving communication and socialization skills in hearing-impaired elders?

4 What environmental modifications can COTAs suggest to reduce background noises in an elder's home?

5 What environmental modifications in an institution might be used to reduce confusion caused by hearing impairments?

6 Why might an elder prefer not to use a hearing aid?

7 Explain how a cochlear implant would improve the hearing of some elders?

8 How might a COTA use an assisted listening device to help an elder in a clinic setting?

REFERENCES

Canadian Transportation Agency. (1997). A look at barriers to communication facing persons with disabilities who travel by air [WWW page]. URL http://www.cta-otc.gc.ca/air-aerien/mdex_e.html

Cherney, L. R. (2002). The effects of aging on communication. In C. B. Lewis (Ed.), Aging: The health care challenge, (4th ed.). Philadelphia: FA Davis.

Christenson, M. A., & Taira, E., (1990). Aging in the designed environment. New York: Halworth Press.

Commission on Education of the Deaf. (1989). Toward equity: Education of the deaf. Washington, DC: US Government Printing Office.

Corso, J. F. (1990). Sensory-perceptual processes and aging. In K. W. Schaie, & C. Eisdorfer (Ed.), Annual review of gerontology (2nd ed.). New York: Springer.

Garstecki, D. C., & Erler, S. F. (1998). Hearing and aging. Topics in Geriatric Rehabilitation, 14(2), 1-17.

Hooper, C. R. (2001). Sensory and sensory integrative development. In B. R. Bonder & M. B. Wagner (Eds.), Functional performance in older adults. Philadelphia: FA Davis.

Janken, J. K., & Cullinan, C. L. (1990). Auditory, sensory and perceptual alteration: Suggested revision of defining characteristics. Nursing Diagnosis 1(4), 147.

Kane, R. L., Ouslander, J. G., & Abrass, I. B. (1989). Essentials of clinical geriatrics (4th ed.). New York: McGraw-Hill.

Kinderknecht, C. H., & Garner, J. D. (1993). Living productively with sensory loss. In J. D. Garner, & A. A. Young (Eds.), Women and healthy aging: living productively in spite of it all. New York, NY: Halworth.

Lichtenstein, M. J., Bess, F. H., & Logan, S. A. (1991). Screening the elderly for hearing impairment. In D. Ripich (Ed.), Handbook of geriatric communication disorders. Austin, TX: Pro-Ed.

Mann, W. C. (1994). Environmental problems in homes of elders with disabilities. Occupational Therapy Journal of Research 14(3), 191.

Rieske, R. J., & Hostege, H. (1996). Growing older in America. New York: McGraw-Hill.

Stach, B. A., & Stoner, W. R. (1991). Sensory aids for the hearing impaired elderly. In D. Ripich (Ed.), Handbook of geriatric communication disorders. Austin, TX: Pro-Ed.

Stoneham, M. A. (1994). Technology and disability. Andover Medica, 13(1), 47.

Tobis, J. S., Block, M., Steinhaus-Donham, C., Reinsch, S., Tamaru, K., & Weil, D. (1990). Falling among the sensorially impaired elderly. Archives of Physical Medicine and Rehabilitation, 71(2), 144.

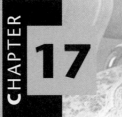

CHAPTER 17

Strategies to Maintain Continence in Elders

KRIS R. BROWN

KEY TERMS

urinary incontinence, fecal incontinence, behavioral techniques, environmental modifications

---

CHAPTER OBJECTIVES

1. Determine the prevalence and cost associated with incontinence.
2. Indicate common causes of incontinence.
3. Review the normal anatomy and physiology of urination and defecation.
4. Identify the different types of urinary and fecal incontinence.
5. Explain the effect of the Omnibus Budget Reconciliation

Act in dealing with the problem of incontinence in nursing homes.
6. Specify the role of each team member, emphasizing the importance of an interdisciplinary approach.
7. Identify the certified occupational therapy assistant's role in the management of incontinence.
8. List suggestions for the management of incontinence.

Incontinence of urine and stool is a common problem many elders face. Incontinence is often considered part of the normal aging process and is therefore accepted but not treated. Society's acceptance of this condition is manifested by the availability of absorbent products and high-fiber foods found in local stores. Some elders afflicted with this problem may feel ashamed and embarrassed, which may lead to psychological conditions such as depression and avoidance of social relations or activities. Other elders may think the problem will correct itself, or they may fear that it will lead to a surgical procedure.

Prolonged hospitalizations are common when incontinence is left untreated. Incontinence may even be a primary reason caregivers decide to place elders in long-term care facilities.

During the normal aging process, bladder capacity and the ability to delay urination and defecation decrease. These changes can increase the risk for incontinence, especially with medical conditions such as pneumonia and chronic heart failure. Often, fecal incontinence results from changes in sphincter musculature and hormonal imbalances.

223

URINARY AND FECAL INCONTINENCE
Prevalence

The prevalence of **urinary incontinence** in the nursing home setting is as high as 55%, as reported in 2001 by Centers for Medicare & Medicaid Services (CMS, 2001). For noninstitutionalized older adults, the range is 15% to 37% (U.S. Department of Health and Human Services [DHHS], 1999). Women are twice as likely as men to experience this problem.

Cost

The estimated total annual cost of health care in nursing homes for elders with urinary incontinence is estimated at 5.2 billion dollars (Agency for Health Care Policy and Research [AHCRP], 1996). This cost can be itemized to include routine care such as labor, supplies, laundry, and diagnostic and medical evaluation; treatment such as surgery and pharmacy and drug costs; incontinent consequences such as skin erosion, urinary tract infection, and falls; and added admissions resulting from incontinence (Hu, 1990). The total cost of managing urinary incontinence for those living in the community is 11.2 billion dollars (AHCRP, 1996).

Private insurance companies and government programs will usually only pay for urodynamic evaluation, surgical procedures, catheterization (Hu, 1990), and sacral nerve stimulation (DHHS, 1999). Consequently, management of incontinence is routine care. Elders and their families may feel financially strained if incontinence is the only reason for institutionalization. Therefore, poor reimbursement encourages management of incontinence rather than determination of the underlying problem and provision of the most effective treatment.

ANATOMY AND PHYSIOLOGY

The anatomic structures of the male lower urinary tract primarily responsible for normal urination include the bladder neck, prostate gland, pelvic floor musculature, and urethra. In women, the structures include the bladder neck, proximal urethra (internal sphincter), and the pelvic floor muscles that provide the strength needed to maintain the pelvic floor tone and urethra resistance.

The bladder fills and empties. The normal bladder capacity averages between 400 and 600 ml. The urinary bladder can normally hold between 250 and 350 ml of urine before the individual feels the urge to void. As the urinary bladder reaches its holding capacity, the bladder becomes strong enough to activate the stretch receptors, which in turn send a message to the nervous system, the pelvic floor and sphincter sense the increased pressure and the individual feels the urge to void (Newman, 2002). The urethra then relaxes, allowing the bladder to empty.

The anatomic structures involved with normal defecation include the pelvic floor muscles, anal sphincter mechanisms (internal and external), colon, rectum, and anal canal.

A stool of an appropriate consistency is delivered to the rectum and anal sphincter through the gastrointestinal (GI) tract and colon. The normal sensory system acknowledges that the rectum is filling and alerts the structures of the type of rectal content (that is, solid, liquid, or gas). Once the stool passes the rectum, the internal sphincter relaxes, allowing the stool to pass.

ETIOLOGY

Causes of urinary and stool incontinence may be pathologic, anatomic, or physiologic. The most common potential causes of urinary incontinence are transient or reversible. These include delirium, infection such as symptomatic urinary tract infection or vaginitis, and psychological factors such as depression. Excessive urine production, hypercalcemia, hyperglycemia, diabetes insipidus, chronic heart failure, lower extremity venous insufficiency, and drug-induced ankle edema are other causes of transient incontinence (DHHS, 1999).

Pharmaceutical causes of transient incontinence are sedative hypnotics (that is, benzodiazepines); diuretics, leading to polyuria; calcium channel blockers; anticholinergic agents (that is, antihistamines, antidepressants, antipsychotics, antiparkinsonian agents, and alpha-adrenergic agents); sympathomimetics; and sympatholytics. Potential causes of **fecal incontinence** include abnormal delivery of feces to the rectum, which may be drug-induced, metabolic, or caused by infection; sphincter dysfunction from trauma, diabetes mellitus, or inflammation; reduced rectal compliance such as rectal ischemia or fecal impaction; and anatomic derangement such as from a tumor or from third-degree hemorrhoids or injury. Other causes of fecal incontinence include muscular and neuromuscular disorders such as congenital or hereditary myopathy, behavioral and developmental dysfunction such as mental retardation or psychiatric disorders, and neurologic impairment such as with the central nervous system, spinal system, or peripheral nervous system (Doughty, 2000).

TYPES OF URINARY INCONTINENCE
Urge Incontinence

Elders commonly have a combination of types of urinary incontinence. Urge incontinence is defined as the inability to hold urine for a time long enough to reach the bathroom (Newman, 2002). Elders may experience a massive and sudden loss of urine without warning and often strain to empty the bladder. This type of urge incontinence is common at night and is referred to as *nocturnal incontinence.* Urge incontinence may also occur when elders hear water trickling or when they drink small amounts of water. Uncontrolled contraction of the detrusor (bladder muscle), a condition that is also referred to as *detrusor hyperreflexia*, may be part of the problem (Newman, 2002).

Stress Incontinence

Stress incontinence is considered more prevalent in women than in men. Elders with stress incontinence experience uncontrolled loss of urine when intraabdominal pressure is placed on the bladder. This type of incontinence can occur while coughing, laughing, sneezing, exercising, bending, lifting a heavy object, or arising from a chair. A child sitting on an elder's lap may place sufficient pressure on the elder's bladder, which can lead to incontinence. Stress incontinence is usually caused by weakened pelvic floor musculature as a result of the childbirth process in women, or a weakened or damaged sphincter mechanism.

Overflow Incontinence

An individual with overflow incontinence experiences frequent or constant dribbling of urine, voiding only small amounts at a time. The bladder is always full, and the elder is never able to completely empty it. The elder cannot sense its fullness. The cause is often an underactive detrusor muscle. In men this type of incontinence is common when there is a blockage in the bladder.

Mixed Incontinence

Mixed incontinence is a combination of urge and stress incontinence. Most cases of urinary incontinence are in this category.

Functional Incontinence and Other Types

Functional incontinence is related to impaired cognitive functioning and mobility. This type of incontinence often warrants occupational therapy (OT) intervention to help with environmental and other adaptations. Other types of incontinence, which are not as common, include reflex incontinence and detrusor instability. Reflex incontinence is a storage and emptying problem resulting from a spinal cord lesion. Detrusor instability is common in individuals diagnosed with dementia. With this type of incontinence, the bladder contracts before it is full.

FECAL INCONTINENCE

Fecal incontinence often is a result of problems with the GI tract and colon. GI problems cause changes in the consistency and volume of stools, leading to problems such as diarrhea and constipation (Doughty, 2000). Diarrhea is defined as "the frequent passage of loose, watery stools" (Keith & Novak, 2001). Associated symptoms are abdominal pain and cramping. Diarrhea can be a symptom of problems such as dietary intolerance, malabsorption syndromes, inflammatory bowel disease, fecal impaction, gastroenteritis, and GI tumors.

An individual with constipation will complain of abdominal pain and fullness in the rectum. Defecation usually occurs infrequently, and consistency of the stool is hard and dry. Constipation can result from intestinal obstruction, diverticulitis, tumors, dehydration, lack of exercise, and poor diet.

OMNIBUS BUDGET RECONCILIATION ACT AND RELATED RESEARCH

The Agency for Healthcare Policy and Research, currently referred to as the Agency for Healthcare Research and Quality (AHCRQ), was created as a result of the Omnibus Budget Reconciliation Act (OBRA) to conduct research on diseases and disorders. The following are the initial guidelines for information on urinary incontinence developed as a result of studies conducted by the AHCRQ panel:

1. Improve education and dissemination of urinary incontinence diagnosis and treatment alternatives to the public and to health care professionals.
2. Educate the consumer to report incontinence problems once they occur.
3. Improve the detection and documentation of urinary incontinence through better history taking and health care record keeping.
4. Establish appropriate basic evaluation and further evaluations.
5. Reduce variance among health care professionals.
6. Encourage further biomedical, clinical, and cost research on prevention, diagnosis, and treatment of urinary incontinence in the adult (Hood, 2002).

This special panel concluded that most elders were improperly diagnosed for urinary incontinence and ineffectively treated. Both urinary and fecal incontinence are areas that surveyors look at closely during their annual inspections because of the secondary complications such as skin erosion and falls associated with these problems (Fig. 17-1). (See Chapter 6 for a review of the Minimum Data Set.) According to OBRA guidelines, the goal with incontinence is to encourage the nursing home staff to use a rehabilitative model (NovaCare, 1993).

INTERDISCIPLINARY TEAM STRATEGIES

Only half of the elders residing in the community actually relate their incontinence problems to their physicians to receive treatment (Doughty, 2000; National Institutes of Health Consensus Development Conference, 2000). When the problem is reported, many health care professionals treat incontinence as a disease rather than determine the underlying cause.

Health care providers involved in the treatment of incontinence in elders include urologists, gynecologists, psychiatrists, nurses, psychologists, social workers, dietitians, pharmacists, and enterostomal therapists

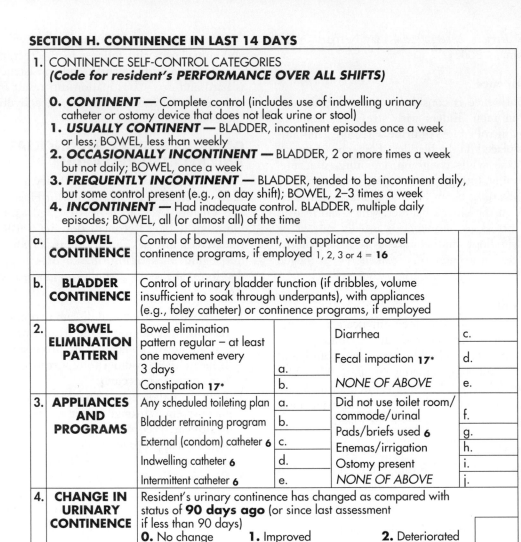

SECTION H. CONTINENCE IN LAST 14 DAYS

1.	CONTINENCE SELF-CONTROL CATEGORIES *(Code for resident's PERFORMANCE OVER ALL SHIFTS)* **0. CONTINENT** — Complete control (includes use of indwelling urinary catheter or ostomy device that does not leak urine or stool) **1. USUALLY CONTINENT** — BLADDER, incontinent episodes once a week or less; BOWEL, less than weekly **2. OCCASIONALLY INCONTINENT** — BLADDER, 2 or more times a week but not daily; BOWEL, once a week **3. FREQUENTLY INCONTINENT** — BLADDER, tended to be incontinent daily, but some control present (e.g., on day shift); BOWEL, 2–3 times a week **4. INCONTINENT** — Had inadequate control. BLADDER, multiple daily episodes; BOWEL, all (or almost all) of the time						

a.	**BOWEL CONTINENCE**	Control of bowel movement, with appliance or bowel continence programs, if employed 1, 2, 3 or 4 = **16**					
b.	**BLADDER CONTINENCE**	Control of urinary bladder function (if dribbles, volume insufficient to soak through underpants), with appliances (e.g., foley catheter) or continence programs, if employed					
2.	**BOWEL ELIMINATION PATTERN**	Bowel elimination pattern regular – at least one movement every 3 days		Diarrhea	c.	
				Fecal impaction **17***	d.	
		Constipation **17***	a. b.	NONE OF ABOVE	e.	
3.	**APPLIANCES AND PROGRAMS**	Any scheduled toileting plan	a.	Did not use toilet room/ commode/urinal	f.	
		Bladder retraining program	b.	Pads/briefs used **6**	g.	
		External (condom) catheter **6**	c.	Enemas/irrigation	h.	
		Indwelling catheter **6**	d.	Ostomy present	i.	
		Intermittent catheter **6**	e.	NONE OF ABOVE	j.	
4.	**CHANGE IN URINARY CONTINENCE**	Resident's urinary continence has changed as compared with status of **90 days ago** (or since last assessment if less than 90 days) **0.** No change **1.** Improved **2.** Deteriorated				

FIGURE **17-1**   Minimum Data Set (MDS; 2.0) form section H. Form is used by nursing staffs to rate incontinence. (From Briggs' Health Care Products, Des Moines, IA, 1995.)

(ET nurses). Other health professionals include OT practitioners and physical and speech therapists. All members of this team work together to determine the most effective plan of care, and each provides a unique role in the interdisciplinary team.

Physicians begin care of elders with incontinence by taking a thorough medical history, performing a physical examination, and scheduling laboratory tests. They may refer the client to a specialist such as a urologist or gynecologist if the problem is recurrent. However, a conservative approach is usually initiated. The primary preference is the use of **behavioral techniques** followed by pharmacologic approaches. Because of potential complications, surgery is considered the last resort. Surgery for stress incontinence in women, which requires repositioning the bladder neck, has a success rate of 78% to 92%. The success rate of surgery in men with overflow incontinence,

which requires removal of the cause of blockage, is similar (DHHS, 1999; CMS 2001). Surgery for fecal incontinence is indicated for traumatic, idiopathic, neurogenic, congenital, and medical problems. Surgery may consist of a bowel resection, sphincter repair, or gracilis muscle transfer (Doughty, 2000).

Medications are often prescribed to improve incontinence by treating infection, replacing hormones (estrogen), decreasing abnormal bladder contractions, and tightening sphincter muscles. This type of treatment is effective primarily with urge incontinence resulting from detrusor hyperactivity. Anticholinergics such as atropine, antispasmodics, tricyclic antidepressants, and calcium channel blockers are the drugs commonly prescribed. Antidiarrheal agents such as loperamide, and fecal softeners and lubricants are common medications used to treat problems with defecation (Doughty, 2000).

The dietitian can determine hydration or nutrition patterns in the elder's diet that may be contributing to both urinary and stool incontinence. Recommendations such as a high-fiber diet and liquid intake of 48 to 64 oz per day help to maintain proper functioning of bowel and bladder (Beers & Berkow, 1997). Caffeine intake should be limited because it acts as a diuretic.

A nurse should complete a bowel and bladder profile indicating the length of time that incontinence has been present and the frequency and timing of episodes (Figs. 17-2 and 17-3). The nurse usually initiates behavioral approaches.

Social service specialists and psychologists are important in determining the family dynamics and support available to elders. They may help to determine the effect that incontinence has on the involvement of elders in social activities and relationships. They may also provide counseling to assist elders in expressing feelings about their incontinence problems.

Speech and language therapists are involved in evaluating elders' abilities to communicate either verbally or nonverbally to make their needs known in a timely and effective manner. These professionals assist elders in compensating for impaired communication by providing instruction in the use of gestures and communication aids. Specific training also is provided to the caregiver to ensure proper carryover.

Physical therapists (RPTs) are involved in completing a comprehensive musculoskeletal and functional mobility assessment to ascertain range of motion, muscle strength, bed mobility, sitting balance, and gait. The treatment provided by RPTs may also include teaching and instruction on the use of an assistive device such as a walker, cane, or brace to improve the elders' abilities to ambulate to the bathroom. Caregiver training by RPTs may include the proper use of a Hoyer lift or sliding board with transfers or encouraging elders to carry over a program involving range of motion and strengthening exercises. Electrical stimulation to strengthen the muscles in stress incontinence, biofeedback, and Kegel exercises may all be part of the physical therapy. These approaches also can be applied by OT with demonstrated competency.

COTAs work closely with the other disciplines to determine the cause of incontinence and to develop an effective treatment plan. The following treatment techniques can be provided by members of the treatment team, including COTAs, to help increase voiding.

Timed Voiding and Habit Training

Timed voiding and habit training consist of establishing a fixed schedule that requires the client to void every 2 hours. Toileting is adjusted according to the client's normal pattern and is determined after approximately 2 weeks of monitoring. Attempts are made to increase the intervals between voiding. This habit training often is used in the nursing home setting and is successful with neurologically impaired residents.

Prompted Voiding

Prompted voiding is commonly used in the nursing facility and is recommended for frail or cognitively impaired individuals. Caregivers are responsible for documenting whether the client is wet or dry on a regular basis, usually every 1 to 2 hours. Caregivers are encouraged to ask whether elders have a need to void.

Name_____ Date_____

Time toilet is offered	Leakage (yes or no)	Was client aware of urge? (yes or no)	Did client void? (yes or no)	Comments
0800				
1000				
1200				
1400				
1600				
1800				
2000				

(2200 and so forth)

FIGURE 17-2   Bladder record. (From Doughty, D.B. [2000]. *Urinary and fecal incontinence nursing management.* St. Louis, MO: Mosby.)

Date and Time	Stimulus to evacuation (digital, suppository, or none)	Response (amount and consistency of stool)	Incontinent episodes (time, amount, and type of leakage)

FIGURE 17-3   Simple diary of bowel function. (From Doughty, D.B. [2000]. *Urinary and fecal incontinence nursing management*. St. Louis, MO: Mosby.)

Bladder Training

Bladder training is recommended with stress and urge incontinence. Studies have shown a 10% to 15% improvement rate in urinary continence using bladder training (CMS, 2001; DHHS, 1999). The goal is to decrease the frequency of voiding and lengthen the intervals between voiding. Caregivers instruct elders to resist the urge to urinate and to follow a planned time schedule rather than responding immediately to the urge.

Biofeedback

Biofeedback offers elders visual and auditory information to teach voluntary control of certain functions. Most elders are taught to relax the detrusor and abdominal muscles while contracting the sphincter muscle. An improvement rate of 20% to 25% in urinary incontinence has been noted for individuals using this technique (DHHS, 1999). A 70% to 90% success rate is reported with fecal incontinence (Blaivas, Romanzi, & Heritz, 1998).

Pelvic Floor Exercise

Pelvic floor exercises are also known as *Kegel*, or *childbirth*, exercises. Kegel exercises are commonly used and have a 30% to 90% success rate in women with stress incontinence (CMS, 2001; DHSS, 1999). Elders are taught to relax the abdominal muscles while contracting the pelvic floor muscles. After assistance is given to identify the correct muscles, elders are told to complete 40 to 80 contractions of the pelvic floor muscles per day (Schmitz, 2001).

This technique is commonly used to improve fecal incontinence and increase muscle tone in the pelvic floor to prevent stool leakage (Schmitz, 2001). Physical and occupational therapists can initiate these exercises.

ENVIRONMENTAL ADAPTATIONS

When considering problems with functional mobility, COTAs are encouraged to look at the elder's environment to determine whether modifications are necessary to facilitate independence and to ensure safety while toileting (Box 17-1). COTAs should make recommendations for improvement where required (Table 17-1). (See Chapter 14 for more information on fall prevention.)

Many **environmental modifications** can be made in the bathroom. For example, grab bars can be mounted either in a 45-degree horizontal fashion to assist in pushing up or in a vertical position to facilitate pulling up. The length of the bars should be between 24 and 36 inches on the back wall and 42 inches on the side wall (Schmitz, 2001).

Physical restraints can be used by caregivers in the nursing facility to prevent an individual from falling out of bed or the wheelchair. COTAs may be involved in assisting with restraint reduction. Because of the OBRA law, the use of restraints is carefully monitored. Restraints are only recommended to encourage more functional

BOX 17-1

Considerations for Environmental Adaptations to Help with Incontinence

1. Does the client need or use side rails to assist with bed mobility?
2. Is the call light easily accessible to the client?
3. Is the height of the bed appropriate for safe transfers?
4. Is the client restrained in bed or in the wheelchair, which would limit mobility to the bathroom?
5. Is there adequate lighting to and from the bathroom (60-year-old elders require three times brighter lighting than a 20-year-old adult)?
6. Are there any obstacles or clutter that would interfere with safe mobility?
7. Is the client able to manage the door leading into the bathroom?
8. Are the floors highly waxed, which could cause a fall?
9. Is the doorway leading into the bathroom wide enough to allow proper clearance for a wheelchair or walker?
10. Is the height of the toilet appropriate?
11. Are there any grab bars or support to assist with a transfer to the toilet?

TABLE 17-1

Environmental Adaptations to Help with Incontinence	
Room	**Adaptations**
Bedroom, nursing home room, or hospital room	Place a commode near the bed.
	Make a urinal or bed pan available.
	Adjust the height of the bed.
	Add side rail to the bed for ease with transfers.
Bathrooms	Add a night light to increase visibility with mobility.
	Add any combination of a toilet safety frame, elevated toilet seat, and grab bars to facilitate independence and ensure safety with transfers and clothing management.
	Eliminate throw rugs or bath mats.
	Add a nonskid material (Dycem) in front of the toilet or commode.

independence, to decrease the risk for a life-threatening medical problem, or to promote a better anatomic seating position that is minimally restrictive (Health Care Financing Administration, 1995). The use of a restraint may cause increased agitation because the elder will be unable to take care of bathroom needs if call lights are not answered in a timely manner to prevent incontinence. OBRA protects the rights of elders to freedom of movement and access to the body. COTAs must work closely with other staff members in deciding on a restraint program that allows the client to remain continent while minimizing the use of restraints (see Chapter 14).

CLOTHING ADAPTATIONS AND MANAGEMENT

Clothing management before and after toileting is a functional independence measure. This measure is often used to evaluate toileting and bowel and bladder management at admission to and on discharge from inpatient facilities (Uniform Data System for Medical Rehabilitation, 2001). COTAs can help elders improve clothing management by providing activities that use fine motor coordination, such as increasing dexterity with manipulation of zippers or buttons. Range of motion and strengthening exercises may facilitate pulling pants over the feet and hips.

ADAPTATIONS FOR CLIENTS WITH FUNCTIONAL INCONTINENCE

An increased incidence of incontinence is often seen in elders with dementia. In addition to an inability to manage their clothing, these elders also have difficulty locating the bathroom and toilet. Some may have problems with their strength, coordination, range of motion, and sense of balance, which affect their abilities to toilet in a timely and safe manner. They may be seen urinating and defecating in inappropriate places. Allen, Earhart, and Blue (1992) describe this level of functioning as the *Allen Cognitive Level 3* (see Chapter 7 for more information on this theory). Elders with dementia might perform part of the toileting task but become confused at some point and require verbal or physical assistance, or both, to continue. COTAs can encourage maximal functioning by determining what tasks the client can do and by training caregivers to assist with only those tasks that become difficult.

Impaired functional mobility of elders can be addressed by COTAs in conjunction with physical therapy. The goal is to improve functional mobility skills and train caregivers to provide the proper physical and verbal cues needed for elders to become successful with safe mobility.

PREVENTION OF SKIN EROSION

One of the secondary effects of incontinence mentioned earlier is skin erosion. Caregivers must be educated on a bowel and bladder program, a repositioning schedule, and proper wound care. Skin integrity may be improved by placing a special mattress on the bed or an incontinence cushion on the sitting surface.

Nutrition is extremely important in wound healing. COTAs must consider elders' abilities to feed themselves. Elders may need to learn how to use adaptive equipment to aid this procedure. Elders must be able to obtain and drink fluids to maintain hydration.

CASE STUDY

Octavio was recently admitted to a skilled nursing facility (SNF) from his home, where his aging partner Paul was attempting to care for him. Octavio's urinary and bowel incontinence was becoming burdensome, and with little support and inconsistent in-home services, the daily routine had become too much for Paul. The situation also was causing a strain on their relationship.

On admission to the SNF, Octavio was diagnosed with early-stage Alzheimer-type dementia, rheumatoid arthritis, and long-term low back pain. In addition, Octavio had the beginning of a pressure sore forming on his coccyx. The nursing home physician reviewed Octavio's medical history and performed a physical examination. He determined that Octavio's incontinence was not caused from medications, but rather was related to the Alzheimer's disease process and pain associated with movement. OT and physical therapy were ordered to evaluate and provide appropriate treatment for Octavio.

The findings from the OT evaluation were as follows:
1. Working memory deficits
2. Limited mobility and ambulation secondary to pain
3. Limited range of motion
4. Weakness in the upper extremities
5. Ability to follow simple 2-step directions

Stacie, the COTA at the SNF, was assigned to provide OT treatment five times a week. She was to assess bed and wheelchair positioning, adaptive equipment needs, fine motor skills, and toileting tasks and transfers. It was determined through the interdisciplinary team process that nursing would assist with pain management, including appropriate medications. Nursing would also implement scheduled toileting and begin treatment to heal the pressure ulcer. The dietitian would provide suggestions for a proper diet, intake, and suggest nutritional supplements to promote healing of the pressure ulcer. Physical therapy would address bed mobility, sitting and standing balance, and safe ambulation.

By the end of the first week of treatment Stacie recommended a higher bed to ease Octavio's transfer process and to decrease the amount of pain associated with transfers. A bedside commode was placed in Octavio's room until his ability to ambulate to the bathroom in his room could be evaluated. Because of his dementia, Octavio was unable to complete pericare; however, with verbal cueing he was able to assist with clothing management before and after toileting. Stacie also recommended a pull-up incontinent undergarment to be used because Octavio was able to assist with clothing management. She also provided positioning equipment for the bed and wheelchair to assist in the healing of and prevention of further pressure ulcers. This included a bed wedge to help Octavio maintain side-lying during scheduled turning when in bed and a gel cushion with a coccyx cut-out for his wheelchair to decrease heat and shear.

Paul began to make regular visits and the social worker helped them to adjust to the changes in their lives.

■ CASE STUDY QUESTIONS

1 Why would a pull-up incontinence product be the most appropriate recommendation for Octavio?
2 What is the advantage of using a gel cushion?
3 List three possible reasons why a pressure ulcer was developing before Octavio's admission to the SNF.
4 Identify two reasons why an elder in Octavio's situation benefits from scheduled turning.
5 Why would Octavio's incontinence cause strain on his relationship with his partner, Paul?
6 Why is timely pain medication helpful?
7 Identify one reason why improved nutrition is important in Octavio's situation.

■ CHAPTER REVIEW QUESTIONS

1 List the members of any incontinence team.
2 Describe how the Omnibus Budget Reconciliation Act has affected the management of incontinence in the nursing facility.
3 Discuss whether urinary and fecal incontinence are part of the normal aging process.
4 What type of incontinence is more prevalent in women?

5 Describe the effect of incontinence on nursing home placement.
6 Which behavioral technique is commonly used for incontinence training with an elder who has dementia?
7 What are some of the secondary complications associated with incontinence?
8 What is the role of the certified occupational therapy assistant in the management of incontinence?
9 What are some environmental modifications that can improve continence?

REFERENCES

Agency for Health Care Policy and Research. (1996). *Urinary incontinence in adults: Acute and chronic management.* Rockville, MD: The Agency.

Allen, C., Earhart, C., & Blue, T. (1992). *Occupational therapy treatment goals for the physically and cognitively disabled.* Rockville, MD: American Occupational Therapy Association.

Beers, M., & Berkow, A. (Eds.). (1997). *The Merck manual of diagnosis and therapy* (17th centennial ed.). Whitehouse Station, NJ: Merck & Co.

Blaivas, J. G., Romanzi, L. J., & Heritz, D. M. (1998). Urinary incontinence: Pathophysiology, evaluation, treatment, overview, and nonsurgical management. In P. C. Walsh, A. B. Retik, E. D. Vaughan, Jr., & A. J. Wein (Eds.), *Campbell's urology* (pp. 1007-1036). Philadelphia: WB Saunders.

Centers for Medicare & Medicaid Services. (2001). *Deficiency decision-making and severity scope determination (draft).* Baltimore, MD: The Centers.

Doughty, D. (2000). *Urinary and fecal incontinence* (2nd ed.). St. Louis, MO: Mosby.

Health Care Financing Administration. (1995). Omnibus Budget Reconciliation Act. Baltimore, MD: The Administration.

Hood, F. J. (2002). Coverage of urinary incontinence. *Southern Medical Journal, 95*(2), 198-201.

Hu, T. W. (1990). Impact of urinary incontinence on health-care costs. *Journal of the American Geriatric Society, 38*(3), 292-295.

Keith, J., & Novak, P. (Eds.). (2001). *Mosby's medical, nursing, and allied health dictionary* (6th ed.). St. Louis, MO: Mosby.

National Cancer Institute. (2003). Surveillance, Epidemiology, and End Results Program (SEER) [WWW page]. URL http://seer.cancer.gov/canques

National Institute on Aging. (2000). Age page, urinary incontinence [WWW page]. URL http://www.aoa.gov/

National Institutes of Health Consensus Development Conference. (2000). *Urinary incontinence in adults.* Bethesda, MD: NIHCDC.

Newman, D. (2002). *Managing and treating urinary incontinence.* Baltimore, MD: Health Profession Press.

NovaCare, Inc. (1993). *OBRA guidelines for occupational therapy and physical therapy clinicians.* (Pamphlet). King of Prussia, PA.

Schmitz, T. (2001). Environmental assessment. In S. B. O'Sullivan, (Ed.), *Physical rehabilitation: Assessment and treatment* (4th ed.). Philadelphia: FA Davis.

Uniform Data System for Medical Rehabilitation. (2001). *Guide for the uniform data set for medical rehabilitation (Adult FIM).* Buffalo, NY: Uniform Data System for Medical Rehabilitation.

U.S. Department of Health and Human Services. (1999). *Urinary incontinence in adults.* Rockville, MD: U.S. Department of Health and Human Services.

CHAPTER 18

Dysphagia and Other Eating and Nutritional Concerns with Elders

DEBORAH MORAWSKI AND TERRYN DAVIS

KEY TERMS

oral intake, undernourishment, malnutrition, dehydration, institutionalized, nutrition, hydration, bolus, velum, compensations, dysphagia, aspiration pneumonia, positioning, alternative means, contraindicated

CHAPTER OBJECTIVES

1. Discuss the increased incidence of swallowing, eating, and nutritional problems occurring with elders.
2. Identify the basic anatomic structures related to swallowing and the swallow sequence.
3. Relate the physiologic changes and the onset of increased age-related medical conditions with the increased incidence of swallowing problems.
4. Identify treatment strategies and precautions for improving oral intake and nutrition.
5. Discuss the roles of the team members and the importance of teamwork in addressing swallowing and nutritional concerns.
6. Relate ideas for managing different types of feeding problems.
7. Discuss the psychological and ethical concerns that are present when swallowing problems develop.

Eating is basic to survival and is an activity of daily living (ADL). As the elder population continues to increase, the incidence of swallowing, eating, and nutritional problems is increasing. Death and illness resulting from impaired **oral intake** is now considered a major health problem of elders (Feinberg, Knebl, Tully, & Segall, 1990).

Most elders have at least one chronic medical condition and many have multiple conditions. These conditions include arthritis, hypertension, heart disease, hearing impairments, orthopedic impairments, sinusitis, diabetes, and vision impairments. These chronic conditions can influence elders' abilities to effectively and independently perform ADL, such as eating, self-care, transfers, going outside, and instrumental ADL, such as meal preparation, shopping, money management, and housework. The need for individuals to receive help increases with age (Association for Retired Persons, 2002). When such help is unavailable, this lack of assistance can lead elders to social isolation and depression, which may lead to decreased oral intake. In addition, many elders often take multiple medications, which may affect oral intake (Rubin, 2002). This decrease in oral intake can result in **undernourishment, malnutrition**, and **dehydration**.

Among **institutionalized** elders, the prevalence of undernourishment and malnutrition may be as high as 85%. This high prevalence may be explained by the increased numbers of elders who need assistance with feeding and the lack of sufficient staff to assist them. In nursing homes, government statistics show that 21% of residents are reported to need total feeding assistance and 47% require some feeding assistance. In these settings, it has been reported that a nursing assistant may feed from 5 to 20 individuals an hour, with research showing that it may take up to 40 minutes for a nursing home resident to complete a meal (Rubin, 2002).

These statistics clearly reflect the growing need for occupational therapy (OT) involvement with elders to help them maintain optimal independence in a home, hospital, or nursing home setting. OT assistance may include training in self-feeding, safe swallowing, positioning, mobility, meal preparation and cleanup, shopping, money management, provision of assistive equipment, and caregiver and nursing instruction. All these activities are essential for elders to adequately maintain **nutrition** and **hydration**.

THE ROLE OF THE CERTIFIED OCCUPATIONAL THERAPY ASSISTANT

The certified occupational therapy assistant (COTA) works in partnership with an OTR to collect data to identify the strengths and weaknesses of elders and establish and implement treatment plans to attain their goals. Ongoing assessment and communication between the COTA and the occupational therapist (OTR) is necessary for program and goal changes. The COTA is involved in individual and group treatment and in staff and caregiver instruction. Providing quality care is the function of the entire health care team. The amount of involvement of the COTA with elders with swallowing problems depends on the COTA's level of experience. An entry-level COTA may work on activities that reinforce good nutrition and hydration such as meal preparation, money management, shopping, oral-facial exercises, instruction in assistive devices, and energy conservation during activities. An experienced COTA, who has demonstrated competence in this area, may participate in videofluoroscopic swallow studies and assist tracheostomized and ventilator-dependent elders with self-feeding and swallowing. It is recommended that the COTA review the article "Specialized Knowledge and Skills for Eating and Feeding in Occupational Therapy Practice," developed by the American Occupational Therapy Association (AOTA, 2000a).

NORMAL SWALLOW

The swallow response requires a rapid interplay between the brain, 6 cranial nerves, 48 pairs of muscles,

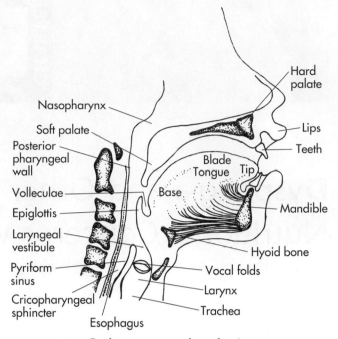

FIGURE **18-1**   Oral structures and mechanisms at rest.

the salivary glands, and cartilaginous structures (Fig. 18-1). The COTA working with elders who have dysphagia must clearly understand the anatomy and physiology of swallowing (Nelson, 1998).

Four phases of swallowing have been defined: oral preparatory, oral, pharyngeal, and esophageal (Logeman, 1998) (Fig. 18-2, *A* to *E*).

1. *Oral preparatory phase:* The oral preparatory phase includes seeing, smelling, reaching for the item, bringing it to the mouth, and putting it in the mouth. Once the item is placed in the mouth, the lips close to maintain a seal, and the tongue and cheek muscles move the **bolus** (that is, the food or liquid) around the mouth in preparation for swallowing. The base of the tongue and the **velum** (soft palate) also make a seal to prevent the bolus from entering the pharynx prematurely. Saliva mixes with the bolus to aid in swallowing. Taste, temperature, and texture receptors of the tongue also play a part in preparing for the action of swallowing.

2. *Oral phase:* The oral phase occurs once the bolus is prepared and formed by the tongue. The bolus is then propelled by the tongue to the back of the mouth and over the base of the tongue.

3. *Pharyngeal phase:* The pharyngeal phase occurs when the bolus passes over the base of the tongue and enters the pharynx. At this time, the soft palate elevates to seal the entrance to the nose, the hyoid bone and larynx elevate upward and anteriorly, the vocal folds close, the epiglottis tilts downward, and the

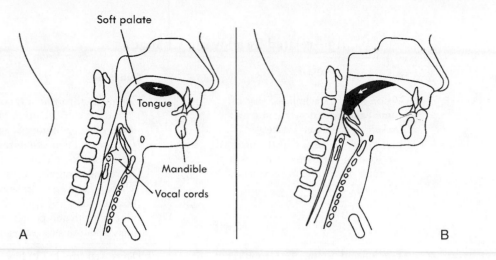

FIGURE 18-2 Lateral view of bolus propulsion during the swallow. **A,** Oral preparation of the bolus and voluntary initiation of the swallow by the oral tongue. **B,** Bolus moves from oral cavity to pharynx, pharyngeal swallow is triggered. **C,** Bolus enters the valleculae and the airway is protected. **D,** The tongue base retracts to the anteriorly moving pharyngeal wall. **E,** Bolus enters the cervical esophagus and cricopharyngeal area. (From Logeman, G. [1998]. *Evaluation and treatment of swallowing disorders* [2nd ed.]. Austin, TX: Pro-Ed, Inc.)

cricopharyngeal sphincter opens to allow the bolus to enter the esophagus.

4. *Esophageal phase:* The esophageal phase occurs when the bolus passes into the esophagus and is propelled to the stomach.

Changes of Swallowing Structures

When individuals eat and swallow, the oral and pharyngeal structures adapt easily to different liquid and food consistencies and to the texture, temperature, and volume of the bolus. These structures also adapt to the different positions that the head and body may assume while swallowing. As individuals age, changes in these swallowing structures occur naturally (Sheth & Diner, 1988). Individuals develop

compensations to these changes spontaneously and often unknowingly. These compensations allow them to eat safely and efficiently, such as with smaller bites, longer chewing time, and softer food (Buccholz, 1985). However, if individuals also develop a medical or neurological disorder, these compensations may no longer be effective and may result in increased swallowing problems (Table 18-1) (Cherney, 1994; Jaradeh, 1994). In addition to understanding the physical changes that occur, COTAs must be aware of the psychological effect of swallowing problems on individuals who can no longer eat as they once did. COTAs should acknowledge elders' and caregivers' feelings about certain types of liquids or favorite foods being eliminated from their daily diet.

TABLE 18-1

Age-related Swallowing Changes		
Swallowing phase	**Healthy elder**	**Frail elder**
Oral preparatory	Vision may be declining. Sense of smell and taste decrease and may result in decreased intake. Elder may be missing teeth and need to wear full or partial dentures and require more time to chew food.	Cognitive impairment (poor memory and decreased attention may exaggerate the influence of normal aging changes). Isolation and depression result in decreased food intake and weight loss. Decreased endurance may interfere with chewing and result in slow eating and low intake. Missing teeth and poor-fitting dentures may result in slow eating and poor intake.
Oral	Tongue and lip muscles atrophy, and elder may take smaller bites and require softer food. Elder may require longer time to form bolus in mouth.	Decreased strength in lips and tongue and jaw muscles may result in drooling, decreased chewing, and problems moving the bolus in the mouth.
Pharyngeal	Phase becomes mildly prolonged. Muscle tone decreases and may delay clearing of food residuals. Bolus moves more slowly through the pharynx. Upward movement of hyoid and larynx becomes delayed. Epiglottis may become smaller and move more slowly. Cricopharyngeal sphincter remains open for shorter time.	Time of passage of bolus increases. Structures move more slowly and may put elder at greater risk for aspiration.
Esophageal	Decreased strength of muscles results in increased time for passage of bolus to stomach.	Increased time needed for bolus to reach stomach. Food contents may reflux from stomach and reenter esophagus and pharynx.

Adapted from Cherney, L. (1994). *Clinical management of dysphagia for adults and children.* Rockville, MD: Aspen.

ETIOLOGY OF DYSPHAGIA

Dysphagia is the inability to swallow. This condition is often seen in elders and may have a variety of causes. These causes may be neurologic (for example, from a cerebrovascular accident, brain tumor, or head injury), neuromuscular (for example, from Parkinson's disease, multiple sclerosis, or amyotrophic lateral sclerosis), dementia (such as with Alzheimer's disease), multiinfarct structural (for example, from cancer), and systemic (for example, from diabetes, rheumatoid arthritis, and scleroderma). Dysphagia may also result from prolonged illnesses or from the side effects of medications. If swallowing problems are not identified, they can result in **aspiration pneumonia**, malnutrition, dehydration, and death (Cherney, 1994; Logeman, 1998; Nelson, 1998).

INTERVENTION STRATEGIES

Elders achieve a sense of empowerment, control, and motivation when they are successful at self-feeding and swallowing. To achieve this success, COTAs should implement individually planned interventions to resolve swallowing problems and promote functional self-feeding. The COTA must first establish a therapeutic relationship with the elder. This will enhance the interventions affecting empowerment and quality of life during mealtime. Treatment of swallowing disorders entails focusing attention on every aspect of the mealtime experience, including preparation, the dining environment, **positioning** of the elder, assistive devices, direct intervention, dietary concerns, precautions, and caregiver training (Box 18-1).

BOX 18-1

Preparation Checklist for Dysphagia and Self-feeding Interventions

1. Collect information
   - Evaluate dysphagia
   - Review medical chart
   - Consult nursing staff
   - Assess changes in medical status
   - Assess changes in diet
2. Inform elder
   - Give evaluation results
   - Recommend treatment
   - Discuss treatment goals with client
   - Provide input
3. Create environment
   - Ensure that environment is positive and appropriate
   - Ensure that environment is conducive to eating
4. Ensure proper fit
   - Eyeglasses
   - Hearing aides
   - Partial and full dentures
5. Assess
   - Arousal and alertness
   - Safety for eating
6. Position safely
   - Trunk
   - Lower extremities
   - Upper extremities
   - Head
   - Height of table surface
7. Complete oral preparation as prescribed by OTR
   - Have client perform oral exercises
   - Have client perform sensory stimulation
   - Have client perform tone facilitation or reduction techniques
8. Check food tray
   - Correct diet consistency
   - Provide needed assistive equipment

Environmental Concerns

In American society, people usually eat 3 meals each day, or about 1092 meals each year, excluding snacks. Eating is a vital part of socialization and greatly adds to the quality of an individual's life. To promote an enjoyable dining experience, pleasant surroundings and personal comfort should be provided to elders during meals. Aesthetics of the dining area should include tablecloths, centerpieces, flowers, and cleanliness. If elders are institutionalized, food items should be taken off serving trays and put directly on the table to help establish a homelike atmosphere. Deficits in visual acuity, light sensitivity, and color perception are common in elders. Poor lighting can

greatly exaggerate these problems; therefore insufficient light and glare should be avoided. Natural light without glare or soft, diffused overhead lighting is best. A quiet, calm environment excludes television, but may allow for age-appropriate dining music. Television may be distracting and detract from social interaction. Compatible table mates in small groups around a table can add to a positive dining experience (Fig. 18-3). COTAs and other service providers should maintain a therapeutic attitude by allowing elders plenty of time to eat a meal. Lengthy waiting periods before being served may decrease the elder's interest in food and may increase fatigue. The table height should be between 28 and 30 inches to accommodate both regular chairs and wheelchairs. The distance between the table surface and an elder's mouth should be between 10 and 15 inches (Hotaling, 1990). Adopting these suggested environmental factors can help to provide a pleasurable experience during mealtime and possibly assist elders to increase their food and fluid intake.

Positioning Techniques

COTAs must have knowledge of proper positioning techniques with elders who have dysphagia. Proper positioning is important for effective and safe swallowing, correcting mechanical problems with swallowing, and increasing dining pleasure. The trachea, or airway, is next to the esophagus, which is the food pipe. Safe positioning can prevent food from entering the trachea, avoiding aspiration. Proper positioning of elders also increases alertness, normalizes muscle tone, provides comfort, and helps with digestion, while allowing dynamic movement for self-feeding.

The preferred seating position for mealtime is sitting in a dining room chair with armrests rather than sitting in a wheelchair. A wheelchair, however, is preferable to a

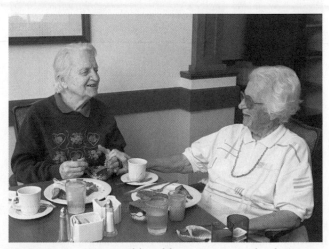

FIGURE 18-3 Compatible table mates can make dining a pleasurable experience.

geriatric chair, which is preferable to sitting up in bed. COTAs should transfer an elder to a regular chair if the elder can possibly sit in one. If optimal posture cannot be obtained in a regular chair, use of a wheelchair may be necessary (Fig. 18-4). The elder's head, neck, trunk, and hips should be aligned. First, the pelvis should be positioned in neutral with a slight anterior tilt. The elder should have an erect posture and sit symmetrically with weight distributed equally on each hip. Second, the elder's head should be positioned in midline with the chin slightly tucked. Both upper extremities should be fully supported on a table or lap tray of appropriate height. Finally, the lower extremities should be in a weight-bearing position. Hips and knees should be flexed 80 to 90 degrees, with ankles in neutral position under the knees and the feet flat on the floor. If the feet do not reach the floor, a stool or wheelchair footrests should be used to provide a secure base of support.

If feeding in bed is essential, elders should be as close to the headboard as possible before the head of the bed is elevated to 45 degrees or more (Fig. 18-5). A pillow may be placed behind the elder's back to increase upright trunk posture and hip flexion. To prevent elders from sliding down in the bed, the knees should be flexed and supported from underneath with pillows if necessary (Hotaling, 1990). As with sitting in a chair, elders should be upright and aligned symmetrically for optimal safety while eating and drinking.

Positioning devices are often required to aid elders in maintaining a straight midline for a dynamic, upright posture. Padded solid back and solid seat inserts provide better postural support that offsets the slinging seats and backs of wheelchairs. Lumbar and thoracic support can facilitate increased scapulohumeral control for self-feeding. Elders with low muscular tone may benefit from high-back wheelchairs. Wedges, lateral and forward trunk supports, head rests, pelvic belts, pillows, and towel rolls often are used to obtain proper positioning. Seating systems must be designed to correct or to accommodate postural problems while preventing skin erosion, maintaining comfort, promoting self-feeding, and providing the right position for safe swallowing.

Many variables affect elders' positioning. If an elder is sitting in a kyphotic posture, the COTA should have the elder lean back slightly so the chin is parallel to the floor. Special considerations also are needed for elders with scoliosis, depending on the curvature of the spine. Elders with a hemiplegic arm should have the arm placed on the table. The arm/hand should be incorporated as a gross stabilizer during meals. Those elders who have recently

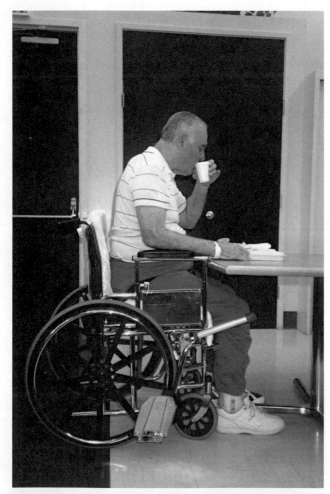

FIGURE 18-4 This gentleman is correctly positioned in his wheelchair for self-feeding. This position promotes dynamic trunk movement. (From Community Hospital of Los Gatos, CA, 1996.)

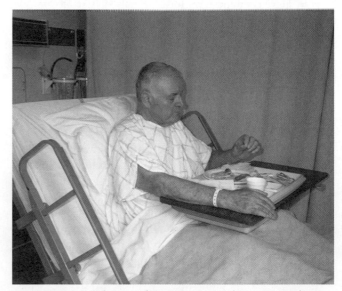

FIGURE 18-5 This gentleman is correctly positioned in bed for self-feeding. (From Community Hospital of Los Gatos, CA, 1996.)

had a lower extremity amputation may also have special positioning needs. COTAs also must consider poor sitting tolerance. Elders with back pain or low endurance need to complete their meal within the time limitations of their upright tolerance. The lower extremities may need to be elevated when sitting up in a chair if edema is present, which often occurs as a result of congestive heart failure. Hearing and visual deficits also should be considered when positioning elders to increase their awareness of their surroundings and to maximize social interaction. The COTA is responsible for following through with the OTR's instructions for positioning while considering the elder's individual needs.

Assistive Devices

An abundance of options for assistive devices is available to assist elders in maintaining independence in self-feeding and safe swallowing. Some devices are prefabricated, whereas others are designed by the creative minds of the COTAs. A hole punched in the plastic lid of a cup can hold a straw and will prevent spilling for elders who have tremors or ataxia. Built-up handles can be used for joint protection or a weak grasp. A universal cuff is available for elders who have no grasp. A swivel spoon or a long-handled spoon is available to assist elders with limited range of motion. Nonslip mats or plates with suction cups can keep items from sliding on the table. Plate guards and plates with lips prevent food from spilling off the plate. Cutout cups and straws can reduce the need for the elder to tilt the head back while drinking, thus protecting against aspiration while swallowing. Straws and cups with spouted lids also can limit the amount of each sip and are helpful for elders with severe dementia who only have a sucking reflex. Small rubber-coated spoons can help control bite size and prevent elders from hurting themselves when biting down on utensils. Rocker knives can be used for one-handed cutting. Mobile arm supports can provide stabilization and assist in hand-to-mouth movement.

Assistive devices should be issued if elders experience a decrease in function. However, elders should be encouraged toward further independence rather than to continue using assistive devices. Before assistive equipment is issued, the COTA should consult with the OTR regarding his or her recommendations.

Direct Intervention

Various feeding strategies may be used to help elders with dysphagia to feed themselves and to swallow safely. To ensure that mealtime is a pleasurable experience, the COTA should avoid making parental comments or giving parental cues (for example, use the word *napkin* rather than *bib*). A method of communication must be established with nonverbal elders so they can indicate when they are ready for another bite or drink. All team members, including family and other caregivers, should use this method consistently. Examples may be nodding of the head or raising a finger. In addition, the COTA should sit next to the elders rather than standing over them during meals.

As noted in the preparation checklist in Box 18-1, oral exercises, sensory stimulation, and tone facilitation or reduction techniques are often needed before eating. Slow, deep pressure on facial and jaw muscles in the opposite direction to the pull of increased muscle tone may help to reduce it. Tongue and facial exercises can increase strength and tone for bolus manipulation. Sensory stimulation may include brushing teeth and icing the cheeks and tongue to increase oral tone and sensation. Brushing teeth also stimulates the salivary glands and helps elders with dry mouths manipulate the bolus easier. After using these necessary strategies, elders are ready to begin eating.

These and many other general strategies help elders with eating and should be enacted before food enters the mouth. Hand-over-hand guiding can provide tactile cueing while bringing food to the mouth and is especially helpful for elders with perceptual difficulties. Proximal upper extremity stabilization techniques can compensate for tremors, ataxia, and weakness. To help with weakness, elders may also use the opposite hand to assist in the movement of the dominant hand when bringing food to the mouth. The "clock method" is helpful for blind elders or those with other visual deficits to orient them to the position of the plate, cup, eating utensils, and food in front of them. Items should be positioned consistently for this method to be most effective. Elders who are impulsive may require cues for both bite size and pacing of bites. Elders can be guided or instructed to put the eating utensil down between bites to pace the amount of food entering the mouth. Presenting elders with one food item at a time may also be helpful. Large food items should be cut into bite-sized portions. Using a spoon for liquids is often helpful. COTAs should coordinate eating with breathing for elders on ventilators or those with other breathing difficulties. Energy conservation may also be indicated, including limiting conversation during mealtime. For elders with low endurance, alternating food textures during the meal, ordering foods that are easy to chew, and/or having six small meals available during the day may be helpful.

Several strategies may be helpful to use with elders who have severe dementia. Frequent small feedings and finger foods are useful for elders with low attention spans or who pace constantly and cannot sit still long enough to complete a meal. Decreasing environmental stimulation, maintaining consistency in feeding helpers, and reducing verbal communication during the meal may help to decrease distractions and permit elders with dementia to focus longer on eating. When such elders refuse a particular food item, a helpful strategy is to place that food item on a plate of a different color, reheat it, and serve it again. With this particular elder population, COTAs should be careful that elders do not eat nonedible items placed on the table such as plants and napkins. Removing the knife from the place setting of such elders may also be necessary for safety (Hall, 1994).

Several interventions may be used during the oral phase. Tongue sweeps prevent oral pocketing of food. Alternating solids and liquids helps to clean the mouth and to remove any food residue in the mouth, but may be **contraindicated** when dysphagia is present. Food should be placed in the center of the tongue. Varying food temperatures with each bite may promote a safer swallow by stimulating the mouth and increasing awareness of the bolus. Occasionally, elders with hypertonicity need food to remain at a consistent temperature to avoid increasing muscle tone. Asking elders to increase the number of times they chew a bite of food helps to break down the bolus and reduce the pace of eating. Elders may need to be cued to close the lips to prevent spillage. The oral cavity should be checked for any residue after each meal. Dentures must fit well and should be thoroughly cleaned after each meal to prevent ulcers from developing in the mouth, to prevent chipping of the dentures from hardened food, and prevent risk for aspiration from food residue under the dentures (Good Samaritan Medical Center, 1995).

Problems during the pharyngeal phase of swallowing may require many treatment strategies. Elders should be given sufficient time to swallow between bites. COTAs should learn to observe and palpate swallowing and be able to recognize delays in the swallow response. These skills help in the ongoing assessment of elders. Individuals with hemiplegia may benefit from turning the head toward the hemiplegic side or tilting the head toward the nonhemiplegic side to protect the airway while swallowing (O'Sullivan, 1990). Elders should be checked for voice clarity after a swallow to make sure that there is no food or liquid residual on the vocal folds. Coughing or clearing the throat followed by a dry swallow may help to eliminate a wet-sounding voice after a swallow. Multiple swallows after each bite may also be encouraged. The COTA should work closely with the OTR when feeding elders with tracheostomies. If approved by the physician, the tracheostomy may or may not be plugged and the cuff can be deflated during feeding to increase air pressure for a stronger swallow.

Several advanced techniques, including the supraglottic swallow, Valsalva maneuver, and Mendelsohn maneuver, may be required, for which close instruction and supervision from the OTR is essential (Logeman, 1998). Advanced training is necessary for the implementation of these strategies and the COTA should demonstrate competency in their application because they are not entry-level skills. Because of the wide range of individual dysphagia problems, the strategies presented

here can be modified as necessary. When interventions are planned and carried out with the elder's quality of life in mind, as well as his or her safety while swallowing, the elder's motivation for food intake and sense of empowerment will prevail.

Dietary Concerns

Research into the nutritional needs of elders has increased as the elderly population grows. COTAs should understand elders' nutritional requirements. Elders often prefer to eat softer, sweeter, and easy-to-prepare foods, and also often drink less fluids. These habits may result in the elder becoming undernourished or malnourished. If elders become ill and are institutionalized, undernourishment or malnutrition can lead to other health problems and delay recovery. It may be important for the elder to be referred to a dietitian to obtain information about optimal nutrition and hydration that does not interfere with medications.

Diet modifications are frequently needed for elders with dysphagia. These modifications may include different consistencies of liquids (for example, thin like water, semithick like nectar, and thick like honey) and different methods of preparing solid foods (for example, pureed, minced, chopped, and soft). If oral intake is limited or impossible, elders with dysphagia may receive nutrition and hydration through **alternative means** (such as a nasogastric tube, a gastrostomy, a jejunostomy, or parenteral nutrition). The entire treatment team is responsible for monitoring intake and ensuring that elders consume the appropriate amounts of protein, fiber, vitamins, minerals, and fluids (Axen & Schou, 1995; Kerstetter, Holthausen, & Fitz, 1993; Howarth, 1991). Misinterpretations regarding intake may occur when intake is being monitored if food sources are not also recorded together with calories consumed.

Food preferences, food allergies, and any diet restrictions resulting from medical conditions such as diabetes and congestive heart failure should be considered when food and liquid selections are being made with elders and their families. Cultural issues regarding food also must be considered when planning for an elder's care. Increased discussion has occurred regarding the ethical and legal issues associated with permitting elders to consume unsafe liquid or solid food consistencies or imposing alternative means for feeding. Ultimately, the physician is responsible for finalizing a decision regarding this issue with elders and their families. This issue, however, requires much input from the team regarding the benefits, risks, alternatives, and prognoses. If the decision is made to allow elders to consume unsafe food items, discontinuation of OT intervention is recommended (Groher, 1990).

Precautions

When working with elders with feeding and swallowing problems, COTAs should consider many factors concerning the safety of oral intake. Some of these factors include level of alertness, orientation and cognitive status, positioning, general endurance, and the ability to self-feed. The presence of a delayed swallow, food pocketing, effortful chewing, coughing, choking, a runny nose, and a wet-sounding voice all indicate swallowing difficulties with the food or liquid being consumed. The COTA should either discontinue the troublesome food or liquid or modify it to a safer consistency. The OTR should be informed of this as soon as possible so that the elder can be further evaluated.

Other indicators of swallowing and nutritional problems may include an increased temperature, lung congestion, and poor intake. Increased temperature and lung congestion may be a sign that the elder has aspirated food or liquid and that pneumonia is developing. Poor intake may indicate an inability to swallow rather than a poor appetite. All personnel working with elders with possible swallowing problems must be aware of these indications and be trained in how to assist someone who is choking and in cardiopulmonary resuscitation in the event that an elder chokes.

Many elders receive medications for various conditions. Medications must be taken with the correct liquid or semisolid consistency. More than 1 oz (30 ml) liquid should be taken after each pill to ensure adequate transport to the stomach. Elders should be sitting up and should be prevented from reclining for 20 minutes after a meal or after taking medication to ensure the safe passage of the food or pill to the stomach. Pills should be taken as specified by the physician. COTAs should consult with the physician or pharmacist to check if the pills can be halved or crushed, because some pills work through time release and crushing them may result in too much medication being absorbed at once. Nursing staff should be present while the medications are taken to ensure swallowing has actually occurred.

Many elders are at greater risk for aspiration when using straws and taking serial swallows with liquids. The OTR should alert the COTA if an elder is safe to drink fluids in these ways. Many elders who are impulsive require close supervision to prevent overfilling the mouth or eating too fast, activities that may result in choking. The COTA should gain extensive knowledge and experience with the swallowing process before attempting to work with elders who have tracheostomies or are on ventilators. Again, service competency in this are should be established with the OTR before the COTA implements any treatment.

Nursing/Caregiver Instruction

COTAs have a vital role in training caregivers to assist elders with self-feeding and dysphagia management. Caregivers may include spouses, partners, family members, friends, hired attendants, and other health care workers such as nurses and nurse's aides. COTAs must consider the caregiver's culture and lifestyle when making decisions about the most beneficial type of teaching technique to use. Some individuals learn best through observing the COTA. Others may learn best by doing it themselves under the direction of the COTA, and others may perform best with verbal instruction. Written information and instructions should be provided to elders and caregivers whenever possible. In general, all these techniques should be used with each caregiver to assure the best follow-through. COTAs must be aware of their verbal tone when teaching the caregiver, taking care not to sound condescending.

The education of caregivers must include training in many aspects of self-feeding and swallowing. First, caregivers should understand the feeding strengths and weaknesses of elders. The need for quality time during the meal and for presentation of a positive attitude to promote elder motivation and independence should be stressed. Thorough instruction should be given on proper body mechanics required by caregivers when assisting elders with feeding. Additional instruction should be provided regarding safe positioning, environmental concerns, use and care of assistive equipment, specific intervention techniques, appropriate verbal and nonverbal cueing, dietary modifications, and signs of possible food or liquid aspiration. Caregivers may take some time to develop good observation and problem-solving skills. Caregivers must understand the importance of communicating any problems or changes in an elder's status to the appropriate team member. Caregivers also should be familiar with choking prevention maneuvers and emergency suctioning procedures. Problem solving together with caregivers is useful when dealing with elders who have difficult feeding behaviors. COTAs may share with caregivers their anecdotal successful experiences in cueing and obtaining desirable behaviors and eliminating undesirable ones with a particular elder.

An integral part of caregiver training is monitoring the food and fluid intake of elders, together with considering nutritional value and maintaining a modified diet. Family and friends may occasionally present a problem by not complying with the dietary restrictions of their loved one. The possible negative consequences of not following through with the prescribed feeding program should be stressed. COTAs should work with dietitians and caregivers in helping families plan meals. COTAs may also ask the caregivers of institutionalized elders to bring a meal from home and modify it with the assistance of a COTA.

Instructing caregivers on the swallowing and self-feeding protocols set up for elders helps COTAs to promote continuity and quality of care. Caregivers should be integrated as soon as possible in the treatment and care of elders. Training several family members and nursing staff helps spread the responsibility of assisting elders during the meal. As with any intervention given to elders, all training of caregivers should be thoroughly documented. By fulfilling these principles, the COTA abides by the Code of Ethics developed by the AOTA (2000b).

Ideas for Managing a Feeding Program

Residents of skilled nursing facilities who are fed in their rooms are frequently positioned poorly, spend most of their day in bed, are often rushed, and often cannot finish their meals. Consequently, their intake, nutrition, and body weight decrease (Axen & Schou, 1995). A well organized facility-wide feeding program helps get elders out of bed, changes their environment, provides social stimulation, ensures good nutrition and hydration, and increases safety. This type of program also helps to maximize their functional abilities and enhances the quality of the mealtime for institutionalized elders. Although many feeding program formats designed for a variety of settings are available, the following is a generic program that requires adjustments to fit the needs of particular elders and particular facilities.

An interdisciplinary approach is the most beneficial in a feeding program. Usually the elder, the OTR, COTA, speech and language pathologist, dietitian, kitchen staff, physician, nursing staff, and family are involved. The physical therapist may also be included to assist with positioning, and the respiratory therapist may be included to assist with issues of pulmonary hygiene or coordination of tracheostomy or ventilator equipment. Elders with self-feeding and dysphagia difficulties are evaluated and referred to a dining group by the OTR or the speech and language pathologist, or both. These elders then are placed in one of several groups organized by the amount of assistance they require. The ratio of elders to COTAs varies depending on the needs of the group. COTAs should always have a group size that can be safely managed. A written protocol should exist that includes information on the purpose of the program and the format, staffing, size, and site of the group. There also should be criteria for referral to, continuation in, and discharge from the program. Timelines, goals, and responsibilities of the COTA or other leader should be made explicit, and documentation and equipment protocols should be explained. There should also be an established system to maintain communication with the entire team to ensure a successful program.

The feeding program should address all meals. In some settings, COTAs are unable to be present at each meal. In other settings, a COTA may not be needed to assist higher-level groups that require minimal assistance or supervision. In these situations, nursing aides, restorative aides, family members, and volunteers may be best used. However, before volunteers are used in this capacity, the guidelines from regulatory agencies should be consulted. For all individuals to perform effectively and safely, they must receive formal training on leading groups, on therapeutic interventions, and on safety.

CASE STUDY

Eric is a 68-year-old, right-hand dominant man who experienced a left cerebrovascular accident and now has right hemiplegia. He has impaired movement and sensation on the right side. In addition, he has apraxia, aphasia, right hemianopsia, and right neglect. One week after his stroke Eric was transferred to a skilled nursing facility's rehabilitation unit.

A dysphagia evaluation and videofluoroscopy were done and the following observations were noted: decreased muscle tone with impaired movement and sensation of the face, tongue, and soft palate on the right side, resulting in facial droop, poor lip seal, minimal drooling and food spillage, slurred speech, and a nasal quality to his speech. The videofluoroscopy revealed impaired oral control of the bolus and spillage of food and liquid into the pharynx before the swallow was initiated. Initiation of the swallow was delayed up to 5 seconds. Residual pooling was observed in the valleculae and pyriform sinuses after the swallow. Spontaneous clearing of the throat with additional swallows was impaired. Eric required verbal cueing to initiate clearing swallows. Aspiration into the trachea was observed while Eric swallowed thin and semi-thick liquids by spoon and thick liquids by cup and a mixed consistency bolus (liquid and solid combination, such as soup). Eric did cough spontaneously when aspiration occurred. He had difficulty chewing dry, hard solids and did better with moist, soft solids and semisolids, although oral pocketing and spillage from the mouth was observed with these consistencies. When Eric used the compensation method of turning his head to the right, decreased pooling in the right valleculae and pyriform sinus resulted.

Therapeutic recommendations included one-on-one assistance at meals for self-feeding and a modified diet of thick liquids by spoon. Semisolids and minced, soft solids with no mixed consistencies also were recommended. Further suggestions were to provide verbal and tactile cues for Eric to turn his head to the right side during the initial swallow and to follow up the initial swallow with two dry swallows. In addition, Eric's caloric and fluid intake were to be closely monitored.

Before the meal, the COTA reviewed the chart for any recent orders and nursing and therapy progress notes to understand how the elder's day had gone thus far. The COTA arranged to meet Eric's family in the dining room for them to observe this meal. When Eric arrived in the dining room, the COTA observed that he was not sitting erect in his wheelchair and that he needed to be repositioned. When Eric was sitting erect, the COTA brought him to the table, locked the wheelchair, positioned Eric's feet on the floor, and placed his hemiplegic arm forward on the table.

Before the meal the COTA directed Eric through several oral-facial exercises. Icing also was used to increase tone and sensation in his right cheek and throat. The COTA iced the outside of Eric's mouth with ice wrapped in a washcloth and then iced the inside of his cheeks and tongue with a cold metal spoon that was dipped in a cup of ice. Icing also would be done on the cheek, the anterior part of the neck, and inside his mouth on the right side during the meal.

When the tray with Eric's meal arrived, the COTA checked to ensure that the consistencies of both solids and liquids were correct. The liquid on the tray was semi-thick, therefore the COTA thickened it with a thickening agent. No other modifications were needed. A plate guard was put on the plate to prevent food from spilling.

Because Eric requires assistance with tray setup and self-feeding, the COTA guided Eric's left hand (nonhemiplegic) using the hand-over-hand method to remove the container lids, butter the bread, cut the food with the rocker knife, and bring the food to his mouth. When Eric was able to integrate the movement and its rhythm and was able to feed himself independently, the COTA stopped providing hand-over-hand guiding. However, when Eric moved too quickly and took too large a bite, the COTA resumed the guiding. When Eric drooled, the COTA guided him to wipe his face with a napkin. With each bite the COTA directed Eric to double swallow and felt Eric's throat for the swallow. The COTA asked Eric to speak occasionally to check his vocal quality, and when it was wet-sounding, the COTA asked Eric to clear his throat. Whenever Eric was unable to clear his throat, the COTA asked him to dry swallow. Finally, the COTA periodically checked Eric's mouth for food pocketing and directed him to clear residuals in his right cheek by using his tongue or left index finger.

After the meal, the COTA guided Eric to use a toothette to clean his oral cavity of the food residue. The COTA instructed Eric to remain upright for at least 20 more minutes. A nurse then arrived with medications, which were crushed and mixed with the thick liquid and given to Eric with a spoon. After he swallowed the medication, Eric was given additional thick liquid by spoon to ensure that the medication passed to the stomach.

The COTA then asked the family if they had any questions and provided them with additional instructions. Finally, the COTA documented what and how much Eric ate; the level of assistance that was required; how long it took to complete the meal; the presence of any coughing, wet-sounding voice, or choking; and the food consistency given him when these events occurred. In addition, the COTA documented all instructions given to the family.

As Eric progressed during meals, he needed less and less hand-over-hand guiding and verbal instruction from the COTA. The COTA began supervising family members as they assisted Eric with meals. Eric progressed to a group dining situation, and when Eric seemed to have a little problem with a wet-sounding voice, food pocketing, follow-through with compensatory techniques, duration of the meal, caloric intake, and spiking temperatures, the COTA requested that the OTR reevaluate him. A follow-up videofluoroscopy was done to rule out aspiration of thin liquids and mixed consistencies, and it showed that Eric had improved but still had impaired oral control of the bolus and pooling in the pharynx. However, Eric now clears this pooling spontaneously, no aspiration is noted, and these items were added to his diet.

Because Eric can now set up his tray with minimal assistance, cut the food with a rocker knife, bring the food to his mouth, eat slowly, and check for pocketing independently, he no longer requires OT supervision at meals.

▮ CHAPTER REVIEW QUESTIONS

1 What is the definition of *dysphagia?*
2 What are the four phases of swallowing?
3 What are the three liquid consistencies?
4 Name four signs that may indicate the presence of swallowing problems.

5 Name three common changes that occur during the phases of swallowing as an individual ages.
6 Identify at least two psychological issues that may have an effect on oral intake.
7 Explain why the certified occupational therapy assistant (COTA) should be concerned about nutritional balance and amount of oral intake.
8 Why is the dining environment important for nutritional intake?
9 What should the COTA do if an elder coughs continuously during a meal?
10 Describe how an individual's body should ideally be positioned during a meal.

REFERENCES

Administration on Aging. (2002). *A profile of older Americans: 2002.* Washington, DC: U.S. Department of Health and Human Services.

American Occupational Therapy Association. (2000a). Specialized knowledge and skills for eating and feeding in occupational therapy practice. *American Journal of Occupational Therapy, 54*(6), 641-648.

American Occupational Therapy Association. (2000b). Occupational Therapy Code of Ethics (2000). *American Journal of Occupational Therapy, 54*(6), 614-616.

Axen, K., & Schou, R. (1995). Nutritional issues in the frail older person. *Topics in Geriatric Rehabilitation, 11*(2), 1.

Buccholz, D. (1985). Adaptation, compensation and decompensation of the pharyngeal swallow. *Gastroenterology Radiation, 10,* 235-239.

Cherney, L. (1994). *Clinical management of dysphagia for adults and children.* Rockville, MD: Aspen.

Feinberg, M. J., Knebl, J., Tully, J., & Segall, L. (1990). Aspiration and the elderly. *Dysphagia, 5,* 61-71.

Good Samaritan Medical Center. (1995). About dysphagia. In S. Di Lima & S. Weavers (Eds.), *The stroke and rehabilitation manual.* Gaithersburg, MD: Aspen.

Groher, M. E. (1990). Ethical dilemmas in providing nutrition. *Dysphagia, 5,* 102-109.

Hall, G. (1994). Chronic dementia challenges in feeding a patient. *Journal of Gerontological Nursing, 20*(4), 21.

Hotaling, D. (1990). Adapting the mealtime environment: Setting the stage for eating. *Dysphagia, 5,* 77.

Howarth, C. (1991). Nutritional goals for older adults: A review. *Gerontologist, 31,* 811.

Jaradeh, S. (1994). Neurophysiology of swallowing in the aged. *Dysphagia, 9,* 218.

Kerstetter, J., Holthausen, B., & Fitz, J. (1993). Nutrition and nutritional requirements for the older adult. *Dysphagia, 8,* 51.

Logeman, G. (1998). *Evaluation and treatment of swallowing disorders* (2nd ed.). Austin, TX: Pro-Ed, Inc.

Nelson, K. (1998). Treatment of dysphagia. In L. Early (Ed.), *Physical dysfunction practice skills for the occupational therapy assistant.* St. Louis, MO: Mosby.

O'Sullivan, N. (1990). *Dysphagia care—team approach with acute and long term patients.* Los Angeles, CA: Cottage Square.

Rubin, H. (2002). Undernourishment in the elderly: Part I, rehabilitation strategies unlimited [WWW page]. URL www.therubins.com

Sheth, N., & Diner, W. (1988). Swallowing problems in the elderly. *Dysphagia, 2,* 209.

CHAPTER 19

Working with Elders Who Have Had Cerebrovascular Accidents

DEBORAH L. MORAWSKI AND RENÉ PADILLA

KEY TERMS

cerebrovascular accident, aphasia, midline alignment, muscle tone, hypotonicity, hypertonicity, subluxation, shoulder-hand syndrome, hemiplegia, transfers, edema, weight bearing, functional activities

CHAPTER OBJECTIVES

1. Discuss cerebrovascular accidents by describing the major features of strokes affecting the main arteries of the brain.
2. Discuss at least three considerations in the occupational therapy evaluation of elders who have had a stroke.
3. Describe the sequence of facilitating midline alignment while elders are supine, sitting, and standing, and explain the steps to follow when transferring elders from a supine position to the edge of the bed or from a sitting to a standing position.
4. Explain precautions for handling an elder's hemiplegic upper extremity.

Virtually every human endeavor is the result of the brain's unceasing activity. The brain is the organ of behavior, cognition, language, learning, and movement. The sophistication of the brain's circuitry is remarkable, if not baffling. Billions of neurons interact with each other to do the brain's work. To appreciate the aging process, certified occupational therapy assistant (COTAs) must have an understanding of the way the brain works (DeArmond, Fusco, & Dewey, 1989; Pansky, Allen, & Budd, 1988; Umphred, 1995). Implications of neuropathologic disorders for occupational therapy (OT) intervention with elders are described in this chapter.

The many biologic and behavioral changes that accompany normal aging are explained in other chapter in this book.

Effects of normal age-related changes in the nervous system vary greatly among individuals and are not generally associated with specific diseases. These changes clearly have little detrimental effect on many elders. Senility is not an inevitable aspect of aging. However, a number of conditions can be devastating to elders because they present serious obstacles to the process of normal, healthy aging. Some of these conditions are related to **cerebrovascular accidents** (CVAs). (Chapter 20 presents the issues related to Alzheimer's disease, which is another disorder affecting the brain.)

CEREBROVASCULAR ACCIDENTS

CVAs, or strokes, are lesions in the brain that result from a thrombus, embolus, or hemorrhage that compromises the blood supply to the brain. This inadequate supply results in brain swelling and ultimately in the death of neurons in the stroke area.

Strokes are the third leading cause of death in the United States and the leading cause of disability among adults. Approximately 700,000 individuals experience strokes each year, and nearly 167,000 die as a result, whereas 4 million individuals live with varying degrees of neurologic impairment after strokes (Centers for Disease Control & Prevention, 2002; National Institute of Neurological Disorders and Stroke [NINDS], 1999). The incidence of strokes increases with age, with the rate doubling every decade of life after 55 years of age, and two thirds of all strokes occur after the age of 65 years. Recurrent strokes account for 25% of yearly reported strokes and usually occur within 5 years. Black individuals have a greater risk for disability and death from stroke than other racial and ethnic groups (NINDS, 1999). Men experience strokes more frequently than women until age 55 years, when the risk for women equals that for men; however, more women die of strokes at all ages (American Stroke Association, 2002).

Ischemic strokes, caused by both thrombus and embolus, account for about 80% of strokes. Intracerebral and subarachnoid hemorrhagic strokes account for about 20% of strokes (National Institute of Neurological Disorders and Stroke [NINDS], 1999). Mortality rates associated with stroke have been declining steadily since the 1950s and are reported to be between 17% and 34% during the first 30 days after a stroke, 25% and 40% within the first year, and 32% and 60% during the first 3 years. Consequently, about half the patients with first strokes live for 3 or more years, and more than one third of individuals live for 10 years (U.S. Department of Health and Human Services [DHHS], 1995).

Risk factors for stroke can be separated into modifiable and unmodifiable. Modifiable factors are those that can be altered by changes in lifestyle or medications, or both. These factors include hypertension, carotid artery stenosis, coronary artery disease, atrial fibrillation, congestive heart failure, cigarette smoking, alcohol and other drug consumption, obesity, diabetes mellitus, and high serum cholesterol, among others. The most preventable of these risk factors is hypertension. Unmodifiable, or fixed, risk factors include prior stroke, age, race, sex, and family history of stroke. Among these unmodifiable factors, increasing age is by far the most significant, because **two thirds** of strokes occur in people age 65 years and older (National Institute of Neurological Disorders and Stroke [NINDS], 1999).

In elders, stroke can result in various neurologic deficits (Table 19-1). Neurologic and functional recovery occurs most rapidly in the first 3 months after a stroke; most elders continue to progress after that time but at a slower rate (Bear, Connors, & Paradiso, 1996). For this reason, predicting functional recovery after stroke and which elders will benefit from rehabilitation is difficult. The World Health Organization (1989) proposes that prognosis for recovery and successful rehabilitation should be indicated in the following order: (1) clients who spontaneously make good recovery without rehabilitation; (2) clients who can make satisfactory recovery only through intensive rehabilitation; and (3) clients with poor recovery of function regardless of the type of rehabilitation. Other factors that complicate prediction of recovery include comorbidity and depression.

The outcome of a stroke depends greatly on which artery supplying the brain is involved (Table 19-2). Medical treatment of a stroke depends on the type, location, and severity of the vascular lesion. In the acute stages, medical intervention is focused on maintaining an airway, rehydration, and management of hypertension. Measures are often taken to prevent the development of deep venous thrombosis (DVT)—that is, blood clots that form in the veins of the lower extremities after prolonged periods of bedrest or immobility. If such clots are released, they can become lodged in the lungs and *can* cause death. The COTA must be alert to any sign of DVT and should request and carefully follow mobilization and activity guidelines set by the physician. Localized signs in the lower extremity that suggest the presence of DVT include abnormal temperature, change in color and circumference, and tenderness. In addition to the use of medications, elders can

TABLE 19-1

Incidence of Neurologic Deficits After Stroke	
Neurologic impairment	**Incidence (%)**
Sensory deficits	53
Dysarthria	48
Right hemiparesis	44
Left hemiparesis	37
Cognitive deficits	36
Visual-perceptual deficits	32
Aphasia	30
Bladder control	29
Hemianopsia	26
Ataxia	20
Dysphagia	12

Adapted from U.S. Department of Health and Human Services. (1995). *Post stroke rehabilitation: Practice guideline no. 16.* Rockville, MD: The Department.

TABLE 19-2

Impairments Resulting from Cerebrovascular Accidents of Specific Arteries

Artery	Impairment
Middle cerebral artery	Contralateral hemiplegia ■ Contralateral sensory deficits ■ Contralateral hemianopsia ■ Aphasia ■ Deviation of head and neck toward side of lesion (if lesion is located in dominant hemisphere) ■ Perceptual deficits including anosognosia unilateral neglect, visual spatial deficits, and perseveration (if lesion is located in nondominant hemisphere)
Internal carotid artery	Contralateral hemiplegia ■ Contralateral hemianesthesia ■ Homonomous hemianopsia ■ Aphasia, agraphia, acalculia, right/left confusion, and finger agnosia (if lesion is located in dominant hemisphere) ■ Visual perceptual dysfunction, unilateral neglect, constructional dressing apraxia, attention deficits, topographic disorientation, and anosognosia (if lesion is located in nondominant hemisphere)
Anterior cerebral artery	Contralateral hemiplegia ■ Apraxia ■ Bowel and bladder incontinence ■ Cortical sensory loss of the lower extremity ■ Contralateral weakness of face and tongue ■ Perseveration and amnesia ■ Sucking reflex
Posterior cerebral artery	Homonomous hemianopsia ■ Paresis of eye musculature ■ Contralateral hemiplegia ■ Topographic disorientation ■ Involuntary movement disorders ■ Sensory deficits
Cerebellar artery	Ipsilateral ataxia ■ Nystagmus, nausea, and vomiting ■ Decreased touch, vibration, and position sense ■ Decreased contralateral pain and thermal sensation ■ Ipsilateral facial paralysis
Vertebral artery	Decreased contralateral pain, temperature, touch, and proprioceptive sense ■ Hemiparesis ■ Facial weakness and numbness ■ Ataxia ■ Paralysis of tongue and weakness of vocal folds

prevent DVTs by wearing elastic stockings and intermittent compression garments, and through early mobilization. Because of DVT and other potential complications of stroke, the COTA should check the elder's medical record and communicate with other team members before initiating each treatment session. By doing this, all team members are fully informed and can modify the interventions with the elder to best serve the elder's needs.

Bowel and bladder dysfunction is common during the initial phases of recovery from a stroke. Usually, a specific bowel and bladder program that includes fluid intake, stool softeners, and other remedies is ordered by the physician. The COTA may be involved in structuring a scheduled toileting program for the elders, which is essential for success. (Chapter 17 presents a more detailed discussion about bowel and bladder training programs.) Other complications during the early phases of recovery from a stroke may include respiratory difficulties and pneumonia caused by the decreased efficiency of the muscles involved in respiration and swallowing. Good pulmonary hygiene, use of antibiotics, and early mobilization are effective prevention measures. Dysphagia, or problems with swallowing, also must be addressed to prevent aspiration pneumonia (see Chapter 18).

OCCUPATIONAL THERAPY EVALUATION

Research evidence and expert opinion suggest that stroke rehabilitation should begin in the acute stage and continue long-term extending several years after onset (DHHS, 1995; Pitkanen, 2000). OT is an essential component in this rehabilitation process. The COTA is an active participant in the evaluation process under the supervision of the occupational therapist (OTR) (Moyers, 1999). As with any client, OT evaluation is an ongoing process that occurs during each treatment session. This is particularly true for elders who have had a stroke, because they may experience many changes during the first few months of recovery. These changes may be noted especially during treatment. Although motor, visual, perceptual, sensory, and cognitive deficits may all contribute to functional impairments, the psychosocial skills and performance of elders and the environment in which they live and perform are critical components of any OT assessment. In addition, assessment should always consider elders' abilities, not just their deficits.

Assessment of motor, sensory, visual, perceptual, and cognitive functions is done simultaneously during performance of an activity. Although the evaluation of each discrete area may be conducted separately, the interaction of these functions and their effects on meaningful activity are of primary importance to OT. Typical impairments are discussed in the section on treatment, but areas of necessary assessment for COTAs are discussed in the following paragraphs.

In the context of motor assessment, the COTA must have an understanding of the elder's ability to maintain the body in an upright position and in the midline against gravity (postural reactions). To do this, the COTA must observe the elder's degree of hypertonicity or hypotonicity, the presence of abnormal movement patterns, primitive reflexes, righting and protective reactions, equilibrium, coordination, and range of motion. The COTA should remember that all these performance components may be, and often are, affected by posture and endurance, and that the optimal assessment will occur when elders are upright and not too fatigued. Alignment of the trunk, pelvis, and shoulder girdle, and any voluntary motor control should be

noted. Assessment of strength has limited benefit in the presence of hypotonicity or hypertonicity and can possibly increase the degree of hypertonicity.

The sensory assessment should include evaluation of light touch, pressure, pain, temperature, stereognosis, and proprioception. The visual and perceptual areas to be assessed include tracking (smooth pursuits), visual fields, inattention to the right or left sides, spatial relations, figure ground, motor planning, and body scheme. In addition, elders may have other visual impairments that may affect their performance (see Chapter 15 for a review of this topic). Cognitive skills often assessed include attention, initiation, memory, planning, organization, problem solving, insight, and judgment. The ability to do calculations and make abstractions may also be tested. COTAs should remember that posture can have a significant effect on sensory, visual, perceptual, and cognitive functioning, and assessment of these areas should occur when elders are upright.

Assessment of swallowing ability and safety is crucial for all elders who have experienced a stroke. Swallowing is a complex behavior that results from the simultaneous performance of motor, sensory, perceptual, and cognitive skills, and deficits in any of these areas may result in elders being at a greater risk for aspirating food into the lungs and subsequent development of pneumonia (see Chapter 18 for a review of this topic).

Depending on the elder's ability to communicate, evaluation of psychosocial skills of elders may need to be completed by interviewing their family or other significant people. Knowledge of the occupations or pursuits the elder was involved in before the stroke and of the elder's values and interests is crucial in the selection of treatment strategies. Occupational task considerations should be made at every stage of OT intervention.

OCCUPATIONAL THERAPY INTERVENTION

The long-range goal of OT intervention for dysfunction caused by stroke is to facilitate maximal independence in all contexts of the elder's life. To reach this goal, intervention is focused on restoration of neuromuscular, visual-perceptual-cognitive, and psychosocial skills that support the elder's ability to perform self-care and engage in productive and leisure occupations. The degree to which each of these areas is emphasized is determined by the previous physical and social environments of elders and their plans after hospitalization. Because each elder's context is unique, the OT intervention plan is tailored specifically to that individual. By recognizing all these areas of an elder's being, the COTA is adhering to the Occupational Therapy Code of Ethics (American Occupational Therapy Association, 2000).

CASE STUDY

The need for tailored intervention programs is illustrated by the cases of Rose and Maria. Both women are in their late seventies and had strokes that have left them with a hemiplegic right side and difficulty verbally expressing themselves **(aphasia)**. Their visual, perceptual, and cognitive functions appear to be intact. Rose is a widow and lives in a senior community that provides one meal a day and assists her with laundry and cleaning. Her two sons live in other states. Maria lives at home with her husband and 2 of her 8 adult daughters; 10 grandchildren, whose ages range from 3 to 18 years, also live in her home. Both Rose and Maria want to return to their previous living environments. The OT program for both women will address all their needs, but the emphasis in Rose's program will be on self-care, meal preparation, and light home management tasks, because she must be independent in these areas to maintain her apartment at the senior community. Maria, however, is counting on family assistance for her self-care and is more interested in cooking again for her extended family; therefore her program will focus more on meal preparation, light home management, and social skills. The OT programs for both women will address their neuromuscular, visual-perceptual-cognitive, and psychosocial skills, but the activities chosen as therapeutic media should reflect their life contexts.

The cases of Rose and Maria illustrate another important principle in stroke rehabilitation: the more familiar the individual is with the activities selected for intervention, the more spontaneous and unconscious are the motor, visual, perceptual, cognitive, and psychosocial reorganization; consequently, changes will last longer (Warren, 1991). Conscious, attention-focused learning often is necessary in rehabilitation, especially when the likelihood of recovery is small and compensation strategies are more viable. However, these strategies may also slow the rehabilitation process because of the mental effort they require. To illustrate this, COTAs should do the following exercise with partners. Have your partner time you writing your full name on a piece of paper using your dominant hand, then have your partner time you writing your name again, but this time with your nondominant hand. Focus carefully on your body while you write your name and on the amount of mental control this task requires. The experience of rehabilitation after a stroke is similar to your experience of writing with your nondominant hand. Although clients who are recovering from stroke may not be learning to use their nondominant hand, they are relearning task accomplishment with a different body. The more these clients must concentrate on the task they are attempting, the longer it may take them to complete it. Engagement in automatic activities may take less time and may reinforce the automatic postural adjustments that support all actions. Consequently, whenever possible, the COTA should approach the intervention for stroke impairments with strategies designed to restore lost function in ways that use the learning and work experiences of elders before they experienced the stroke. Compensation strategies, particularly those related to the use of assistive equipment or alternative motor patterns, should be evaluated carefully because they require conscious attention and may create habits that may be difficult to break later.

Motor Deficits

Several sensorimotor approaches exist for the treatment of motor dysfunction resulting from stroke. Some of these include Brunnstrom (1970), Bobath's neurodevelopmental therapy and proprioceptive neuromuscular facilitation (Davies, 1985; Voss, Ionta, & Meyers, 1985), and constraint-induced movement therapy

(Morris & Taub, 2001). Regardless of the approach, the goal of intervention is to facilitate normal voluntary movement and use of the affected side of the body. Thus, normal postural mechanisms also must be developed, and abnormal reflexes and movements must be inhibited.

Although hypertonicity is often the most visible sign that a person has a motor dysfunction, this problem is best addressed in the context of postural control rather than in isolation. Abnormal tone in any extremity may drastically change depending on whether the individual is lying, sitting, or standing. Therefore, motor dysfunction should be treated when the individual is in alignment. Alignment means that the individual's pelvis is in a neutral position with no anterior or posterior tilt, that the spine is in **midline alignment**, and that the upper and lower extremities are in a neutral position.

The correct positioning while the elder is reclining can have a dramatic effect on **muscle tone** and pain, especially in the presence of **shoulder-hand syndrome**. (Specific issues with the **hemiplegic** upper extremity are discussed later in this chapter.) Having elders lie on the more affected side is most helpful in inhibiting abnormal tone and pain because of the heavy pressure exerted on that side (Fig. 19-1). However, caution must be taken to determine that the shoulder girdle is correctly aligned, the scapula is slightly abducted, and the humerus is in external rotation. The position of the bed should be rearranged (unless the elder finds the change too disorganizing) so that the elder can lie on the affected side and face the side of the bed from which **transfers** will occur. An added advantage of lying on the affected side is that it frees the less involved upper extremity for functional use while the elder is in this position (Fig. 19-2).

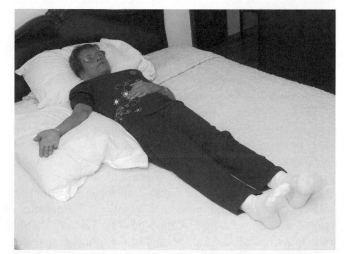

FIGURE 19-1   In the supine position, the trunk and upper extremities should be aligned. The hemiplegic upper extremity should be supported on pillows with the palm facing up.

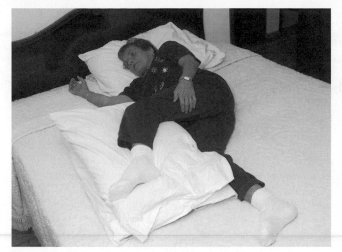

FIGURE **19-2** Lying on the hemiplegic upper extremity frees the less involved arm for functional use.

Body alignment also should be maintained during transitional movements, such as changing from a side-lying position to sitting at the edge of the bed and back to side lying; transferring to and from a chair, wheelchair, toilet, or car; changing from a sitting to a standing position and back to sitting; and while walking. COTAs should follow established sequential procedures when assisting elders to change from a supine position to sitting at the edge of the bed or when doing transfers (Boxes 19-1 and 19-2). In all these circumstances, COTAs must remember *not* to pull on the affected upper extremity to assist elders. COTAs should assist by holding the elder from the shoulder with the COTA's hand on the elder's scapula. Pulling the arm or supporting the elder from the axilla can easily cause or worsen any shoulder pain or glenohumeral subluxation. Shoulder subluxation can occur inferiorly, anteriorly, and

superiorly. Alignment of the humerus in the glenohumeral fossa is evaluated by the OTR. The COTA needs to determine if the alignment is correct before range of motion of the shoulder. Shoulder pain is a frequent problem and can occur from malalignment of the trunk, shoulder girdle, and humerus; subluxation; adhesive capsulitis; and trauma (Pitkanen, 2000). Shoulder subluxation and pain can lead to other complications such as increased hypertonicity, contractures, edema, nerve injury, and shoulder-hand syndrome. Before the COTA attempts any intervention for these conditions, service competency should be established with the OTR.

COTAs must pay constant attention to the elder's body alignment during sitting because this is often the elder's position during most activities, especially during the initial stages of rehabilitation. If the elder must sit fairly still for long periods, the therapist must ensure that the elder's pelvis is in a neutral position and is as far back in the chair as possible. Hips should be flexed at no more than 90 degrees. Greater hip flexion will cause posterior pelvic tilt and lumbar and thoracic spine flexion, inhibiting breathing and active upper extremity control and requiring greater cervical spine extension for the person to look straight ahead. Placing a folded towel or thin pillow in the small of the back to maintain alignment may be helpful. However, too thick a pillow or support can push the lumbar spine into hyperextension, causing anterior pelvic tilt and encouraging the elder to use back extension as the primary means of posture control. When back hyperextension is the base from which the elder begins movement in the extremities, hypertonicity throughout the body is likely to increase.

Another concern when the elder is in the sitting position is lateral pelvic tilt, or lateral flexion of the spine. Because of sensory and tone changes, half of the trunk muscles may not be working well; consequently, the

BOX **19-1**

Sequential Procedures for Changing from a Supine Position to Sitting at Edge of Bed

1. Plan to have elder exit bed toward hemiplegic side.
2. Gently provide passive abduction to hemiplegic scapula and extend hemiplegic arm at side of body so that humerus is in external rotation and palm is facing up; an alternative is to have elder clasp hands and hold arms in 90-degree flexion with straight elbows and roll toward side of bed.
3. Have elder hook less affected leg under hemiplegic ankle and slide both legs toward edge of bed.
4. Have elder roll on to hemiplegic side, facing side of bed.
5. Have elder cross less affected upper extremity in front of body and place on bed at a level slightly below chest.
6. As the elder lowers legs at the side of the bed, have elder push up with less affected hand and hemiplegic elbow (if able).
7. Once sitting at edge of bed, have elder scoot forward by alternating **weight bearing** on each thigh and scooting the free thigh forward until both feet are flat on floor.

BOX 19-2

Sequential Procedures for Transfers

1. If transferring from wheelchair to another chair, toilet, or bed, place wheelchair at no more than 45 degrees (perpendicular) from destination surface; elder should transfer toward hemiplegic side whenever possible.
2. Make sure wheelchair is locked and footrests and armrests are out of the way.
3. Place both feet flat on floor.
4. Have elder sit upright so back is not against back rest.
5. Have elder scoot forward to front edge of chair by alternately shifting weight onto one thigh and scooting other thigh forward; do not permit elder to push off back of chair using back extension, because this will increase abnormal muscle tone throughout the body.
6. Position elder's feet so tips of toes are directly below knees; make sure feet remain flat on floor; if ankle dorsiflexion is limited, toes may be placed somewhat anterior to knees.
7. Have elder lean forward until shoulders are directly above knees.
8. Have elder push off from knees with both hands if elder is able.
9. As elder leans forward, have elder stand up; if unable to stand up fully, guide elder's body toward target chair, toilet, or bed while elder is partially weight bearing on both feet.

other side of the trunk may be overworking. The resulting misalignment causes the spine to flex toward one side. Because of this lateral flexion, the spine is no longer in midline, and weight bearing on the elder's thighs is unequal. Pelvic tilt upward toward one side results in shortening of the trunk on the same side and elongation of the trunk on the opposite side. Weight bearing occurs primarily on the side of the elongated trunk. The COTA must help to actively or passively align the spine toward the midline, rather than to simply build up one side of the sitting surface.

When pelvic and spine alignment are achieved, the COTA can focus on placing the feet flat on the floor or on footrests so that knee flexion and ankle dorsiflexion of no more than 90 degrees is present. The COTA should take care that the femurs are in neutral rotation (that is, there is no external or internal rotation) and that there is little or no hip abduction or adduction. Thus, the heels will be resting directly below the knees, and the knees will be aligned with the hips. Unless the elder is being pushed in a wheelchair, both feet should be placed on the floor so that they bear weight more evenly. Consequently, hemi-wheelchairs, the seats of which are slightly lower than standard wheelchairs, are recommended so that the elder's feet can comfortably reach the floor. The use of a padded seat and backboards placed in the wheelchair also improves the elder's sitting position and midline orientation, thus preventing the problems that may occur from poor positioning in a wheelchair.

After attending to the pelvis, spine, and lower extremities, the COTA can align the elder's hemiplegic upper extremity. The strategies for positioning are similar for both hypotonic and hypertonic arms. The elder should be placed in front of a table or outfitted with a full or half

lapboard so that the hand can be placed facedown on a flat surface to benefit from the normalizing effects of weight bearing. To accomplish this, the COTA should ensure that the elder's scapula is slightly abducted, the shoulder is flexed so the elbow is anterior to the shoulder, the humerus is in neutral or slight external rotation, the elbow is resting lightly on the lapboard to provide support for the shoulder, the forearm is pronated and positioned away from the trunk, and the hand is resting on the support surface. This permits the hand to bear weight normally. The normal weight-bearing surface of the hand includes the lateral external surface of the thumb, fingertips, lateral border of the hand, and thenar and hypothenar eminences. The COTA should maintain the arch formed by the metacarpophalangeal joints so that the hand is not flattened. The hand should not be fastened in any way to the lapboard except in extreme cases in which clear evidence indicates that the elder may be hurt otherwise. Restricting normal, spontaneous weight bearing inhibits normalization of muscle tone. In cases of extreme hypertonicity in the hand, the COTA can place a soup bowl or a ball cut in half face down on a square of nonslip material on the lapboard, thus permitting some weight bearing against a hard surface (Fig. 19-3). However, the elder's hand should never be placed on nonslip material. Such material can contribute to shoulder pain or subluxation, because the hand cannot move when repositioning of the shoulder or body occurs. Caution must be used when a lapboard is used with an elder, because it may be considered a form of restraint unless the elder is independently able to remove it. (See Chapter 14 for a detailed discussion on this topic.)

During intervention sessions that do not require sitting for long periods, the elder should sit in a chair, on a

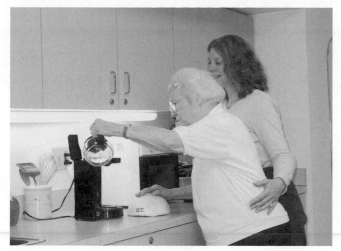

FIGURE 19-3   In cases of hypertonicity, the hemiplegic hand can be placed on an inverted soup bowl or ball cut in half to bear weight more comfortably.

stool, or at the edge of a mat. The concerns with alignment in this position are similar to those described earlier for sitting, but the focus of intervention will be on the elder moving into and out of alignment while participating in activities. Sitting on a stool or at the edge of the mat forces active trunk control because there are no back or armrests for support and the base of support under the thighs is reduced. Concerns regarding lower extremity placement are the same as described previously. However, as the elder's ability to control the trunk increases, the height of the mat can be increased, thus gradually increasing and challenging the amount of active weight bearing on the lower extremities. This gradation prepares the elder for the trunk and postural control required during standing activities. If the elder has little or no active movement of the hemiplegic upper extremity, the elder should position the limb on a table, following similar guidelines as those described previously. As the height of the mat increases, so should the height of the table or surface that supports the hand.

Although standing and ambulation training does not traditionally fall into the realm of OT, it should be considered a transitional movement that permits elders to perform and maneuver from one task or occupation to another. For example, elders may need to ambulate from the bed to the bathroom and stand to complete toileting tasks, or ambulate from the sink to the stove to the refrigerator and stand to complete a meal preparation task. Consequently, COTAs should assist in maintaining alignment in the same way as described previously. During standing and ambulation, the person's midline shift toward the less affected side is most obvious. This often is accentuated when elders are taught to walk using a broad-based cane, and they establish the habit of maintaining the

midline in the middle of the less affected side rather than in the middle of the body. Because there is less motor control, or less sensory feedback, elders may hesitate to bear weight equally on each leg as they stand or take a step. The COTA should coordinate intervention with the Registered Physical Therapist to understand what standing and ambulation pattern to reinforce with elders during OT intervention.

Special attention should be given to the hemiplegic upper extremity. This extremity should be purposefully included in any activity early during the course of intervention, even if little or no active motor control is present, because this will keep the elder's attention on the extremity and will reduce its neglect and the development of learned nonuse (Morris & Taub, 2001). Before any active or passive motion is expected of the elder, the COTA must first passively mobilize the elder's scapula to ensure that it glides when the arm is moved. The scapula may not glide sufficiently or may stop altogether because of muscle paralysis or hypertonus. Consequently, the COTA should never flex or abduct the shoulder of elders more than 90 degrees unless the COTA can be sure that the scapula is gliding properly. If elders do not have active scapular control, the COTA can passively move the scapula while ranging the shoulder. When the shoulder is flexed more than 90 degrees, the scapula glides downward on the posterior wall of the rib cage. In addition, the inferior border, or angle, of the scapula rotates slightly upward. When the shoulder is abducted more than 90 degrees, the scapula glides toward the vertebral column and the inferior border rotates slightly downward.

If elders have minimal or no active movement in the hemiplegic upper extremity, they should be instructed to move it by holding their hands together in one of two ways. If the elder has any active movement in the hand, clasping the hands with the thumb of the hemiplegic hand on top is recommended (Fig. 19-4). If there is no movement in the hand, the uninvolved hand should be placed on the ulnar side of the hemiplegic wrist and hand and the uninvolved thumb in the palm of the hemiplegic hand. This method will protect the small joints of the hemiplegic hand and will maintain the arches in the palm. While holding onto the hands using either method, elders should be instructed to extend the elbows and hold the shoulders flexed at approximately 90 degrees. With the arms in this position, elders can go from a supine to a side-lying position, from a sitting to a standing position, or they can hold on to the knee of the hemiplegic lower extremity to cross it during dressing and bathing and during other **functional activities**. The COTA's imagination and creativity are essential in assisting elders to use this two-hand technique to perform numerous functional activities such as picking up a mug to drink and mixing a cake. In addition, elders can flex or abduct the hemiplegic shoulder themselves by guiding the arm when

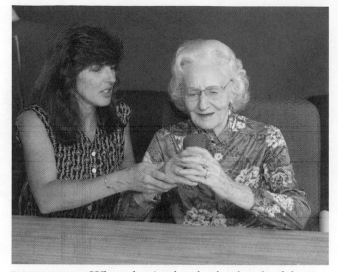

FIGURE 19-4   When clasping hands, the thumb of the hemiplegic hand should be on top.

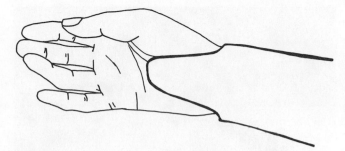

FIGURE 19-5   A modified cock-up splint holds the wrist in slight extension and helps to reduce fluid buildup in the hand.

the hands are held together. This bilateral integration assists with normalizing tone and encourages elders to actively care for the hemiplegic upper extremity (Davies, 1985).

Elders may develop shoulder-hand syndrome if the hemiplegic upper extremity is not managed appropriately. This syndrome is characterized by swelling or edema that is usually observed in the hand but may also be present in the forearm and upper arm, tenderness, loss of range of motion, and vasomotor degradation. Pain and subluxation of the glenohumeral joint may not necessarily be present. The COTA should address all these problems immediately to avoid irreversible atrophy of bones, skin, and muscles (Davis, 1990). The swelling is best decreased by filling a bucket or pail two-thirds full with crushed ice and adding cold water to the level of the ice. Elders should sit, while maintaining good alignment, with the bucket in front of them, which is placed on the floor, and should lean forward to place the hemiplegic hand and wrist in the water. The edematous hand should be kept in the water for 3 to 5 seconds, and this process should be repeated three times. The COTA should dry the hand gently with a towel. The COTA should ask the elder to flex the fingers if possible, or the COTA should provide gentle passive ranging of the fingers and hand. The whole procedure should be done repeatedly during the day until swelling subsides. While the COTA is providing the range of motion exercise, retrograde massage while the limb is elevated also can be done, and a simple cock-up splint can be used to hold the wrist in extension (no more than 30 degrees) to help reduce the buildup of fluid in the hand when elders are not receiving therapy (Fig. 19-5). Swelling also occurs from decreased muscle

activity to move the fluid from the limb, dependent positioning, and trauma.

COTAs can use graded activities to facilitate voluntary control of an elder's hemiplegic upper extremity. Such activities should be geared toward developing control in a progression from shoulder to elbow to hand. Elders may develop control in the hand before the more proximal parts of the arm. Despite the apparent control in the hand, the COTA should first facilitate active movement in the shoulder by engaging elders in activities that emphasize the body moving on the arm while the hand is maintained in weight bearing. The weight-bearing surface of the hand is limited to the lateral surface of the thumb, the thenar eminences, and the fingertips. In this position the palm of the hand is free and not in contact with the weight-bearing surface. Weight bearing on the hand does not need to be forceful, and elders should *never* have the hand completely flattened. Placing weight on a flat hand can lead to loss of the normal and functional arches of the hand and, consequently, can interfere with elders' abilities to develop grasp later. Placing weight on the hand can be done in both sitting and standing positions. In a sitting position, for example, an elder's affected hand can be placed in a weight-bearing position on the table or on a stool placed next to the elder. In a standing position, the elder should be taught to place the affected hand on a weight-bearing surface such as a table or countertop while performing functional tasks such as putting away dishes or groceries or folding laundry (Fig. 19-6). As control of the shoulder increases, activities should be introduced that emphasize free movement of the hemiplegic extremity on the more stable part of the body. During all these activities, the COTA should continue to ensure that good body alignment is maintained and that elders are not using abnormal movements in one part of the body to obtain control in another.

COTAs should instruct elders in proper one-handed dressing techniques to protect the hemiplegic upper extremity and to avoid falling. Dressing should be done while sitting in a chair and, in general, the hemiplegic extremity should be dressed first and undressed last to avoid

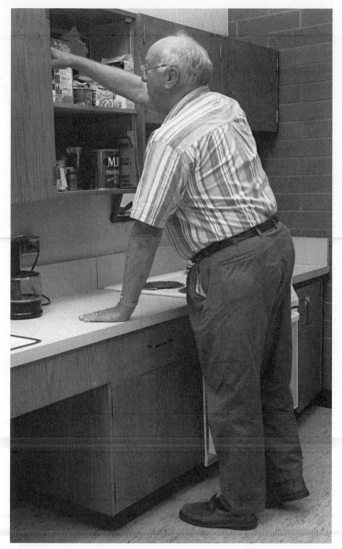

FIGURE 19-6   Bearing weight on the hemiplegic hand can be done while standing at a counter.

pulling on it or twisting it unnecessarily. Front-buttoned shirts or blouses are easiest to don by dressing the hemiplegic arm first and then draping the shirt over the shoulders by holding on to the shirt collar with the other arm. When the shirt is draped over the opposite shoulder, the elder can reach into the sleeve with the unaffected arm. This procedure is reversed when taking the shirt off. The process is similar when putting on pants, with the exception that the elder should cross the hemiplegic leg over the opposite leg to dress the hemiplegic leg first. If the elder is able to stand to pull up the pants, the elder may do so when both legs are clothed. If standing is not possible, the elder can shift weight to each side while sitting in the chair and gradually can pull the pants up over the buttocks.

All the principles mentioned previously should be considered when training elders in functional activities or selecting assistive equipment. Although progress may seem slower at the beginning, following these principles can make a marked difference in the quality of movement elders develop. When tasks are too difficult, elders are more likely to use abnormal movement patterns, become fatigued quickly, and become discouraged. The COTA must use good observation and clinical reasoning skills in selecting activities that challenge elders at the appropriate levels.

Visual-Perceptual-Cognitive Deficits

Although the motor deficits resulting from a stroke are the most easily observed, many less visible problems can severely hinder the rehabilitation process if not appropriately addressed. Depending on the type of brain lesion, the individual may have sensory disturbances that range from a total absence of sensation to a heightened perception of pain and other distorted sensations. These problems are accentuated when the individual has a body scheme disorder or difficulties planning motor actions, which is known as *apraxia*. Consequently, the individual has difficulty integrating and using any perceptual input from the hemiplegic side. Visual–perceptual deficits common in strokes include hemianopsia, poor figure ground perceptions, and difficulty with spatial relationships. Unilateral neglect results from a unique constellation of these symptoms when elders have no sense that the hemiplegic side of the body even exists, and they fail to visually scan toward that side. All these disorders should be addressed simultaneously during intervention, using bilateral functional activities that encourage the use of the hemiplegic side of the body. The use of normal movement will provide repeated sensory stimulation to the hemiplegic side and relay information that will be processed in the brain and used as feedback in determining where each body part is and what it is doing. Consequently, the COTA should grade a variety of motor and sensory activities so that they maximize the elders' abilities to control movement independently and provide increased sensory input. However, the activities should not be so overwhelming that they cause withdrawal reactions or increases in abnormal tone. Various textures, smells, colors, distances, and depths can be graded during most functional activities. In addition to these remedial approaches, the COTA should teach elders to compensate for deficits by providing repeated practice in establishing habits of visually scanning the hemiplegic side and methodically protecting and integrating the hemiplegic extremities in whatever activity they may be involved.

Other areas of concern for the COTA include elders' abilities to comprehend and produce language and to plan and safely perform activities. As a result of stroke, elders may not be able to understand what others are saying, a condition known as *receptive aphasia*, or may not be able to produce the words they intend to utter, a condition known as *expressive aphasia*, or both disorders may be present, which is known as *global aphasia*. These disorders may also extend to nonverbal language, as elders may be unable to interpret or appropriately use gestures. Language deficits are usually treated by the speech language pathologist, but strategies must be reinforced during OT intervention. When talking to elders, COTAs should keep instructions and explanations simple and concrete and should state them in an empathetic, patient way. Demonstration is usually helpful (Fig. 19-7). The best way to ensure elders have understood the instructions is to observe their performance (Pedretti, Smith, & Pendelton, 1995).

Cognitive dysfunction is often believed to be a major cause for failure of elders to reach rehabilitation goals and must be considered, particularly when planning for discharge (Woodson, 1995). Safety may be compromised if elders cannot plan activities, make judgments, solve problems, or express verbally their needs for emergency care. For example, limited memory may cause elders to overmedicate themselves or not turn off the stove after cooking. Being unable to remember all the steps involved in a task may mean that elders can often be surprised by the outcome. Elders may get stuck on a step and may be unable to determine what to do next or may neglect to realize that something dangerous could happen if an inappropriate action is taken. OT intervention, as mentioned earlier, should involve graded repetition of procedures until elders can routinely perform them safely. Emphasis should be placed on varying the context or

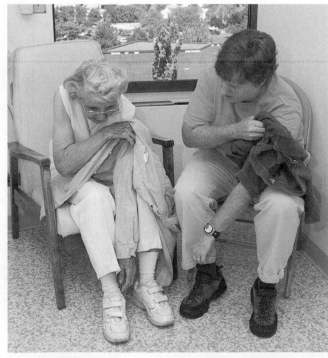

FIGURE **19-7**   Demonstration is a valuable teaching technique especially if the elder is aphasic.

situation in which the procedure is practiced to enhance learning (Toglia, 1991).

Emotional Adjustment

COTAs should consider the emotional adjustment of elders to the disability caused by the stroke. Depression, a common reaction to any catastrophic event, is one of the most undiagnosed and untreated responses to stroke (National Institute of Mental Health, 2002). Depression may be caused from natural grief trying to cope with the loss of function, but also may be caused by the location of the lesion in the brain, previous or family history of depression, and social functioning before the stroke. Mild or major depression can develop from 2 months to 2 years after the stroke in up to 53% of clients (National Institute of Mental Health, 2002; Pitkanen, 2000). Anxiety, poor frustration tolerance, denial, anger, and emotional lability are all signs that elders are struggling to deal with the reality of their condition. COTAs must listen empathetically and supportively, while sensitively maintaining the focus on areas of realistic recovery. Permitting elders to control choices in intervention as much as possible can reinforce the sense that they can affect their environments. Although a complete recovery cannot be guaranteed, neither can a lack of recovery. COTAs must honestly explain to elders that residual limitations will probably be present, but the best chance for recovery will occur by the practice of skills. COTAs should use their creativity and ingenuity skills to help elders adapt tasks or environments that elders consider lost, thus instilling new hope and motivation in the rehabilitation process. As with any area of intervention, family and social involvement is crucial for elders to accept residual limitations and maximize their residual abilities. Ultimately, elders must see that they can continue to be effective in some measure and can still actively pursue activities and ideals they valued highly before the stroke.

■ CHAPTER REVIEW QUESTIONS

1 Sit at the edge of a bed or chair and lift up the left side of your pelvis. What happens with your spine and trunk when you do this? What occurs with the imaginary midline of the body when you sit in this position? Where on your thighs do you feel the most pressure while sitting in this position? Can you tell any difference in how your arms work while sitting this way? How would you feel after sitting in this position for 10 or 15 minutes?

2 Sitting on a firm chair, make sure that your pelvis is as far back in the chair as possible and your back is well supported. From that position, without moving forward, attempt to stand. What did you do with your arms while attempting to stand? How much work did your trunk have to do to get you to a standing position? Now repeat the activity but first scoot to the edge of the chair before you stand. Did you notice any differences in the amount of work your upper trunk and arms had to do to get you upright? From which position was it easier to stand?

3 Sitting at the edge of a chair with your trunk well aligned, move your feet as far forward as you can, making sure that they are flat on the floor. From that position, attempt to stand. Were you able to do so? How much work did your upper trunk and arms have to do? Return to sitting at the edge of the chair, and now attempt to stand again, but first place your feet as far back behind your knees as possible. Was standing from this position more or less difficult than your first attempt? Did you fall forward? Now return to sitting at the edge of the chair, and this time place your feet so that your toes are directly aligned below your knees and are flat on the floor. Did this help to keep your midline where it should be, even during movement?

REFERENCES

American Occupational Therapy Association. (2000). Occupational Therapy Code of Ethics (2000). *American Journal of Occupational Therapy, 54*(6), 614-616.

American Stroke Association. (2002). *Stroke: are you at risk?* Washington, DC: American Heart Association (Brochure).

Bear, M., Connors, B., & Paradiso, M. (1996). *Neuroscience: Exploring the brain.* Baltimore, MD: Williams & Wilkins.

Brunnstrom, S. (1970). *Movement therapy in hemiplegia.* New York: Harper & Row.

Centers for Disease Control and Prevention. (2002). *Deaths from strokes fact sheet.* Washington, DC: U.S. Department of Health and Human Services.

Davies, P. (1985). *Steps to follow: A guide to the treatment of adult hemiplegia.* New York, NY: Springer-Verlag.

Davis, J. (1990). The role of the occupational therapist in the trea. of shoulder-hand syndrome. *Occupational Therapy Practice, 1* (30).

DeArmond, S., Fusco, M., & Dewey, M. (1989). *Structure of the brain: A photographic atlas* (3rd ed.). New York, NY: Oxford University Press.

Morris, D. M., & Taub, E. (2001). Constraint-induced therapy approach to restoring function after neurological injury. *Topics in Stroke Rehabilitation, 8*(3), 16-30.

Moyers, P. A. (1999). The guide to occupational therapy practice. American Occupational Therapy Association. *American Journal of Occupational Therapy, 53*(3), 247-322.

National Institute of Mental Health. (2002). *Depression and stroke.* Bethesda, MD: The Institute.

National Institute of Neurological Disorders and Stroke. (1999). *Stroke: Hope through research.* Bethesda, MD: The Institute.

Pansky, B., Allen, D., & Budd, G. (1988). *Review of neuroscience* (2nd ed.). New York: Macmillan.

Pedretti, L., Smith, J., & Pendelton, H. (1995). Cerebral vascular accident. In L. Pedretti (Ed.), *Occupational therapy: Practice skills for physical dysfunction* (4th ed.). St. Louis, MO: Mosby.

Pitkanen, K. (2000). Stroke rehabilitation in the elderly: A controlled study of the effectiveness and costs of a multidimensional intervention. Ph.D. diss., Departments of Neurology and Medicine, University of Kuopio, Kuopio, Finland.

Toglia, J. (1991). Generalization of treatment: A multicontext approach to cognitive perceptual impairment in adults with brain injury. *American Journal of Occupational Therapy, 45,* 505-516.

Umphred, D. (1995). *Neurological rehabilitation* (3rd ed.). St. Louis, MO: Mosby.

U.S. Department of Health and Human Services. (1995). *Post stroke rehabilitation: Practice guideline no. 16.* Rockville, MD: The Department.

Voss, D., Ionta, M., & Myers, B. (1985). *Proprioceptive neuromuscular facilitation* (3rd ed.). New York, NY: Harper & Row.

Warren, M. (1991). Strategies for sensory and neuromotor remediation. In C. Christiansen, & C. Baum (Eds.), *Occupational therapy: Overcoming human performance deficits.* Thorofare, NJ: Slack.

Woodson, A. (1995). Stroke. In C. Trombly (Ed.), *Occupational therapy for physical dysfunction.* Baltimore, MD: Williams & Wilkins.

World Health Organization. (1989). Recommendations on stroke prevention, diagnosis, and therapy: Report of the WHO Task Force on stroke and other cerebrovascular disorders. *Stroke, 20,* 1460.

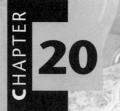

CHAPTER 20

Working with Elders Who Have Dementia and Alzheimer's Disease

CARLY R. HELLEN

KEY TERMS

Alzheimer's disease, activity-focused care, personhood, person-centered care, "therapeutic fibs," creative reality, rescuing, chaining, bridging

CHAPTER OBJECTIVES

1. Understand that elders with Alzheimer's disease (AD) are persons first; they are not their disease. Therefore, person-centered care (personalized) focuses on overall well-being, reflecting the elders' remaining strengths and abilities.
2. Describe person-centered care and personhood.
3. Gain awareness and sensitivity to the cognitive, physical, and psychosocial needs of elders with AD.
4. Describe activity-focused care.

5. Relate suggestions to promote wellness through task simplification and modification.
6. Identify caregiving techniques, approaches, and interventions that can be used to help empower elders who have AD to participate in daily living tasks.
7. Suggest appropriate communication responses to elders with AD.
8. Problem solve antecedents and approaches to refocus unwanted behavioral responses.

Travis is a certified occupational therapy assistant (COTA) who works in a skilled nursing facility. One of his responsibilities is consulting with staff at a special care unit for persons with **Alzheimer's disease (AD)**. John, the charge nurse on the unit, contacts Travis. "We are having problems with Grace. She is wandering in and out of other's rooms and taking their possessions, which is irritating the other residents. She is also having difficulty communicating her needs. Her performance with ADL functions seems variable. We are also having problems

with increased agitation with Grace and all of our residents, especially at shift change. Do you have any ideas?"

Hilde is a COTA working on a subacute unit. Ruth, one of the elders, was admitted after a total hip replacement. After reviewing her chart, Hilde finds out that Ruth has a history of AD. Both Travis and Hilde can provide practical suggestions to better help these elders with AD function. This chapter provides background information about AD and occupational therapy (OT) treatment interventions.

The dementia syndrome includes confusion, forgetfulness, decreased judgment, "Dementia is a loss of intellectual functions (such as thinking, remembering and reasoning) of sufficient severity to interfere with daily life" (Alzheimer's Association, 1999), and loss or failure of mental abilities. Depression, medications, and metabolic dysfunction may cause a reversible dementia. Causes of nonreversible dementia include small strokes (vascular dementia), dementia with Parkinson's disease, dementia with Lewy bodies, frontal lobe dementias, and AD. AD affects 4 million elders in the United States and is projected to affect up to 6 million by 2010 (Evans, 1990). It is a progressive, degenerative disease of brain tissue that leads to memory loss and problems with thinking and carrying out daily life activities. Performing routine tasks, using good judgment, being aware of surroundings, communicating effectively, and coping become more difficult as the disease progresses. The problems start gradually and become more severe over time, leading to a total inability to perform self-care. Although the rate of change varies, the usual stages are mild, moderate, severe, and terminal (Box 20-1).

AD can last 2 to 20 years. Most people die after 8 years, often from pneumonia or other systemic problems. Causes of AD are not known, but current research suggests the involvement of brain chemicals, amyloids, and genetic factors (Alzheimer's Association, 1999). With the help of standardized diagnostic criteria, physicians can now diagnose AD with an accuracy of 85% to 90% once symptoms occur (Alzheimer's Association, 1999). Treatment is based on medical and psychosocial support. The disease currently has no known cure.

Aronson (1994) reported that of the 1.5 million residents of nursing homes in the United States, more than half have AD or some form of dementia. COTAs work with elders who have AD and related dementia in nursing homes, as well as in homes, assisted living facilities, adult day programs, and hospitals. COTAs often provide therapy to elders with AD on special care units or as part of their regular caseload. OT treatment for these elders usually focuses on activities of daily living (ADL) functions, communication, strengthening, and adaptations of purposeful activities.

PERSON-CENTERED AND ACTIVITY-FOCUSED CARE FOR ELDERS WITH ALZHEIMER'S DISEASE

An elder with AD or related dementia continues to seek meaning and connectedness with life. The person is not the dementia (Hellen, 1998). **Personhood** as described by Kitwood and Bredin (1992) refers to one's sense of self, the "I am" within each person. Kitwood and Bredin described 12 indicators of personhood and well-being for individuals with dementia including: the assertion of desire or will, the ability to experience and express

BOX 20-1

Four Stages of Alzheimer's Disease

Early/Mild impairment stage
Average 1 to 3 years, possibly longer
Memory loss, especially with recent events
Difficulty with complex cognitive tasks
Difficulty with decision making and planning
Decreased attention span and concentration
Lack of spontaneity and lessening of initiative
Impaired word-finding skills
Preference for familiar settings

Mid-/Moderate impairment stage
Average 5 to 7 years, possibly longer
Chronic recent memory loss
Difficulty with written and spoken language
Tendency to ask questions constantly
Tendency to experience visual-spatial perceptual problems
Possible delusions, hallucinations, and agitation
Increasing difficulty with familiar objects and tasks
Assistance with ADL functions necessary
Ability to respond to multisensory cueing
Tendency to wander, pace, and rummage
May get lost at times even inside the house

Late/Severe impairment stage
Average 2 to 3 years
Dependence on others for ADL functions
Ability to respond to hand-over-hand activity
Decreased interest in food
Difficulty with chewing and swallowing
Incontinence
Decreased vocabulary
Misidentification of familiar objects, persons
Impaired ambulation/gait, increased falls
Repetitious movement or sounds

Terminal stage
Average 3 months to 1 year
Usually in bed or wheelchair
Limited ability to track visually
Mute or few incoherent words
Little spontaneous movement
Loss of appetite, severe weight loss

Difficulty in swallowing
Tendency to utter sounds rather than words
Total dependence on others for care
Possible development of contractions, skin breakdown
Possible reaction to music and touch, fleeting attention span

a range of emotions, initiation of social contact, self-respect, humor, creativity, and self-expression. They found that person-specific or **person-centered care** daily supported elders with dementia and enhanced and promoted their life's meaning and personhood (Hellen, 1998).

The COTA developing a therapeutic program for elders with dementia individualizes care that supports wellness, strengths, and abilities. This personalized or person-centered care also supports the components of activity-focused care that recognizes that all of life is an activity of being and doing. The tasks of life, therefore, are interconnected. The objectives of activity-focused care include focusing on abilities, not limitations; promoting the purposeful and meaningful use of time; supporting sense of belonging and enabling verbal and nonverbal communication skills. **Activity-focused care** also encourages positive behaviors and the development of interventions to refocus unwanted behaviors (Hellen, 1998).

Activity-focused care redefines interventions, especially in long-term care settings and special care units. Success is achieved through augmenting the client's strengths by reframing expectations and relating to all of daily life tasks as activities. It involves the willingness to enter the client's world with sensitivity and flexibility and the provision of holistic support.

COMMUNICATION: UNDERSTANDING AND BEING UNDERSTOOD

Communicating with people who have AD is often challenging. As the disease progresses, verbal abilities decrease and communication continues through nonverbal gestures and sounds. Verbal and nonverbal communication reflect the same objectives: expressing thoughts and needs, supporting the elders' self-image and a sense of worth. Other objectives for communication include improving socialization, maximizing quality of life, increasing involvement in a supportive community, understanding others, and promoting safety and comfort. COTAs must care enough to listen carefully. During the early stages of AD, changes that occur in language and communication include the onset of difficulty with using nouns. Substituted words are sometimes used for the noun. For example, Mary was asked to identify an object (a comb). Her response was, "Oh, honey, you know," as she ran her hand through her hair. She was unable to use the noun "comb" (Fig. 20-1).

Reality orientation is usually embarrassing for elders with AD because of their inability to remember and retrieve words to answer questions. One type of response that maintains the dignity of elders with disorientation is to refrain from confronting them with corrections, especially if the confrontation would increase agitation. Caregivers should use **creative reality** with elders by focusing on the emotions being expressed and responding appropriately by validating feelings.

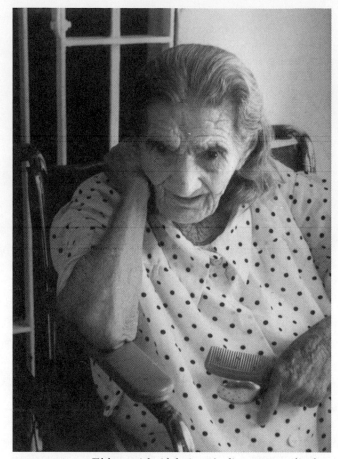

FIGURE 20-1   Elders with Alzheimer's disease may display difficulty identifying and verbalizing the names for common objects. (Courtesy Yolanda Griffiths, OTD, OTR/FAOTA, Creighton University, Omaha, NE.)

A strategy called **"therapeutic fibs"** can be used as illustrated by the following story. Jim states "My wife is taking me home in 5 minutes." In reality, the treatment session has an additional 30 minutes remaining. Sue, the COTA, agrees with him, stating that he and his wife will soon be together and that he has a wonderful, caring wife. Sue realizes that a discussion of the amount of remaining time would increase Jim's agitation. Sue, having validated Jim's desire for his wife, can then redirect him to do a meaningful task. Elders asking for their mothers or wanting to go home may be seeking acceptance and the need to feel connected. They may also be expressing the need for safety, purposeful use of time, or the company of others. Telling them that their mother is dead or the facility is now their home can upset them. Instead, the COTA may say, "You are safe with me and I will be here today with you. If you are like your mother, she must have been wonderful. I miss my mother too; we used to have fun folding the laundry; perhaps you and I can work together."

As the disease progresses, the ability to speak and understand decreases. Some of these elders become more intuitive, often with increased awareness of people's attitudes and the environment (Hellen, 1998). Therefore, caregivers should be aware of their nonverbal messages such as acting rushed, looking at the clock, sighing, or raising one's voice. In time, elders with AD lose almost all language skills, but they may still occasionally utter a perfectly appropriate statement (Kovach, 1996). For example, Juan talked a lot, but his words were just sounds that made no sense. When a caregiver impatiently spoke to him in an abrupt and firm tone, saying "Juan, time out; go to your room," Juan responded, "In the military, I was in solitary confinement and I can do that standing on my head." The family later confirmed that Juan had indeed been in the military and the story was true. The caregiver's "drill sergeant" tone and body posture triggered Juan's response.

People with AD need to experience acceptance and success, especially as their language skills diminish. COTAs can keep the dialogue going even when the words are few (Box 20-2).

BEHAVIOR AND PSYCHOSOCIAL ASPECTS

People with dementia are not "stupid"; they are forgetful and often maintain an inner wisdom. Like anyone else, they have needs and should be approached and cared for with respect. They also should have opportunities for proud and meaningful involvement. Knowledge of the elders' life story often becomes the basis for COTAs to plan and carry out therapy. A "Life Story" book can be used for this purpose. This book can include pictures with captions, lists, favorite recipes, family traditions, schools attended, and military history. Using the book is an excellent tool for connecting with elders and as an intervention to refocus difficult behaviors and to reduce agitation (Hellen, 1998).

The behaviors of people with dementia are often attempts to communicate. For example, increased agitation may be the client's way of communicating illness. Rapid pacing might be a sign of an inability to cope with others, escape from excessive noise, or environmental factors.

Some of the typical behaviors displayed by people with AD include wandering, pacing, and rummaging or redistribution of personal belongings (Fig. 20-2). Combativeness and aggression also can occur. Catastrophic reactions are explosive responses to distress. These reactions result from the inability to understand, interpret, and cope with real or imagined situations, people, the environment, or oneself. "Sun-downing" results from a combination of increased behavioral responses occurring in the mid-to-late afternoon. These responses often reflect physical problems such as dehydration and physical/emotional exhaustion. Screaming, yelling, and calling often reflect fear, a need for acceptance, and a lack of active participation and connectedness during the day. Other behavioral

BOX 20-2

Suggestions for Improving Communication and Connectedness

1. Attract the client's attention by using touch and talking **to him or her** at eye level.
2. Use short, simple sentences to express one thought at a time. Be willing to repeat as needed, allowing time for the elder to respond. Do not appear rushed; offer the elder your full attention. Assess and limit distractions from the environment, such as the TV, vacuum cleaners, and loud nearby conversations (Hellen, 1998).
3. Be aware that asking questions often can be embarrassing for people with AD, who often have difficulty finding the right words for the answer. Instead, help them respond by giving as many multisensory verbal or nonverbal cues as possible. If asking a question, offer two choices. For example, ask Ella if she would like to shower before breakfast or after breakfast, showing her the towel and clean clothing that you are holding.
4. Do not try to apply logic or to give long explanations. Ignore the need to be right, to argue, or to confront. At times having information written down for elders helps them to focus and understand, especially when they ask the same question repeatedly. For example, providing Richard with a business type letter with his name on it that states that his apartment has been paid in full and that he has a place to spend the night helps him to retain the information. Be willing to supply this letter as often as he needs for reassurance of having a place to stay.
5. State requests with positive words ("Please sit here" rather than "Don't sit there").
6. Listen carefully to all the words, gestures, and facial expressions the person uses. Validate feelings behind the words. For example, if Henry's words seem to make no sense but sound angry and upset, say, "You sound upset, Henry. I know when I feel that way I like a hug. Can I give you a hug?" However, be aware that some people are tactile defensive and become agitated when touched.
7. Realize that elders with AD often respond literally to words (because the fire alarm says "pull," Hazel pulls it).
8. Be aware that elders with AD often revert to their primary language. COTAs may have to learn appropriate key words in that language to encourage therapy.

manifestations may include inappropriate sexual conduct, hitting or pushing staff or other elders, accusing or demanding speech, withdrawal from activities, and apathy. Elders with AD might also show perseveration in their

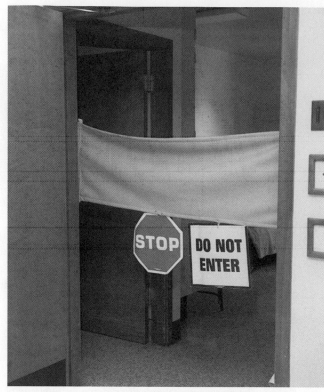

FIGURE 20-2 Environmental adaptations should help restrict elders with Alzheimer's disease from wandering into other people's rooms without restricting access to corridors.

actions by repetitious movement or sounds, such as wiping or patting the table surface, pulling on clothing, and shouting.

Difficult behaviors are usually not done on purpose as a method of making care more difficult; rather, they are often part of the disease. At times, behaviors can be a problem to others but not to the elder. For example, Betty, who lives in a special care unit, goes into other people's rooms. She looks through their closets and takes clothing and items from their drawers. This behavior suggests that Betty likes to feel in control and is "cleaning up the house." Whose problem is it? Carmen, the owner of these possessions, is angry and feels that her privacy has been invaded. The facility staff meets the challenge of working with both people in a supportive way by identifying acceptable places for Betty to rummage, such as a bureau or desk in the social center and "busy boxes" or baskets filled with safe items. Examples of items to include in a "busy box" are balls of yarn, greeting cards, small scrapbooks, car brochures, maps, catalogs, fabric pieces, and carpet samples. Having Betty participate in the purposeful activity of carrying safe items can help address her need to feel connected.

A respectful response exists for every behavior. In some cases, attempting to reason with people with AD may not work, especially if they mistake others for people that they do not like. Logic also may not work, especially with people who are having visual or auditory hallucinations. Usually, COTAs can identify the event that precipitated the unwanted behavior and make adjustments that might prevent it, stop it, or decrease the likelihood of recurrence. Three problem-solving tools can help to refocus unwanted behavior: the Behavioral Profile, the Behavioral Analysis, and the Behavioral Observation Form.

The Behavioral Profile is a tool used to examine the situation. COTAs can ask themselves the following thought-provoking questions: WHAT exactly is happening? WHY has the behavior happened, and WHAT was the antecedent? WHO is involved, and WHERE is the behavior exhibited? WHEN does the behavior usually occur? WHAT now?

The Behavioral Analysis outlines the specific behavior by focusing on the client's actions and defining the antecedent or possible causes. In addition, it outlines acceptable approaches and interventions with attention to the impact on the family, environment, and activity (Box 20-3).

The Behavior Observation Form is used to determine a behavioral pattern involving the time of day and possible antecedents. This form can help COTAs and other health care workers make appropriate changes for reducing or refocusing difficult behaviors (Fig. 20-3).

The challenge of identifying the source of the difficult or unwanted behavior and a solution to the problem also requires critical reasoning. The following are some questions that COTAs can ask themselves to help with the critical reasoning process: What is this behavior "saying"? Whose problem is it? What are some environmental factors that might be contributing to the behavior?

The story of Alfonso, an elder in an AD special care unit, illustrates the importance of critical reasoning in addressing difficult or unwanted behaviors. Alfonso tries constantly to go out the door because he thinks it is time to go to work. Possible reasons for his attempts to leave include the time of day, that he sees visitors leaving with their hats and coats, and lack of involvement in meaningful activities. The staff may not be trained to redirect him when his anxiety and agitation increases, the day room may be too noisy, or he may believe that the intercom voice is calling him to the phone. The COTA might consider the following options: asking him to help with a project (he might forget his need to leave), painting the exit door the same color as the walls on either side so it appears less obvious, involving Alfonso in a meaningful activity (drawing ideas from his life story), and spending some quality time with Alfonso.

Audrey is another person in the same unit. She often becomes combative when performing ADL functions, especially showering. In fact, she strikes the COTA during an assessment of showering. The COTA considers possible causes for this behavior: Did Audrey formerly

BOX 20-3

Problem: Pacing, or Wandering, or Both

Behavior Analysis Approach

Behaviors exhibited
- Pacing with increases in speed, intensity, and length of time; unable to respond to normal fatigue
- Trying to exit area without supervision
- Displaying increased agitation, anxiety, frustration, pushing, or kicking
- Seemingly lost; packing and leaving
- Searching behavior for something unattainable (for example, mother)
- Inappropriately going into areas/rooms not their own

Possible cause or antecedent
- May have feelings of fearfulness, insecurity
- May be reflecting on a past life role such as being in the workforce or being a parent
- May want to escape
- May be feeling out of control or sensing overmanipulation by others
- May be searching for something familiar or something lost
- May be acting consistent with former habits (always "on the go") or doing a stress-reducing activity
- May reflect need for self-stimulation as a method to reestablish sense of well-being
- May be expressing a physical need such as hunger, constipation, or illness
- May result from anxiety, boredom, hyperenvironmental or hypoenvironmental stimulation

Interventions with the resident
- Ask what the wandering is "telling" you: whether the client is hungry, needs to void, feels uncomfortable, is really lost.
- Identify positive aspects of the pacing/wandering.
- When attempting redirection, use a calm approach with eye contact.
- Use distraction techniques to break up the pacing pattern (offer to sit with the elder, have a glass of juice).
- Monitor elders for unwanted weight loss and excessive fatigue.
- Monitor elders for increased risks for falls and compromised safety.
- Have elders wear Medic-Alert ID bracelet of Alzheimer's Association's "Safe Return" program.
- Take photographs for the police, if elopement is a factor.
- Avoid stressful situations such as excessive environmental stimulation, too many people present, or overwhelming demands.
- Provide regular and consistent routines with familiar staff and caregivers.
- Develop a "Head Count" system for elders at high risk for elopement.

Family/Caregiver focus
- Discuss treatment approaches.
- Provide information on policies and procedures.
- Provide information such as the phone number of the local Alzheimer's Association chapter and their "Safe Return" program.
- Instruct not to contradict the elder's stories; instead, they should assure the elder that everything will be all right. This helps to facilitate a sense of security and reduces feelings of fearfulness.
- Recommend to not overdramatize entrances, exits, and promises to return.
- Encourage walks with the elder and usage of walking areas, "discover" paths, or fitness trails.
- Inform of possible risks for elopement even when the treatment area has a security system.
- Encourage use of local support groups for discussions with others.

Facility adaptations
- Provide environmental changes and sensory stimulation to decrease stress and restlessness, and to increase physical well-being, gross motor skills, appetite and healthy fatigue.
- Allow for environmental changes that promote purposeful ways to spend time.
- Remove environmental cues that suggest leaving the facility, such as coats and suitcases.
- Use familiar objects in rooms that facilitate a sense of comfort and security.
- Install Dutch doors, if permitted by regulations.
- Design walking areas, "discover" paths, or fitness trails within the care setting that offer safe, monitored spaces for pacing.

(Continued)

BOX 20-3

Problem: Pacing, or Wandering, or Both—cont'd

Behavior Analysis Approach

- Develop procedures to follow such as periodic unit safety checks and checks for missing persons.
- Provide routine orientation and escorts for new admissions.
- Alert visitors to facility procedures. For example, when leaving an area visitors should turn around and check that wandering elders have not followed them out of the door.
- Employ experienced, trained staff who know the elders.
- Introduce the elder to all staff, especially those near the doors (for example, switchboard operators and receptionists).
- Write problems/interventions on a kardex after identifying any positive aspects from the physical activity of pacing and wandering.

Activity
- Support physical exercise to promote overall wellness.
- Offer to walk with the elder as a meaningful activity. Suggest that the elder help out by taking letters to be mailed, visiting a friend, or picking up laundry.
- Establish a walking club, keep track of miles walked, and provide club t-shirts.
- Provide supervised outings with a focus on safety and the reduction of elopement risks.
- Offer expressive arts that include large muscle groups and movement or dancing activities.
- Present routine, familiar, normalized activities that promote sense of connectedness, respect, and meaningfulness.
- Set up a fitness trail that includes repetitive upper and lower extremity movements such as doing pulley activities, finger climbing ladders, and deep knee bends. Train volunteers and family members to involve the elders with the trail's activities.

Name:						
Date	Time	Observed activity and behavior	Behavior			Observer
			Trigger (What started it)	Intervention (What stopped it)	Time elapsed • Before stopping • Stayed stopped	

FIGURE 20-3   Behavioral Observation Form.

take baths, and is she unhappy with the change in her routine? Is Audrey a very private person, and is she embarrassed that someone is helping her? Did she react to the COTA's tone of voice? Is Audrey getting sick and unable to report it? Is she too tired when the shower is scheduled? Is she experiencing chronic pain such as arthritis, which may be upsetting her? Does she feel rushed? Has the showering task been simplified enough so that she can participate and feel in control? The COTA then considers the following behavioral interventions: asking Audrey to help wash down the shower, singing Audrey's favorite hymn with her while she showers, postponing the shower for another time, and allowing Audrey to bathe with some of her clothes on or wrapping her in a bath blanket during the bathing process.

As illustrated by the preceding examples, handling the behavioral difficulties of elders who have AD can be a trial and error process until COTAs identify solutions that work. Each elder will respond differently. Different techniques, based on the person's abilities, can succeed one time and fail the next. Even when COTAs cannot ascertain the exact reason for the behaviors, they can try the following intervention techniques. Distraction is a helpful technique, especially if the person is agitated. COTAs can be creative with ideas for distraction that involve the person in a meaningful activity, such as listening to music or offering a snack. **Rescuing** is another distraction technique: When one caregiver is in conflict with the client, a second caregiver responds by "rescuing" that person. This technique is illustrated by the following example. Sally, a nursing assistant, says to Theresa, the resident, "Don't go out the door." If Amy, the COTA, approaches Theresa in the same fashion, Theresa might feel outnumbered. Conversely, if Amy says, "Sally, Theresa and I want to be alone; please leave us," Theresa might feel "rescued" and go with Amy.

Inappropriate timing, attempts to manipulate the elder to fit a schedule, and unrealistic performance expectations can cause negative behavior such as hitting. Consequently, caregivers must be aware of the elder's mood before approaching with an ADL or social event.

TREATMENT
Observations, Screening, and Assessment

The COTA/occupational therapist (OTR) team may collaborate in the administration of the following evaluations. The Folstein Mini-Mental State is a short and simple quantitative measure of cognitive performance. This measure is a questionnaire in five areas of cognition, including orientation, registration (memory), attention, and calculation, as well as recall and language (following oral and written instructions) (Folstein, Folstein, & McHugh, 1975). The Global Deterioration Scale measures clinical characteristics at seven levels based on the progressive stages of AD (Reisberg et al., 1982).

The Allen Cognitive Performance Tests and the Routine Task Inventory examines cognitive function through completion of tasks (Allen, 1985). The levels of function help predict behavior and effects on ADL functions. These levels range from the ability to use complex information and perform ADL functions accurately and safely to severe deficits in recognition and use of familiar objects. This assessment includes information on communication, response to tasks, and need for task simplification. It also addresses the role of the therapist during treatment. (See Chapter 7 for a more detailed explanation of these tests.)

The Cognitive Performance Test is a standardized functional assessment instrument designed for the evaluation of Allen cognitive levels (Burns & Mortimer, 1993). Six functional tasks—dressing, shopping, making toast, making phone calls, doing laundry, and traveling—comprise the test. This test also looks at the person's abilities to process information in relation to functional performance.

The importance of the COTA being an integral part of the overall treatment team with other disciplines cannot be stressed enough (Lane, Trudeau, Hewitt, Bloom-Charette, Morris, & Volicer, 2000). The continuous development of dementia-specific assessments provides the treatment team with sensitive, appropriate tools that not only bring together information about the elder's challenges but encourage the recognition of the client's personhood and how to build on current strengths and abilities. For example, the Person, Environment, Occupation measurement model helps to determine how AD affects the function of both the person with disease and his or her family (Baum, Perlmutter, & Edwards, 2000).

Treatment Planning

OT for people with AD involves attention to self-care skills, communication, mobility, and safety. Areas to address in treatment planning include decreased attention span, inability to initiate tasks, difficulty with sequencing tasks, impaired judgment, and overall wellness. Therefore, in a special care unit, the plan of care should emphasize OT.

Treatment planning begins with establishing a cognitive and functional baseline and includes ability-based goals. These goals should identify functional capacity and needs to restore, maintain, or improve skills. The goals should focus on abilities and opportunities for participation in activities that support cognitive, physical, and psychosocial wellness. These goals should include interventions that enable **person-centered** caregiving and refocus difficult behaviors in a supportive and safe environment.

Treatment planning should include the use of assessment and observation to measure changes in functional status. The process of treatment planning includes providing and suggesting continuous modifications and adaptations of approaches, such as task simplification and cueing.

The elder's life story may be used as the basis for treatment that focuses on past (and present) wisdom and experiences. Treatment planning also involves assessing all aspects of treatment support and factors that lead to negative responses, including environmental components. For example, Andrew's limited attention span prohibited him from eating more than a few mouthfuls of each meal. He was seated in a large dining room with five other people at his table. Music was played on the tape deck, and the staff often talked loudly with each other. When the COTA suggested relocating Andrew to a small dining area where the tables seated two and reducing the environmental stimulation, he was able to focus on his food and complete his meal.

Treatment Intervention

OT treatment interventions consider the effects of dementia on the elder's cognitive abilities and well-being. Success with treatment interventions entails many crucial components, including the COTA's flexibility and creativity. Success may need to be redefined, as exemplified by Beverly a resident of a special care unit. Beverly liked to wear a yellow floral blouse and her favorite orange and black plaid skirt. She was proud of her ability to select and dress independently, although some disapproved of her choices.

Equally important for successful treatment intervention is the COTA's nonverbal approach. It should reflect acceptance and respect for the elder with AD. To ensure success, treatment interventions should not place elders in situations in which their inabilities may lead to failure. For example, Clara had always been a talented knitter of lovely sweaters. Her ability to do intricate stitches became impaired as her dementia progressed. The COTA set up the stitches on large needles and helped her get started knitting squares using a basic stitch. Clara was able to knit the simple squares for a baby blanket and was delighted in the recognition of her success. This activity could be further adapted by involving Clara in winding yarn as her knitting abilities diminish.

Applying life history and experiences to functional abilities also is meaningful. For example, Sara, a 78-year-old mother of five, responds to normalization activities such as washing dishes, hanging laundry, and sweeping floors. These activities provide tactile stimulation, lower and upper body range of motion, strengthening, trunk stabilization, and fine hand motor skills.

COTAs can use their skills in analyzing activities to identify steps toward task simplification. Harry was able to dress himself independently when each item of clothing was placed on his bed in the appropriate sequence for dressing. Successful treatment interventions also should focus on working with elders to promote active participation and collaboration. Charles had lost interest in feeding himself but accepted the COTA's suggestion to have the caregiver place a hand over his hand. That way

he could continue to feed himself with assistance rather than being fed by others.

When possible, treatment interventions should be provided in appropriate and familiar settings. For example, Millie was unable to experience success with simple dressing tasks when she attempted them in the clinic. However, when the COTA arrived at Millie's bedside early each morning, Millie was able to use visual cues found in her bedroom, including the bureau and closet, to trigger self-dressing skills.

Activities of Daily Living

COTAs can make a significant contribution to the well-being of elders with AD and enhance their quality of life by supporting ADL functions. Understanding task breakdown, task simplification, and appropriate treatment approaches enables these elders to become involved in performing these familiar skills. This understanding can be facilitated by using one-step commands and visual cueing, including objects or gestures. The use of the Allen's stage levels can be a helpful measure of the elder's level of functioning (Allen, 1985).

Difficulties with ADL functions associated with dementia include decreased attention span, limited ability to follow directions, and increased length of time to complete tasks. Other difficulties include problems with sequencing, perception, and body awareness. Emotional responses of fear, paranoia, and reactions to excessive environmental stimulation that are real or imagined also can influence ADL functioning. Beck, Baldwin, Modlin, and Lewis (1990) described how the caregivers' perceptions of aggressive behavior in nursing home residents with cognitive impairments affect ADL outcomes.

COTAs working on ADL functions will be most successful when they use creative problem solving. Therapy requires working *with* elders, not doing *to* or *for* them (Hellen, 1998). COTAs should do everything possible to make ADL functions meaningful. The use of distraction techniques (for example, singing and holding items such as costume jewelry, scarves, and neckties) should be part of daily care. The COTA's attitude, approach, and direct involvement are key components in supporting the elder's quality of life.

COTAs should consider the timing when working on ADL functions. Often, these decisions are based on knowing the elder and responding to nonverbal language that suggests the best and worst times for these activities. Sometimes, COTAs must come back several times because many elders with AD are sensitive to being rushed. For example, Charles appeared agitated when the COTA wanted to work on dressing skills. After several attempts the COTA decided to return later. At that time, Charles was calmer and accepting of the activity.

Assisting with ADL functions can also provide opportunities for COTAs to monitor the elder's physical well-being and safety. Elders with AD often do not report bruises, rashes, and blisters. Decreased cognitive ability and judgment, combined with an unawareness of perceptual difficulties, may lead to unsafe situations. Elders may eat dirt or plants, walk on wet floors, put their shoes on the wrong feet, forget necessary items such as glasses, misjudge a chair seat and fall, or scald themselves in the shower because they do not know how to turn on the cold water—all these are examples of potential dangers.

When working with elders on ADL functions, COTAs should always focus on abilities by encouraging active involvement. The techniques of hand-over-hand guidance, chaining, and bridging can be used. Hand-over-hand guidance may help the elder complete the ADL task. With **chaining,** the caregiver begins a task by putting one hand over the elder's hand and continuing until the elder can take over and complete the task. For example, Astrid had no idea what a toothbrush was or how to use it. However, when the COTA placed it in her hand and guided it to her mouth to start the brushing action, Astrid was able to complete the task independently (Fig. 20-4). With these techniques the palmar surfaces of the hand or the surface receiving touch during a handshake can be a more "accepting" surface than the back of the hand. COTAs should establish contact with the elder's palm before moving their hand around to the dorsal surface if needed for assisting the elder during activities.

With **bridging,** elders who are unable to perform any part of the daily living task can focus their attention by holding the same object the caregiver is using. This technique

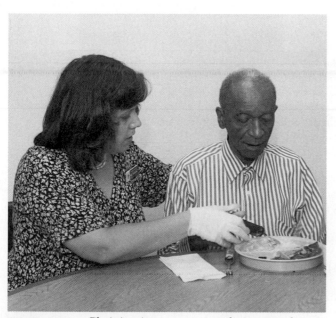

FIGURE 20-4 Chaining is a common technique used to facilitate participation in activities of daily living.

also can help to decrease anxiety. For example, Allan could not shave. The COTA demonstrated to the caregivers a bridging technique to try with Allan. She placed a turned-on electric razor in his hand so he could feel the vibration while she shaved him with another electric razor. By holding a razor, Allan was better able to focus attention on the task (Hellen, 1998).

The creativity and flexibility of COTAs can promote the remaining abilities of elders and their willingness to be actively involved in daily life tasks (Box 20-4). Knowledge of the client's past routines is helpful during ADL functions.

Using Adapted Equipment

Elders with AD often refuse or misuse adapted equipment. Improper use may affect the elder's safety, especially if the item does not look familiar. For example, a plate guard may appear so strange that the elder with AD might spend the mealtime trying to remove it from the plate. Sometimes, large, built-up handles on eating utensils may feel so different that clients do not use them. Reachers and other metal devices used for ADL functions can be used as weapons. Flatware with large handles and scoop dishes can be helpful because they closely resemble their ordinary counterparts. Adapting the environment by using color contrast between objects, pictures, words, labels, and arrows is often the best way to cue for successful involvement in ADL functions.

Using Activities to Promote Well-Being

Activities can be adapted for individuals and groups. The objectives of therapeutic activities are enhancing meaning, encouraging active participation, and ensuring success. All of life's activities can be used as treatment modalities. Suggestions for cognitive activities are adapted trivia games, word puzzles, rhyming games, singing of familiar songs, and reminiscence. Others include spelling games, simple crafts, clothes-sorting, cards, and Life Story "book clubs." Suggestions for physical activities include parachute exercises; dancing; and tossing, hitting, and kicking balls and balloons. An exercise program may include use of handheld wands, light weights, scarves, and fabrics. Psychosocial activities include parties, service projects, grooming tasks, celebrations of special days, field trips, and pet care. Worship and related spiritual activities may offer elders with dementia a sense of the familiar, well-being, and security. Recommendations for normalizing activities are folding and hanging up laundry, dusting and sweeping, sorting silverware, and shining shoes (Hellen, 1998).

Communication with and Teaching Caregivers

OT treatment of elders who have AD focuses on maintaining functional abilities and preventing secondary complications. These objectives can be achieved by

BOX 20-4

Suggestions for Provision of Activities of Daily Living Support for Elders with Alzheimer's Disease

Bathing

1. Know whether client prefers a bath or shower; use handheld shower head.
2. If privacy is an issue, elder can bathe with some clothing on or with a bath blanket.
3. If needed, elder may wash one part of the body per day until able to accept total bathing.
4. Consider safety by using adaptations such as bath seats, grab bars, and floor mats.
5. Create a warm and homelike bathing environment. Placing colorful beach towels on the walls can help reduce the room's echo and loud water sounds. The towels also can be used to wrap elders if they become agitated during clothing removal.
6. Consider alternatives such as having a family member present to assist with bathing to help reduce the elder's anxiety.

Shaving

1. Use a mirror unless elders do not recognize themselves or feel that they are being "watched."
2. Use a bridging technique with elders incapable of actually shaving. Have them hold an electric razor that they can see, feel, and hear while shaving them with another electric shaver.

Oral care

1. Use a child-sized tooth brush.
2. Pretend to be brushing your own teeth and encourage elders to mirror the activity.
3. Use bridging technique of asking the elder to hold an extra set of dentures while removing the elder's dentures.
4. Set up a simulated dental chair and announce that the dentist has sent you to assist with dental care.
5. Set up a monitor system so that presence of dentures are checked after each meal in case elders have wrapped them up in a napkin for disposal.

Dressing

1. Suggest clothing one size larger for dressing ease. Keep the clothes appropriate to the elder's past lifestyle.
2. Use verbal and visual cues to simplify each step, and always thank the elders for helping.
3. If elders become anxious, ask them to show you how the clothing items are put on.
4. If possible, use washable shoes with Velcro closures.
5. Use 100% cotton clothing because it does not retain the odor of urine.
6. Ask the elder to sit when dressing, especially if balance is a concern.

Toileting

1. Be aware of elder's past toileting routines and habits.
2. Use pictures of toilets with the word "toilet" on the bathroom doors.
3. Determine whether the bathroom mirror prohibits elders from using the toilet because they do not recognize their image and think someone else is there.
4. Be sure the toilet seat color contrasts with the floor. Change the seat or use a washable rug around the toilet base.
5. Use key words to remind the elder about the task. Often, the words they used when toilet training their children work well.
6. Offer the elder something (for example, a magazine) to hold or do while seated on the toilet.
7. Never refer to pads for incontinence as "diapers" (use terms such as panties or shorts).
8. Have different types of incontinence products available. Don't assume that a full-sized item is needed immediately. For example, a pad placed within a panty can be used if urine is leaked.
9. Use suspenders to keep full-sized incontinence products in place.

Eating*

1. Observe eating for safety problems such as overstuffing the mouth, not chewing before swallowing, and eating nonedibles (napkins, foam cups). If the elder is storing food in the mouth, check for a clear swallow. Obtain a swallowing evaluation if a problem is apparent.
2. Offer the meal in a quiet area to decrease distractions and to improve attention span. If the food needs to be set up, always do that out of the elder's sight. This prevents reinforcement of the elder's inability to perform certain simple tasks.
3. Provide color contrast between the food and the plate and the plate and the table.
4. Avoid plastic utensils, which are easily bitten and broken.

*See discussion of dysphagia in Chapter 18 for more specific information about safe eating.

(Continued)

BOX 20-4

Suggestions for Provision of Activities of Daily Living Support for Elders with Alzheimer's Disease—cont'd

5. Obtain, if appropriate, a dietary order for variation in food textures.
6. Simplify the meal by serving one item and one utensil at a time.
7. If elders will not sit to eat, use finger foods or have a small bowl that can be easily carried.
8. Incorporate food into a sandwich. Pureed food can be put into an ice cream cone to assist elders who want to continue self-feeding.
9. If elders are not eating and no medical reasons prohibit it, use sugar or honey on the food to increase palatability.
10. After a swallowing evaluation, if deemed appropriate, provide non-salty chicken or beef broth that can be poured over the food for a more "slurpy" consistency to facilitate an appropriate swallow.
11. If the elder needs to be fed, bridge the task by having the elder hold a spoon or plastic cup.
12. If the elder is disinterested in eating, alternate bites of hot and cold foods and sweet and nonsweet food.
13. When the elder appears to stop eating or has lost all interest in food, ask the family to identify the elder's "comfort foods" to facilitate reinterest in eating.
14. Foods such as mashed potatoes and gravy, pizza, and macaroni give a sense of well-being.
15. If weight loss is a problem, double the elder's breakfast.
16. Try to avoid commercial food supplements if possible by allowing time for the meal to be eaten and providing protein-enriched foods such as milkshakes.
17. Sit with the elders. Have something to eat or drink to reduce elders' anxiety that you don't have anything to eat and therefore must have some of theirs.

If elders refuse to eat because of not having money, provide a letter stating that their dues to your association (the name of your facility or place of practice) have been paid in full and meals are included in their membership.

tailoring communication and education to caregivers. Caregivers benefit from a variety of techniques, including written instruction and demonstration. The instructional method of requiring a "return demonstration" allows COTAs to observe first-hand that caregivers follow through with activities. Afterwards, the COTA can make necessary suggestions or corrections.

The COTA and OTR team can formulate a maintenance program (American Occupational Therapy Association, 1993). Contributing to a maintenance program may require COTAs to sensitize caregivers to the nature and progression of AD. An understanding of task breakdown and simplification, activity modification, behavioral interventions, supportive communications, and the need for flexibility is essential in maintenance programs.

TERMINAL STAGE ISSUES

Severe dementia, or terminal stage, is exhibited when the elder is oriented only to person and depends entirely on others for self-care. Defining the exact time of terminal, or end-stage, AD is difficult because of changes and variations in the disease process. For example, Vernon appeared to have entered the terminal stage because he had been refusing food for 2 weeks. When offered

familiar "comfort" foods from his past and sweet foods, he suddenly started to eat again.

Many elders at the terminal stage of AD are kept in bed or positioned in wheelchairs or recliners. Unfortunately, those kept in bed often lie in the fetal position. These elders are dependent on others for basic life functions and display an almost total loss of communication skills or the ability to express pain. To help make them more comfortable, COTAs may provide positioning suggestions and passive range-of-motion exercises. A caring touch, hand-over-hand movement, and various sensory activities may produce a response. Some people become ill with symptoms leading to pneumonia or other systemic problems shortly before death. This is an important time for supporting family members and staff caregivers.

REIMBURESEMENT FOR SERVICES

A functional outcome must be meaningful, utilitarian, and sustainable over time. Currently, maintenance of remaining abilities of elders with dementia, or any chronic illness, is not usually covered by third-party payers such as Medicare unless there is a need for "skilled" therapeutic coverage. Elders on Medicare Part A in Skilled Nursing Facilities under the Prospective Payment System (PPS) may qualify for therapy on the basis of their determined level of resources needed with the Resource Utilization Groups (Centers for Medicare and Medicaid Services [CMS], 2001) (see Chapter 6 for more details on the PPS system). For elders on Medicare Part B, the COTA/OTR team may address cognitive and physical impairment related to functional performance. Medicare will reimburse for cognitive disabilities that require "complex and sophisticated knowledge to identify current and potential capabilities" (CMS, 2001, p. 10). All levels of assistance from total to standby address both physical and cognitive components. Table 20-1 outlines only the cognitive components. Behavioral issues with cognitive impairment can be focused on if they require skilled OT services (CMS, 2001).

The COTA/OTR team may suggest a short-range program on the basis of continuous functional support, especially if a change in functional status has occurred. Often, elders with AD who receive Medicare reimbursement for care have an initial evaluation from OT. A maintenance program is then developed by the therapists and carried out by facility staff. Medicare will reimburse if skilled OT is needed to evaluate a "complex" patient to increase function or safety, and then to train staff to carry out the program (CMS, 2002; K. Warchol, personal communication, July, 2003). The OTR evaluates the elder and establishes the plan of care. The COTA may train caregivers to carry out the plan. OT practitioners may manage the elder for reevaluation when significant changes occur in functional status. As discussed in Chapter 6, recent memorandums from Medicare prevent automatic denials just because a person has the diagnosis of AD and mention benefits for therapeutic

TABLE 20-1

Medicare Cognitive Levels of Assistance	
Assistance level	**Cognitive assistance**
Total assistance	"Total assistance is the need for 100 percent assistance by one or more persons to perform all cognitive assistance to elicit a functional response to an external stimulation." "A cognitively impaired patient requires total assistance when documentation shows external stimuli are required to elicit automatic actions such as swallowing or responding to auditory stimuli. Skills of an occupational therapist are needed to identify and apply strategies for eliciting appropriate, consistent automatic responses to external stimuli."
Maximal assistance	"Maximum assistance is the need for 75 percent … cognitive assistance to perform gross motor actions in response to direction." "A cognitively impaired patient, at this level, may need proprioceptive stimulation and/or one-to-one demonstration by the occupational therapist due to the patient's lack of cognitive awareness of other people or objects."
Minimum assistance	"Moderate assistance is the need for 50 percent assistance by one person … or constant cognitive assistance to sustain/complete simple, repetitive activities safely." "The records submitted should state how a cognitively impaired patient requires intermittent one-to-one demonstration or intermittent cueing (physical or verbal) throughout the activity. Moderate assistance is needed when the occupational therapist/care-giver needs to be in the immediate environment to progress the patient through a sequence to complete an activity. This level of assistance is required to halt continued repetition of a task and to prevent unsafe, erratic or unpredictable actions that interfere with appropriate sequencing."
Standby assistance	"Standby assistance is the need for supervision by one person for the patient to perform new procedures adapted by the therapist for safe and effective performance. A patient requires such assistance when errors are demonstrated or the need for safety precautions are not always anticipated by the patient."
Independent status	"Independent status means that no physical or cognitive assistance is required to perform functional activities. Patients at this level are able to implement the selected courses of action, demonstrate lack of errors and anticipate safety hazards in familiar and new situations."

Data from Centers for Medicare and Medicaid Services (CMS). (2002). Medicare program integrity manual [WWW page]. URL http://cms.hhs.gov/manuals/108_pim/pim83c06.pdf
The Physical Levels of Assistance are not included in this chart.

intervention with this diagnosis (CMS, 2001, 2002). (See Chapter 6 for a more in-depth discussion of Medicare policy.)

CONCLUSION

COTAs can make a unique contribution to elders with AD. COTAs can treat these elders from the initial stages of forgetfulness and poor judgment by offering strategies for continuing independence. COTAs may also provide advice about late-stage care by focusing on positioning, feeding, and responses to sensory activities. Understanding the changes that occur as dementia progresses challenges elders, caregivers, and families to pursue creative and supportive solutions for daily care. The holistic programs and care provided by COTAs support the abilities and well-being of elders. When offered activity-focused care, elders with dementia can have meaningful lives.

CASE STUDY

Mildred is 78 years of age and has mid-stage AD. Mildred was formerly a teacher and experienced a happy family life with her husband of 58 years and their two sons. She has been widowed for the last 5 years. Mildred was originally brought to the special care unit where she currently resides when she was found wandering outside during the cold winter months.

At the special care unit the COTA helped to assess Mildred's functional status. The COTA identified the following abilities: Mildred follows one-step directions, responds to multisensory cueing, maintains strong socialization skills, and refers to her former profession by often mentioning her past role as a teacher. She also mentions her past interest in the activities of cooking and sewing.

Mildred functions at Allen's Cognitive Level 3. The COTA observed that she was forgetful, with limited instructional carryover. Mildred experiences problems with sequencing ADL functions. She often becomes anxious, which leads to combativeness during ADL functions, especially bathing. Other assessment findings included the inability to toilet independently and use multiple utensils with meals. Communication challenges included receptive and expressive understanding of words, especially nouns.

The COTA instructed all staff members who work with Mildred to consider her strengths, as well as her attention span deficits and feelings of depression, as she attempts to cope with her disease.

CASE STUDY QUESTIONS

1 Considering Mildred's case, how can visual triggers and written phrases be used to help Mildred be as independent as possible?
2 What anxiety-reducing approaches can be explored? What specific interventions can be used during bathing?
3 How can the COTA develop a system for sequencing Mildred's clothing?
4 What environmental issues might need to be addressed, especially in the bath/shower room?
5 What suggestions can be incorporated as mealtime interventions for promoting successful dining?

6 If Mildred can find the toilet, what strategies can enable her to remain continent?
7 How can the COTA use ADL functions as therapeutic modalities for reducing feelings of depression and helplessness?
8 How can the COTA make Mildred's care "person centered" and "activity focused"?

CHAPTER REVIEW QUESTIONS

1 In reference to the entire chapter, what are the basic symptoms of Alzheimer's disease (AD) and how do they affect elders with the disease and their caregivers?
2 Identify six ways to facilitate communication with elders who have dementia.
3 How can a functional assessment be used to develop treatment goals?
4 List three guidelines for the provision of activities of daily living support to elders functioning at the mid-stage level of AD.
5 Outline six specific mealtime adaptations for elders with a short attention span.
6 List steps for getting dressed using task simplification.
7 What are possible antecedents and appropriate interventions for agitation?
8 Why do people with dementia wander, and how can the risk for elopement be decreased?
9 Give specific examples of ways activity-focused care supports certified occupational therapy assistants' treatment interventions.
10 Describe strategies to adapt the activity of folding laundry to address the elder's cognitive, physical, psychosocial, and normalization needs.

REFERENCES

Allen, C. K. (1985). *Occupational therapy for psychiatric diseases: Measurement and management of cognitive disabilities.* Boston: Little Brown.

Allen, C. K. (1999). *Stage one workshop Allen's cognitive levels.* Allen Conferences, Inc. [WWW page]. URL http://www.allen-cognitive-levels.com/products.htm

Alzheimer's Association. (1999). Fact sheet. Chicago: The Association.

American Occupational Therapy Association. (1993). Occupational therapy roles. *American Journal of Occupational Therapy, 47*(12), 1087.

Aronson, M. K. (1994). *Reshaping dementia care.* Thousand Oaks, CA: Sage Publications.

Baum, C., Perlmutter, M., & Edwards, D. (2000). Measuring function in Alzheimer's disease. *Alzheimer's Care Quarterly, 1*(3), 44-61.

Beck, C., Baldwin, B., Modlin, T., & Lewis, S. (1990). Caregivers' perceptions of aggressive behavior in cognitively impaired nursing home residents. *Journal of Neuroscience Nursing, 6*(3), 169-172.

Burns, T., & Mortimer, J. (1993). The cognitive performance test: A new approach to functional assessment in AD. *Journal of Geriatric and Psychiatric Neurology, 7*(1), 46.

Centers for Medicare and Medicaid Services. (CMS). (2001). Skilled nursing facility prospective payment system refinements and

consolidated billing quick reference guide [WWW page].
URL http://www.cms.gov/medlearn/refsnf.asp

Centers for Medicare and Medicaid Services. (CMS). (2002). Medicare program integrity manual [WWW page]. URL http://cms.hhs.gov/manuals/108_pim/pim83c06.pdf

Evans, D. A. (1990). Estimated prevalence of Alzheimer's disease in the United States. *Milbank Quarterly, 68,* 267.

Folstein, M. F., Folstein, S. E., & McHugh, P. R. (1975). Mini mental state: A practical method for grading the cognitive state of patients for the clinician. *Journal of Psychiatric Research, 12,* 189.

Hellen, C. R. (1998). *Alzheimer's disease: Activity focused care.* Boston: Butterworth-Heinemann.

Kitwood, T., & Bredin, K. (1992). Towards a theory of dementia care: Personhood and well-being. *Ageing and Society, 12,* 269-287.

Kovach, C. (Ed). (1996). *Late stage dementia care: A basic guide.* Washington, DC: Taylor & Francis.

Lane, P., Trudeau, S. A., Hewitt, S., & Bloom-Charette, L. (2000). Interdisciplinary assessment of persons with Alzheimer's Disease and other progressive dementias. Alzheimer's Care Quarterly, *1*(3), 28.

Working with Elders Who Have Psychiatric Conditions

L. MARGARET DRAKE

KEY TERMS

deinstitutionalization, nursing homes, mood disorders, anxiety disorders, agoraphobia, panic disorder, social phobia, posttraumatic stress disorder, acute stress disorder, schizophrenia, hypochondriasis, drug abuse, dual diagnosis, personality disorder, psychotropic medication, group treatment

CHAPTER OBJECTIVES

1. Understand the prevalence of mental illness among elders.
2. Become acquainted with psychiatric diagnoses common among institutionalized elders.
3. Describe the importance of considering both mental health and medical conditions when working with elders.
4. Identify assessments commonly used by occupational therapy practitioners with elders who have mental illness.
5. Describe treatment approaches commonly used with elders who have mental illness.

In most health care settings, elders are treated for all types of medical diagnoses. Often, these diagnoses are accompanied by less obvious psychiatric conditions. For example, an elder who sustained a recent stroke and does not want to attend or participate in occupational therapy treatment may be experiencing depression, as well as an elder with cancer who does not seem to care about his or her appearance. Although mental health problems are strongly associated with disability and poor performance, few people identify mental health problems as the reason for poor functional performance (Sadavoy,

Lazarus, Jarvik, & Grossberg, 1996; Stahl, 1996). Many researchers suspect that institutionalized elders often have untreated mental illness (Smith, 1994). If certified occupational therapy assistants (COTAs) are not aware of the need to monitor and address mental health conditions, they may overlook treating the whole person. Elders who have mental health conditions often are found in nonmental health settings because they need additional assistance after discharge from other care facilities. **Deinstitutionalization,** or the release of elders with mental illness from state hospitals, also contributes problem. Elders who have mental illness should be approached in the same way as any other occupational therapy client. Therefore, the COTA must recognize and address mental health conditions in elders in all treatment settings, not merely in mental health facilities. This chapter considers primary mental health conditions of elders and suggests strategies for occupational therapy treatment.

CARE OF ELDERS WITH MENTAL ILLNESS
General Facts

The deinstitutionalization movement of the 1960s and 1970s led to the closing of many state mental hospital wards that previously cared for many elders with mental illness. Before deinstitutionalization, each state received funding to pay for this care. When officials in state governments realized that this financial burden could be shifted to the federal government, they began referring these elders to **nursing homes**. A consequence of this situation is that more elders with mental illness live in nursing homes than in mental hospitals (Wagenaar, Mickus, Gaumer, & Colenda, 2002). In addition, because of the trend toward shorter stays in acute inpatient mental health care units, many elders with mental illness are sent to nursing homes for stabilization of medications. These situations have made nursing homes the major caregivers for elders with mental illness.

Consumer groups such as The National Alliance for the Mentally Ill have lobbied for legislation to make mental health treatment more accessible and equitable. Mental Health Parity legislation (P.L. 104-204) has been passed in Congress to provide more equitable insurance benefits. Provider groups such as psychiatrists, mental health nurses, social workers, and occupational therapists (OTRs) also have lobbied for such legislation. Despite this situation on a national public policy level, which reflects a societal concern for mental illness, on a local level many staff members of nursing homes have little or no training in mental health (Wagenaar, Mickus, Gaumer, & Colenda, 2002). Failure to recognize depression is a continuing problem in nursing home care (Wagenaar, Mickus, Gaumer, & Colenda, 2002). Consequently, COTAs educated in psychosocial care can be important advocates for elders and a tremendous help to other staff members at the facility.

Many medical conditions coexist with psychiatric disorders. Because this is such a common occurrence, a whole chapter is devoted to this problem in the fourth edition of the *Diagnostic and Statistical Manual of Mental Disorders (DSM-IV)* (American Psychiatric Association, 1994). This manual of mental illness categorizes and defines all known mental disorders in the United States. By using this manual, clinicians can easily find diagnoses and symptoms of each disease. The manual includes scales to measure the severity of each dysfunction, as well as the disturbance of relationships. Mood, psychotic, and anxiety disorders caused by medical conditions are among the diagnostic categories discussed in this manual.

The functional performance of many elders is severely handicapped by mental disabilities (Sadavoy, Lazarus, Jarvik, & Grossberg, 1996; Stahl, 1996). Limitations may occur in any of the performance areas or contexts relevant to occupational therapy. For example, the memory deficits that occur with depression may affect the ability of elders to follow their medication schedule. The following sections discuss specific mental health conditions of the elder population and suggested treatment interventions for COTAs.

DEPRESSION

The term **mood disorder** describes various kinds of depression. Two basic types of mood disorders exist: those that involve a depressed mood only and those that involve fluctuation in mood. Major depression is the most severe form of mood disorder. It involves only a depressed state. A less severe form of this disorder is known as *dysthymic disorder*. The most severe mood fluctuation disorder is bipolar disorder. A less severe form of this disorder is cyclothymic disorder (American Psychiatric Association, 1994).

Researchers report varied statistics on the prevalence of depression among the elder population. Some studies show that approximately 5% to 15% of those older than 65 years have active, current mood disorders (Sadavoy, Lazarus, Jarvik, & Grossberg, 1996). Other studies indicate that 25% of elders experience a form of depression (Johnson, 1995). By 70 years of age, approximately 6% of elders have a mood disorder (Kales & Valenstein, 2002). Depression and all other forms of mental illness are reported to be more prevalent among institutionalized elders than among those in the community (George, 1993). Moreover, depression usually lasts longer in elders than in younger people. Female elders are more likely than male elders to be depressed. Even though the elder population contains many more females than males, figures on the prevalence of depression are calculated proportionally (Busse & Blazer, 1996). Since 1980 the rate of suicides among elders has increased from 9% to 13%. One elder commits suicide in the United States approximately every 90 minutes. This amounts to 18 elder suicides a day, or about 6500 a year. Almost 75,000 elder Americans killed themselves between 1980 and 1995. These elders account for one out of every five suicides committed in the United States (Sajatovic, 2002; Wagenaar, Mickus, Gaumer, & Colenda, 2002). Between 1980 and 1998, the rate of suicides for people between the ages of 80 and 84 years increased more than any other elder cohort. Firearms are the most common method for all suicides of people older than 65 years. Divorced or widowed elders are at much greater risk for suicide (Centers for Disease Control, 2003).

Major Depression

The symptoms most often associated with major depression are sadness, tears, feelings of emptiness and worthlessness, changes in eating and sleeping habits, slowed movements, complaints of fatigue, decreased concentration, and suicidal thoughts. For a diagnosis of major depression, these symptoms must last at least 2 weeks. Recognizing depression among elders is often difficult because other symptoms may mask this diagnosis. Often, elders blame dysfunction on physical problems rather than depression. However, certain symptoms are common (Box 21-1).

Depressed elders are more likely to neglect their personal hygiene. Because elders are more successful than other people when they attempt suicide (Scocco & De Leo, 2002), COTAs should be especially aware of this risk. Major depression can occur as a result of life events, such as the loss of a mate, home, and professional role. Consequently, the depression may be called *reactive* because the person is reacting to the event in an exaggerated way. If no apparent event or situation provoked the depression, it may be called *endogenous* (coming from within the person). The symptoms of reactive and endogenous depression are identical.

Mild Depression, or Dysthymic Disorder

Although symptoms of major depression are the ones most commonly recognized, those associated with mild depression, or dysthymic disorder can interfere with socialization and enjoyment of life. Elders with dysthymia have many symptoms associated with major depression, albeit in a less debilitating form. Symptoms of dysthymia are considered personality characteristics because they have been present for many years (American Psychiatric Association, 1994). Depressive symptoms become part of a diagnosis only when they impair function to the extent that the elder is unable to perform necessary tasks (Busse & Blazer, 1996). For example, an elder with Parkinson's disease who lacks the motivation to attempt activities of daily living (ADL) functions in treatment might be diagnosed as clinically depressed.

Bipolar Disorder

Fluctuating mood disorders are less common in elders. The mania occurring in bipolar disorder is much less common in elders than in younger people. Bipolar disorder is less likely to develop later in life if the individual did not experience his or her first manic episode before the age of 40 years (Sajatovic, 2002). The hyperactivity, impulsiveness, euphoria, and grandiosity usually associated with manic episodes of bipolar disorder in a younger person are more likely to be displayed as confusion, irritability, and increased suspiciousness in elders. Although elders with bipolar disorder may be treated with lithium like younger people, they are at increased risk for experiencing toxic effects, although there is a new low-dose lithium therapy that works better for many elders (Wilkinson, Holmes, Wollford, Stammers, & North, 2002). Consequently, COTAs must recognize the symptoms of lithium toxicity to identify it early in treatment, including nausea, cramping, vomiting, thirst, and polyuria or excessive urination. If symptoms are not identified early enough, tremors may develop, and elders may experience convulsions or go into a coma. Few outcome studies describe the treatment of elders with bipolar disorder (Busse & Blazer, 1996).

Cyclothymia

A less severe fluctuating disorder, cyclothymia, has symptoms that are similar to those of bipolar disorder but milder. For a diagnosis of cyclothymia, the person must have experienced these symptoms for more than 2 years. The onset of cyclothymia usually occurs early in life, and its symptoms are reflected in the person's personality; elders with cyclothymia may be described as moody or unpredictable (American Psychiatric Association, 1994).

BOX 21-1

Symptoms of Depression Among Elders

- Sad facial expression, poor posture, deep sighing, and frequent tears
- Inability to enjoy activities that previously brought pleasure
- Neglect of personal hygiene (for example, unwashed hair, unpleasant body odor, ragged fingernails)
- Weight change—usually associated with loss of appetite
- Increased preoccupation with physical problems
- Sleep difficulties such as frequent wakefulness at night and fatigue during the day
- Slowed movement in ambulation and self-care activities
- Fatigue that prevents initiation and completion of tasks
- Low self-esteem as demonstrated by self-deprecatory statements such as "I'm just not good at that anymore"
- Increased confusion as demonstrated by the tendency to get lost easily and forget dates and scheduled times
- Difficulty concentrating that interferes with ability to read and solve problems
- Indecisiveness as expressed by difficulty making simple choices between two options
- Suicidal thought as expressed by statements such as "I wish I were dead" and "Life is just too difficult. I want to end it all"

Causes of Late-Life Depression

Late-life depression, a term used by some gerontologists, may result from bereavement or a reduced activity level. In addition, physical and chemical changes such as gradual metabolic slowing of and decreased viability of the endocrine and neurotransmitter systems may contribute to the onset of late-life depression (Wagenaar, Mickus, Gaumer, & Colenda, 2002).

Complaints about changes in sleep patterns increase with aging. The amount of time spent sleeping decreases naturally in elders. Some theorists attribute this change to the decreased production of melatonin in the aging brain. Rapid eye movement sleep, which is associated with dreaming and completion of the sleep cycle, decreases in elders (Sadavoy, Lazarus, Jarvik, & Grossberg, 1996). COTAs should recommend traditional methods known to enhance sleep such as warm baths, darkness, relaxing music before sleep, and even guided imagery. However, the short attention span of many depressed clients may make some of these activities difficult.

A medical illness can itself cause reactive depression in elders. Once the cycle of depression starts, it tends to spiral downward. A reactive depression provoked by life events or losses may exacerbate other diseases. COTAs may be the first to recognize this secondary depression and recommend referral for psychiatric evaluation. Some medications also contribute to depression. When reviewing the medication section of the medical record, COTAs should pay particular attention to medications associated with depression (Box 21-2). If elders are taking any of these medications, the COTA should discuss this matter with the physician.

Treatment Intervention for Elders with Depression

In the assessment of elders with depression, both physical and social functioning are important considerations. Knowledge of traditional psychiatric symptoms also is important. If elders have poor social support before the diagnosis of depression, they will have this problem after discharge (Sadavoy, Lazarus, Jarvik, & Grossberg, 1996).

COTAs play an important role in differentiating depression from dementia. The term *pseudodementia* is sometimes used to describe a person who exhibits cognitive symptoms associated with dementia but actually caused by depression. A clue that may help COTAs differentiate between true organic dementia and depression is that elders with depression complain of cognitive problems (such as diminished memory, problem-solving difficulties, and the ability to concentrate), whereas elders with organic dementia usually deny that they have such problems. In addition, elders with depression appear sad, whereas elders with dementia usually appear indifferent or apathetic. When asked a question, elders with depression often say, "I don't know," whereas elders with dementia may attempt to cover the cognitive deficits by manufacturing a story in response (Sadock & Sadock, 2000).

Mental stimulation is an important part of treatment for depression. Remotivation therapy has been used successfully for a number of years to get depressed people involved again in daily activities (Ireland, 1972). Gradually over the years, it has been included in what is called "reality orientation therapy" (Mosey, 1986; Stein & Cutler 1998). This kind of therapy is usually done in a group. The therapist uses objects, pictures, pets, and holiday symbols to stimulate discussion and memories (Box 21-3).

Some general considerations for group work include avoiding rushing, which may increase stress and lower functional performance outcomes; allowing time for elders to focus on details; reducing irrelevant noise; and speaking loudly and clearly with regular pauses for those who process information slowly. Activities such as moving to music increase oxygen in elders' blood and consequently raise their mood. Music, particularly the blues, can be used to assist clients in expressing their feelings of depression (Pedersen, 1986) (Fig. 21-1).

BOX 21-2

Medications That Contribute to Depression
Analgesics Antianxiety drugs Sedatives and hypnotics Antihypertensive agents Antipsychotics Cancer chemotherapy agents Cortisone

BOX 21-3

Phases of Remotivation Groups
1. Greeting phase 2. Introduction to the discussion topic (by using various objects or media) 3. Open-ended questions for discussion, such as "What is your earliest memory of …?" 4. Discussion of the memories and ideas presented by the participants 5. The COTA expresses appreciation for the contributions of the group members

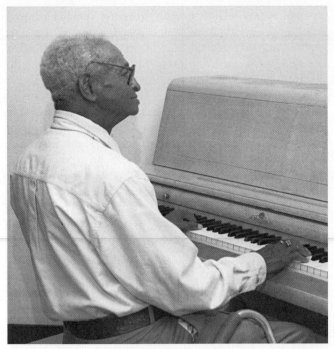

FIGURE **21-1** Music, especially the blues, can help elders to express their feelings.

Each elder who has depression reacts to the illness differently, and COTAs must interact with clients as individuals and focus treatment on what is meaningful to the elder—that is, be client centred (Law, 1998). In working with elders who have depression, COTAs obtain better results by speaking slowly and using the elder's name frequently. COTAs should be warm but not overly solicitous. In some cases, telling elders what to do may be more helpful than asking them to choose; people with depression often have difficulty making decisions. However, COTAs should permit elders to guide the intervention when they are ready to make choices. Interpersonal contacts with these clients should be frequent but short. COTAs should praise the elders' projects rather than the elders themselves, who are apt to reject personal praise. Some precautions include watching for signs of fatigue and supervision in the use of sharp tools to prevent accidents and suicide attempts. The number of therapists working with each elder should be limited. In addition, elders should be advised well in advance when a change is necessary.

Recommended activities include short-term projects that provide repetitive, structured, and well-defined routines, with few possibilities for frustration. Competitive activities and those that require high levels of concentration are best avoided until some improvement is apparent. COTAs should be aware of community resources such as support groups, which give a voice to the elder population. The role of COTAs may involve helping elders find addresses and telephone numbers of such organizations. Support groups have been identified as strong factors in the recovery of some patients (National Alliance for the Mentally Ill, 1995). Elder females may be referred to organizations such as the Older Women's League.

ANXIETY DISORDERS

Anxiety disorders are no more prevalent in elders than in younger people. However, elders tend to experience specific types of anxiety, including the fear of being a victim of crime or elder abuse. The fear of going out after dark is one of the main phobias experienced by elders. Nursing home residents who frequently witness the deaths of other residents may develop anxiety related to the fear of death. Other common anxieties involve the fear of cognitive problems such as memory loss and fear of injury or sickness. These anxiety disorders manifest themselves in elders with the same symptoms as in younger people (Box 21-4).

Anxiety disorders include agoraphobia, panic attacks, social phobia, and posttraumatic stress disorder (Sadavoy, Lazarus, Jarvik, & Grossberg, 1996).

Agoraphobia is a fear of specific situations from which the person cannot escape (Fig. 21-2). These fears may make elders afraid to leave their houses. Other common agoraphobic fears include being in crowds of people, crossing a bridge, and using various modes of travel, such as flying or being on a boat. An elder might be unwilling to go to the laundromat for fear of not being able to put the correct coins in the washing machine and being embarrassed.

Panic disorder is characterized by recurrent panic attacks. These attacks include symptoms such as heart palpitations, shaking, excessive sweating, shortness of

BOX **21-4**

Symptoms of Anxiety Among Elders

- Excessive worry about loved ones, personal health, and impending catastrophes
- Restlessness demonstrated by inability to stay seated or attentive
- Difficulty with concentration and tendency to be distracted by everything in environment
- Muscle tension that may cause pain, especially in the neck, and headache
- Irritability with those nearby (especially the health care workers) that may be expressed as a refusal to participate in treatment sessions
- Sleep disturbance that leaves elders so fatigued the following day that they decline to participate in therapy sessions
- Panic attack that may be expressed as acute fear of dying

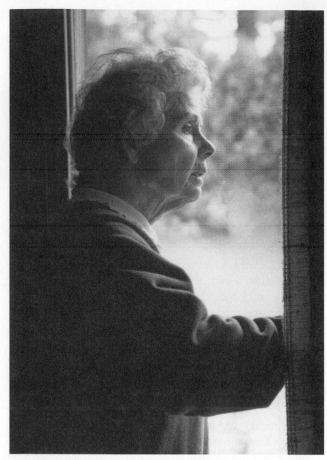

FIGURE 21-2 Elders may fear leaving home and restrict their social interactions because of mental conditions.

breath, chest pains, nausea or other digestive distress, light-headedness, feelings of unreality, fear of mental imbalance or death, and bodily sensations for which no cause is apparent. COTAs who work with these elders should involve them in activities and occupations. This involvement frequently alleviates feelings of panic. COTAs also should reassure elders that they are not dying or "going crazy."

People with **social phobia** fear that they will not be able to act appropriately in public. These people are often afraid that they will embarrass themselves by doing something unacceptable. A common manifestation of social phobia is the fear of being unable to talk to other people. The fear of offending others while dining in public also is common (American Psychiatric Association, 1994). For example, elders may avoid going to restaurants or become anxious when served food for fear that they will drop some on the tablecloth or their clothes. COTAs should grade involvement in anxiety-producing tasks.

Posttraumatic stress disorder and **acute stress disorder** result from exposure to an event that is outside the realm of usually human experience. Examples of these

types of events include a natural disaster such as a hurricane or an accident in which loved ones are hurt or exposed to danger. In the acute form of the stress disorder, the symptoms occur within a month after the event. In posttraumatic stress disorder, months or years may elapse before symptoms appear. The three main symptoms of these disorders are reliving the traumatic event, avoiding reminders of the event, and experiencing symptoms of anxiety similar to those of panic disorder (Hyer & Sohnle, 2001). Encouraging elders to talk about the event, describe the experience, and express their feelings are typical strategies of COTAs. Some ways to facilitate the process include expressive arts activities, structured group interaction sessions, and video presentations that deal with similar events. After viewing such videos, COTAs can facilitate a group discussion.

Treatment Interventions for Elders with Anxiety Disorders

Some suggested interventions for elders with anxiety disorders have already been discussed. Successful occupations and activities have some additional characteristics. Although avoidance of situations causing anxiety may appear helpful, treatment of these disorders often involves exposing elders to controlled simulations of the original event and helping them to gradually overcome the desire for avoidance. For COTAs, this help may involve asking elders to use expressive therapies such as movement, drawing, and making a collage to describe anxiety (Fig. 21-3). Expression of these feelings may provide some relief. Repetitive motions such as those in needlework soothe some clients. Acceptance, reassurance, encouragement, and praise are appropriate for these elders. After elders have expressed their anxiety, COTAs can assist them in gradually confronting the anxiety-producing situation.

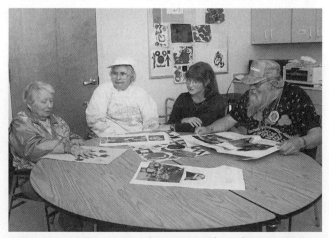

FIGURE 21-3 Expressive therapies such as drawing or making a collage can help elders to express their feelings.

SCHIZOPHRENIA

The major form of psychosis in the Western world is **schizophrenia**. The first symptoms of this disabling disease usually appear before age 30 years (Box 21-5). Approximately 28% of elders 60 years or older who are admitted to psychiatric units for psychosis developed it late in life (Barry, Blow, Dornfeld, & Valenstein, 2002). Discoveries in the dopamine receptor system have made many forms of schizophrenic symptoms treatable, but the symptoms of Parkinson's syndrome may increase (Birren, Sloane, & Cohen, 1992).

In schizophrenia, symptoms that make a person more animated or active, such as delusions, hallucinations, suspiciousness, and disorganized language and behavior, are called positive symptoms. Symptoms that subtract from a person's essential personality are called negative symptoms and include restricted emotions, decreased speech and interaction, and diminished behavior of all types. It was previously thought that people who have late onset of schizophrenia are more likely to have positive symptoms of the disease (Birren, Sloane, & Cohen, 1992). More recent research shows that as people with schizophrenia age, they maintain both positive and negative symptoms. About one quarter to one third of elderly people with schizophrenia show some improvement of their symptoms as they age (Barry, Blow, Dornfeld, & Valenstein, 2002). Some people with schizophrenia who show symptoms of the disease in old age may have been considered "odd" throughout their life. A number of studies show that the majority of elders with schizophrenia have been single throughout their lives (Sadavoy, Lazarus, Jarvik, & Grossberg, 1996). This means that these elders probably have little family support.

Many people with early onset of schizophrenia commit suicide (Birren, Sloane, & Cohen, 1992). However, many others live to old age and can be found in the nursing home population and in the geriatric wards of mental hospitals. These elders are especially vulnerable to the side effects of neuroleptic drugs. A common side effect is tardive dyskinesia, a movement disorder that includes involuntary blinking, tongue thrust, foot tapping, jerking, and twisting. The "Pisa syndrome" may also develop in elders, in which they lean to one side. Elders with schizophrenia are more likely to experience faintness from neuroleptic medication than younger people (Birren, Sloane, & Cohen, 1992). Because COTAs work with elders soon after these symptoms appear, they must share this important information with the team. Because COTAs see elders performing daily activities, they are able to notice any abnormal movement. Other health care workers may not see elders during routine activities and therefore may not recognize abnormalities. The sooner COTAs report abnormal movements resulting from neuroleptic drugs, the sooner the drug can be adjusted to prevent a potentially permanent impairment. (See Chapter 13 for a more detailed discussion about the side effects of medications.)

Treatment Interventions for Elders with Schizophrenia

COTAs can assist elders who have schizophrenia by addressing the functional areas of their lives. COTAs can make sure that elders can perform ADL functions as independently as possible. COTAs also can involve these elders in concrete projects such as simple crafts, cooking, gardening, or whatever other meaningful activities have been identified by the elder. Projects should be structured with clear guidelines for accomplishing the tasks. Projects should be successfully finished in a short time. Because schizophrenia is primarily associated with sensory distortions, COTAs may first need to verify elders' feelings and perceptions. It is particularly important not to argue with elders about the reality of their hallucinatory or delusional perceptions. Unless these elders want to discuss their feelings about the symptoms or the way their illness interferes with occupational performance, COTAs should redirect them to a concrete activity that may help orient them to reality.

HYPOCHONDRIASIS

Hypochondriasis is a disorder characterized by the individual's preoccupation with personal health. The person is overly concerned about disease and usually does

---

BOX 21-5

Symptoms of Schizophrenia Among Elders

- Delusions: false beliefs that have no basis in reality
- Hallucinations: most commonly auditory (in which voices direct persons to do things they would not normally consider doing, such as harming themselves or others) or tactile (in which elders might feel as if something were crawling on their skin); hallucinations involving all the senses also are possible
- Disorganized speech in which the speaker has no logical sequence or coherent theme to statements
- Lack of meaningful speech in which the elder speaks without providing information
- Disorganized behavior such as appearing to start an action but suddenly dropping it and changing to another with no apparent sense of purpose
- Lack of emotion: sometimes called *flattened affect* (voice is monotonous, and face shows no feelings)
- Lack of motivation: often demonstrated by apathetic responses to requests to participate
- Lack of self-care: often demonstrated by unruly, uncombed hair; food spills on the clothes; and unpleasant body odor

not realize that this concern is unreasonable. Concerns are considered unreasonable after the physician has ruled out physical illness and finds no evidence of disease. The person with hypochondriasis, however, continues to believe that the illness is real (American Psychiatric Association, 1994). Many complaints focus on specific organ systems, particularly the digestive tract. Hypochondriasis is common in elders, but it should not be considered normal (Sadavoy, Lazarus, Jarvik, & Grossberg, 1996). Approximately half of the elders diagnosed with depression also have hypochondriasis (Birren, Sloane, & Cohen, 1992). Individuals with hypochondriasis use their bodies as a way to communicate messages they are unable to express otherwise. For example, instead of directly asking someone for attention, elders with hypochondriasis may complain at length about their aches and pains. Naturally this behavior often results in alienating others, which just increases their social isolation and their need for attention.

Health care workers sometimes discount reports of bodily illness among elders. However, aging often does produce physical pain as arthritis and other degenerative diseases take their toll. COTAs must know elders well enough to distinguish among physical complaints, those caused by degenerative disease, and those resulting from a mental disorder. Complaints must be believed until proven false (that is, the physician has exhausted medical tests to rule out disease).

If COTAs determine that a complaint is an attention-seeking behavior, the best response is to direct attention to positive qualities in the elder. Behavioral studies demonstrate that positive attention, such as a reward, changes, or maintains behavior more efficiently than negative attention, such as punishment and criticism (Early, 2000). Although 95% of clients blame their illnesses on physical problems, physicians find that these physical problems are often symptomatic of psychosocial problems (Stahl, 1996). For this reason, COTAs should encourage interaction and participation in group activities and meaningful occupations in home and institutional environments.

SUBSTANCE ABUSE

Historic events such as Prohibition (when alcohol was forbidden) and World War II (when many young adult women had the opportunity to smoke and drink) have affected the attitudes of elders toward these substances. The increased use of sedatives in the 1960s may also play a part in elders' attitudes toward drug use (Birren, Sloane, & Cohen, 1992). Alcohol abuse is common among elders, and many are hospitalized for alcohol-related dysfunction after coming to the hospital for other reasons (Adams, 1993). For example, an elder may be admitted for a fracture that resulted from falling while intoxicated.

Any mind-altering drug may affect elders more intensely than predicted because their mechanisms of neutralizing and eliminating the drug are diminished. Therefore, elders are often more sensitive to drug treatments. This sensitivity is compounded by the fact that most elders take more than one kind of medication. These medications often create unintended interactions. **Drug abuse** often is part of a **dual diagnosis** in which the elder is both depressed and addicted to alcohol or drugs. (See Chapter 13 for a more thorough discussion of this topic.)

The contribution of COTAs in cases of substance abuse is to notify the physician of the problem and join the team in confronting the elder. Although elders with substance abuse problems require individual assessment to determine specific performance deficits, most need guidance in time management. COTAs can provide elders with schedule sheets and assist them in planning better use of leisure time. Many elders substitute alcohol for other entertainment when they are housebound. Drinking may also be a mechanism for coping with bereavement and loneliness. COTAs should develop plans to help elders find ways to socialize. Most communities have special transportation services available to senior citizens. Many local agencies provide programs and information on aging. Awareness of substance abuse problems is crucial if COTAs are providing home health services.

PERSONALITY DISORDERS

That elders do not have new **personality disorders** is a common assumption. However, some research shows the contrary (Sadavoy, Lazarus, Jarvik, & Grossberg, 1996). The elder may have suppressed the behavior earlier in life, or the personality disorder may indeed be a new development. Elders are more likely to cover up personality traits that are undesirable. Some elders who are diagnosed as paranoid, schizoid, or schizotypal may have been considered strange even during youth. Sensory losses and changes may exacerbate elders' paranoia because the interpretation of stimuli becomes more difficult. Characteristics such as suspiciousness and inflexibility tend to remain stable throughout life.

The most common personality disorders found in elders are the dependent, avoidant, and compulsive types. People who have a primary diagnosis of depression are most likely also to have a personality disorder (Agronin, 1994). Antisocial personality disorders are less common in later years. Elders are usually less impulsive and less likely to commit violent crimes. They are more likely to exhibit behaviors such as exposing their genitals and being drunk in public (Agronin, 1994). People who have the overly dramatic disorders of narcissistic, borderline, or histrionic types are more prone to experience transference, in which the patient or client perceives the COTA as someone they have known previously and begins to behave toward the COTA in that way (Kennedy, 2000).

Because of their long- or short-term behaviors, elders with personality disorders often lack social support systems.

The COTA/OTR team, therefore, should include building social support as part of the treatment plan (Agronin, 1994) on the basis of meaningful activities identified by the elder. This could mean encouraging the elder to contact old friends or attend a class or social group in the facility, adult day program, church, or other community organization. Most local newspapers publish lists of support groups and their meeting times and places.

People who are overly dependent need approval, reassurance, and support. They should be provided with opportunities to make their own decisions and gradually establish their independence in a context where the opportunities for failure are minimal. Some elders may never overcome their dependency. In such cases, COTAs can create situations in which reasonable dependence is part of an activity, such as the COTA reading the instructions while the elder assembles a project. Activities such as group singing allow elders to participate while depending on others to set the volume and rhythm of the music.

Unpredictable situations are best avoided with elders who show obsessive–compulsive tendencies. Such situations sometimes provoke obsessive thoughts and compulsive behaviors in affected elders. The objective with these elders is to involve them in constructive activities that replace compulsive rituals. They should be given encouragement, praise, and approval for effort.

PSYCHOTROPIC MEDICATIONS

Polypharmacy is the term used when a patient is taking a variety of drugs for different purposes. This is especially hazardous for the elderly because their diminished capability to excrete excess medication makes them vulnerable to adverse drug interactions. (See Chapter 13 for a more thorough discussion of this topic.) There are four main categories of psychotropic medications that elders with mental illness use: antipsychotics, antidepressants, anxiolytics, and hypnotics (Linjakumpa, et al., 2002). Antipsychotics are to reduce psychologically painful experiences such as hallucinations and delusions. They are not only used for people with schizophrenia but also for those with major depression. Antidepressants are for elevating a person's depressed mood. There are a number of new drugs in this category, called selective serotonin reuptake inhibitors, or serotonin and norepinephrine reuptake inhibitors; this category includes brand name drugs such as Prozac (Eli Lilly and Co, Indianapolis, IN), Paxil (Glaxo Smith Kline, Research Triangle Park, NC), Zoloft, and Effexor. They are prescribed often because they usually do not have the side effects of nausea, dry mouth, and constipation, which are associated with older antidepressants or tricyclic antidepressant and monoamine oxidase inhibitor medications. There are other atypical antidepressants as well. Almost all antidepressants cause drowsiness. Many also cause sexual dysfunction, which may exacerbate a problem that is common to some elderly. Anxiolytics are to reduce symptoms of nervousness and anxiety. Hypnotics are sleeping medications used by many elderly because insomnia often increases with age. Because functional problems resulting from overmedication or negative drug interactions are often observed first in occupational therapy, it is extremely important for COTAs to become familiar with symptoms of overmedication or drug interaction problems (Early, 2000).

EVALUATION STRATEGIES

COTAs participate in the evaluation process once service competency has been established. Among the assessments that can be administered by COTAs in nursing homes and mental health settings is the Canadian Occupational Performance Measure (COPM). This assessment is an outcomes measure that is client centred as the elder (or significant other if the elder is not at the level to complete the assessment) identifies and prioritizes problems in occupational performance to work on in treatment (Law, et al., 1998). Another assessment is the Allen Cognitive Levels (ACL) (Allen, Earhart, & Blue, 1992). The Routine Task Inventory is an assessment of ADL functions that COTAs may administer (Allen, 1985; Early, 2000). COTAs help clients to reassess their interests and values through a variety of interview and checklist techniques. The Neuropsychiatric Institute (NPI) Interest checklist (Early, 2000; Matsutsuyu, 1969) is commonly used in assessment by COTAs. Behavioral checklists are another way COTAs provide valuable assessment information. The Comprehensive Occupational Therapy Evaluation Scale (Brayman, Kirby, Misenheimer, & Short, 1976; Early, 2000) is one such checklist in which 25 behaviors are scored according to a scale from 0 for normal to 4 for severely impaired. This numeric score allows COTAs to identify improvement and deterioration (Early, 2000).

GROUP TREATMENT STRATEGIES

Socialization is one of the most important parts of treatment for mentally ill elders. Their losses of hearing, sight, and mobility often impinge on their self-esteem. Listening to and being listened to are some of the most therapeutic experiences for all people, and especially for the elderly. Group treatment offers the opportunity for elders to communicate in an accepting environment.

Mosey's Developmental Groups (Hopkins & Smith, 1983) have six levels of group function. The COTA may find this way of thinking about patients helpful. The lowest function group level involves people who are capable of simply sitting in the group, working alone, and interacting with only the COTA. In the next level, individuals in the group are aware of the others in the group but have minimal interaction with them. The third level involves more interactions with group members in a short-term activity. At the next level, group members may cooperate on long-term efforts. The fifth level involves having people work to help each other. Finally, the sixth level provides opportunities to share leadership and contribute to the greater good of everyone.

Group work involves careful planning to choose an appropriate activity that can be done by all participants. With elders it is better to have fewer participants, because it is too distracting to have so much activity when sensory systems are diminished (Banks, 2000). The sessions need to be structured. The following discussion includes one way to structure a group. First there is an introduction and some kind of warm-up to draw participants into the feeling of belonging to the group (see Box 21-3). A warm-up using some common memory such as meals in childhood and the first train or boat ride will be inclusive for almost everyone. It is good to relate the warm-up to the task the group will do next—for example, a baking memory prepares the group members to be involved in a baking activity. This is followed by a task such as an art or craft, cooking, or a discussion of a certain topic. Next, there is a time to finish the activity and wind down. The final step in this progression is for the COTA to do a short evaluation of the session, mentioning the various things people contributed such as interesting things they said or products of their activity that they might want to display. This is a time to enhance self-esteem and reinforce good ideas that were expressed (Creek, 2002).

CASE STUDY

Louise is a 75-year-old woman diagnosed with depression. After being stabilized on an antidepressant at an acute care hospital, she was placed in a group home that specializes in the care of elders with mental illness. The residents are taken daily to a day treatment program, where a COTA provides the major part of the service. An OTR visits the center twice a week.

Louise is a widow and has three married daughters and eight grandchildren. Sewing clothes for her daughters and grandchildren has always been important to Louise. She also has been a member of the same quilting club since the birth of her first child. A homemaker until age 45 years, she experienced the "empty-nest syndrome" after all her daughters left for college or got married. She had been depressed then, but not severely enough to require hospitalization. Her husband, a farmer, encouraged her to visit her sister, who lived in a large city. The change of scenery seemed to help her overcome the loss she felt. She returned from her visit to her sister's home and enrolled in a technical program for office workers. From age 45 to 65 years she worked as a secretary at the local high school. At 65 years, she retired but continued to work as a substitute. Her husband lost their farm as a result of bank foreclosure and eventually accepted a position on a corporate farm. When Louise was 68 years old, her husband died of a sudden heart attack. She began to show symptoms of depression within a year. She reduced her activities, turning down jobs to fill in at the school, refusing to go out with her friends, declining to baby-sit her grandchildren, and quitting her quilting group. Her daughters did not become worried until they realized she was hoarding medication and planning suicide. They persuaded Louise to admit herself to the psychiatric unit of the regional hospital.

Although her medication was working at the time of her discharge from the acute care inpatient psychiatric unit, she had residual dysfunction in several self-care, socialization, and cognitive areas. Because all the daughters lived more than 3 hours away, they agreed that Louise would stay in a group home until the family felt she could adequately take care of herself again. Fortunately, they were able to place her in a local group home with 24-hour supervision.

The schedule of the group home included chair aerobics, weekend outings to the mall, a reminiscence group, and a crafts group that made stuffed toys for children with developmental disabilities. Louise also participated in a day treatment program 3 days a week. The family hoped that when Louise recovered sufficiently, she could resume her life in one of the assisted living units in a nearby housing development operated by her religious denomination.

Soon after Louise's arrival in the day treatment program, the COTA completed the COPM (Law, et al., 1998) with her. Louise identified priorities of some activities that she missed doing. Louise began crying as she discussed her grandchildren and her quilting group. She also discussed her difficulty with some ADL and especially with homemaking tasks. After consulting with the OTR, the COTA left a copy of the NPI Interest checklist (Matsutsuyu, 1969) for Louise to fill out on her own. The COTA returned a day later and gave Louise the ACL test (Allen, Earhart, Blue, 1992). Louise scored at cognitive level 4.1 on the ACL, which meant that although she recognized an error, she could not correct it. Two days later, the COTA administered the Routine Task Inventory-2 (Allen, 1985). Louise also scored at Cognitive Level 4 on this test of ADL functions. This score meant she initiated grooming tasks and completed most of them; however, she neglected the back of her hair and neglected to clean up the bathroom after she bathed herself (Allen, Earhart, & Blue, 1992).

Louise was able to find the mailbox in the group home when she wanted to mail letters to her daughters. However, she got lost easily when she attempted to walk unsupervised in the neighborhood. She was independent in toileting but got anxious when she had to use any restroom other than the one in her room or the occupational therapy clinic. She usually remembered to ask the nurse for her medications. She was able to fix a sandwich in the kitchenette at the day treatment program, but she often burned the soup. The last time this happened she stated, "I can't do anything right anymore. I am just a burden to my daughters. They would be better off not having to worry about me." Although she could dress herself in the morning, she did not pay attention to whether her clothing matched or was appropriate for the weather.

After discussion with the OTR, the COTA explained her findings to Louise and one of her daughters. The OTR, COTA, daughter, and Louise then planned for her participation in a daily ADL group session with the COTA to work on self-care and homemaking occupations. The plan included the use of self-cueing devices such as timers, environmental aids such as a neighborhood map, and a medication check-off sheet. These adaptations would be useful after discharge. Louise also would participate in the remotivation group.

■ CASE STUDY QUESTIONS

1 Considering the case study above, which of Louise's behaviors might cause the therapist to think she was experiencing depression rather than dementia?

2 What other activities in the group home schedule might the COTA want to encourage Louise to attend?

3 Which of Mosey's Developmental Group levels might be most appropriate for Louise?

4 What community resources could be used in guiding Louise's recovery?

■ CHAPTER REVIEW QUESTIONS

1 Identify three or more common causes of late-life depression.

2 Describe types of activities recommended for elders experiencing auditory hallucinations.

3 How should you structure occupational therapy intervention for an elder who refuses to leave home because he believes he will fall whenever he walks on cement?

REFERENCES

Adams, W. L. (1993) Alcohol-related hospitalizations of elderly people. *Journal of the American Medical Association, 270*(10), 1222.

Agronin, M. E. (1994). Personality disorders in the elderly: An overview. *Journal of Geriatric Psychiatry, 27*(2), 151.

Allen, C. K. (1985). *Occupational therapy for psychiatric diseases: Measurement and management of cognitive disabilities.* Boston, MA: Little, Brown and Company.

Allen, C. K., Earhart, C. A., & Blue, T. (1992). *Occupational therapy treatment goals for the physically and cognitively disabled.* Rockville, MD: American Occupational Therapy Association.

American Psychiatric Association. (1994). *Diagnostic and statistical manual of mental disorders* (brochure) (4th ed.). Washington, DC: The American Psychiatric Association.

Banks, B. W. (2000). *Activities for older people: A practical workbook of art and craft projects.* Oxford, UK: Butterworth-Heinemann.

Barry, K. L., Blow, F. C., Dornfeld, M., & Valenstein, M. (2002). Aging and schizophrenia: Current health services research and recommendations. *Journal of Geriatric Psychiatry & Neurology, 15*(3), 121-127.

Birren, J. E., Sloane, R. B., & Cohen, G. D. (Eds.), (1992). *Handbook of mental health and aging.* San Diego, CA: Academic Press.

Brayman, S. J., Kirby, T. F., Misenheimer, A. M., & Short, M. J. (1976). Comprehensive occupational therapy evaluation scale. *American Journal of Occupational Therapy, 30*(2), 94-100.

Busse, E. W., & Blazer, D. G. (1996). *Geriatric psychiatry.* Washington, DC: American Psychiatric Press.

Centers for Disease Control. (2003). Suicide in the United States [WWW page]. http://www.cdc.gov/ncipc/factsheets/suifacts.htm

Creek, J. (2002). *Occupational therapy and mental health* (3rd ed.). London: Churchill Livingston.

Early, M. B. (2000). *Mental health concepts and techniques for the occupational therapy assistant* (3rd ed.). New York: Lippincott William & Wilkins.

George, L. K. (1993). Depressive disorders and symptoms in later life, *Generations, 17*(1), 35.

Hopkins, H. L., & Smith, H. D. (1983). *Willard and Spackman's occupational therapy* (6th ed.). Philadelphia: Lippincott Williams & Wilkins.

Hyer, L. A., & Sohnle, S. J. (2001). *Trauma among older people: Issues and treatment.* Philadelphia: Brunner-Routledge.

Ireland, M. (1972). Starting reality orientation and remotivation. *Nursing Homes, 21*(4), 10.

Johnson, C. (1995). *Depression workshop.* Unpublished monograph.

Kales, H. C., & Valenstein, M. V. (2002). Complexity in late-life depression: Impact of confounding factors on diagnosis, treatment and outcomes. *Journal of Geriatric Psychiatry & Neurology, 15*(3), 147-155.

Kennedy, G. J. (2000). *Geriatric mental health care: A treatment guide for health professionals.* New York: The Guilford Press.

Law, M. (Ed.). (1998). *Client-centered occupational therapy.* Thorofare, NJ: Slack.

Law, M., Baptiste, S., Carswell, A., McColl, M. A., Polatijko, H., & Pollock, N. (1998). *The Canadian Occupational Performance Measure (COPM)* (3rd ed.). Ottawa, Ont: CAOT Publications ACE.

Linjakumpa, T., Hartikainen, S., Klaukka, T., Koponen, H., Kivela, S. L., & Isoaho, R. (2002). Psychotropics among the home-dwelling elderly—increasing trends. *International Journal of Geriatric Psychiatry, 17,* 874-883.

Matsutsuyu, J. S. (1969). The interest checklist. *American Journal of Occupational Therapy, 24*(4), 32.

Mosey, A. C. (1986). *Psychological components of occupational therapy.* New York: Raven Press.

National Alliance for the Mentally Ill. (1995). *NAMI families just like yours, families like yours, learning to live with severe mental illness.* Arlington, VA: The Alliance.

Pedersen, I. D. (1986). Treatment of depression in institutionalized older persons. *Physical & Occupational Therapy in Geriatrics, 5*(1), 77.

Sadavoy, J., Lazarus, L. W., Jarvik, L. F., & Grossberg, G. T. (1996). *Comprehensive review of geriatric psychiatry—II* (2nd ed.). Washington, DC: American Psychiatric Press.

Sadock, B. J., & Sadock, V. A. (2000). *Kaplan & Sadock's comprehensive textbook of psychiatry* (7th ed.). Philadelphia: Lippincott Williams & Wilkins.

Sajatovic, M. (2002). Aging-related issues in bipolar disorder: A health service perspective. *Journal of Geriatric Psychiatry & Neurology, 15*(3), 128-133.

Scocco, P., & De Leo, D. (2002). One-year prevalence of death thoughts, suicide ideation and behaviors in an elderly population. *International Journal of Geriatric Psychiatry, 17,* 842-846.

Smith, M. (1994). Evaluation of a geriatric mental health training program for nursing personnel in rural long-term care facilities. *Issues in Mental Health Nursing, 15*(2), 149.

Stahl, C. (1996). Psychosomatic illness and function. *Advances in Occupational Therapy, 12*(4), 14.

Stein, F., & Cutler, S. K. (1998). *Psychiatric occupational therapy: A holistic approach.* San Diego, CA: Sinclair Publishing Group.

Wagenaar, D. B., Mickus, M. A., Gaumer, K. A., & Colenda, C. C. (2002). Late-life depression and mental health services in primary care. *Journal of Geriatric Psychiatry & Neurology, 15*(3), 134-140.

Wilkinson, D., Holmes, C., Wollford, J., Stammers, S., & North, J. (2002). Prophylactic therapy with lithium in elderly patients with unipolar major depression. *International Journal of Geriatric Psychiatry, 17,* 619-622.

CHAPTER **22**

Working with Elders Who Have Orthopedic Conditions

BRENDA **M.** **C**OPPARD, **T**YROME **H**IGGINS, AND **K**AROLINE **D.** **H**ARVEY

KEY TERMS

orthopedic, fracture, osteoarthritis, compound fracture, transverse fracture, spiral fracture, comminuted fracture, closed reduction, open reduction, internal fixation, external fixation, delayed union, nonunion, malunion, Hemovac, total hip replacement, arthroplasty, antiembolus hosiery, rheumatoid arthritis, wrist subluxation, ulnar drift, swan-neck deformity, boutonnière deformity, Nalebuff type I deformity, joint protection, work simplification, energy conservation

CHAPTER OBJECTIVES

1. Identify the causes of fractures in the elder population.
2. Identify terminology related to fractures and their management.
3. Describe the precautions required after a hip pinning and implications of such a procedure relative to occupational performance.
4. Describe the precautions required after a total hip replacement and the implications of such a procedure relative to occupational performance.
5. Identify adaptive equipment and modified methods of performance that benefit elders with hip fractures.
6. Identify the signs and symptoms of osteoarthritis, rheumatoid arthritis, and gout.
7. Describe the effects of osteoarthritis, rheumatoid arthritis, and gout on occupational performance.
8. Explain the principles of joint protection, work simplification, and energy conservation.

The two weeks I spent in rehab were tough, but I had to learn how to walk all over again, just like a baby! Not only did the physical therapist teach me how to walk, the occupational therapist taught me how to dress, and how to do things around the house. They presented me with all sorts of new gadgets that would help me in my daily living.

—Linda

Orthopedic problems are prevalent among elders. For example, an estimated 850,000 **fractures** occur annually in persons 65 years or older (Centers for Disease Control [CDC], 1996); one of every two women and one in eight men older than 50 years will experience an osteoporosis-related fracture (National Institute of Arthritis and Musculoskeletal and Skin Diseases [NIAMS], 2000).

Orthopedic problems may result in elders being hospitalized for a surgical procedure, rehabilitation, and possibly being placed temporarily or permanently in a long-term care facility.

The role of the certified occupational therapy assistant (COTA) and occupational therapist (OTR) team is to help maximize the occupational performance of elders who have orthopedic problems. Elders who would otherwise need to enter an extended care facility are often able to go home as a result of occupational therapy (OT) treatment. COTAs must be familiar with orthopedic conditions and their effects on occupational performance to ensure that appropriate evaluation and treatment are carried out. This chapter addresses orthopedic problems and conditions that contribute to these problems.

FRACTURES

Causes of Fractures

Causes of fractures include falls, trauma from automobile accidents, **osteoarthritis**, and metastatic carcinoma (Holley, 2002). Other factors such as current or previous smoking habit (Forsen, et al., 1998), alcohol abuse, diabetes (Wallace, et al., 2002), and decreased level of physical activity also correlate with the incidence of fractures (Black & Cooper, 2000).

The majority of fractures in elders result from falls (Gillespie, Gillespie, Robertson, Lamb, Cumming, & Rowe, 2002). Factors associated with falling include poor vision, orthostatic hypotension, poor balance, diminished mobility, side effects of medication, muscle weakness, neurologic diseases, reduced alertness, urge incontinence (Brown et al., 2000), cluttered home environment (Cumming et al., 1999; Salkeld, et al., 2000), and dementia (Connell & Wolf, 1997). (An in-depth examination of the causes of falls in elders is provided in Chapter 14.)

The number of elder drivers is increasing. For example, in 1983, 1 of every 15 drivers in the United States was older than 70 years. In 1995, the ratio rose to 1 of every 11 drivers. It is estimated that by 2020, 20% of all people who drive will be older than 65 years (National Institute on Aging [NIA], n.d.). According to the U.S. Department of Transportation (1997), elders have greater rates of fatal crashes than younger drivers, and they do not deal well with complex traffic situations. Trauma resulting from auto accidents accounts for a portion of the fractures seen in the elder population.

Elders are more likely to sustain fractures after a fall because of osteoporosis, osteomalacia, and diminished ability to repair microfractures (Haverstock, 2001; Maenpaa, Soini, Lehto, & Belt, 2002; Patel & DeGroot, 2001). Stress fractures also can occur in elders who, for example, suddenly increase their levels of activity by jogging, walking farther than usual, or walking on a different terrain (Mehta & Nastasi, 1993).

Fractures may also be caused by cancer that has metastasized to bone. Although any cancer may metastasize to bone, metastases from carcinomas, particularly those that arise in the breast, lung, prostate, kidney, and thyroid, are most common. Metastatic lesions weaken the strength of bones and may lead to fractures (Patel & DeGroot, 2001).

Types of Fractures

A fracture is a break in a bone. Although radiographs are used to diagnose the fracture, it does not reveal damage to soft tissues or cartilage. Fracture sites can disrupt the intraarticular, epiphyseal, metaphyseal, or diaphyseal portions of the bone. If a fracture occurs and dislocates a joint, it is a fracture-dislocation (Altizer, 2002).

Various terms are used to categorize fractures. A fracture is considered to be "**compound**" or "open" if the bone protrudes through the soft tissue and skin. If the soft tissue and skin are undamaged, the fracture is considered to be "closed" or "simple." Different physical forces can result in certain types of fractures. A **transverse fracture** occurs as a result of a direct force, whereas a spiral fracture results from a circular or twisting force. A fracture that results in more than two bone fragments is a **comminuted fracture**. Figure 22-1 shows these various types of fractures.

Medical Intervention for Fractures

The goals of medical management of a fracture are to reduce pain and align the fracture for proper healing. The fracture can be aligned with or without surgery. The process of manually realigning (sometimes using traction devices) and then casting a fracture is termed **closed reduction.** The **open reduction** is a surgical procedure that is used to internally fixate the fracture site.

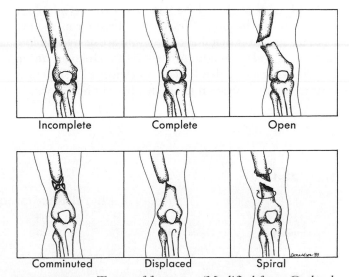

FIGURE 22-1 Types of fractures. (Modified from Garland, J. J. [1979]. *Fundamentals of orthopaedics*. Philadelphia: WB Saunders.)

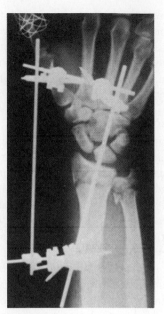

FIGURE 22-2   External fixator in place to maintain reduction. (From Hunter, J., Mackin, E., & Callahan, A. [Eds.]. [1995]. *Rehabilitation of the hand: Surgery and therapy* [4th ed.]. St. Louis, MO: Mosby.)

Internal fixation is performed with use of orthopedic nails, screws, pins, rods, or plates. When **external fixation** is used to align or reduce a fracture, the fixator device is attached with pins or wire, which is inserted through the soft tissues and into the bone (Fig. 22-2). This device usually involves the use of screws and rods that are removed after the fracture has healed. The skin around placement sites of the rods or screws must be kept clean to prevent infection (see Table 22-1 for pin site cleaning instructions).

COTAs also should be familiar with terminology relating to the healing of fractures. Three terms used to describe fractures that do not heal well are delayed union, nonunion, and malunion (Altizer, 2002). **Delayed union** describes a fracture that heals at an abnormally slow rate. **Nonunion** describes a fracture that has not healed within 4 to 6 months. **Malunion** describes a fracture in which the bone heals in a normal length of time, but with an unsatisfactory alignment.

Complications After Fractures

Several complications can occur after a fracture (Altizer, 2002). Edema can lead to joint stiffness, and joint contractures often are caused by adhesions or prolonged immobilization. After a fracture, posttraumatic arthritis can occur in joints associated with or near the fracture site. Reflex sympathetic dystrophy is a syndrome that often occurs after minor injuries. The condition is believed to be related to the sympathetic nervous system and presents with severe pain, edema, stiffness, muscle atrophy, muscle spasms, contractions, and loss of bone mineralization. Myositis ossificans is the formation of heterotopic ossification near a traumatized area. The most common joints where heterotopic ossification forms are the arms, thighs, and hips.

Factors Influencing Rehabilitation

Several factors affect the outcome of rehabilitation efforts in elders who sustain fractures. Age is a predominant factor in rehabilitation. Elders may need more time than younger persons to achieve their greatest levels of independence. For example, in elders, a comminuted fracture of the proximal humerus should be immobilized for the shortest period possible to reduce the chances of development of adhesive capsulitis or frozen shoulder. With a younger person, the threat of such a complication may not always be a concern.

The general condition of elders also affects the course of rehabilitation. For example, elders who are in shock or are unconscious require different treatment than those who are alert and oriented. In addition, past and current medical conditions may affect the rehabilitation of elders who have fractures. Elders with congestive heart failure or chronic obstructive lung disease may be limited in their abilities to participate in endurance and strengthening activities. Furthermore, a large percentage of elders with fractures also have associated medical problems such as

TABLE **22-1**

General Recommended Pin Site Care				
Frequency	**Massage**	**Crusts**	**Cleaning solution**	**Dressing**
1-2 times each day	Massage site area gently to prevent abnormal adhesions/scars	Remove from site	Peroxide or saline	Dry dressing, especially if oozing

Adapted from Sims, M., & Whiting, J. (2000). Pin-site care. *Nursing Times, 96*(48), 46.

arthritis, hypertension, hearing impairments, heart disease, cataracts, orthopedic impairments, sinusitis, and diabetes (Administration on Aging, 2002).

The presence of dementia often affects rehabilitation outcomes for elders with fractures. For example, teaching the integration of hip precautions or joint protection methods while engaging in self-care tasks to an elder with short-term memory deficits is difficult. (A detailed discussion of intervention considerations for elders who have dementia is presented in Chapter 20.)

Although hip fractures are the most common type of fracture sustained by elders, fractures of other bones also occur. COTAs should know the common fractures and general recommended treatment techniques (Table 22-2).

TABLE **22-2**

General Recommended Treatment Techniques for Upper-Extremity Fractures			
Fracture location	**Precautions and/or contraindications**	**Acute injury treatment techniques**	**Treatment techniques after repair**
Humeral	Keep elbow, wrist, and finger joints mobile or per physician's order; monitor for signs of edema; position upper extremity above heart if edema occurs and is not contraindicated for cardiac condition; PROM is contraindicated; discontinue immobilizer or brace with physician's order	Use shoulder immobilizer or plaster cast to immobilize; after 5 to 7 days, a humeral cuff brace can be used	Begin AROM when acute pain is subsided to prevent stiffness; PROM is contraindicated; encourage isometric exercises during and after immobilization; Codman's exercises should only be encouraged in the absence of edema
Elbow	Keep shoulder, wrist, and finger joints mobile or per physician's order; monitor for signs of edema; position upper extremity above level of heart if edema occurs and is not contraindicated for cardiac condition; PROM is contraindicated; discontinue immobilizer(s) with physician's order	A plaster cast or elbow conformer can be used to immobilize the elbow in 90 to 100 degrees of flexion; a sling also can be used	Begin gentle, nonresistive AROM after removal of cast; perform AROM in a gravity-eliminated plane; PROM in the early stage is not advised; person may have difficulty regaining full elbow extension, but a functional arc should be regained for ADL
Wrist (scaphoid)	Keep shoulder, elbow, and finger joints mobile or per physician's order; if an external fixator is in place, monitor sites for infection; clean pin sites with hydrogen peroxide; discontinue any splints with physician's order	A plaster cast may be worn for 2 weeks to 2 months depending on the physician; a thumb spica splint can be used after the cast is removed to position the wrist in slight flexion and radial deviation	When stabilized and cast removed, AROM should begin to all wrist motions
Colles' (distal radius)	Keep shoulder, elbow, and finger joints mobile or per physician's order; if an external fixator is in place, monitor sites for infection; clean pin sites with hydrogen peroxide; discontinue immobilizer(s) per physician's order	A volar wrist splint is used for positioning after a plaster cast or internal/external fixation is removed	Begin ROM of wrist and forearm once a bony union has occurred and cast has been removed

Adapted from Daniel, M. S., & Strickland, L. R. (1992). *Occupational therapy protocol management in adult physical dysfunction*. Gaithersburg, MD: Aspen. Physicians may vary these protocols.
ADL, activity of daily living; AROM, active range of motion; PROM, passive range of motion; ROM, range of motion.

TABLE **22-3**

Weight-bearing Terminology	
Term	**Definition**
No weight bearing (NWB)	No body weight is borne on the involved side
Toe-touch weight bearing (TTWB)	No weight is borne on the heel; weight is borne only on the toes
Partial weight bearing (PWB)	A partial amount of the body weight can be borne on the involved side; usually a percentage of body weight (for example, 50% PWB) or pounds (PWB with 50 lb) is stated
Weight bearing at tolerance (WBAT)	Weight bearing is allowed to the extent that it does not cause the elder too much pain; the elder tolerates the weight bearing
Full weight bearing (FWB)	Full body weight is borne on the involved side

Hip Fractures

Approximately 250,000 hip fractures occur annually in people older than 65 years (CDC, 1996). Hip fractures occur more commonly in women than in men (NIAMS, 2000). Fractures of the hip are classified by the type and direction of the fracture line.

Hip fractures usually require an open reduction internal fixation, or pinning procedure. The open reduction internal fixation of the involved hip usually must be protected from excessive force through weight-bearing restrictions (Table 22-3). The open reduction internal fixation site is sutured shut, and a **Hemovac*** may be used for about 2 days (Kim, Cho, & Kim, 1998). A Hemovac, which is connected to a suction machine, is a device that draws and collects drainage from the site. The Hemovac unit should *not* be disconnected for any activity and is usually removed by a registered nurse or a physician.

The amount of time required for a hip fracture to heal depends on the elder, the fracture site, the fracture type, and the severity of injury. Most incisions for hip surgeries are 12 to 18 inches in length; however, some new surgical approaches that involve less cutting of muscle, tendons, and ligaments are being tested in hopes that hospital length of stay will dramatically decrease (Rush University, 2001).

Many health care providers in hospitals follow a protocol or clinical pathway that outlines the timeframe for each professional's rehabilitation tasks (Coleman, 2001). Out-of-bed therapy activities for persons with hip pinnings are usually initiated 2 to 4 days after surgery (Birge, Morrow-Howell, & Proctor, 1994). Most function returns within 6 weeks to 6 months after the fracture

occurs; most persons experience little improvement in function from 6 months to 1 year after sustaining a fracture (Oberg, Oberg, & Hadstedt, 1996).

Weight-bearing restrictions for hip pinnings

Depending on the type and severity of the fracture, the physician may restrict the amount of weight bearing allowed on the involved hip while the person is walking. Most weight-bearing restrictions are observed for 6 to 8 weeks, during which time the person may use crutches or a walker to ambulate. COTAs must be aware of any weight-bearing precautions before initiating therapy and should know the terminology related to weight-bearing restrictions (see Table 22-3).

JOINT REPLACEMENTS
Total Hip Replacements

Total hip replacements (THRs), or total hip arthroplasties (THAs), are often elective surgeries indicated for reducing pain and restoring motion for elders who have severe osteoarthritis, rheumatoid arthritis, or ankylosing spondylosis. Emergency THAs frequently follow traumatic injuries to the hip, such as after a motor vehicle accident or fall. A hip replacement, or arthroplasty, may be full or partial. During a full hip arthroplasty, the hip's ball and socket are replaced with metal or metal and plastic prosthetic implants (Saikko, Ahloroos, Calonius, & Keranen, 2001). During a partial joint replacement, which is commonly used for fractures of the femoral neck and head, the femoral neck and head are replaced with a prosthesis. Hip prostheses last approximately 10 to 15 years or longer in 90% of elders (Capello, D'Antonio, Feinberg, & Manley, 2002; Della-Valle & Paprosky, 2002). When radiographs show evidence of loosening of the cement and the client is experiencing pain, a hip revision arthroplasty may be performed (Stromberg & Herberts, 1994).

The two basic surgical approaches for THRs are the anterolateral approach and the posterolateral approach

*Zimmer Orthopedic Products.

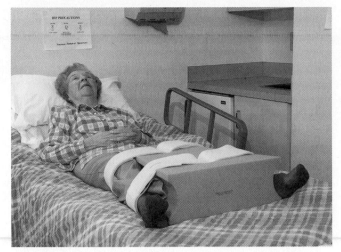

FIGURE 22-3 While the elder is supine, the elder's legs should be abducted with a wedge to prevent hip rotation and adduction.

(Daniel & Strickland, 1992). When an anterolateral approach of surgery is used, elders must avoid adduction, external rotation, and extension of the operated hip. If a posterolateral surgical approach is used, elders should avoid flexion beyond 60 to 90 degrees, adduction, and internal rotation of the operated hip (Lewis, 2003). COTAs must be aware of which type of surgical approach was used to properly carry out OT treatment (Fig. 22-3). COTAs also should note the position precautions for each surgical approach.

The movement precautions are usually observed for 6 to 12 weeks as indicated in a physician's order (Brander, Mullarkey, & Stulberg, 2001) (Table 22-4). Cemented THRs usually have no weight-bearing restrictions. When cement is not used, bony ingrowth is used to secure the prosthesis to the elder's bone. Often 6 to 12 weeks of weight-bearing restrictions are required when this type of prosthesis is used (Brander, Mullarkey, & Stulberg, 2001).

TABLE **22-4**

Motion Precautions for Clients Who Have Had a Total Hip Replacement

Approach	Position precautions
Anterolateral approach	1. Hip external rotation 2. Hip adduction 3. Hip extension
Posterolateral approach	1. Hip flexion beyond 90 degrees 2. Hip internal rotation 3. Hip adduction

After THA surgery, physicians often instruct clients to wear **antiembolus hosiery.** These thigh-high hose are worn 24 hours a day and removed only during bathing. Clients are instructed to wear this hosiery because it assists with blood circulation, prevents edema, and reduces the risk for deep vein thromboses. If an elder has not been instructed to wear these hose and complains of pain or swelling in the affected leg, the physician should be consulted immediately because this could be a sign of the presence of a thrombus. COTAs should be skilled in donning and doffing antiembolus hosiery because they may need to assist elders before bathing. If the hose are to be worn for a length of time, caregiver training should occur because it is often difficult for elders to perform this task independently.

Researchers show that there are several milestones during rehabilitation, including adherence to hip precautions; ambulating 100 feet with a mobility aid; independence with home exercise program; and requiring only supervision with toileting, transfers, and activities of daily living (Brander, Mullarkey, & Stulberg, 2001).

Three areas reported in research studies that are important concerns for clients with THA are sexual activity, driving, and work return (Brander, Mullarkey, & Stulberg, 2001). In a study of 86 clients with THA, 50% of preoperative clients reported experiencing difficulties with sexual activities because of hip problems, and 90% of these clients reported a desire for more information about sexual functioning after THA. The majority of clients (55%) resumed sexual activity within 2 months of the THA with physician approval and following positioning precautions. Most people report that the supine position during intercourse is the most comfortable (Brander, Mullarkey, & Stulberg, 2001). (A detailed discussion of addressing sexuality with elders is presented in Chapter 12.)

After surgery, driving reactions normalize between 3 and 8 weeks if elders resume good leg control. Return to work activities is dependent on the amount of stress and torque on joints. Typically, elders must take off from work for 3 to 6 weeks after surgery.

A number of studies exist on appropriate leisure activities after a THA (Brander, Mullarkey, & Stulberg, 2001). A survey of 28 orthopedic surgeons from Mayo Clinic* recommended that activities such as cycling, golfing, and bowling are acceptable after a THA. Generally, many physicians counsel well elders to avoid participation in sports that impart high torque or stress on the hip joint, such as jogging. Often, active elders resume activities and athletics regardless of physician or therapist warnings.

Psychosocial issues after total hip replacement
A number of psychosocial issues may surface during an elder's rehabilitation after a hip replacement. Dealing with a chronic condition such as arthritis can be stressful

*Rochester, MN.

and frustrating; many elders are required to deal with pain, swelling, and mobility limitations on a daily basis. Providing information on support groups may be beneficial to the elder.

After a THR, some elders find it difficult to abide by the position precautions. They may view these precautions as impediments to resuming the lifestyles they had before the procedure, especially when they had no predisposing medical conditions that limited activities. COTAs should be empathetic to the elder's concerns, but they must also help elders to understand the rationale for adhering to hip precautions (Figs. 22-4 and 22-5). The COTA also should address the consequences of not following these precautions. COTAs may need to reassure elders that healing takes time and that involvement in activities may continue, but usually with some modifications.

Many elders feel guilty or become anxious when they require assistance from family or friends (Murphy, Williams, & Gill, 2002; Roe, Whattam, Young, & Dimond, 2001). Elders who are temporarily placed in an extended care facility while they heal may also find it difficult to accept assistance from nursing staff in the facility. Feelings of guilt are sometimes accompanied by financial worries about the cost of care. In addition, relocation to a new environment such as a hospital, extended care facility, or long-term care facility can be stressful (McKinney & Melby, 2002). COTAs should encourage elders to talk about their feelings. When possible, discussing the situation with elders before they are moved to a new facility is beneficial. In addition, the elder should be thoroughly oriented to the new facility.

Occupational therapy interventions

The specific intervention strategies and techniques used with an elder who has had a THA vary depending on whether the anterolateral or posterolateral surgical approach was used (Box 22-1; Fig. 22-6). Provision and use

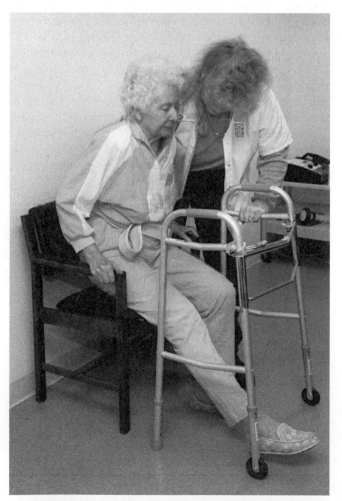

FIGURE 22-4 The elder should extend operated leg and bear weight on arms when coming into a standing position.

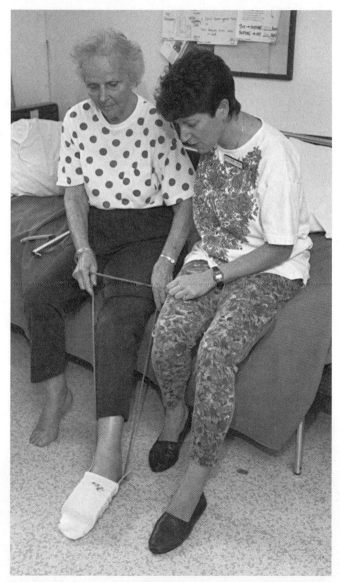

FIGURE 22-5 A sock aid is used to don socks while following hip precautions.

286

BOX 22-1

Occupational Therapy Interventions for Posterolateral and Anterolateral Approaches to Total Hip Replacement

Bed mobility

For both approaches

- Abduct legs with wedge or pillows to prevent hip rotation and adduction.

Walking

For both approaches

- Avoid pivoting on the leg that has been operated on.
- When approaching corners, take small steps in a circular fashion.
- If possible, take 10- to 15-minute walks 4 times per day 6 to 8 weeks after the operation.
- Walk at a slow, comfortable pace.

Chair transfers

For both approaches

- Sit on chairs with firm seats, preferably with arm rests.
- Avoid low, soft chairs and rocking chairs.
- Extend leg that has been operated on, reach for arm rests, and bear some weight through arms when trying to sit down.

Commode chair transfers

For posterolateral approach

- Use a chair with a height that accommodates for hip flexion precaution.
- Wipe between legs while seated or wipe from behind while standing with caution to avoid internal rotation.
- Stand and face the toilet to flush.

For anterolateral approach

- An over-the-toilet commode is usually used initially in the hospital and on discharge; elders usually have enough hip mobility to use a standard toilet seat.
- Avoid external rotation while wiping.
- Stand and face the toilet to flush.

Shower stall transfer

For both approaches

- Use a nonskid mat to avoid slips and falls.
- Use a shower chair and grab bars.

Car transfer

For both approaches

- Avoid bucket seats in small cars.
- Back up to passenger seat, hold onto a stable part of the car, extend the leg that has been operated on, and slowly sit in the car.
- Increase the seat height with pillows, if necessary.
- Avoid prolonged sitting in the car.

Lower extremity dressing

For both approaches

- Sit on a chair or the bed's edge when dressing.
- Use assistive devices, if necessary, to observe precautions.
- Use a reacher or dressing stick in donning and doffing pants and shoes.
- Dress the leg that has been operated on first using a reacher or dressing stick to bring pants over the foot and up to the knee.
- Avoid crossing the operated lower extremity over the nonoperated lower extremity.
- Use a sock aid to don socks or knee-high nylons and a reacher or dressing stick to doff these items.
- Use a reacher, elastic shoe laces, and a long-handled shoehorn, if necessary.

(Continued)

BOX 22-1

Occupational Therapy Interventions for Posterolateral and Anterolateral Approaches to Total Hip Replacement—cont'd

Lower extremity bathing
For both approaches
- Use a long-handled sponge or back brush to reach the lower legs and feet safely and use soap on a rope to prevent the soap from dropping (drill a hole into a bar of soap and thread a cord through the hole).
- Wrap a towel around a reacher to dry the legs.
- If a bath bench is used, place a damp towel on the seat to avoid sliding off the bench.
- Consider a handheld shower extender.

Hair shampooing
For both approaches
- Shampoo hair while seated until able to shower.

Leisure interests
For both approaches
- Adapt and use long-handled tools when appropriate.
- Use stools when appropriate to avoid bending, squatting, and stooping.

Home Management
For both approaches
- Avoid heavy housework (e.g., vacuuming, lifting, and bed making).
- Practice kitchen activities; keep commonly used items at countertop level.
- Carry items in large pockets, a walker basket, a fanny pack, or a utility cart.
- Use reachers to grasp items in low cupboards or pick up items off the floor.
- Move frequently used items located low in cabinets and shelves to counter level.
- Keep a cordless phone with a belt clip close by at all times.
- Carry a water bottle with a belt holster.
- When initially recovering, place the television remote control, radio, telephone, medication, tissues, wastebasket, and water glass in the most convenient location.
- Before surgery, stock up on food that can be easily prepared or reheated.

of adaptive equipment after THA has been studied with 74 clients (Davidson, 1999). Participants in the study were asked to rate the usefulness of each piece of equipment they received. The most used piece of equipment was the raised toilet seat, and participants reported using it for at least 6 months after their THA. Other pieces of equipment that participants reported to be helpful were the reacher, long-handled shoehorn, and sock aid; however, they did experience some difficulties in using them.

COTAs are involved in educating elders and their caregivers about proper and safe usage of adaptive equipment, observing hip precautions during functional activities, and making environmental adaptations. Laurel is a COTA who works in an acute care hospital and is involved in patient education. Before having a hip replacement, elders and their primary caregivers attend a class to prepare them to return home. Laurel reviews the precautions for both the posterolateral and anterolateral approaches. The elders bring clothing to practice using a

dressing stick, reacher, sock aid, and long-handled shoehorn. Laurel has the elders practice transferring to and from a chair, couch, commode, and raised toilet seat. They also practice using reachers to retrieve items from the floor and cupboards. During one question and answer session several elders expressed an interest in feeding their pets. Laurel asked a volunteer from her church to make pet feeders that could be easily lifted from the floor to the counter so that the elders could fill them with water and food without bending over (Fig. 22-7). Laurel also reviews information in a notebook with elders and their caregivers that will be used as their home programs. After surgery, Laurel works with elders to review the dressing techniques and reinforces the information that they learned earlier in class. Laurel also makes recommendations for bathroom equipment that the elders may need to return home. Some elders have stated that it was helpful to be exposed to the information before surgery because it was harder for them to concentrate after surgery.

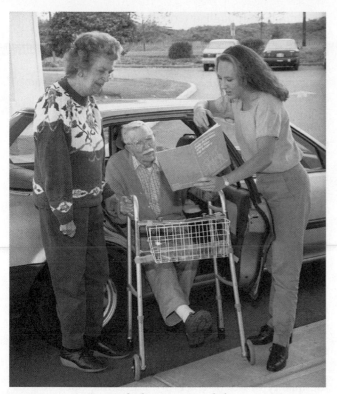

FIGURE **22-6**   A certified occupational therapy assistant provides training on proper techniques for transfers.

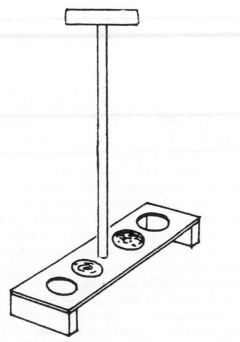

FIGURE **22-7**   This easily constructed pet feeder allows elders to fill the water and food bowls without bending over. (Courtesy Ron Connon.)

Knee Replacements

The knee joint has a large amount of synovium fluid, and thus is one joint often affected by rheumatoid and osteoarthritis (Dowdy, Cole, & Harner, 1998; Guccione, 1994). Chronic knee pain may cause difficulty in ascending and descending stairs, squatting, walking, and jogging, thus affecting one's quality of life.

Nonsurgical intervention may include a variety of approaches including medication, activity modification and exercise, braces, and weight reduction (Dowdy, Cole, & Harner, 1998). Nonsteroidal antiinflammatory drugs (NSAIDs) are often prescribed to reduce swelling and pain. Intraarticular injections are sometimes used when oral NSAIDs are ineffective.

Activity modification is targeted to minimize symptoms by avoiding high-impact activities. Maintaining a healthy body weight is difficult for people with knee pain, because it often decreases their activities without changing their intake of calories. If possible, elders with knee pain should try to maintain a regular exercise program to maximize aerobic conditioning.

Physical therapists may provide braces to help active elders regain a sense of knee stability during activities. Such knee braces are helpful in the short term, but people tend not to use them on a day-to-day basis (Dowdy, Cole, & Harner, 1998).

Surgical intervention includes a total knee joint arthroplasty or total knee replacement (TKR). Knee arthroplasties are best suited for sedentary persons older than 65 years (Dowdy, Cole, & Harner, 1998). Approximately 90% of TKRs are successful up to 10 years after surgery.

Rehabilitation after knee replacement

After a TKR, the knee is bandaged and changed 2 to 4 days after surgery. A Hemovac may be used and discontinued 2 to 3 days after surgery. To promote blood flow and decrease the chance of blood clot formation, the elder will likely wear thromboembolic disease (TED) hose. A knee immobilizer may be prescribed by some physicians. Others will prescribe the use of a continuous passive motion (CPM) machine (Mullarkey & Brander, 2002), which is designed to slowly and smoothly range the knee into flexion and extension. Physical therapists monitor the CPM unit and prescribe exercises to the elder.

Occupational and physical therapy services will work with elders to meet the following goals: transfer independently to and from bed, walk with crutches or a walker on a level surface, independently ascend and descend three stairs, independently carry out one's home exercise program, flex affected knee to 90 degrees, extend knee to neutral. Other rehabilitation concerns of clients with TKRs include sexual activity, driving, and return to work. Many physicians do not discuss sexual activity related to the TKR. However, clients should be counseled to avoid sexual intercourse for 4 to 6 weeks after TKR. (See Chapter 12 for more specific information about resuming sexual activity after a TKR.) Resuming driving can occur as early as 3 weeks for some elders, whereas others are not ready to drive until 8 months after surgery. The ability to return to driving is dependent on exhibiting good leg control, limiting use of narcotic pain relievers, and if the overall recovery is unremarkable (Mullarkey & Brander, 2002). Returning to work is more difficult to predict and is dependent on the type of work. Typically patients return to work 3 to 6 weeks after their surgery (Mullarkey & Brander, 2002). Keep in mind these are generic timeframes; physicians may instruct their clients with different timeframes on the basis of the clients' conditions.

ARTHRITIS

Arthritis affects millions of adults in the United States and is prevalent in nearly half of the elder population (NIA, n.d.). The self-reported prevalence of arthritis is greater among women than men, and for women aged 45 years and older, arthritis is the leading cause of activity limitation (Verbrugge & Patrick, 1995). Arthritis also is a leading predisposing condition for fractures (Gillespie, et al., 2002). Arthritis causes bone demineralization. The pain from arthritis limits people's activity, thus causing weight gain. These factors combined with environmental factors often result in falls/fractures.

More than 100 types of arthritis have been identified (NIA, n.d.). According to the National Institute on Aging, the three most common types of arthritis in the elderly population are osteoarthritis (OA), **rheumatoid arthritis** (RA), and gout (NIA, n.d.). Descriptions, causes, and symptoms of these three forms of arthritis are presented in Table 22-5.

Treatment for arthritis in elders can consist of any combination of therapy, medication, and surgery. Therapy may consist of the provision of physical therapy and OT. Medications commonly prescribed to elders who have arthritis are NSAIDs and cyclooxygenase-2 inhibitors (similar to NSAIDs but with fewer side effects). Performing surgery to replace joints often is a last resort.

COTAs must be aware of the physical restrictions and limitations that arthritis imposes on elders' activities. Interventions by the COTA/OTR team should focus on helping elders manage their symptoms more effectively in addition to modifying occupational tasks.

Common Problems Associated with Arthritis

Osteoarthritis of the knee affects approximately 60% of people older than 65 years (Buckwalter & Lane, 1996). Limitations caused by knee OA include difficulty using stairs, squatting, and high-impact activities (i.e., running or jumping) (Dowdy, Cole, & Harner, 1998). These activities can be quite painful and can reduce the quality of life for an active elder.

Upper extremity deformities caused by OA can be problematic. Osteophytes form in the fingers and base of the thumb. Although osteophytes are not painful, they are seen at the distal interphalangeal (DIP) (Heberden's nodes) and proximal interphalangeal (PIP) joints (Bouchard's nodes). Such nodes result in difficulty and pain during pinching. In advanced stages, the thumb's carpal metacarpal (CMC) joint can subluxate and result in joint instability.

The hands are the most severely affected joints in RA. Often, the PIP joints present with fusiform swelling or spindle-like shape. Boutonnière and swan-neck deformities also are finger deformities that may result from RA. Nalebuff deformities are common to the thumb when affected by RA. Ulnar drift often is present in the metacarpophalangeal (MCP) joints of the hand, and the wrist may volarly sublux.

Gout commonly affects the toes, ankles, elbows, wrists, and hands. Swelling can cause the skin to become taut around the joint and make the area appear red or purple and be tender. These presentations in turn reduce joint mobility (NIA, n.d.).

Occupational Therapy Intervention

The primary goal of OT intervention is to improve the quality of life of elders with arthritis. Specific goals may include maintaining joint mobility or joint stability, preventing joint deformity, maintaining strength, maintaining or improving functional ability, maintaining a healthy balance of rest and activity, modifying performance of activities, and improving psychosocial acceptance and coping mechanisms.

Maintenance of joint mobility and stability

COTAs may develop an exercise program for the elder to keep arthritic joints moving. Such an exercise program should seek to minimize stress to all involved joints. Elders with arthritis often find that taking a warm bath or shower after waking up in the morning relieves joint stiffness, thereby making it easier to exercise and engage in other activities. Elders with arthritis may also find it helpful to use a paraffin bath before engaging in wrist and hand exercises. COTAs should demonstrate service competency when using Physical Agent Modalities.

Joints requiring stability may warrant orthotic intervention. A carefully designed splint may provide stability to a joint and improve function. For example, discomfort in the CMC joint may be reduced by fabricating a hand-based thumb spica splint to support the CMC joint in a functional position (Riley, Lohman, Berger, Cavanaugh, & Coppard, 2001).

Prevention of joint deformity

COTAs must be aware of the common types of joint deformities that may develop as a result of arthritis. Deformities include **wrist subluxation**, **ulnar drift** of the MCP joints, **swan-neck deformity**, **boutonnière deformity**, and **Nalebuff type I deformity** of the thumb (Fig. 22-8).

TABLE 22-5

Description of Osteoarthritis and Rheumatoid Arthritis

Name	Definition	Cause	Symptoms
Osteoarthritis (degenerative joint disease)	A degenerative disease of cartilage with a secondary degeneration involving underlying bone	Possible biomechanical, inflammatory, and immunologic factors; secondary factors include congenital defects, trauma, inflammation, endocrine and metabolic disease, and occupational stress	Progressively developing pain, stiffness, and enlargement with limitation of motion; crepitus with PROM; commonly affects weight-bearing joints (hips, knees, cervical and lumbar spine, PIPs [enlargements or osteophytes in PIPs are often referred to as Bouchard's nodes], DIPs [enlargements or osteophytes in DIPs are often called Heberden's nodes], CMCs, and MTPs); joints appear red, tender, swollen; asymmetrical presentation; deformities of joints; pain often follows periods of overuse or extended inactivity
Rheumatoid arthritis	Chronic, systemic disease characterized by inflammation of the synovial tissue of joints; may involve the heart, lungs, blood vessels, or eyes	Unknown; seems to be of an unknown immune reaction in synovial tissue	Characterized by exacerbations and remissions; commonly affects weight-bearing joints (hips, knees, cervical and lumbar spine, PIPs, DIPs, CMCs, and MTPs); joints appear red, tender, swollen, and hot; usually a symmetrical presentation; deformities of joints (i.e., swan-neck, boutonnière); fusiform swelling in PIPs
Gout	Painful rheumatic disease affecting connective tissue, joint spaces, or both, caused by uric acid	Caused by deposits of needle-like crystals of uric acid in the connective tissue, joint spaces, or both	Characterized by swelling, redness, heat, pain, and joint stiffness; commonly affects the toes, ankles, elbows, wrists, and hands

CMC, carpometacarpal; DIP, distal interphalangeal; MTP, metatarsophalangeal; PIP, proximal interphalangeal; PROM, proximal range of motion.

Volar subluxation of the wrist frequently occurs in elders who have arthritis. A wrist cock-up splint may aid the elder in maintaining better wrist alignment, which will promote function and reduce pain (Lohman, 2001b). Ulnar drift, or ulnar deviation, of the MCP joints is another common deformity caused by arthritis. Ulnar drift usually is caused by destruction and loosening of the radial collateral ligaments. Some experts suggest that the use of an ulnar drift splint may prevent further deformity (Riley, Lohman, Berger, Cavanaugh, & Coppard, 2001).

A swan-neck deformity of the finger results in PIP hyperextension with DIP flexion. A boutonnière deformity results in PIP flexion with DIP hyperextension. Both these deformities can be splinted or surgically repaired with varying results. A Nalebuff type I deformity results in the metacarpal joint of the thumb flexed with hyperextension of the interphalangeal joint. A radial gutter thumb spica splint often is used for better positioning (Lohman, 2001a).

To prevent further deformity, elders should be evaluated to determine if they need splints that are appropriate for the deformity and activity level. In addition, elders should be taught joint protection techniques (Box 22-2; Fig. 22-9).

Maintenance of strength
COTAs may be asked to develop graded strengthening programs for elders who have arthritis. These programs should include the principles of joint protection discussed previously. During periods of acute exacerbation of arthritis, elders should *not* engage in strengthening programs.

Improvement of functional ability
Functional ability can be improved through careful collaboration between the COTA, OTR, and elder. This collaboration can help to determine whether assistive equipment works well and is accomplishing the goal for which it was intended. For example, a rocker knife may allow the elder to continue to cut meat during meals.

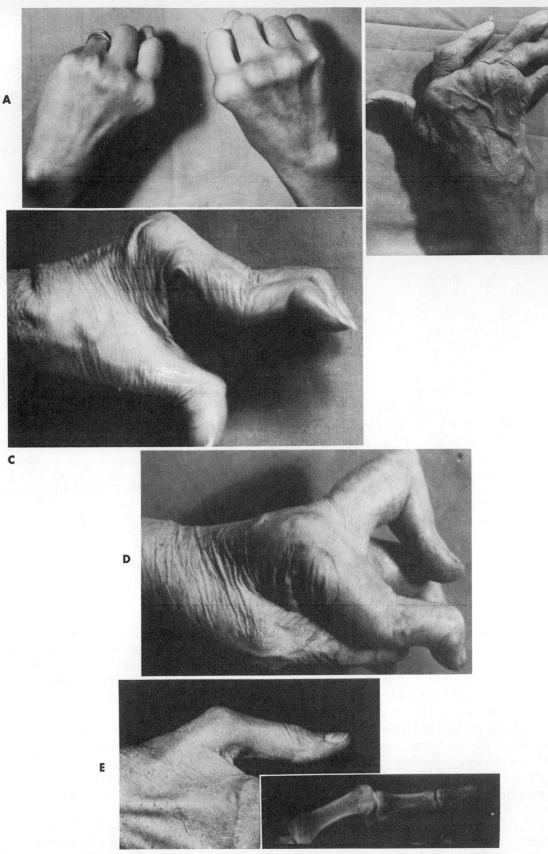

FIGURE **22-8**   Joint deformities that may develop as a result of arthritis. **A,** Wrist subluxation. **B,** Ulnar drift of metacarpophalangeal joints. **C,** Swan-neck deformity. **D,** Boutonnière deformity. **E,** Nalebuff type I deformity of the thumb. (From Hunter, J., Mackin, E., & Callahan, A. [Eds.]. [1995]. *Rehabilitation of the hand: Surgery and therapy* [4th ed.]. St. Louis, MO: Mosby.)

BOX 22-2

Joint Protection Principles

- Respect pain. Monitor activities and stop to rest when discomfort or fatigue develops. For example, if kneeling or stooping to garden causes pain and stiffness, stop and rest. Next time, try sitting on a stool.
- Reduce stresses on joints. Use the largest joint possible for activities. For example, when using hands to push up from a seated position, push up with the palms, not the back of the fingers.
- Wear splints as prescribed to protect joints. For example, wear resting hand splints during exacerbation periods to reduce pain. Movements should be done in the opposite direction of deformity. For example, when wringing out a wash cloth, twist toward the radial side rather than the ulnar side.
- Avoid sustaining a strong, tight grasp. For example, use foam or a cloth wrapped around handles to relax the grip needed to manipulate an object.
- Avoid carrying and lifting heavy objects. For example, use a cart to move heavy objects. Distribute object weight evenly over many joints. For example, use both hands to handle a carton of milk.
- Limit the amount of time spent climbing, walking, and standing. For example, take an elevator or escalators; drive or use a walking aid; sit whenever possible.
- Avoid sustained flexion of the finger joints. For example, use a large sponge for cleaning; work with the fingers extended over the sponge rather than squeezing it.
- Avoid using heavy objects. For example, cook with lightweight pots and pans rather than heavy cast-iron pots and pans.

COTAs must observe how the elder handles the knife to ensure that the involved joints are protected as the knife is used and to ascertain that the knife actually cuts the meat.

Maintenance of life balance

Graded strengthening programs for elders who have arthritis are developed by OTRs and may be administered by COTAs. Assisting elders in achieving a balance between rest and activity is paramount. For example, elders are often tempted to schedule all activities during the morning hours with hopes of resting in the afternoon. However, a better balance is achieved when activities are scheduled throughout the day and an appropriate period of rest is incorporated after each activity. This type of schedule will help to decrease the fatigue of elders and is less likely to lead to an exacerbation of their conditions. In addition, elders will likely accomplish more during the day.

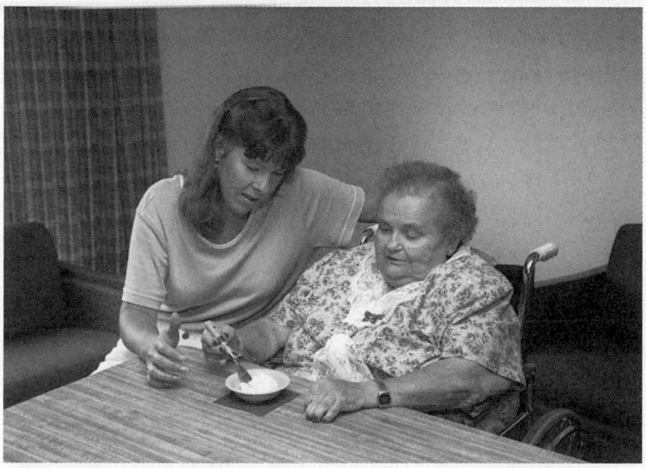

Modification of activity

Work simplification and **energy conservation** techniques often benefit elders who have arthritis (Box 22-3). These elders must attempt to distribute their energy output evenly over the number of tasks to be accomplished. Incorporating energy conservation and work simplification techniques into the elders' daily routines can assist them in maintaining a functional lifestyle.

Improvement of psychosocial well-being and coping mechanisms

The combination of acute and chronic pain, coupled with joint stiffness and immobility, can result in limitations of activities of daily living (ADL) such as dressing, and recreational and social outlets such as dancing. The population of elders who experience pain is challenged daily to use strategies that will enhance productive living. Elders who do not have coping and support systems will need assistance in developing such systems. COTAs may provide assistance by linking elders who have arthritis with community resources that can provide support and help elders to develop coping mechanisms. Self-help courses sponsored by the Arthritis Foundation can provide social interaction. Alternative methods of pain control may include relaxation training, cognitive restructuring and

FIGURE 22-9   Built-up handles help elders with arthritis maintain independence in a variety of activities.

BOX 22-3

Principles of Work Simplification and Energy Conservation

Pace
A moderate, slow pace is most productive; a slower pace is needed in a hot and humid atmosphere.

Rhythm
Working in a rhythmic manner saves energy and increases efficiency.

Eyes
Work in a well-lighted room, with local light for close work, and rest the eyes periodically.

Rest
Plan regular rest periods that are properly spaced during the day.

Body mechanics
Sit to work whenever possible; sit in a seat large enough to give full support; work with the elbows close to the body; if working at a table, the height of the table should be near the height of the elbows when they are bent at 90-degree angles.

Work areas
A place should be designated for all tools, utensils, and materials; materials should be located close to the area where they will be used.

Design of equipment
Handles of utensils and equipment should permit the maximum surface of the hand to come in contact with the handle; handles should be heat-resistant and built up as appropriate; handles that have impressions for the fingers should be used when possible; lightweight equipment should actually be light in weight.

Kitchen storage
Store supplies and utensils within easy reach; arrange the cupboards so that all articles are easy to see, easy to reach, and easy to grasp; store heavy equipment (e.g., stacks of plates and pans) on shelves that are easy to reach; use vertical dividers for dish storage, baking pans, trays, and lids; avoid clutter by eliminating or discarding unnecessary equipment.

Cooking
Use a cart for transporting food and dishes; slide heavy pots from the sink to the stove instead of lifting them; avoid holding containers or mixing bowls when preparing food; select equipment that can be used for more than one job.

Bed making
To avoid numerous trips around the bed, make one side completely and then the next side; if possible, keep the bed away from the wall; have the bed put on rollers if it must be moved.

Cleaning
When cleaning the bathtub, use long-handled brushes and sit on the edge of the bathtub; use a dust cloth on a long-handled stick for dusting baseboards and ceilings; have cleaning equipment available both upstairs and downstairs.

---

modification, medication fading, and social assertiveness training. The process of helping elders cope with arthritis must involve a multidisciplinary approach for chronic pain management to be successful.

CASE STUDY

Ford and Ida are meeting with a builder to design their retirement condominium. In planning the space, they have decided to consult with an agency that provides assistance for home design and modification for elders. They are awaiting a contact from the agency to schedule a meeting to begin plans for the new condominium.

One month previously, Ford fell during the nighttime in an attempt to go to the bathroom and sustained a hip fracture. Subsequently, he underwent an open reduction internal fixation and pinning of his right hip. Also, last year Ida had a TKA. Ida has considerable pain from RA. They hope to plan their ranch-style condominium to meet their current and future needs in relation to their health.

■ CASE STUDY REVIEW QUESTIONS

1 List the precautions that Ford might need to follow after his hip pinning procedure.
2 List the ADL functions that will be directly affected by Ford's hip pinning procedure.
3 Describe the problems that Ida may be dealing with as a result of RA.
4 Name the wrist and hand deformities associated with RA that may be afflicting Ida.
5 Describe some possible causes for Ford's fall that should be investigated.
6 Describe the ways in which Ford's performance of ADL functions and his environment will need to be modified.
7 List appropriate recommendations for the living room, kitchen, bathroom, and bedroom for their new condominium.

CHAPTER REVIEW QUESTIONS

1 Identify the most common causes of fractures in elders.
2 Why do elder women have a greater occurrence of orthopedic problems than elder men?
3 Why is it important for the certified occupational therapy assistant to have an understanding of the anterolateral and posterolateral approaches related to total hip replacements?
4 Identify two psychosocial issues that may have an effect on an elder after a total hip replacement.
5 Using joint protection techniques, explain how you would teach elders with arthritis in their hands to do the following:
   • wash delicate clothing in the sink
   • lift a child from a playpen
   • use a computer
6 Explain how you teach an elder energy conservation techniques during the following activities:
   • removing groceries from the trunk of a car and taking them in the house
   • vacuuming the floor
   • cleaning the kitchen after a meal

REFERENCES

Administration on Aging. (2002). *A profile of older Americans.* Washington, DC: U.S. Department of Health and Human Services.

Altizer, L. (2002). Fractures. *Orthopaedic Nursing, 21,* 51-59.

Birge, S. J., Morrow-Howell, N., & Proctor, E. K. (1994). Hip fracture. *Clinics in Geriatric Medicine, 10,* 589.

Black, D. M., & Cooper, C. (2000). Epidemiology of fractures and assessment of fracture risk. *Clinics in Laboratory Medicine, 20,* 439-453.

Brander, V. A., Mullarkey, C. F., & Stulberg, S. D. (2001). Rehabilitation after total joint replacement for osteoarthritis: An evidence-based approach. *Physical Medicine and Rehabilitation, 15*(1), 175-197.

Brown, J. S., Vittinghoff, E., Wyman, J. F., Stone, K. L., Nevitt, M.C., Ensrud, K. E., & Grady, D. (2000). Urinary incontinence: Does it increase risk for falls and fractures? *Journal of American Geriatric Society, 48,* 721-725.

Buckwalter, J. A, & Lane, N.E. (1996). Aging, sports, and osteoarthritis. *Sports Medicine and Arthroscopy Review, 4,* 276-287.

Capello, W. N., D'Antonio, J. A., Feinberg, J. R., & Manley, M. T. (2002). Hydroxyapatite coated stems in younger and older patients with hip arthritis. *Clinical Orthopedics, 92,* 100.

Centers for Disease Control. (1996). Incidence and costs to Medicare of fracture among Medicare beneficiaries age ≥ 65 years—United States, July 1991-June 1992. *Morbidity and Mortality Weekly Report* [On-line serial], *45*(41), 877-883. URL http://www.cdc.gov/aging/health_issues.htm

Coleman, S. (2001). Hip fractures and lower extremity joint replacement. In L. W. Pedretti & M. B. Early (Eds.), *Occupational therapy practice skills for physical dysfunction* pp. 867-880. St. Louis, MO: Mosby.

Connell, B. R., & Wolf, S. L. (1997). Environmental and behavioral circumstances associated with falls at home among healthy elderly individuals. *Archives of Physical Medicine & Rehabilitation, 78,* 179-186.

Cumming, R. G., Thomas, M., Szonyi, G., Salkeld, G., O'Neill, E., Westbury, C., & Frampton, G. (1999). Home visits by an occupational therapist for assessment and modification of environmental hazards: A randomized trial of falls prevention. *Journal of the American Geriatrics Society, 47,* 1397-1402.

Daniel, M. S., & Strickland, L. R. (1992). *Occupational therapy protocol management in adult physical dysfunction.* Gaithersburg, MD: Aspen.

Davidson, T. (1999). Total hip replacement: An audit of the provision and use of equipment. *British Journal of Occupational Therapy, 62,* 283-287.

Della-Valle, C. J., & Paprosky, W. G. (2002). The middle-aged patient with hip arthritis: The case of extensively coated stems. *Clinical Orthopedics,* 101-107.

Dowdy, P. A., Cole, B. J., & Harner, C. D. (1998). Knee arthritis in active individuals. *The Physician and Sports Medicine, 26,* 43-54.

Forsen, L., Bjartveit, K., Bjorndal, A., Edna, T., Meyer, H. E., & Schei, B. (1998). Ex-smokers and risk of hip fracture. *American Journal of Public Health, 88,* 1481-1483.

Gillespie, L. D., Gillespie, W. J., Robertson, M. C., Lamb, S. E., Cumming, R. G., & Rowe, B. H. (2003). Interventions for preventing falls in elderly people (Cochrane Review). In *The Cochrane Library, 4,* 1507-1514, Chichester, UK: John Wiley & Sons.

Guccione, A. A. (1994). Arthritis. In S. B. O'Sullivan & T. J. Schmitz (Eds.), *Physical rehabilitation assessment and treatment* (3rd ed.). pp. 423-449. Philadelphia: FA Davis.

Haverstock, B. D. (2001). Stress fractures of the foot and ankle. *Clinics in Podiatric Medicine and Surgery, 18,* 273-284.

Holley, S. (2002). A look at the problem of falls among people with cancer. *Clinical Journal of Oncology Nursing, 6,* 217-218.

Kim, Y. H., Cho, S. H., & Kim, R. S. (1998). Drainage versus nondrainage in simultaneous bilateral total hip arthroplasties. *Journal of Arthroplasty, 13,* 156-161.

Lewis, S. C. (2003). *Elder care in occupational therapy.* Thorofare, NJ: Slack.

Lohman, H. (2001a). Thumb immobilization splints. In B. M. Coppard & H. Lohman (Eds.), *Introduction to splinting.* pp. 219-251. St. Louis, MO: Mosby.

Lohman, H. (2001b). Wrist immobilization splints. In B. M. Coppard, & H. Lohman (Eds.). *Introduction to splinting.* pp. 139-184. St. Louis, MO: Mosby.

Maenpaa, H. M., Soini, I., Lehto, M. U., & Belt, E. A. (2002). Insufficiency fractures in patients with chronic inflammatory joint diseases. *Clinical and Experimental Rheumatology, 20,* 77-79.

McKinney, A. A., & Melby, V. (2002). Relocation stress in critical care: A review of the literature. *Journal of Clinical Nursing, 11*, 149-157.

Mehta, A. F., & Nastasi, A. E. (1993). Rehabilitation of fractures in the elderly. *Clinics in Geriatric Medicine, 9*, 717.

Mullarkey, C. F., & Brander, V. (2002). Rehabilitation after total knee replacement for osteoarthritis. *Physical Medicine and Rehabilitation: State of the Art Reviews, 16*, 431-443.

Murphy, S. L., Williams, C. S., & Gill, T. M. (2002). Characteristics associated with fear of falling and activity restriction in community-living older persons. *Journal of American Geriatrics Society, 50*, 516-520.

National Institute on Aging. (n.d.). Arthritis advice [WWW page]. URL http://www.niapublications.org/engagepages/arthritis.asp

National Institute of Arthritis and Musculoskeletal and Skin Diseases. (2000). Osteoporosis: Progress and promise [WWW page]. http://www.niapublications.org/engagepages/arthritis.asp http://www.niams.nih.gov/hi/topics/osteoporosis/opbkgr.htm

Oberg, U., Oberg, T., & Hadstedt, B. (1996). Functional improvement after hip and knee arthroplasty: 6-month follow-up with a new functional assessment system. *Physiotherapy Theory and Practice, 12*, 3-13.

Patel, B., & DeGroot, H. (2001). Evaluation of the risk of pathologic fractures secondary to metastatic bone disease. *Orthopedics, 24*, 612-617.

Riley, M. A., Lohman, H., Berger, S. M., Cavanaugh, M. T., & Coppard, B. M. (2001). Splinting on elders. In B. M. Coppard & H. Lohman (Eds.), *Introduction to splinting.* pp. 359-395. St. Louis, MO: Mosby.

Roe, B., Whattam, M., Young, H., & Dimond, M. (2001). Elders' perceptions of formal and informal care: Aspects of getting and receiving help for their activities of daily living. *Journal of Clinical Nursing, 10*, 398-405.

Rush University. (2003). Pioneering hip replacement surgery sends patients home the day after the operation [WWW page]. http://www.rush.edu/webapps/MEDREL/servlet/NewsRelease?id=274. January 15, 2004.

Saikko, V., Ahloroos, T., Calonius, O., & Keranen, J. (2001). Wear simulation of total hip prostheses with polyethylene against CoCR, alumina, and diamond-like carbon. *Biomaterials, 22*(12), 1507-1514.

Salkeld, G., Cumming, R. G., O'Neill, E., Thomas, M., Szonyi, G., & Westbury, C. (2000). The cost effectiveness of a home hazard reduction program to reduce falls among older persons. *Australian & New Zealand Journal of Public Health, 24*, 265-271.

Stromberg, C. N., & Herberts, P. (1994). A multi-center 10-year study of cemented revision hip arthroplasty in patients younger than 55 years old. *Journal of Arthroplasty, 9*(6), 595-601.

U.S. Department of Transportation. (1997). *Improving transportation for a maturing society* (DOT-P10-97-01). Washington, DC: U.S. Government Printing Office.

Verbrugge, L. M., & Patrick, D. L. (1995). Seven chronic conditions: Their impact on U.S. adults' activity levels and use of medical services. *American Journal of Public Health, 85*, 173-182.

Wallace, C., Reiber, G. E., LeMaster, J., Smith, D. G., Sullivan, K., Hayes, S., & Vath, C. (2002). Incidence of falls, risk factors for falls, and fall-related fractures in individuals with diabetes and a prior foot ulcer. *Diabetes Care, 25*, 1983-1986.

CHAPTER 23

Working with Elders Who Have Cardiovascular Conditions

TONYA BARTHOLOMEW, JANA K. CRAGG, JEAN T. HAYS,
AMY MATTHEWS, AND CLAIRE PEEL

KEY TERMS

cardiac rehabilitation, cardiovascular diseases, heart rate, blood pressure, maximum
heart rate, metabolic equivalents, energy conservation, work simplification

CHAPTER OBJECTIVES

1. Identify the signs and symptoms of cardiac dysfunction.
2. Describe the phases of cardiac rehabilitation.
3. Recognize the role of occupational therapy in cardiac rehabilitation.
4. Describe assessments, treatment techniques, and precautions used with elders who have cardiac conditions.
5. Describe treatment approaches for elders with cardiac conditions in various treatment settings.

...I have seen a woman who seemed catatonic suddenly came to life and shout out lines from an almost-forgotten song. There is an electricity generated by a skilled professional which is not usually equaled by even the most sincere amateur.

—Jennifer Davis
Executive Director,
Area Agency on Aging

Some certified occupational therapy assistants (COTAs) may specialize in cardiac rehabilitation, and others may work in settings with elders who have cardiac conditions as primary diagnoses or accompanying other diagnoses. Joan is a COTA who specializes in **cardiac rehabilitation.** She works closely with the cardiac team as she provides occupational therapy (OT) treatment. Mark is a COTA employed by a skilled nursing facility. He treats elders with a variety of conditions. Many of the elders are admitted for specific reasons such as rehabilitation after a total hip replacement or stroke. Most have accompanying chronic illnesses, including cardiac conditions. Mark often informally consults with Joan when he has a treatment question about cardiac conditions because he does not have the same specialty experience that she has and values her expertise. This chapter primarily focuses on the role of COTAs in cardiac rehabilitation settings. However, treatment of elders with cardiac conditions in other settings also is addressed.

Heart disease is one of the most frequent chronic conditions that occur among elders (American Heart Association, 2002; Centers for Disease Control [CDC], 2002), and the leading cause of morbidity and mortality in the United States, accounting for "84% of deaths in men and women in adults over 65" (American Heart Association, 2004). "Heart failure is the most common discharge diagnosis for hospitalized Medicare patients in the United States" (Department of Health and Human Service, 2003; Casper et al., 2003). According to the CDC (2002), heart trouble is the third leading cause of disability in the United States. **Cardiovascular diseases** include disorders of the heart and vascular system. These diseases can be categorized as the following: (1) diseases that primarily affect the heart such as coronary artery disease and congestive heart failure, (2) circulatory problems involving peripheral vessels such as peripheral vascular disease, and (3) circulatory problems involving the cerebral circulation. This chapter primarily focuses on diseases in the first category: the heart.

BACKGROUND INFORMATION

During the aging process, the body experiences gradual changes. Although many of these changes are inevitable, studies show that some of the changes are less pronounced in elders who do not have cardiovascular diseases and associated risk factors (Pate et al., 1995). This is especially true for elders who have lifestyles that include regular physical activity. However, most elders experience age-related changes in their cardiovascular systems, including changes in the heart muscle and vessels, peripheral vascular disease, and an increase in systolic pressure, which makes the heart work harder (Lakatta & Yin, 1982; Schwartz, 1999). Most coronary diseases are related to lifestyle and family history, as well as age. Chronic cardiac conditions include hypertension, angina pectoris, congestive heart failure, and peripheral vascular disease. Heart disease often accompanies other illnesses or conditions such as diabetes or chronic obstructive pulmonary disease; therefore, the COTA should be aware of any additional precautions or contraindications associated with these diagnoses and cardiovascular disease.

Medical treatment varies according to the condition and other individual health factors. Thrombolytics are used to prevent muscle damage from heart attacks. Other common drugs are those used to treat hypertension, angina, heart failure, and dysrhythmias. The COTA should be aware of the medications the patient is taking and the associated side effects. If conservative treatments involving medications are not effective, then surgical interventions may be necessary. Surgical treatments may include angioplasty or bypass for damaged arteries. In rare cases, treatment may involve a heart transplant to replace heart muscle that is irreversibly damaged. Cardiac management may include electromechanical devices such as pacemakers to achieve a normal **heart rate (HR)** and rhythm.

Heart disease may begin with a loss of elasticity in the small vessels, causing the heart to work harder to maintain blood flow to organs. A change in the temperature in the extremities, cyanosis, or an increase in systolic blood pressure may indicate circulatory insufficiency. Atherosclerosis is a condition in which lipid deposits accumulate on the walls of large and medium vessels (Andereoli, Bennett, Carpenter, & Plum, 1997). This narrows the lumen of these vessels, which restricts blood flow. Atherosclerosis of coronary vessels can produce ischemia, which causes angina (chest pain), a myocardial infarction (MI), or both, which damages the heart muscle. Atherosclerosis of cerebral vessels can lead to a cerebrovascular accident, or stroke. A change in the structure of the heart valves, either from viral illness or aging, may result in heart failure, a condition in which the heart cannot deliver enough oxygen to peripheral tissues.

Valvular disease may be heard as a murmur during a routine examination. When the left side of the heart fails, fluid accumulates in the lungs, causing exertional dyspnea, orthopnea, paroxysmal nocturnal dyspnea, dyspnea at rest, pulmonary edema, weakness, and fatigue (Andereoli, Bennett, Carpenter, & Plum, 1997). When the right side of the heart fails, blood backs up in the periphery, causing systemic venous congestion, dependent edema, upper right quadrant pain, anorexia, nausea, bloating, and fatigue (Andereoli, Bennett, Carpenter, & Plum, 1997). Many elders with cardiovascular disease lose the ability to perform physical activities and lose independence in their daily skills (CDC, 2002).

PSYCHOSOCIAL ASPECTS OF CARDIAC DYSFUNCTIONS

Cardiac dysfunction can have profound psychosocial implications on elders and their significant others. All elders react differently to a cardiac event, experiencing a wide range of emotions including anxiety, depression, denial, and helplessness (Fuster, 2002), but most progress through many stages of adjustment. Initially, the anxiety produced by fear of death, discomfort, dependence, and disability can have a profound effect and produce overwhelming feelings. Some elders demonstrate this anxiety in behavioral changes and may act out or become agitated. This level of anxiety places a physiologic demand on the cardiac system at a time when rest is important. Elders experiencing a rapid change in their care status may also have difficulty with anxiety; as a result, antianxiety medications often are used to assist them. However, antianxiety medications can have unwanted side effects and lead to additional stress. Elders should be encouraged to voice their feelings and work with the health care team to alleviate their fears about the course of events. Good communication and supportive staff members are the key elements in reducing elders' anxiety levels.

Fear of another cardiac event can impair functional levels, especially in the early rehabilitation phase. Education and therapeutic intervention can help to alleviate these fears. Once stable, elders should be encouraged to begin ambulation and self-care activities following the guidelines established by the occupational therapist (OTR). This helps to eliminate the helplessness elders may feel after a cardiac event. The longer these two elements are delayed, the more helpless elders may feel, which can reinforce the disability (Mathews, Foderaro, & O'Leary, 1996; Fuster, 2002). (Chapter 12 includes a discussion of ways to address the sexual concerns of elders with heart disease.)

As elders begin to regain some strength and control over their activity, denial of risk related to the disease may become evident. Denial gives some elders the mechanism necessary to cope with the cardiac event. This particular phase may be more prevalent in elders with coronary disease because the symptoms and characteristics associated with this disease are vague. COTAs must not try to break through the denial phase too soon. Facing the realities of the situation may be overwhelming and may create stress-related physical and emotional complications. COTAs can help elders by instructing them to monitor their performance carefully, thus reducing the risk for another cardiac event.

Some elders become depressed after a cardiac event. Inactivity and anxiety may trigger depression. Depression and anxiety combined can have a long-term effect on the elder's physical and emotional well-being. Patients with depression are less likely to resume normal activity and are at an increased risk for death (Fuster, 2002).

COTAs can play a strong role in addressing the psychosocial aspects of cardiac disease by educating elders about the expected outcomes after a cardiac event. Relaxation training and lifestyle education are key elements in achieving emotional well-being. Informing the family of risks and precautions can assist elders in the transition to the home environment and ensure that elders have the best chance to regain their status in the home and community.

EVALUATION OF ELDERS WITH CARDIAC CONDITIONS

COTAs working with elders who have had cardiac events or who have chronic cardiac conditions should be able to monitor vital signs. It is important that COTAs accurately determine HR and take **blood pressure (BP)** during activities (Fig. 23-1). Guidelines for HR and BP responses are typically written as treatment precautions. To determine the HR, COTAs should palpate the elder's pulse at the wrist, count the number of beats felt for 15 seconds, and then multiply this number by 4. This will provide a baseline HR in beats per minute (bpm) before the elder engages in activity. Although HRs vary, a normal baseline HR ranges between 60 and 100 bpm (Mathews, Foderaro, & O'Leary, 1996). **Maximum HR** corresponds with performing maximal levels of exertion that involve large muscle groups in rhythmic activities such as walking and cycling. One method of predicting maximum HR is by subtracting the elder's age from 220. This figure is

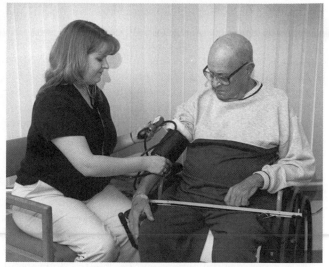

FIGURE **23-1**   Elders with cardiac conditions should be monitored for heart rate, blood pressure, and respiratory rate responses to activity.

multiplied by 0.6 to predict the appropriate HR response for normal activity (American College of Sports Medicine, 1991). For example, a 78-year-old woman's predicted maximum HR would be 142 bpm (220 − 78 = 142). Her HR appropriate for activity would be 85 (0.6 × 142 = 85 bpm). Signs and symptoms, such as dyspnea, must be considered when using formulas to predict activity HR values. Elders should perform activities in a symptom-free range. Some medications (beta-blockers, verapamil, and diltiazem) blunt the usual HR in response to exercise, especially in elders; therefore, watching symptoms is especially important (Taylor, 2000). In phase I, patients are often on continuous pulse oximetry. The COTA should be careful to ensure the patient is maintaining pulse and oxygen saturation levels within the range set by the physician.

Likewise, BP should be taken if a physician has so ordered or if the elder has symptoms of distress such as shortness of breath, dizziness, weakness, or cyanosis. Elders with hypertension should be monitored for excessive increases in BP or orthostatic hypotension, which may occur as a side effect of medications. BP values greater than 140/90 mm Hg indicate mild hypertension, and those greater than 160/100 mm Hg indicate moderate hypertension (Joint National Committee on Detection, Evaluation and Treatment of High Blood Pressure, 1993). BP is considered hypotensive if the systolic BP is less than 90 mm Hg. Hypotension can be associated with dizziness and light-headedness or, in severe cases, circulatory inadequacy of the extremities (Mathews, Foderaro, & O'Leary, 1996). In the presence of a shunt for renal dialysis, the BP should be read on the opposite limb. Renal shunts are fragile and cannot withstand the pressure produced by the BP cuff (sphygmomanometer) during BP monitoring.

For training, COTAs should practice monitoring HR and BP with an instructor before performing care.

The COTA/OTR team should be able to perform basic bedside activities of daily living (ADL) evaluation as part of the initial evaluation. This might include having the elder perform oral care, grooming tasks, washing of the upper body, and dressing. COTAs working with elders who have decreased endurance and low activity tolerance caused by cardiac disease may use **metabolic equivalents** (METs) as a basis for estimating the energy expended when performing an activity. The MET table provided along with HR and BP responses can help COTAs to determine the cardiovascular stress and amount of work performed for specific tasks (Table 23-1). Further areas to be assessed are grip strength, muscle strength, and bed mobility. The OT also should assess the patient's cognitive abilities to ensure the patient will be able to comprehend the education and interventions the COTA is teaching.

INTERVENTIONS, GOALS, AND STRATEGIES

For interventions to be effective, COTAs must understand the functional levels that are used to classify elders with cardiac disease. There are four functional categories for cardiac disease (Box 23-1). Knowing the categories allows COTAs to make adjustments in elders' rehabilitation programs. The four phases of cardiac rehabilitation describe where the elder is in the recovery process (Box 23-2).

COTAs need to be aware of activities that can be stressful to the heart. Such activities include isometric and upper extremity activities, especially if performed at a level above the heart. The stress on the heart is reflected by the elder's HR and BP responses, as well as other signs and symptoms. Consequently, any activity that produces excessive increases in HR and BP may overstress the heart.

The primary goal of any cardiac rehabilitation program is to return elders to their maximum functional capacities.

TABLE 23-1

Santa Clara Valley Medical Center's Metabolic Equivalents after Myocardial Infarction and after Open Heart Surgery	
Stage	**OT**
In ICU or on ward	General mobility (bed mobility, transfers to the commode, and position changes) with energy conservation techniques (environmental setups, equipment, and pacing)
1-2 METs	Sedentary leisure tasks with arms supported (reading, writing, playing cards) Standing tasks (seconds to 2 minutes) Simple hygiene, semi-recline sitting position Standing tasks (3 to 5 minutes) Bedside bathing (assist with feet and back) Bathroom privileges Light leisure tasks such as keyboarding at a computer
2-3 METs	Standing tasks (5-30 minutes) Sustained upper extremity (UE) activity (2-30 minutes) Total body bathing at sink Total hygiene, bathing, dressing at sink Total body mobility: bending for small objects, retrieval training Moderate leisure tasks
3-4 METs	Shower transfers Total showering task (hair washing, total body washing, drying, and dressing) Simple homemaking tasks such as meal preparation Energy conservation techniques with activity such as cleaning windows
4-5 METs	Pushing a light power mower Dance Raking leaves
5-6 METs	Digging in a garden Sex Fishing

Reed, K. L. (2001). *Quick reference to occupational therapy* (2nd ed.). Gaithersburg, MD: Aspen.
ICU, intensive care unit; MET, metabolic equivalent.

BOX 23-1

The Four Functional Categories of Cardiac Disease

Class I
Elders with cardiac disease but without resulting limitations of physical activity. Ordinary physical activity does not cause undue fatigue, palpitation, dyspnea, or anginal pain.

Class II
Elders with cardiac disease resulting in slight limitation of physical activity. They are comfortable at rest. Ordinary physical activity results in fatigue, dyspnea, palpitation, or anginal pain.

Class III
Elders with cardiac disease resulting in marked limitation of physical activity. They are comfortable at rest. Less than ordinary physical activity causes fatigue, dyspnea, palpitation, or anginal pain.

Class IV
Elders with cardiac disease resulting in inability to perform any physical activity without discomfort. Symptoms of cardiac insufficiency or of anginal syndrome may be present even at rest. If any physical activity is undertaken, discomfort increases.

From New York Heart Association. (1979). *Nomenclature and criteria for diagnoses of diseases of the heart and great vessels* (8th ed.). Boston: Little, Brown.

The COTA/OTR team must design an individualized rehabilitation program for each elder. Although the phases of rehabilitation follow certain key steps, each elder's progress will be different. Psychosocial aspects, family support, age, and medical status, as well as the desire to participate in the rehabilitation program, affect treatment progression. A rehabilitation treatment plan for OT with MET allowances for specific activities is useful (see Table 23-1).

Phase I

Phase I consists of the period of inpatient hospitalization. Most referred elders are in the acute phase after undergoing surgery or experiencing MI. Other elders are referred for atypical chest pain. Beginning in phase I, elders are evaluated by an OTR. During the evaluation, the COTA/OTR team reviews the medical chart to obtain information on medical history and current cardiac status, and they interview the elder to determine lifestyle

BOX 23-2

The Four Phases of Cardiac Rehabilitation

Phase I
This phase occurs in the acute phase of hospitalization for the cardiac event. Elders qualifying for cardiac rehabilitation must be stable after event as determined by physician(s).

Phase II
Occurs during subacute period after event. Instituted once elder leaves the hospital and continues for 6 to 12 weeks. Elder is followed up by home health or outpatient service.

Phase III
Elder enters a program designed to regain former functional and performance level. Focus is on increasing duration and intensity of physical activity to achieve health benefits and to increase cardiorespiratory fitness.

Phase IV
Elder enters a maintenance phase of cardiac rehabilitation. This phase is indefinite in length and involves periodic evaluations.

Modified from Kloner, R. (1984). *The guide to cardiology.* New York: Wiley & Sons.

and personal goals for rehabilitation. During phase I, OT practitioners and elders work toward developing a discharge plan on the basis of the elder's individual needs and lifestyles. Goals for meeting each of the stages in phase I are discussed (see Table 23-1). Activities and educational information are introduced as the rehabilitation process begins. Activities and exercises are initially low level. Early in phase I, COTAs educate elders regarding the need for balancing their lifestyles, which includes stress reduction techniques (Fig. 23-2). Elders also are educated to accommodate for changes in their health status. Using the occupational behavioral model of work, rest, and play, COTAs can introduce the concepts of **energy conservation** and **work simplification** while providing bedside treatment (Gibson, 1993). This gives elders the ability to regain some of their self-care and dignity while learning to work with their limitations after a cardiac event. COTAs can build rapport and support continued rehabilitation by carefully monitoring physiologic responses, signs, and symptoms and structuring activities to prevent elders from feeling fatigue.

METs help to establish parameters for functional activities. One MET, the oxygen consumed by the body at rest, is equal to approximately 3.5 ml O_2/kg body mass per minute. To translate this concept into an activity level, it takes 1.5 METs to write a letter in bed with the arms supported (Mathews, Foderaro, & O'Leary, 1996). Most self-care activities range from 1.5 to 3.5 METs, and although this may seem to be light work, it can be physically demanding for some elders. In some rehabilitation settings, OT does not intervene in cardiac rehabilitation until the elder is able to perform light work (1.5 to 2 METs) without symptoms of dyspnea, palpitation, or angina during or after activity. Once elders are at this level, they can attempt activities required to return home and can independently perform most self-care activities. During phase I, elders are reevaluated to determine whether additional equipment or education is necessary so that they are able to return home and conduct functional activities with safe and appropriate HR, electrocardiogram (ECG), and BP responses.

Phase II

Phase II, often referred to as the *recovery*, or *healing*, *phase*, is the period immediately after hospitalization. Elders receive rehabilitation through home health or outpatient clinic services. An elder's functional performance during self-care activities is evaluated by monitoring the resting pulse and peak pulse during a task and then measuring the recovery time to a resting pulse once the activity is terminated. The elder's status is monitored during the activities by measuring HR, BP, ECG, and respiratory responses before, during, and after task completion. The course of treatment and the elder's progress are determined by the physiologic responses during activities and the estimated MET level for activities. During this phase of rehabilitation, education and training continue for modifications of risk factors and monitoring of the elder's general health.

Phase III

Once elders are able to tolerate increased MET activities at greater than 3.5 METs with safe and appropriate HR, BP, and ECG responses, they are ready to move into phase III of rehabilitation. At this level of function, elders ideally have been under the care of a cardiac rehabilitation team for 2 to 3 months. Goals of phase III programs include increasing activity duration and intensity to a level sufficient to elicit cardiorespiratory training adaptations while assisting elders in making necessary lifestyle changes. Phase III of cardiac rehabilitation requires elders to be more responsible for self-monitoring and to react appropriately if signs or symptoms of a recurring cardiac event become evident. Elders in phase III programs typically attend outpatient programs two or three times per week. These sessions provide opportunities for therapists to evaluate function and performance and to facilitate progression of activity programs. Providing elders with the education and techniques necessary to maintain their new lifestyles allows them to be more successful at self-monitoring. Elders often are counseled to make dietary changes, to stop smoking, and to increase physical activity levels. COTAs are in a position to reinforce lifestyle changes. Continued training in energy conservation and the use of assistive devices is provided to elders at functional levels III and IV. In outpatient clinics, elders also can receive training in a simulated work environment to provide guidelines for returning to a job or for avocational interests.

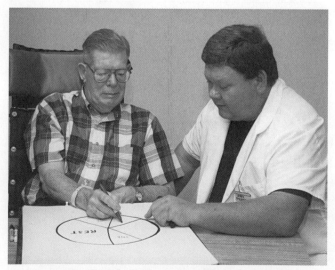

FIGURE 23-2 Certified occupational therapy assistants educate elders regarding the need for balancing their lifestyles.

Energy Conservation, Work Simplification, and other Education

During OT, elders receive education on energy conservation, work simplification, and cardiac status monitoring. Energy conservation is not only important for the elder's well-being, but it also is a safety monitor for routine tasks. In the acute portion of cardiac rehabilitation, this component allows elders to set the pace of their self-care routines. Energy conservation begins with basic task analysis, which includes identifying the main steps in the task, analyzing the way the task is performed, and determining the tools or skills needed to perform the task. Once analyzed, the next component of work simplification is added. Having elders perform basic grooming at the bedside is an example of ADL energy conservation. Using the bedside table, with arms propped for energy conservation, the elder can perform grooming with all the supplies and a basin of water on the table (Fig. 23-3). Elders may need to be educated to take rest breaks during the task if they experience dyspnea or an increase in HR beyond the established parameters. The task can be simplified with a complete setup of supplies, including removal of all caps from grooming supplies and provision of a lightweight electric razor, if appropriate. With the elder in the semi-reclined position in bed, this task can be accomplished with no more than 1.5 METs. Other ADL functions are analyzed in the same manner, with the therapist identifying ways to reduce the energy expenditure (energy conservation) and minimize steps to perform the task (work simplification). The addition of assistive devices may be an added benefit (Table 23-2). (See Chapter 12 to learn about addressing sexuality aspects of ADL with heart disease.)

Elders should be educated to pace themselves during activities to reduce fatigue. The work-rest-work principle is important for elders to maintain in the acute phase,

TABLE 23-2

Assistive Devices and Rationale for Use

Item	Rationale
Long-handle reacher Long-handle shoehorn Sock aid Elastic shoelaces Long-handle bath sponge	These items prevent the need to bend more than 90 degrees forward flexion in trunk. This may be a precaution for bypass surgery to reduce strain over incision. Limiting trunk flexion to 90 degrees facilitates breathing by allowing full excursion of the diaphragm.
Bath bench	Allows patient to sit during bathing.
High stool	Allows patient to sit during household tasks, such as food preparation and ironing.

especially when denial is an issue. Elders in denial about their cardiac disease may want to prove they are well by overworking or pushing themselves, placing unnecessary stress on their damaged hearts.

TREATMENT OF ELDERS WITH CARDIAC CONDITIONS IN OTHER SETTINGS

This chapter has focused primarily on cardiac rehabilitation when cardiac disease is the primary diagnosis. However, COTAs may encounter elders who have cardiac problems, perhaps as one of many chronic conditions, in settings such as nursing homes. Elders with acute cardiac conditions eventually may be transferred from the cardiac rehabilitation setting to another setting for further rehabilitation. In these settings, COTAs who are not formally trained in cardiac rehabilitation need to be aware of treatment approaches and precautions. Elders with cardiac conditions in any setting need to be educated on work simplification and energy conservation. The optimal approach is to demonstrate work simplification and energy conservation during the performance of meaningful tasks.

The primary recommendation for all elders with cardiac conditions is to monitor responses to activity by measuring HR, BP, and respiratory rate at rest, during activity, and during recovery. Activities that elicit excessive increases in HR or BP or that elicit abnormal signs and symptoms should not be performed or should be modified to ensure appropriate responses. Elders who have had coronary artery bypass graft surgery often are given lifting restrictions. Recommendations vary by physician and often

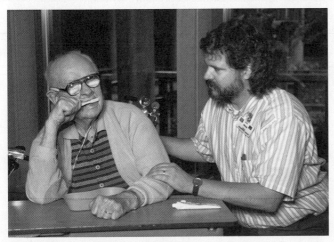

FIGURE 23-3 Elders should perform oral care with arms propped on a table.

include not lifting more than 10 lb for at least 1 month after surgery. Lifting precautions also may be recommended for elders who have had a procedure involving catheterization of the femoral artery, such as angioplasty and stent placement. Lifting guidelines for these procedures, determined by the elder's physician, are based on the elder's lifestyle and physical status and the specific procedures performed.

Recognition of distress signals is vital in any setting when working with elders with cardiac dysfunction. Primary signs and symptoms are chest pain, shortness of breath, cyanosis, sweating, fatigue, weakness, and confusion. Elders with cardiac dysfunction often complain of burning or pressure in the chest or of upper extremity, jaw, or cervical pain. These symptoms may occur with elders who have congestive heart failure, dysrhythmias, or a history of MI or angina. If elders demonstrate or report any of these symptoms, the COTA should monitor their BP, HR, and ECG readings for changes in medical status. Any abnormal sign or symptom should be documented and discussed with the OTR and other health care professionals.

Another key area is the type of medication elders with cardiac or BP problems are taking. Anticoagulants are commonly used for elders who have hypertension or who have had a cerebrovascular accident or hip or knee replacement surgery. Nitroglycerin is a common medication for elders with angina pectoris. Table 23-3 lists commonly prescribed medications. Knowledge of which medications elders are taking and their side effects is important to any therapist, but especially to those who perform therapy services through a home health agency or in a community setting.

CASE STUDY

Adelle, who is 79 years old, is being managed with occupational therapy in an acute care hospital setting after a coronary bypass graft. Her medical history includes type II diabetes mellitus, hypertension, peripheral vascular disease, and iron deficiency anemia. Her occupational history includes interests in growing tomatoes and volunteering at her church, where she answers the telephone and sends welcome letters to new members. She lives alone in a home with three stairs. Some adaptations have been made in the home environment such as a tub/shower combination on the main level next to her bedroom. Adelle would like to

TABLE 23-3

Examples of Common Medications and Potential Side Effects

Condition	Medication category: examples	Side effects
Angina pectoris	Nitrates: nitroglycerin, isosorbide dinitrate Beta-blockers: atenolol, propranolol Calcium channel blockers: verapamil, diltiazem	Headache, orthostatic hypotension, dizziness Bradycardia, depression, fatigue Peripheral edema
Heart failure	Cardiac glycosides: digitalis, digoxin Diuretics: furosemide Ace inhibitors: enalapril, captopril	Cardiac dysrhythmias, GI distress, CNS disturbances Electrolyte disturbances, volume depletion Skin rash
Hypertension	Beta-blockers: atenolol, metoprolol Diuretics: hydrochlorothiazide Calcium channel blockers: verapamil, diltiazem Ace inhibitors: enalapril, Alpha-blocker: prazosin Centrally acting SNS antagonists: clonidine Vasodilators: hydralazine	Bradycardia, depression, fatigue Volume depletion, electrolyte imbalance Peripheral edema Skin rash Reflux, tachycardia, orthostatic hypotension. Dry mouth, dizziness, drowsiness Reflux, tachycardia, dizziness, orthostatic hypotension, weakness, headache
Dysrhythmias	Sodium channel blockers: quinidine, lidocaine Beta-blockers Drugs that prolong repolarization: amiodarone Calcium channel blockers: verapamil	Cardiac rhythm disturbances Bradycardia Pulmonary toxicity, liver damage Bradycardia, dizziness, headache
Acute MI	Narcotic analgesic: morphine Platelet-aggregation inhibitors: aspirin Thrombolytics: streptokinase, tissue plasminogen activator	Sedation, respiratory depression, GI distress GI distress Excessive bleeding

ACE, angiotensin-converting enzyme; CNS, central nervous system; GI, gastrointestinal; MI, myocardial infarction; SNS, sympathetic nervous system.

remain independent with doing self-care and light homemaking tasks, managing her health, and gardening. Her son and daughter live nearby and drive her to appointments, shopping, and social activities. Her friends from her church visit weekly and they tend to her garden together. Adele's niece helps her with vacuuming and cleaning the bathroom.

Trina, the COTA, has been educating Adelle on energy conservation and work simplification techniques. They have practiced pacing self-care activities in bed and have discussed techniques for gardening and cooking simple meals when she returns home. Trina also has provided Adelle with handouts and a home program. Adelle will be receiving home health OT and Trina will be communicating with the home health OT to update her on Adelle's progress and goals in the acute care hospital program.

■ CASE STUDY REVIEW QUESTIONS

1 Describe how the HR for activity should be determined in Adelle's case.
2 How would Adelle's endurance for dressing be calculated? Discuss when it can be increased.
3 What tools or equipment could be provided to simplify her self-care and home-making tasks?
4 What are three activities Adele should avoid? Why are these activities contraindicated?
5 What would be important for Trina to report to the home health OT?
6 What recommendations should the COTA make for home health?
7 How does Adelle's support affect her overall health?
8 What health management techniques would be important for Adelle to engage in?

■ CHAPTER REVIEW QUESTIONS

1 Describe the impact anxiety may have on an elder's ability to perform occupations.
2 Explain the role certified occupational therapy assistants (COTAs) play in addressing the psychosocial aspects of cardiac disease.
3 Describe how maximum heart rates (HRs) and activity HRs are determined.
4 Describe what is involved in evaluation of elders with cardiac conditions.
5 Describe why evaluating cognition is important.
6 Describe the four functional categories of cardiac disease.
7 Describe the four phases of cardiac rehabilitation.
8 What is a metabolic equivalent (MET) and how can the MET system be used in cardiac rehabilitation?
9 Describe how energy conservation and work simplification are used in elders with cardiac conditions.
10 What should COTAs do for elders who report symptoms of angina pectoris while washing their hair?

11 Identify a method of energy conservation for elders while dressing their lower extremities.

REFERENCES

American College of Sports Medicine. (1991). *Guidelines for exercise testing and prescription* (4th ed.). Philadelphia: Lea and Febiger.

American Heart Association. (2002). 2002 Heart and stroke statistical update [WWW page]. URL http://www.americanheart.org/presenter.jhtml?identifier=2011.2004. Dallas, TX: The Association.

Andereoli, T. E., Bennett, J. C., Carpenter, C. J., & Plum., F. (1997). *Cecil essentials of medicine* (4th ed). Philadelphia: WB Saunders.

Casper, M. L., Barnett, E., Williams, I., Halverson, J., Braham, V., Greenlund, K. The Atlas of Stroke Mortality: Racial, Ethnic, and Geographic Disparities in the United States, 1st ed. Atlanta, Georgia: U.S. Department of Health and Human Services, CDC, February 2003.

Centers for Disease Control. (2002). National Center for Chronic Disease Prevention and Health Promotion. Chronic disease overview [WWW page]. URL http://www.cdc.gov/nccdphp/overview.htm

Comoss, P. M., Froelicher, E. S., Smith, L. K., & Wenger, N. K. (Eds.). (1999). *Cardiac rehabilitation: A guide to practice in the 21st century*. New York: Marcel Dekker.

Department of Health and Human Services Centers for Disease Control and Prevention (2003). Atrial Fibrillation as a Contributing Cause of Death and Medicare Hospitalization. Vol. 52. 7. [WWW page] URL http://216.239.41.104/search?q=cache:_wnoN_n_B80J:www.cdc.gov/mmwr/PDF/wk/mm5207.pdf+Wegner,+2000+medicare+cardiovascular&hl=en&ie=UTF-8#4. 2004.

Gibson, D. (1993). The evolution of occupational therapy. In H. L. Hopkins & H. D. Smith (Eds.), *Willard and Spackman's occupational therapy* (8th ed.) (pp. 525-543). Philadelphia: JB Lippincott.

Joint National Committee on Detection, Evaluation and Treatment of High Blood Pressure, National High Blood Pressure Education Program, Coordinating Committee. (1993). *Report of the Joint National Committee on Detection, Evaluation and Treatment of High Blood Pressure.* Bethesda, MD: National Heart, Lung and Blood Institute, National High Blood Pressure Program.

Lakatta, E. G., & Yin, F. C. (1982). Myocardial aging: Functional alterations and related cellular mechanisms. *American Journal of Physiology, 242*(6), H927.

Mathews, M. M., Foderaro, D., & O'Leary, S. (1996). Cardiac dysfunction. In L. W. Pedretti (Ed.), *Occupational therapy: Practice skills for physical dysfunction* (4th ed.) (pp. 693-709). St. Louis, MO: Mosby.

Pate, R. R., Pratt, M., Blair, S. N., Haskell, W., Macera, C. A., Bouchard, C., Buchner, D., Ettinger, W., Heath, G. W., King, A. C., Kriska, A., Leon, A. S., Macus, B. H., Morris, J., Paffenbarger, R. S., Patrick, K., Pollock, M. L., Rippe, J. M., Sallis, J., & Wilmore, J. H. (1995). Physical activity and public health: A recommendation from the Centers for Disease Control and Prevention and the American College of Sports Medicine. *Journal of the American Medical Association, 273*(5), 402-407.

Schwartz, J. (1999). Cardiovascular Function and Disease in the Elderly [WWW page]. URL http://www.galter.northwestern.edu/geriatrics/chapters/cardiovascular_function_disease.cfm.2004.

Taylor, G. J. (2000). *Primary care management of heart disease.* St. Louis, MO: Mosby.

CHAPTER 24

Working with Elders Who Have Pulmonary Conditions

ANGELA M. PERALTA AND SHERRELL POWELL

KEY TERMS

chronic obstructive pulmonary disease, chronic pulmonary emphysema, chronic bronchitis, bronchiectasis, energy conservation, work simplification

CHAPTER OBJECTIVES

1. Define chronic obstructive pulmonary disease.
2. Identify common symptoms of chronic obstructive pulmonary disease.
3. Identify the psychosocial effect of chronic obstructive pulmonary disease on elders.
4. List conditions that effect the sexual functioning of elders with chronic obstructive pulmonary disease.
5. Describe assessment and treatment intervention for elders with chronic obstructive pulmonary disease.

Denise is a certified occupational therapy assistant (COTA) who works in a large rehabilitation hospital in the South Bronx section of New York City. Her clients are from lower socioeconomic backgrounds. Many of them are factory workers and manual laborers. Denise has noticed a marked increase in the number of referrals to occupational therapy (OT) of elders who have **chronic obstructive pulmonary disease (COPD)** as a secondary diagnosis. These elders are finding it difficult to carry out their activities of daily living (ADL) because of the debilitating effects of COPD. On reviewing their social histories, Denise found that many of these elders worked with a variety of chemicals and that many of them were heavy smokers. Some of the major problems these elders must deal with include difficulty engaging in self-care activities,

a decreased level of endurance, chronic fatigue, and an inability to engage in leisure activities. Many elders with COPD report a fear of not being able to breathe because of frequent episodes of shortness of breath.

COPD also is seen in elder residents of nursing homes, usually as a secondary diagnosis. Regardless of the setting, COTAs working with elders who have COPD must be aware of the causes, symptoms, and OT interventions for this disease.

CHRONIC OBSTRUCTIVE PULMONARY DISEASE

COPD is a general disease that can include **chronic pulmonary emphysema, chronic bronchitis,** and chronic severe asthma. Chronic bronchitis and emphysema affect the upper and lower respiratory tracts and are characterized by cough, expectoration, wheezing, and dyspnea. These symptoms occur first with exercise and later when the elder is at rest. Asthma, which is characterized by an increased responsiveness of the bronchi to various stimuli, results in bronchoconstriction, inflammation of the mucosa, and an increased amount of secretions (Pauwels, 2000). COPD is associated with airflow obstruction, which may be accompanied by airway hyperreactivity and may be partially reversible (Baum, 1997). Clinical symptoms of COPD vary depending on the severity and duration of the diseases.

Chronic Bronchitis

Chronic bronchitis is defined as the presence of a chronic productive cough and sputum production for at least 3 months out of a year for a 2-year period. One symptom of chronic bronchitis is hypersecretion of mucus in the respiratory tract in individuals for whom other causes, such as infection, have been ruled out (Keith & Novak, 2001). The sputum of a person with chronic bronchitis is usually thick yellow to gray. A deep productive cough is the main symptom of this disease. Other symptoms include shortness of breath, wheezing, a slightly elevated temperature, and pain in the upper chest that is aggravated by cough.

A person may have a mild form of chronic bronchitis for many years. Individuals with mild chronic bronchitis may have only a slight cough in the morning after being inactive at night. This cough can become aggravated after the person has an acute upper respiratory tract infection. As the condition progresses, obstructive and asthmatic symptoms appear, together with dyspnea. Chest expansion becomes diminished, and scattered rales and wheezing are frequently heard (Petty, 2001).

Bronchiectasis, a permanent dilation of the bronchi, is the most common complication of bronchitis. Bronchiectasis often is associated with bronchiolectasis, a dilation of the bronchiole. Such dilation occurs as a result of persistent inflammation inside the airways. The dilated bronchi and bronchiole are filled with mucopurulent material that stagnates and cannot be cleared by coughing. Infection then spreads into the adjacent alveoli, and recurrent episodes of pneumonia are common. Clubbing of the fingers often develops in elders with this condition (Damjanov, 2000).

Chronic Pulmonary Emphysema

Emphysema is a chronic condition characterized by permanent enlargement of the air spaces distal to the terminal bronchioles. Emphysema is accompanied by destruction of the alveolar walls and causes the lungs to lose elasticity, resulting in decreased airflow (Pauwels, Buist, Calverley, Jenkins, & Hurd, 2001). This decreased airflow results in dyspnea. Elders with emphysema have no bronchial obstruction or irritation that would cause them to expectorate (Petty, 2001). The inability to exhale the carbon monoxide that is trapped in the lungs causes the chest to overexpand, a condition referred to as *barrel chest.* The elder must hunch forward while holding onto a stable object to engage the auxiliary respiratory muscles during breathing. These elders manage to oxygenate their blood by hyperventilating, which prevents cyanosis and anoxia (Pauwels, Buist, Calverley, Jenkins, & Hurd, 2001).

Asthma

Asthma is defined as a reversible airway disease characterized by an increased responsiveness of the trachea and the bronchi to various stimuli. Asthma is displayed by a widespread narrowing of the airways that changes in severity either spontaneously or as a result of therapy. During an acute attack, pronounced wheezing occurs because of difficulty in inhaling and exhaling air. Dyspnea, tachypnea, and chest tightness may also occur. The elder experiencing an asthmatic attack may also perspire profusely (Baum, 1997).

PSYCHOSOCIAL EFFECT OF CHRONIC OBSTRUCTIVE PULMONARY DISEASE

Rehabilitation of elders with COPD should include both medical management and assistance in coping with the debilitating effects of this chronic condition. As with any chronic condition, elders adapt in different ways. Some elders accept and adapt to the changes in energy level and other accompanying symptoms of COPD. For other elders, coping with symptoms of COPD may be a frustrating and depressing experience. Furthermore, elders with COPD often have additional stressors in their lives, such as the loss of a spouse and close friends, changes in living situation, a decrease in financial status, loss of productivity, lack of family support, inability to perform ADL functions, and loss of general body function (Bonder & Wagner, 2001; Pauwels, Buist, Calverley, Jenkins, & Hurd, 2001).

Weakness and fatigue associated with COPD may require changes in living situations including a move to a higher level of assistive living. As with any move, emotional adaptations are required. Often elders with COPD seek to live in a different environment where they believe the air is cleaner or they can breathe better; however, they may find that such a move is not the solution to their problem because it cuts them off from a social support network. A sense of isolation may cause an increase in anxiety and may lead to depression.

Additional problems related to decreases in finances may arise for elders. The primary source of income for many elders is Social Security payments. Funds obtained from this source may not be sufficient to pay for medications or home health services if needed. The situation can be particularly frustrating for elders with COPD who are insured by Medicare, because they will not be reimbursed for rehabilitation care unless they have a change in functional status.

In addition, elders with COPD may have a sense of loss of productivity if they are unable to engage in activities that provided enjoyment in previous years. Social isolation because of concerns about a decreased energy level, shortness of breath, oxygen usage, coughing, and sputum production may contribute to depression. Elders may become afraid that engaging in any type of physical activity may cause an increase in shortness of breath. This can lead to a cycle of fear and ultimately a need for more oxygen. Some elders with COPD also experience frustration because of a decline in their abilities to perform ADL functions as a result of a decreased level of endurance. Finally, some elders with COPD may have other chronic problems such as decreased vision, or perhaps a general decline in other body systems. All these stressors could contribute to anxiety and depression.

Over time some elders with COPD begin to realize that a change in emotional status, whether positive or negative, has a direct effect on the respiratory system. Fear of expressing any type of emotion becomes a reality. This situation can further perpetuate a state of isolation. These elders may rationalize, "If I cannot express my emotions, then I will stay by myself." This position may be misinterpreted by others as hostility or aloofness, thereby creating more isolation.

SEXUAL FUNCTIONING

Elders with COPD may experience some loss of sexual functioning. Factors that may affect sexual functioning are shortness of breath, a decreased level of endurance, and a lack of desire. Changes in self-concept also can affect sexuality. Some men may have difficulty maintaining or obtaining an erection, perhaps because of fears of sexual failure. However, impotence can be the result of many causes, including side effects of medication. Therefore, elders who are impotent should contact their physicians. Fear of sexual failure because of shortness of breath is one of the most common causes of sexual inactivity among elders with COPD. Engaging in sexual activity involves an increase in the breathing rate. For many elders a fear of suffocation or not being able to increase the depth of breathing inhibits their abilities to engage freely in sexual activity (Hodgkin, Bartolome, & Gerilynn 2000). COTAs can address some of the sexual functioning concerns of these elders by being open to discussing these concerns during treatment. Providing energy conservation suggestions such as encouraging elders to have sexual relations when they are most rested may be beneficial. (A more in-depth discussion of ways to address sexual concerns with elders is provided in Chapter 12.)

Occupational Therapy Assessment and Treatment Planning

COTAs contribute to the evaluation process of elders with COPD and collaborate with occupational therapists (OTRs) in treatment planning. ADL functions and productive and leisure activities often are the primary areas of concern. Elders may experience the most disabling symptoms of COPD, such as dyspnea and fatigue, when engaging in these activities. These symptoms, together with anxiety and depression related to the chronic illness, perpetuate the vicious cycle of inactivity. The deconditioning and muscle weakness that occur from inactivity make it increasingly difficult for elders to perform necessary ADL functions to be independent in the home and community (Bonder & Wagner, 2001)

The OTR and COTA assess many performance components to determine the effects of COPD on function. Performance components such as sensory awareness are assessed to determine tactile impairment. Perceptual skills are assessed to determine an elder's response during episodes of dyspnea, particularly if they become dizzy. Neuromuscular components are assessed to determine physical tolerance and endurance, shortness of breath on exertion, muscle strength, range of motion, and posture. Cognition is assessed to determine the elder's knowledge of the disease and accompanying problems. In addition, the elder's judgment, problem-solving skills, ability to generalize learning, and awareness of safety hazards are evaluated. Psychosocial ability is assessed to determine the elder's psychological, social, and self-management skills. Elders with COPD may experience feelings of hopelessness, depression, withdrawal from social activities, and dependency on a spouse or caregiver (American Psychiatric Association, 2000). Impairment in any of these areas directly affects the elder's ability to engage in self-care, work, and leisure activities.

COTAs must be aware of certain precautions during treatment. Knowing the various symptoms associated with COPD, such as shortness of breath and asthma, as well as the environmental irritants that can affect the elder's ability to breathe, is important. These irritants can include cigarette smoking, dust from woodworking activities, and fumes that arise from activities such as copper tooling. Other irritants include talcum powder, certain perfumes, and poor air quality in the clinic.

OT intervention is geared toward increasing independence in functional activities by improving strength and endurance through resistive activities. Reconditioning programs such as the metabolic equivalents (METs) that are used with individuals who have cardiac conditions often are also used with patients with COPD (Bonder & Wagner, 2001). (A more in-depth discussion of the use of METs to guide activity prescriptions is provided in Chapter 23.) Low-impact exercise places minimum stress on joints and is easier to perform than high-impact activities. Exercise programs should include functional activities that target the upper body, and they should be designed to increase the strength of respiratory muscles.

Activities should be stopped if nausea, dizziness, fatigue, increased shortness of breath, or chest pain develops.

Energy conservation and **work simplification** techniques are used with elders who are predisposed to fatigue (Fig. 24-1). COTAs should actually try these techniques with elders rather than simply providing them with education sheets. Energy conservation and work simplification techniques should include scheduling rest periods in between activities, sitting whenever possible, reducing or eliminating steps, pushing rather than pulling, and analyzing an activity before starting it. Having all supplies for ADL functions within easy reach to avoid unnecessary trips also is beneficial. Time management is a technique that teaches elders to plan daily activities so that rest periods are "built in" to avoid some of the complications of COPD. Good time management skills may make the difference between a full, active life and a sedentary one.

Elders must develop the problem-solving skills needed to identify that they are no longer able to perform a task in the customary way and when to change the process. Adaptive equipment such as a reacher, a cart to carry heavy items, and a motor scooter for outdoor activities can assist with function. In addition, COTAs can encourage elders to become involved in social activities. Teaching stress reduction techniques can help encourage elders to have a sense of independence.

The COTA/OTR team may also reinforce breathing techniques taught in the respiratory therapy program, such as pursed-lip breathing and diaphragmatic breathing (Fig. 24-2). According to Spencer (1993), "Pursed-lip breathing creates a resistance to the flow of air out of the lungs and slows down the breathing rate. This technique is used with stressful activities to avoid shortness of breath. Diaphragmatic breathing decreases the cost of breathing and enables the elder to engage in purposeful activities" (p. 653). COTAs working with elders who have COPD must become efficient at administering oxygen and must be prepared to assist with controlled coughing, breathing, and other procedures.

CONCLUSION

COPD is a common disease in the United States, especially among elders. COTA/OTR teams are becoming increasingly proactive in the treatment of this debilitating disease. They provide intervention to elders with COPD in a variety of settings. OT intervention is geared toward restoration of self-care skills, instruction in pacing of daily activities, and the restoration of physical capabilities. COTAs are instrumental in teaching compensatory techniques to be used in the performance of ADL functions and in the selection and use of assistive devices and adaptive equipment. COTAs may also become involved in teaching energy conservation and work simplification techniques. Addressing stress management may be a part of therapy; this may also help to reinforce respiratory therapy breathing techniques. Ultimately, the goal of OT with elders who have COPD is to maximize their level of independence as they adjust to living with a chronic condition.

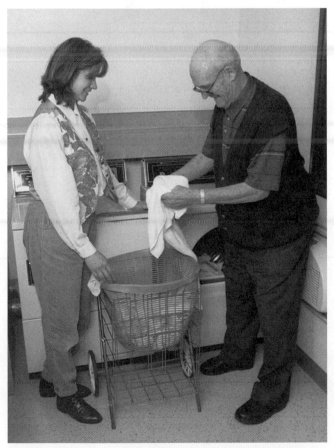

FIGURE 24-1 A certified occupational therapy assistant observes an elder practice energy conservation and work simplification techniques as he does laundry.

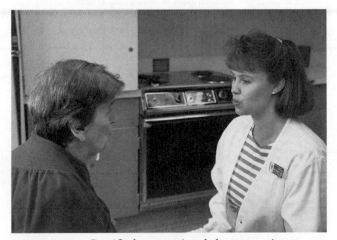

FIGURE 24-2 Certified occupational therapy assistants often must reinforce techniques such as pursed-lip breathing during activity.

CASE STUDY

Lily is a 70-year-old woman who was recently discharged from the hospital after being treated for pneumonia. She has a 20-year history of COPD. Lily's most current hospitalization compromised her health greatly. Lily has been a widow for 25 years. She has one son who lives in the area but is not very involved in her life. "He is afraid that I may need him to fix something. I wish that I would see him more often as I do enjoy his company," Lily stated.

Lily enjoys needlework and her concern for the environment is evident in the extensive recycling she does in her home. She previously went out into the community three or four times a month for doctor appointments, shopping, and socializing with friends. She does not drive and relies on others for transportation.

Lily was independent in ADL and IADL before her hospitalization. Her primary care physician ordered home health at discharge and the OTR completed the initial evaluation. Maritza is a COTA who has been working in home health for 5 years and will manage Lily twice a week for 3 weeks. Initially, Lily is concerned about how she will be able to complete her daily routine now that she is on oxygen 24 hours a day and her endurance is severely limited.

Maritza and Lily discuss the occupational tasks that Lily wants to complete independently. They identify that it would be best to start with basic self-care activities incorporating energy conservation. Maritza reviews handouts on energy conservation for Lily to refer to later. She then has her practice the techniques while engaged in activities. For example, she places a chair in the bathroom for her to sit in while undressing, dressing, and for resting. Martiza instructs Lily in using pursed-lip breathing techniques during self-care tasks. Maritza saw photos of Lily posted in her home and observed that she took pride in her appearance. Low endurance and a fixed income have prevented Lily from visiting the beauty salon, so Maritza suggests that she purchase a wig. Lily embraces the idea.

Maritza provides a commode that Lily can use over the toilet and next to her bed at night. Other bathroom equipment includes a handheld shower and a tub transfer bench. The shower doors are removed and replaced with a shower curtain to help Lily transfer to the tub safely.

Lily becomes independent in ADL using energy conservation techniques. She figures out ways to get around her home safely while managing the oxygen hose. She reports difficulty with food preparation and the desire to address that area in treatment. Subsequently, Maritza completes a kitchen evaluation and finds that cooking is difficult and unsafe. Lily tires easily, forgets about food in the oven, and leaves food out to spoil. She has lost interest in eating nutritious meals. Maritza suggests that Lily receive Meals on Wheels.

Lily expresses an interest in continuing her recycling activities. The recycling bins are located on the porch floor and she has difficulty reaching them. Maritza moves a small picnic table close to the door, places the recycling bins on top of it, and labels the bins for easy identification. The picnic table allows Lily to work at a proper work height. A neighbor boy who visits frequently volunteers to take them to the curb on a weekly

basis. At discharge Lily is able to function in her environment safely and plans to pursue public transportation so she can move about the community because she is interested in taking a needlepoint class at a local craft store.

◼ CASE STUDY QUESTIONS

1 Why did Maritza instruct Lily in pursed-lip breathing techniques while transferring?
2 What are the physical and psychological benefits of Lily wearing a wig?
3 Why is it important to practice energy conservation techniques during activities?
4 Describe how Lily could use energy conservation during two other activities.

◼ CHAPTER REVIEW QUESTIONS

1 Describe some physiologic factors that may affect elders with COPD.
2 Describe precautions to be aware of when working with elders with COPD.
3 Describe community resources that would be useful for elders with pulmonary conditions.

REFERENCES

American Psychiatric Association. (2000). *Diagnostic and statistical manual of mental disorders* (4th ed.). Washington, DC: The Association.

Baum, G. (1997). *Textbook of pulmonary diseases*. Philadelphia: JB Lippincott.

Bonder, R., & Wagner, B. (2001). *Functional performance in older adults*. Philadelphia: FA Davis.

Damjanov, I. (2000). *Pathology for the health-related professions* (2nd ed.). Philadelphia: Elsevier.

Hodgkin, J. E., Bartolome, R., & Gerilynn, L. (2000). *Pulmonary rehabilitation: Guidelines to success*. Boston: Lippincott Williams & Wilkins.

Keith, J., & Novak, P. (Eds.). (2001). *Mosby's medical, nursing, and allied health dictionary* (6th ed.). St. Louis, MO: Mosby.

Pauwels, R. A. (2000). National and international guidelines for COPD: The need for evidence. *Chest 117*(Suppl 2), 20S-22S.

Pauwels, R. A., Buist, A. S., Calverley, P. M., Jenkins, C. R., & Hurd, S. S. (2001). Global strategy for the diagnosis, management, and prevention of chronic obstructive pulmonary disease. NHLBI/WHO Global Initiative for Chronic Obstructive Lung Disease (GOLD) Workshop summary. *American Journal of Respiratory and Critical Care Medicine, 163*, 1256-1276.

Petty, T. L. (2001). *Early diagnosis of COPD: National Lung Health Program in the United States*. Program and abstracts of 67th Annual Scientific Assembly of the American College of Chest Physicians.

Spencer, E. A. (1993). Functional restoration: Implementation of occupational therapy with adults. In H. L. Hopkins & H. D. Smith (Eds.), *Willard and Spackman's occupational therapy*. Philadelphia: JB Lippincott.

CHAPTER 25

Working with Elders Who Have Oncological Conditions

LESLIE BRUNSTETER-WILLIAMS

KEY TERMS

cancer, metastasis, pathological fracture, myelosuppression, cachexia

CHAPTER OBJECTIVES

1. Identify common oncological diagnoses.
2. Discuss incidence of cancer as it relates to elders.
3. Define the role of occupational therapy in cancer care.
4. Understand the importance of the interdisciplinary team in cancer care.

The constant improvements in **cancer** treatment produced by ongoing clinical trials have resulted in better survival rates for people with cancer. Surgery, radiation, cytotoxic chemotherapy, and hormone therapy are all currently being used in cancer treatment. However, elders with cancer appear to be at a disadvantage because of their age. Clinical trials of treatment protocols are used to develop the most effective form of cancer treatments, and subjects are generally younger than 65 years of age (Hutchins, Unger, Crowley, Coltman, & Albain, 1999). Elders are often considered rigid and untreatable, with comorbid conditions that cannot be reversed. Although comorbidity does occur with age, increasing evidence suggests that elders tolerate cancer treatments as well as their younger counterparts do (Cova, Beretta, & Balducci, 1998). It is hoped that in the future elders will be included in cancer treatment trials, and improved treatment options will be made available on the basis of physiologic rather than biologic age.

GENERAL OVERVIEW OF COMMON CONDITIONS

This chapter discusses four types of cancer that are associated with aging: breast, colorectal, lung, and prostate (Table 25-1). Lung cancer continues to be the leading cause of death, accounting for almost one third of cancer deaths in men and about one fourth of cancer deaths in women. Colorectal cancer is the second leading cause of cancer death, followed by breast and prostate cancer. The "Annual Report to the Nation on the Status of Cancer, 1973–1999, Featuring Implications of Age and Aging on the U.S. Cancer Burden" published in May 2002 (Edwards et al., 1999) reveals that death rates for all cancers combined continued to decline. However, the number of

TABLE 25-1

Common Malignancies in Individuals 65 Years or Older		
5-Year relative survival rates for common malignancies (1992-1999)		**Impact of age on cancer incidence**
Site	**All races 65 and older**	**Median ages for four most prevalent cancers**
All sites	63%	68 yr
Lung/bronchus	14.9%	70 yr
Colon/rectum	62.3%	72 yr
Breast	86.6%	63 yr
Prostate	98.4%	69 yr

Adapted from National Cancer Institute. Seer Cancer Statistics Review 1975-2000 tables and graphs retrieved from the National Cancer Institute (SEER) [WWW page]. URL http://www.seer.cancer.gov

cancer cases can be expected to increase because of the growth of the general and the aging population in coming decades. Therefore, the need for rehabilitation of elders with cancer must be recognized. Certified occupational therapy assistants (COTAs) have a unique and valuable role in the interdisciplinary treatment of elders with cancer. Methods for improving overall function and quality of life are described later in this chapter.

Breast Cancer

The incidence of breast cancer has been increasing for 40 years, with a dramatic increase occurring in the 1980s (Landis, Murray, & Bolden, 1999). Earlier screening through the use of mammography may account for this increase. The National Health and Medical Research Council (1999) asserted that 1 in 8 women in the United States will experience development of carcinoma of the breast during her lifetime and 1 in 28 women in the United States will die of the disease. As with many other cancers, the incidence of breast cancer increases with age. Researchers estimate that more than 43% of all patients with newly diagnosed breast cancer will be older than 65 years, with 52% of related deaths expected from this age group (Silva & Zurrida, 2000). As a woman ages, her risk for development of breast cancer increases. The risk for breast cancer developing in a 40-year-old woman by age 50 years is 1 in 63, but by age 60 years, the risk increases to 1 in 26, and by age 70 years, the risk becomes a startling 1 in 14 (Edwards et al., 1999). In a report published by the American Association of Retired Persons (U.S. Department of Health and Human Services [DHHS], 2001), the population of elders older than 65 years has grown more than eightfold since the beginning of the twentieth century.

The report also noted that in 1994, the ratio of women to men in this age group was 146 to 100. As the average length of life and the number of older women increase, researchers predict a corresponding increase in the number of elders being treated in health care settings for breast cancer.

Because breast cancer is increasingly being diagnosed at an early stage, the person is often asymptomatic at the time of diagnosis. The diagnosis is made when a breast mass is found to be malignant. Whether the surgical approach involves a lumpectomy with lymph node dissection or a modified radical mastectomy with removal of the entire breast and axillary lymph nodes, the elder must deal with important decisions. These decisions concern the future course of treatment and the psychological ramifications of dealing with a life-threatening illness.

Colorectal Cancer

Colorectal cancer is the second leading cause of cancer death, accounting for 10% of deaths in the United States (National Cancer Institute [NCI], 2002). Individuals have a 1 in 20 risk for development of colorectal cancer, and this risk increases with age (Bond, 1999; National Institutes of Health [NIH], 2002a). From 1987 to 1991 the incidence of colorectal cancer was 18.1 per 100,000 for individuals younger than 65 years, but increased to 323.1 per 100,000 for those 65 years and older (Ries, 2002). In examining the impact of age on cancer incidence, the median age for colorectal cancer is 77 years, which indicates the propensity of colorectal cancer to be present in later years (Cancer, 2000).

Initial symptoms of colorectal cancer may include changes in bowel habits, the presence of blood in stools, and progressive weight loss. The primary tumor may be localized in the rectum, distal colon, or proximal colon areas. Surgery may be used as a curative treatment. If surgery is indicated, a colostomy may be necessary. The elder's adjustment to this situation will need attention. Local invasion of colorectal cancer is evaluated at the time of diagnosis, and the course of treatment is outlined. Depending on the extent of tumor spread, treatment to control distant metastases may include surgery, radiation, and chemotherapy.

Lung Cancer

Cancer of the lung is the most prevalent cancer in the Western world, and its incidence among women has increased significantly in recent years. This increase probably corresponds to the increase in the number of women who smoke. Lung cancer is now the leading cause of cancer-related death among women in the United States (American Lung Association [ALA], 2001). The frequency of lung cancer increases up to the age of 70 years, with more than 40% of deaths attributable to lung cancer in people older than 65 years (ALA, 2001). In the United States, between 1973 and 1991, a 16.2% increase occurred in deaths caused by lung cancer in individuals younger than 65 years. The mortality rate increased sharply (67%) in those patients 65 years and older with the same disease (Ries, 2002). From 1987 to 1991, the incidence rate in individuals 65 years or older was estimated to be an average of 317 per 100,000 cases (ALA, 2001).

The majority of lung malignancies have an infiltrative pattern of growth, which means that the tumor spreads within the mucosa of the lung and then through the lymphatic system (Bruderman, 1997). Because of the aggressive nature of this disease, it metastasizes early, frequently by the time of diagnosis (Bruderman, 1997). Because many patients with lung cancer are or were smokers, the presence of cough or dyspnea (shortness of breath) may be nonspecific and usually is not the presenting symptom. Hemoptysis, or the presence of blood in the sputum, may be the symptom that brings the elder to the doctor for evaluation. If metastasis has occurred, chest pain in the midline of the chest or on the side of the tumor may be described as severe and debilitating.

Prostate Cancer

The NCI identified carcinoma of the prostate as the fourth leading cause of cancer death in the United States (NCI, 2002). This cancer most often affects men older than 70 years (NIH, 2002b). As with breast cancer, the recent trends in prostate cancer may reflect improved screening practices. Diagnosis is made through blood tests, specifically the prostate-specific antigen test (Stanford et al., 1999). This test is widely available and appears to be responsible for increased early detection and treatment.

If prostate cancer is diagnosed early and the tumor has a well differentiated cytology, the disease can be slow and progressive. However, the cancer can be aggressive if poorly differentiated. Treatment involves surgical removal of the prostate gland and hormonal therapy. In cases of advanced metastatic disease, radiation therapy may be used as a palliative measure (Ries, 2002).

Metastases

Metastases occur when malignant or cancerous cells spread from the primary site of origin to other organs or systems of the body. This spread may be local, occurring in tissues surrounding the primary tumor site, or distant, traveling to another site in the body. This migration occurs through the blood vessels or the lymphatic system. Common sites of **metastasis** include breast cancer to bone, lungs, or brain; lung cancer to brain, liver, or bone; prostate cancer to bone; and colorectal cancer to liver or lungs.

Lung metastasis is commonly seen secondary to breast cancer but may also be found in progressed colorectal cancer. When lung metastasis occurs or lung cancer is the primary disease, pulmonary functions may change.

This alteration may limit functional capacity and respiratory potential. Rehabilitation efforts can be beneficial in these situations. Rehabilitation works to maximize functional abilities through adaptation, pacing, and correct body mechanics.

Skeletal, or bone, metastasis may be seen secondary to breast, prostate, and colorectal cancers. When weight-bearing or long bones are affected by metastases, they become weakened in structure and susceptible to easy breaking or **pathological fractures.** A pathological fracture may occur with the placement of very little weight or pressure on the bone. For example, if an elder's humerus has a metastatic lesion, an activity such as taking out the trash or picking up a carton of soda could actually precipitate a fracture at that site. When upper extremities are affected by a fracture, immobilization, surgical reduction, and radiation therapy may be used alone or in combination. During this period, the elder can use only one hand and may require training in self-care tasks. Should the hip or femur be affected, partial or total hip replacement surgery may be performed to restore integrity and return weight-bearing potential to the hip joint (see Chapter 22 for details on this type of surgery). After surgery, rehabilitation efforts should include instruction in total hip precautions during activities of daily living (ADL) functions, including adaptive equipment to allow for limited hip flexion and adduction. If healing does not occur after surgery and the joint remains unstable, use of a walker during ADL functions and avoidance of weight-bearing on the affected hip joint may be necessary. If metastasis involves the spinal column, pain can be a major problem. Medical treatment includes epidural nerve blocks to the spinal area, radiation treatments, and surgical stabilization of the spine. During rehabilitation, emphasis should be placed on use of correct body mechanics in functional tasks to protect the spine and to prevent further damage.

PSYCHOSOCIAL ASPECTS OF ONCOLOGICAL CONDITIONS

When dealing with cancer, elders have varying emotional needs depending on the stage of the illness. Stages include initial diagnosis, treatment, disease recurrence, and the terminal stage of the illness. The elder's reaction(s) to the diagnosis may include anxiety, denial, worry, anger, and depression (NIH, 2002a,b). Helplessness, uncertainty, and fear also are common. Fear may be related to a loss of control. It may also originate in a fear of pain, which has been associated with cancer. For example, in the case of early-stage lung cancer, pain may be caused by the chest tumor or metastatic areas in the bone. Lack of sufficient pain control may exacerbate fears of dying (Bernhard & Ganz, 2000). COTAs can help by actively listening to elders, allowing them to express feelings and fears, and providing emotional support. The diagnosis of cancer suggests images of death and dying to most people, but with improved screening and more effective treatments, many elders can continue to lead productive, satisfying lives.

During the early phase of diagnosis and treatment, the establishment of trust between the elder and health professional is essential in helping the elder adjust to treatment and maintain compliance (Bernhard & Ganz, 2000). When elders and families are given information regarding treatment and potential toxicities, fear of the unknown may decrease.

The successful treatment of cancer, whether it includes chemotherapy, radiation, surgery, or a combination of any of these, often brings adverse side effects with which the elder must deal. Elders often have one or more chronic conditions already present, such as arthritis, heart disease, orthopedic impairments, diabetes, and visual impairments (DHHS, 2001). These comorbid conditions may compound the problematic side effects of cancer treatment. Alopecia, or hair loss, may occur as a side effect of certain chemotherapeutic drugs. Total-brain irradiation for brain cancer may also cause alopecia. This change in body image can negatively affect elders' self-esteem, sometimes causing them to avoid social activities that were once important to them. Social support is important for elders with cancer. If elders neglect previously important activities, they also lose opportunities for emotional assistance. Women may have difficulty adjusting to the loss of a breast after a mastectomy and experience changes in their feelings about femininity and sexuality. In both cases, losses have occurred that will precipitate the grieving process (National Health Medical Research Council [NHMRC], 1999).

Cytotoxic drugs can affect the bone marrow by impairing its ability to produce needed white blood cells, red blood cells, and platelets. This phenomenon is called **myelosuppression.** Myelosuppression renders elders susceptible to infection, anemia, and easy bruising. Elders may need to limit their contacts with others during this period to prevent infection. This may decrease the emotional support available, adding to feelings of isolation. COTAs can encourage solitary activities such as putting photos in albums, which promotes reminiscence; rewriting recipe cards; and communicating with friends through letter writing or e-mail.

During the course of cancer treatment, fatigue is common. Performing everyday tasks such as bathing and dressing may be difficult and may require assistance. Adjustment to this loss of independence may be difficult for elders, and a profound feeling of loss of control may surface. Social support and referral to community resources that provide assistance with ADL can be beneficial during this period.

During cancer treatment, the chronic nature of the disease may become evident. Routines include regular medical appointments for treatment and blood work. Periodic radiographic scans also are necessary to assess response to treatment. Transportation to and from clinics may present a problem for many elders. This stress, compounded with anxiety about the possible recurrence of cancer, may result in emotional difficulties.

If the cancer recurs, initial feelings of denial and anger may resurface. At this point, uncertainty about the future becomes a real concern (NHMRC, 1999). If recurrence results in loss of function or strength, family roles may change, and family education and support by the health care team are essential. Cancer has been called a "family affair," and its effect on the family is evident throughout all stages of the illness (NHMRC, 1999). According to a report published by the DHHS (2003), 68% of elders lived in a family setting in 1994. An example of the effects of cancer on the family follows. An active man with lung cancer is no longer able to meet the physical demands of meal preparation and homemaking, duties that he previously performed. Although his wife might need to assume these duties, he can still participate in menu planning and grocery shopping, thereby contributing to the family needs.

Many community cancer support and self-help groups exist. Both elders with cancer and their caregivers may find these groups beneficial. Meeting others who are dealing with similar changes and problems can help to alleviate fear and anxiety. The health care team should facilitate referrals to these community groups when the need is identified. Examples of available support organizations are Reach to Recovery (for people who have undergone breast surgery), the American Cancer Society, the local YMCA or YWCA (for indoor exercise or swim programs), and hospital-based support groups.

Quality of life is an elusive term, one that continues to be studied by many professionals with diverse perspectives. The four areas generally included in defining quality of life are physical, functional, emotional, and social status (Balducci & Extermann, 2000). The ultimate goal in the rehabilitation of elders with cancer is to maintain quality of life. Because these different areas overlap, each area must be thoroughly explored. However, functional status is likely to influence all other domains (Balducci & Extermann, 2000). The way elders perceive their functional status influences emotional adjustment and ultimately affects their abilities or desires to seek out needed social support. Therefore, maintaining functional status becomes the primary goal in treatment.

When elders reach the terminal stage of the cancer process, family support and education are critical. The identification of needed home care services, such as a homemaker, hospice intervention, and occasional respite care, becomes the primary focus of the health care team. Measures provided should alleviate suffering while maintaining dignity. All home care services should be coordinated to promote the emotional adjustment and support of the entire family. (Chapter 26 contains further information regarding the hospice philosophy and approach.)

OCCUPATIONAL THERAPY TREATMENT
Evaluation and Treatment Plan

Elders who have cancer require a holistic approach to treatment. Intervention should be tailored to all stages of the disease: diagnosis, treatment, recurrence, and in the terminal stage, for palliation of symptoms. The first step in the occupational therapy (OT) evaluation of elders with cancer is a thorough review of the client's medical record. Particular attention should be paid to radiographic studies in the event of known skeletal metastasis and laboratory blood studies, which may reveal myelosuppression.

After reviewing the medical record, the occupational therapist (OTR) and COTA collaborate in the evaluation of the elder. The elder's functional status should remain the focus of assessment, with both deficits and functional capabilities identified. Sensorimotor performance should be assessed, particularly the elder's functional endurance and strength. During the evaluation process, communication with the family is especially important. The family can describe the elder's functional status before admission. COTAs should ask about adaptive equipment at home and whether the elder has received previous instruction in adaptation so that this information can be incorporated into the treatment plan.

COTAs then develop a treatment plan, which includes problem areas that can be improved through adaptation, strengthening, and education. The goals of treatment must be objective and measurable and should reflect the elder's personal values and goals. At this point, communication with other team members is important to provide the most beneficial and comprehensive plan. During the treatment process, the COTA and OTR should meet regularly to discuss complications and the elder's tolerance of treatment and improvements. The medical record must be periodically checked to monitor the elder's response to medical treatment, progression of the disease, and changes in blood counts. Treatment is adapted to meet the changing needs of the elder. During the treatment process, the family or primary caretaker should be included in treatment and education. This participation enables them to understand the capabilities of the elder, as well as the type and amount of assistance that will be necessary after discharge. If changes in family roles or duties are necessary, COTAs can provide support and assistance in renegotiation of role functioning (Lloyd & Coggles, 1990). As the date of discharge approaches, important topics for discussion include home care needs, equipment needs, and assistance required in the client's care (see "Discharge Planning" for further discussion).

Treatment Goals and Strategies

The primary purpose and ultimate goal of OT intervention is to maximize the elder's functional independence within the limits of the disease. The desired outcome is that elders gain an increased sense of control over the environment, have an improved sense of self-esteem, and take more responsibility for their lives (Balducci, Lyman, & Ershler, 1998). To meet this goal, COTAs work to improve the elder's abilities in independent living skills through training in dressing, bathing, feeding, homemaking, functional ambulation, transfers, and leisure activities. If needed, adaptive equipment can provide a means to complete activities. COTAs should instruct clients in the use of this equipment and encourage them to practice using it. The family also should be included in the education process. If weakness or deconditioning limits elders' functional independence, COTAs may suggest some general strengthening exercises to increase functional capacity.

As noted, fatigue is a common problem among elders with cancer. Conservation of energy becomes an important aspect of preventive OT. COTAs can provide instruction in energy conservation and work simplification in ADL functions (Fig. 25-1). These techniques may include learning to prioritize daily tasks, use improved body mechanics, organize work centers, and rest frequently. To understand elders' feelings and to help address them, families also must understand the effects of fatigue and the purpose of energy conservation techniques (Balducci, Lyman, & Ershler, 1998). In the case of an elder man with prostate cancer that had metastasized to his spine and pelvis, adapting his position during bathing by use of a shower bench allowed him to be independent. This change kept him from bending, thus limiting stress on his spine, while conserving energy and helping to prevent

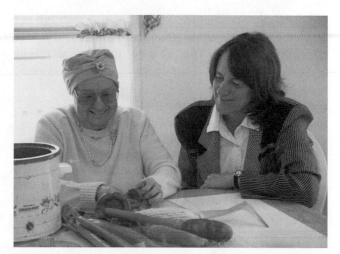

FIGURE 25-1   Certified occupational therapy assistants provide instructions in energy conservation and work simplification during meal preparation tasks.

a fall. COTAs may provide written materials on body mechanics and energy conservation to elders and family (Boxes 25-1 and 25-2).

OT treatment may include various orthotic devices designed to protect and support joints, maintain functional position, relieve pain, promote healing, support fractures, reduce deformities, and improve functioning (Larson, Steven-Ratchford, Pedretti, & Crabtree, 1996). Examples of devices frequently seen are lumbosacral supports, arm elevators, slings, and braces. COTAs may need to fabricate an upper or lower extremity splint to provide needed joint support and to maintain the joint in a functional position. Once the orthotic device is in place, treatment should include instruction of elders and their families regarding purpose, proper positioning, methods of donning and doffing, wearing schedule, and care of the device or support.

Cancer affects the entire family, and as physical and functional changes occur, alterations in family roles may become necessary. The loss of a contributory role may be difficult for elders to accept, and COTAs can help in this adjustment by suggesting alternative roles that may be more practical. Rather than being involved in the physical jobs of homemaking or yard work, for example, elders may now become involved in balancing the checkbook and other decision-making roles. Inclusion of the family in discussion and planning is important to determine the amount of assistance needed and to fully understand the elder's abilities (Balducci, Lyman, & Ershler, 1998).

OT practitioners should address both the emotional and physical needs of elders. Ideally, treatment goals for elders who have cancer should combine these needs with recognition of the psychological effects of cancer. COTAs need to maintain and communicate respect for the client, as well as demonstrate empathy. Maintaining eye contact and listening carefully convey the message that the elder with cancer continues to be valued as a human being (Balducci, Lyman, & Ershler, 1998). If elders are extremely anxious, COTAs may suggest relaxation exercises such as visual imagery and deep breathing. Music has been shown to decrease anxiety, depression, and feelings of isolation (Ezzone, Baker, Rosselet, & Terepka, 1998). The appropriate use of therapeutic touch also is helpful in treatment and reminds elders that they will not be rejected because of their illness (Balducci, Lyman, & Ershler, 1998). As mentioned earlier, alopecia may cause decreased self-esteem. In the case of an elder woman with lung cancer who loses her hair after chemotherapy, the COTA may provide or suggest a turban, scarf, or wig. The COTA may also coordinate a facial or makeover, which could help to restore the elder's self-esteem.

BOX 25-1

Body Mechanics to Decrease Stress on Bones and Skeletal System

1. Pain may arise from sitting in one position for prolonged periods; therefore, change positions frequently.
2. While working at a desk or table, make sure the work surface is the correct height so that your shoulders are not raised or lowered and your neck is not bent forward.
3. While sitting for activities, place a small pillow or rolled towel at your lower back for added support. Also, keep your knees higher than your hips by using a low stool to slightly raise your feet.
4. Stooping and bending are not advised, but if you must perform an activity in a bent position, interrupt the position at regular intervals **before** the pain starts. This may be done by standing upright or sitting down briefly.
5. Avoid bending your neck backwards; you may need to rearrange your kitchen to prevent reaching and looking up for items on high shelves.
6. While driving, move the seat forward enough to keep your knees bent and back straight. Using a small pillow or supportive roll behind your lower back may be helpful while sitting in the car.
7. When moving from a lying position to a sitting position, first roll on your side and bring your legs up toward your chest; then, as you swing your legs off the bed, push up with your arms.
8. Usually a good firm bed with support is desirable. If your bed is sagging, slats or plywood supports between the mattress and base will help add firmness.
   Whenever lifting, follow these rules:
   - Stand close to the object.
   - Concentrate on using the small curve, or lordosis, in your lower back.
   - Bend at your knees and keep your back straight.
   - Get a secure grip and hold the load as close to you as possible.
   - Lean back slightly to stay in balance and lift the load by straightening your knees.
   - Take a steady lift, and do not jerk.
   - When upright, shift your feet to turn and avoid twisting the lower back.

BOX 25-2

Work Simplification Techniques to Decrease Stress on Bones and Skeletal System

1. Avoid stairs whenever possible. Use ramps or elevators. When you must use stairs, take them one at a time to decrease stress on your joints.
2. Whenever possible, sit rather than stand while working. Any activity that lasts longer than 10 minutes should be done from a seated position.
3. Avoid sitting or lying on low surfaces such as beds or chairs. Use foam or pillows to raise the seat.
4. Avoid kneeling or squatting. If you absolutely must squat, use heavy objects nearby to help pull yourself up.
5. Slide objects rather than lifting or carrying, and push rather than pull objects whenever possible.
6. Do not reach up high for an object; instead, use a stool or long-handled reacher.
7. Never start an activity that cannot be stopped immediately if it proves too strenuous.
8. When performing a daily activity with equipment or tools, use lightweight tools. Stand near the work rather than reaching.

Special Considerations in Treatment Planning and Implementation

The treatment of elders with cancer requires awareness of certain considerations unique to this population. Because of the abnormal resting energy expenditures found in hospitalized patients with cancer, attention must be given to the effect of fatigue on rehabilitation (NIH, 2002a,b). **Cachexia,** or general ill health and malnutrition, is manifested in overall weakness, generalized muscle atrophy, and loss of body mass. Cachexia occurs when energy intake decreases because of biochemical abnormalities or loss of appetite. Progressive activity is difficult to promote in elders with cachexia. The elder's physical tolerance to the treatment provided and current nutritional intake should be considered when working toward functional achievement.

Elders with cancer who are experiencing depression and fatigue may show a lack of interest in participating in treatment. The combination of depression and fatigue makes ongoing emotional support by all team members essential. Involving elders in identifying meaningful goals of treatment may help to increase their motivation. If additional supportive care is needed, formal psychosocial interventions may be necessary.

One of the greatest challenges in working with elders who have cancer occurs when physical changes take place or when functional abilities are lost because of disease progression (Fig. 25-2). At this point, COTAs should reassess clients' capabilities and develop new, realistic goals with them. They also should provide frequent encouragement and reassurance during this process.

Complications Related to Cancer and Cancer Treatment

Complications of inactivity may occur as a result of fatigue. Metabolic and physiological changes occur secondary to prolonged bed rest (Duthie, 1998). Reports also indicate changes in cardiovascular functions, muscle wasting, joint stiffness, and ligament weakness when inactivity is continuous (Balducci, Lyman, & Ershler, 1998). These problems can complicate the rehabilitation process and require a carefully monitored progressive treatment program. Complications from cytotoxic (cell-damaging) chemotherapeutic drugs require ongoing monitoring. If myelosuppression occurs, changes in the daily treatment plan may become necessary. For example, with decreased normal white blood cells, or granulocytopenia, resistance to infection decreases. Therefore, keeping elders away from potential sources of infection (for example, other elders) is important. Good hand-washing techniques and frequent cleaning of equipment also are essential. If the normal production of platelets is decreased (thrombocytopenia), sharp objects should be avoided during treatment. Decreasing the amount of physical resistance used in exercise may be necessary. These strategies lessen the risk for unnecessary bleeding, which further compromises the

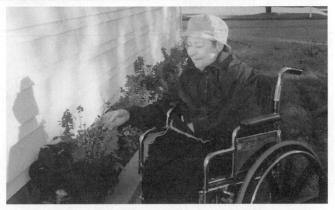

FIGURE 25-2 This elder in the late stages of lung cancer is physically unable to garden, but can enjoy the flowers she planted earlier in the year. (Photo courtesy Sue Byers-Connon, Mt. Hood Community College, Gresham, OR.)

elder's status. Other complications may occur secondary to cancer treatment or the disease process itself (Table 25-2). The COTA must be aware of potential complications and modify treatment accordingly if complications occur.

Lymphedema, or swelling that results from an abnormal collection of protein-rich fluid, is sometimes seen after lymph node removal or radiation treatment for breast cancer (Beaulac, McNair, & LaMorte, 2002). If the lymph nodes are absent after dissection or are rendered ineffective after radiation, the normal pathway for fluid removal in the affected upper extremity is interrupted.

The fluid accumulates, and the upper extremity swells (Fig. 25-3). Lymphedema also can occur in the lower extremities if the inguinal lymph nodes are involved. This condition may also be accompanied by chronic inflammation, pain, and fibrosis (Beaulac, McNair, & LaMorte, 2002). Lymphedema can be a major problem, interfering with the ability to wear certain types of clothing, negatively affecting body image, and hindering the performance of daily activities. Rehabilitation approaches include applying pressure to the extremity with compression garments or bandages, exercise, massage therapy (known as

TABLE 25-2

Complications Related to Cancer and Its Treatment

Complication	Clinical symptoms	OT treatment implications
Granulocytopenia (decreased white blood cells)	Increased susceptibility to infection	Good hand-washing technique, frequent cleaning of equipment, wearing of mask if in reverse isolation; treatment in client's room
Thrombocytopenia (decreased platelets)	Easily bruised, potential for bleeding, CNS bleeding	Avoidance of sharp objects, resistive exercises, participation in less strenuous activities
Anemia (decreased red blood cells)	Easy fatiguing, shortness of breath	Frequent rest periods, client monitored for fatigue, treatment modified according to client's tolerance
Hypercalcemia (excessive calcium in blood; normal level: 8-10.5 mg Ca)	Confusion, giddiness, mental status changes, drowsiness, polyuria, polydypsia	Consultation with physician before beginning activity, reality orientation
Hyperkalemia (abnormally high level of potassium)	Weakness, paralysis, ECG changes, renal disease if severe	Decrease in physical demands of treatment
Airway obstruction (emergent situation caused by tumor impingement on trachea)	Coughing, SOB, acute difficulty breathing	Immediate notification of medical staff
Increased intracranial pressure (caused by primary tumor or metastatic lesion in the brain)	Headaches, blurred vision, nausea or vomiting, seizure	Avoidance of physically active tasks, avoidance of tasks requiring fine vision, quiet environment for treatment
Spinal cord compression (caused by tumor impingement on spinal cord)	Back pain, leg pain or weakness, sensory loss, bowel or bladder retention	Consultation with physician before treatment, avoidance of resistive exercise, extreme care in client transfers, immediate notification of any changes in sensation or strength
Skin desquamation (breakdown of outer layer of skin)	Open ulcers on skin, fragile epidermis	Protection of skin surfaces during treatment, avoidance of abrasive contact
Cardiac toxicity (decreased cardiac output or function)	Limited cardiovascular tolerance, SOB, dizziness	Selection of activities that do not exceed client's tolerance, monitoring of client's pulse and blood pressure during treatment
Peripheral neuropathy (impaired sensory pathways in upper or lower extremities)	Impaired sensation; loss of coordination; unsteady gait, foot-drop	Adaptive equipment, splints, compensation techniques

CNS, central nervous system; ECG, electrocardiogram; OT, occupational therapy; SOB, shortness of breath.

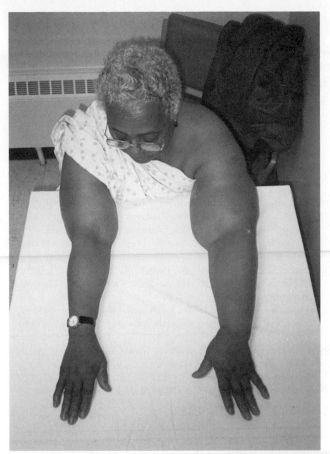

FIGURE 25-3 Lymphedema is swelling that results from the abnormal accumulation of protein-rich fluid. This condition is sometimes seen after lymph node removal or radiation treatment for breast cancer.

manual lymph drainage), and sequential pumps. Treatment can improve skin texture and overall appearance, decrease limb girth, and increase functionality.

Discharge Planning

Because of the short duration of hospital stays and the push for the earliest possible discharge, discharge planning must begin early and continue throughout treatment. This preparation and discussion occurs as an ongoing process among the team members, elders, and their families. A weekly team meeting is a good way to bring all the team members together to share concerns, identify the needs of elders, and develop a comprehensive plan for their discharge.

Necessary home equipment that will improve safety and independence in the home should be discussed. The family should be present to help identify potential problems in daily activities. When equipment needs have been identified, COTAs can assist in the selection of this equipment and provide instruction in its proper use, setup, and care. If a caregiver must assist the elder in using the equipment, the caregiver also should be trained in its use. If assistance is required in any daily activity, COTAs can instruct caregivers and family members in proper methods of care, including proper transfers and bathing assistance.

In some cases, OT treatment at home may be beneficial. An assessment within the home by an OTR/COTA team ensures proper setup of equipment and use of the best space available for ADL functions. The team also can give the caretaker and family needed support in bringing their loved one home.

CASE STUDY

Joyce is a 70-year-old woman who underwent a right modified radical mastectomy, secondary to a diagnosis of infiltrating ductal carcinoma that was detected through an abnormal mammogram and confirmed through biopsy. A postsurgical metastatic workup revealed that metastatic lesions were present in her thoracic spine and pelvis. The axillary lymph node dissection revealed that 12 of the 18 nodes removed were malignant, indicating lymph node metastasis. Postsurgical systemic chemotherapy was recommended, followed by irradiation treatments to her thoracic spine and pelvis. Joyce's medical history includes hypertension and degenerative arthritis of the spine. Before this admission, she lived with her husband of 35 years and performed all homemaking duties, was active in a bridge club and in church activities, and volunteered at a nursing home. Her hobbies included gardening and needlework. Joyce has two grown children, both living in other states.

In the OT assessment, the OTR and COTA found that Joyce was right-hand dominant and had limitations in active range of motion at her right shoulder since her surgery. Active shoulder flexion and abduction were limited to 90 degrees 4 days after surgery, with mild numbness or paresthesia in her axilla. Because of her limited range of motion, Joyce was unable to perform grooming and bathing independently and was fearful of moving her arm. She had previously experienced back pain intermittently as a result of arthritis in her spine; now she has questions regarding ways to move without injuring herself. Joyce was found to have good endurance. She is anxious to return home and resume her previous activities.

▌ CASE STUDY QUESTIONS

1 Consider the case study above and identify independent living skills that could be used to help Joyce in the gradation of shoulder range of motion to facilitate full return of movement.
2 The upper extremity precautions after breast surgery include avoidance of cuts, pinpricks, or infections in the affected arm to prevent the occurrence of lymphedema. During what activities will Joyce need to take particular precautions to avoid lymphedema? What might she do to protect her arm?
3 What principles of body mechanics should the COTA teach Joyce to protect her spine and pelvis? What principles should be covered to prevent falls?
4 What are some examples of adaptive equipment that could help Joyce maintain her independence while protecting her from pathological fracture?
5 When should the COTA include Joyce's husband in the OT treatment?

6 What needs should the COTA communicate to the other team members during discharge planning to ease the transition from hospital to home?

7 What other special considerations in treatment apply to Joyce?

CHAPTER REVIEW QUESTIONS

1 Research has shown an increased incidence of breast cancer and lung cancer among elder women. To what are these increases attributed?

2 If a pathological fracture occurred in the hip, what would the rehabilitation approaches include?

3 Discuss the psychological symptoms that may occur with elders who have cancer at various stages.

4 Why is involvement and education of the client's family important in the treatment process?

5 Describe the role of the certified occupational therapy assistant in discharge planning.

REFERENCES

American Association of Retired Persons. (1999). *Profile of older Americans* (brochure). Washington, DC: The Association.

American Cancer Society. (2000). *Cancer facts & figures 2000*. Atlanta, GA: The Society.

American Lung Association. (2001). Best practices and program services: Trends in lung cancer morbidity and mortality. [WWW page]. URL http://www.lungusa.org/data/lc/lcp1.pdf

Balducci, L., & Extermann, M. (2000). Management of cancer in the older person: A practical approach. *Oncologist, 5,* 224-237.

Balducci, L., Lyman, G. H., & Ershler, W. B. (Eds.). (1998). *Comprehensive geriatric oncology*. Amsterdam, The Netherlands: Harwood Academic Publishers.

Beaulac, S., McNair, L., & LaMorte, W. (2002). Lymphedema and quality of life in survivors of early-stage breast cancer. *Archives of Surgery, 137,* 1253-1257.

Bernhard, J., & Ganz, P. (2000). Psychosocial issues in lung cancer patients. In H. H. Hansen (Ed.), *Textbook of lung cancer.* Zurich, Switzerland: Kluwer Academic Publisher.

Bernstein, C. (Ed.) (2002). *The health care challenge* (4th ed.). Philadelphia: FA Davis.

Bruderman, I. (1997). Bronchogenic carcinoma. In G. L. Baum, J. D. Crapo, R. C. Bartolome, & E. Wolinski (Eds.), *Textbook of pulmonary diseases.* Boston: Little, Brown.

Cova, D., Beretta, G., & Balducci, L. (1998). Cancer chemotherapy in the older patient. In L. Balducci, G. H. Lyman, Ershler & W. B. Ershler (Eds.), *Comprehensive geriatric oncology* (pp. 429-442). Amsterdam, The Netherlands: Harwood Academic Publishers.

Duthie, E. (1998). Physiology of aging: Relevance to symptom perceptions and treatment tolerance. In L. Balducci, G. H. Lyman, & W. B. Ershler (Eds.), *Comprehensive geriatric oncology* (pp. 247-262). Amsterdam, The Netherlands: Harwood Academic Publishers.

Edwards, B. K., Howe, H. L., Ries, L. A., Thun, M. J., Rosenberg, H. M., Yancik, R., Wingo, P. A., Jemal, A., & Feigal, E. G. (2002). Annual report to the nation on the status of cancer, 1973-1999, featuring implications of age and aging on the U.S. cancer burden. *Cancer, 94*(10), 2766-2792.

Ezzone, S., Baker, C., Rosselet, R., & Terepka, E. (1998). Music as an adjunct to antiemetic therapy. *Oncology Nursing Forum, 25,* 1551-1556.

Hutchins, C. F., Unger, J. M., Crowley, J. J., Coltman, C. A., & Albain, K. S. (1999). Under representation of patients 65 years of age or older in cancer treatment trials. *New England Journal of Medicine, 341,* 2061-2067.

Landis, S. H., Murray, T., Bolden, S., & Wingo, P. A. (1999). Articles-Cancer Statistics, 1999- The Surveillance Research Program of the American Cancer Society's Department of Epidemiology and Surveillance Research reports its 33rd annual compilation of cancer frequency, incidence, mortality, and survival data for the United States. *A Cancer Journal for Clinicians, 49*(1), 8.

Larson, O., Steven-Ratchford, R., Pedretti, L., & Crabtree, J. (Eds.). (1996). *ROTE.* Bethesda, MD: American Occupational Therapy Association.

Lloyd, C., & Coggles, L. (1990). Psychosocial issues for people with cancer and their families. *Canadian Journal of Occupational Therapy, 57*(4), 211-215.

National Cancer Institute Surveillance. (2003). Epidemiology, and end results program [WWW page]. URL seer.cancer.gov/canques/

National Council on the Aging. (2000). American perceptions of aging in the 21st century [WWW page]. URL www.ncoa.org

National Health and Medical Research Council. (1999). Psychosocial clinical practice guidelines: Information, support and counselling for women with breast cancer [WWW page]. http://www.health.gov.au/nhmrc/publications/synopses/cp61syn.htm

National Institutes of Health. (2002a). What you need to know about cancer of the colon and rectum (NIH Publication No. 99-1552) [WWW page]. URL http://www.cancer.gov/cancerinfo/wyntk/colon-and-rectum

National Institutes of Health. (2002b). What you need to know about prostate cancer (NIH Publication No. 00-1576) [WWW page]. URL http://www.nci.nih.gov/cancerinfo/wyntk/prostate

Parker, S. L. (1996). Cancer statistics. *A Cancer Journal for Clinicians, 46* (1), 5-27.

Pienta, K., Sandler, H., Shah, N., & Sanda, M. (2002). Prostate cancer. In R. Pazdur, W. J. Hoskins, L. Wagman, & L. R. Coia (Eds.), *Cancer management: A multidisciplinary approach: Medical, surgical and radiation oncology* (4th ed.). Melville, NY.

Stanford, J. L., Stephenson, R. A., Coyle, L. M., Cerhan, J., Correa, R., Eley, J. W., Gilliland, F., Hankey, B., Kolonel, L. N., Kosary, C., Ross, R., Severson, R., & West, D. (1999). *Prostate cancer trends 1973-1995, SEER Program, NIH Pub. No. 99-4543.* Bethesda, MD: National Cancer Institute.

Silva, O., & Zurrida, S. (2000). *Breast cancer—A practical guide.* Oxford: Elsevier Science.

U. S. Department of Health and Human Services. (2003). Administration on Aging: A Profile of Older Americans. [WWW page]. URL http://www.aoa.dhhs.gov

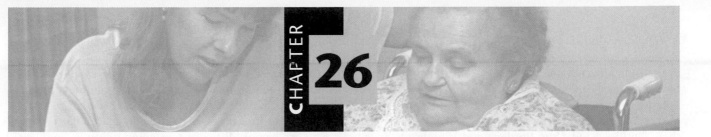

CHAPTER 26

Working with Elders in Hospice

SUE BYERS-CONNON AND JEAN VANN

CHAPTER OBJECTIVES

1. Define and discuss the hospice concept.
2. Define the role of the certified occupational therapy assistant in hospice care.
3. Discuss the role of the hospice team.
4. Explain the fears of the dying person.
5. Relate ways of communicating with the dying person.
6. Discuss ways to teach and communicate with caregivers.

You Matter Because You Are You ...
You Matter To The Last Moment Of Your Life ...
And We Will Do All We Can ...
Not Only To Help You Die Peacefully ...
But Also To Live Until You Die.

—Dame Cicely Saunders,
St. Christopher's Hospice, London

Hospices originated in medieval times as way stations where weary travelers rested. They were usually located in monasteries, and monks set the precedent of nurturing and caring that established the current philosophy of **hospice**.

With a holistic background as a nurse, social worker, and physician, Dame Cicely Saunders began the modern hospice movement in 1969. She established St. Christopher's Hospice in London according to a model of **palliative** care for the dying that provides symptom control and emphasizes quality of life.

The first U.S. hospice opened in 1971 in New Haven, Connecticut. The National Hospice Organization was organized in the 1970s and incorporated in 1978. Medicare hospice guidelines were established in 1982. Soon after, most hospice organizations sought Medicare hospice accreditation (Hamilton & Reid, 1980). In a Medicare-certified hospice, the primary physician must document that the elder has an estimated life span of 6 months or less and is not seeking active treatment.

Care should be provided by a Medicare-participating hospice program, using only palliative, or pain-relieving, treatment. A hospice patient can receive hospice care for two 90-day periods followed by an unlimited number of 60-day periods. At the start of each period the doctor must certify that the elder is terminally ill (Medicare Hospice Benefits, 2002). Occupational therapy (OT) services are available to elders, at least on a contract basis, in Medicare-certified hospice programs (Thiers, 1993).

Hospice no longer refers to a specific place; instead, it suggests a concept of care. Most of this care is provided in the individual's home but may also occur in hospitals, free-standing hospices, group homes, foster care homes, nursing homes, and adult daycare centers. Regardless of the setting, the primary mission is to help dying people and their families handle the burdens and trauma of dying. Maintaining the client's dignity is a major concern.

This chapter provides certified occupational therapy assistants (COTAs) with examples of OT interventions in the hospice setting. The importance of working effectively with family members, caregivers, and members of the hospice team also is discussed. In addition, considerations for COTAs interested in practicing in a hospice setting are covered.

THE HOSPICE PHILOSOPHY

The philosophy statement of the National Hospice and Palliative Care Organization (1995) includes the following:

Hospice provides support and care for persons in the last phases of incurable disease so that they may live as fully and comfortably as possible. Hospice recognizes dying as part of the normal process of living and focuses on maintaining the quality of remaining life. Hospice affirms life and neither hastens nor postpones death. Hospice exists in the hope and belief that through appropriate care and the promotion of a caring community sensitive to their needs, patients and their families may be free to attain a degree of mental and spiritual preparation for death that is satisfactory to them (American Occupational Therapy Association [AOTA], p. 872, 1998).

ROLE OF THE HOSPICE TEAM

The hospice team can include a physician, nurse, social worker, home health aide, OT practitioner, physical therapist, chaplain, volunteer coordinator, well trained volunteers, bereavement counselor, speech-language pathologist, and dietitian. The roles of the hospice team members are defined as follows. A physician serves as the medical director of the team. An elder may also have a personal physician. The medical director is present at staff meetings and is available to the team at all times. One of the medical director's primary roles is to collaborate with the elder's primary physician on medical matters. The elder's primary physician should have the major responsibility for care. The medical director also advises members of the hospice team. Nurses generally direct the hospice team and also serve as the primary team managers. Nurses provide pain management, monitor physical symptoms, dispense medications, and meet the elder's overall medical needs. Nursing services are available on an intermittent basis 24 hours a day through home visits and telephone consultations. Social workers provide information pertaining to resources, counseling, financial assistance, and emotional support for the elder, family

members, and caregivers. Home health aides assist with personal care and bathing and can perform light household tasks. Physical therapists are concerned with safe mobility, equipment needs, and sometimes physical agent modalities for pain relief. Speech-language pathologists may be called on to provide assistance to clients who are having difficulties in communicating and swallowing. Chaplains provide spiritual support or contact a counselor from the elder's own faith if requested to do so. All members of the hospice team provide emotional support for family members and caregivers. The volunteer coordinator recruits and trains volunteers and assigns them to clients as requested by the team or patient. The volunteers provide respite care for families, allowing caregivers to leave home for a few hours. They also can spend meaningful time with elders. The bereavement counselor and staff maintain contact with each family for 1 year after the death of the elder. They may have support programs available or refer to others in the community if needed. Dietitians provide advice about nutrition. Some hospices have alternative or complementary therapy such as acupuncture, massage, and naturopathy.

The role of OT is discussed throughout this chapter. The common thread that links hospice and OT is quality of life. Both hospice and OT use a holistic approach and foster self-actualization (Brown, 1984). Interventions include providing adaptations, teaching energy conservation and relaxation techniques, providing meaningful activities, training caregivers, and helping elders maintain autonomy in their life roles. All team members should communicate regularly and work together for the benefit of the individual. "A degree of role blurring inevitably occurs among the disciplines, and this needs to be permitted" (Hospice Task Force, 1987). According to Flanigan (1982), "to serve the best interests of the patients who are striving for a meaning in a limited life, we must be able to sidestep the defined limits of our traditional roles and cooperate in providing hospice care" (p. 276).

HOW HOSPICE DIFFERS FROM TRADITIONAL SETTINGS

Hospice differs from traditional settings in several ways, and COTAs who have worked in conventional rehabilitation settings must understand the hospice philosophy. The role of COTAs in rehabilitation settings focuses on helping clients become independent. In hospice care, the COTA works with people who have declining abilities. The COTA needs to change their philosophy from cure to care (Table 26-1).

Reimbursement is another area in which hospice differs from traditional settings. Elders who are older than 65 years almost always receive Medicare benefits. In traditional Medicare settings, elders pay a portion of each bill and all medication costs. If elders have other health care needs not related to their terminal illness, they can

TABLE 26-1

	Differences in Treatment Between a Rehabilitation and a Hospice Approach	
	Rehabilitation	**Hospice**
Treatment philosophy	Focuses on adapting to disability and maximizing independent functioning	Focuses on a caring environment, enhancing quality of life and dealing with spiritual, physical, and emotional aspects
Approach to death and dying	Deals with issues related to living and coping with a disability	Deals with issues of life and death, particularly the elder's need to come to terms with dying
Treatment goals	Goals are specific and measurable with functional outcomes	Goals are short term, usually changing from session to session, and focused on enhancing quality of life and finding meaning in dying
Treatment approach	Treatment is fast paced, with a push for discharge within a reasonable period	Treatment is slow, and unhurried, with an emphasis on quality time
Application of activities (occupations)	Used to increase endurance, strength, ROM, coordination, and ADL functions	Used to increase meaning of life
Role of ADL functions	Used to enhance functional abilities	Used to maintain function, if meaningful
Role of exercise	Used to enhance functional abilities	Used only if important to the elder and if it will increase safety and comfort and maintain functional abilities
Role of energy conservation	Some education with certain diagnoses	Strongly emphasized
Role of relaxation training	Varies by practitioner	Used to increase energy and decrease pain and stress
Role of environmental adaptations and adaptive equipment	Used to increase safety and function	Used to increase safety, compensate for functional abilities, maintain function, and improve comfort
Role of caregiver training	Done for safety reasons and follow through with the treatment	Done to improve body mechanics, energy conservation, bed mobility, communication systems, safety, and decrease burnout
Treatment discontinuation	Focus on discharge to another setting or home within a timely period	Focus on maintaining quality of life during the dying process; often includes planning for death

ADL, activities of daily living; ROM, range of motion.

use his or her original Medicare plan. For example, if an elder falls and breaks their hip and requires hospitalization, surgery, and/or therapy, these costs would be covered by Medicare.

Hospice care is covered under Medicare, Part A, for terminally ill persons who are no longer seeking treatment. The physician must certify that the elder is terminally ill and probably has 6 months or less to live. Prescriptions related to the terminal disease may require small copayments. If the elder requires medication for other illnesses (for example, high blood pressure), the elder is responsible for the payment. If the elder requires inpatient respite care for up to 5 days, there may be a copayment (Medicare Hospice Benefits, 2002). All team visits and approved and necessary equipment also are covered. The family is relieved of all Medicare paperwork and billing. Many insurance companies also offer a hospice plan similar to Medicare.

OCCUPATIONAL THERAPY EVALUATION

Most Medicare and insurance regulators, as well as state licensure laws, require that occupational therapists (OTRs) be responsible for the OT evaluation. COTAs contribute to the assessment process under the supervision of OTRs (AOTA, 1999). Ultimately, COTAs, OTRs, and elders collaborate on the evaluation. When seeing the elder for the first time, the OTR should initiate a general functional assessment. Because almost all persons in hospice have limited endurance, the assessment should be done in a timely manner. Included in the assessment are the physical abilities, activities, interests, and roles of the elder; the roles and abilities of the caregiver(s); and the environment in which the elder and caregiver reside.

The role of COTAs in the assessment process is to contribute to the data collection, which involves interviewing elders on past and present interests, occupational roles, and activities to determine what is meaningful. Assessment in engagement in meaningful occupations includes considering emotional, physical, cultural, temporal, and spiritual dimensions (AOTA, 2002). Therefore, COTAs should ask elders about what is important to them and assist them in the functional level at which the elder can participate in occupations. Elders receiving hospice care may not be able to engage in occupations at their current functional level. COTAs also must determine whether activities are possible with or without adaptation.

The role of the elder within the family and community is noted, and the family is treated as a unit of care. The emotional aspect of caring for a dying person should always be addressed by the hospice team. In addition, the living environment is assessed for safety, function, and comfort. The caregiver's role, skills, and abilities are assessed. Most important is the caregiver's ability to safely transfer the elder while using good body mechanics.

After the assessment is complete, the OTR and COTA should collaborate on formulating a treatment plan. The goals should be driven specifically toward the individual, with input from members of the hospice team to ensure that a holistic approach is used. Hospice care is designed on the basis of the dying person's perspective, not a medical diagnosis (Pizzi, 1983).

COTAs must be flexible to adjust to the changing needs of elders and should modify treatment accordingly. COTAs and OTRs regularly discuss treatment and changes in each elder's condition. The treatment plan should reflect these changes. New short-term goals are usually made for each session. Based on the skills and experience of the COTA, supervision occurs along a continuum that includes close, routine, general, and minimal. A plan should be documented

including a log of frequency and the methods of supervision used (AOTA, 1999).

ADDRESSING FEARS AND LOSSES OF THE DYING PERSON THROUGH OCCUPATIONAL THERAPY INTERVENTION

Fear is a common reaction to impending death, and it is apparent in people who are dying and others around them. Losses contribute to fears.

Loss of Abilities

Grief usually accompanies each loss. The loss of physical, cognitive, and psychosocial abilities in daily life affects elders' self-esteem and sense of identity. Relying on others to hold a glass of water, place a bedpan, and perform other routine activities serves as a grim reminder of the loss of self-determination and can lead to sadness, depression, and anger (Tigges & Marcil, 1988). COTAs possess skills to help elders make the most of their remaining physical abilities. They help elders to develop compensatory methods, including use of adaptive equipment. COTAs also teach elders safe alternative bathing methods, suggest ways to conserve energy, and recommend equipment and its placement. Cognitive loss can impair clients' abilities to perform daily living skills. For example, a woman with cognitive deficits may frequently dial the wrong number when attempting to phone her daughter. The COTA could suggest interventions such as using speed dialing or saying the number aloud while dialing it.

The loss of the ability to participate with others in meaningful activities affects psychosocial needs. COTAs can work with elders on activities they find meaningful. This may involve almost any activity, such as cooking simple meals, doing art projects, and writing in a journal. Joe is an elder who receives hospice services. He previously enjoyed fishing and camping and complained because he could no longer participate in these activities. The COTA assessed one of Joe's abilities and graded the activity; the first step entailed planning, and next was the "doing" of the activity. He cooked trout while teaching members of the hospice team his "cooking secrets." The cooking activity gives those involved a "sense of nurturing." Joe's whole demeanor changed and the complaining ceased. Then the COTA worked with the family, teaching them how to care and nurture Joe by demonstrating caring issues through role modeling.

There are many ways to involve elders in meaningful activities while adapting to changes in functional abilities. Labeling and arranging photos in an album could result in a parting gift for a loved one, while also providing the elder with an opportunity for reminiscing. Participation in meaningful activities promotes a sense of competence and mastery, leading to a sense of personal worth (Cusick, Lawler, & Swain, 1987). Kubler-Ross stated that occupational therapy has used arts and crafts projects to show clients that they can still function at a useful level (Dawson, 1982).

Many elders in hospice programs would benefit from the use of energy conservation techniques to help them gain control of their environments. The example of Katie illustrates this point. Katie is a 76-year-old elder in hospice who refused to try energy conservation and exerted herself in the morning hours. Consequently, she quickly became fatigued and was in bed the rest of the day. After learning energy conservation principles, she paced herself better and was able to attend activities such as an evening birthday party for her grandchild. An afternoon nap and cutting back on her activities allowed her to participate in activities that were meaningful to her.

Loss of Relationships and Roles

Dealing with psychosocial loss can be devastating to dying people. Their roles in life and relationships with family members and friends may be totally altered or relinquished. In the book *Tuesdays with Morrie*, the relationship between Morrie and Mitch illustrates the importance of a nurturing, consistent relationship. These two men made spending time together a priority and both benefited from the relationship as they experienced personal growth (Albom, 1997). COTAs can facilitate adjustments to new roles. For example, a terminally ill man had become bed bound. He had a car that would not run and was teaching his teenage granddaughters to repair it. After working on the car the granddaughters would return to him for feedback and further instructions. They were successful in getting the car on the road, and he was able to continue his involvement in their lives. The COTA's expertise in analyzing the role of this grandfather led to this successful outcome. OT is invaluable in a hospice setting because it promotes feelings of self-worth and competence and helps elders to be productive (Tigges, Sherman, & Sherwin, 1984).

Many elders have a strong work ethic. Their self-concept is directly related to their ability to be productive. Men in particular traditionally have been the providers for their families. As their abilities to be productive decrease, so may their self-concept. To improve productivity and self-concept, the COTA may identify an activity that matches the elder's interests and abilities. For example, Sam, who was a carpenter for 40 years, made and sold custom tables. As his disease progressed, he was no longer able to be productive in this manner. The COTA helped Sam use his woodworking skills to make bird houses for the Audubon Society. In addition, they completed a life review to help Sam realize his self-worth apart from his past work role.

Loss of Control

Loss of control is a major concern for most people in hospice programs, possibly because it entails a loss of mastery over themselves and their environment. Encouraging elders to make decisions, if they can be made safely, promotes this sense of control. COTAs also can help dying people regain control of the environment through adaptations and positioning. Touch-on lamps, speaker phones, electronic devices, and ramps are examples of adaptations. This control may include planning a funeral and writing an obituary.

Loss of the Future

"The presence of a terminal illness not only threatens one's immediate life, but also abruptly confronts the future goals one has set in life" (Parad & Caplin, 1960). A **terminal illness** may force a person to reevaluate goals and set more realistic ones. For example, a terminally ill photographer wanted to say goodbye to all the meaningful people in her life. This would mean extensive traveling to several cities, which she was unable to do. The COTA suggested that she use a digital camera and e-mail photographs to these people. This example illustrates a way COTAs can offer suggestions to help clients realize their dreams. Some future goals, such as seeing a grandchild grow up and graduate, may be impossible, and elders need permission to grieve.

Fear of Pain

One of the primary goals in palliative care is the control of pain and relief of other discomforting symptoms (S. Park, 1991, unpublished manuscript). One of the most significant reasons why people choose hospice care is to control the severe and unrelenting pain that often accompanies terminal illness (Tigges & Marcil, 1988; S. Park, 1991, unpublished manuscript). Many clients with terminal illnesses fear pain. Physical pain can be decreased and controlled with medication in almost all cases, allowing clients to remain alert and functional. It is important that the client is informed of the benefits of medication, and that any fears they may have related to taking specific medications are addressed. For example, Alice was dying of lung cancer and asked her family not to give her morphine because she viewed it as a drug used by addicts. This drug would not only relieve her pain, but would also assist her in breathing. Don't underestimate the elder's pain; it is real and valid. The individual's perception of pain is important. A study published in *Official Journal of the American Society of Pain Management Nursing* found that a patient's verbal description of pain is equally important (Duggleby, 2002). This verbal description can be valuable to the COTA when planning an activity. Pain sensation may be localized or appear to occupy the entire body. The COTA should report the client's pain level to the hospice team for medication adjustment if needed. COTAs also help to alleviate pain by using relaxation techniques such as tapes of nature sounds or music.

Emotional and Spiritual Pain

Emotional and spiritual pain can be overwhelming and is, therefore, as important as physical pain (Brown, 1984). Elders may confuse deep emotional and spiritual pain with physical pain. The fears they experience and the anticipated loss of everyone and everything is painful. Dame Cicely Saunders distinguished emotional and spiritual pain from physical pain, claiming that the former is often more severe and longer lasting. Emotional and spiritual pain encompasses the loss of one's own life and separation from not only loved ones but all humanity. This pain exists regardless of the presence or absence of religious values (Carr, 1995). One woman often wept and said, "You will cry over the loss of me, but I am crying over the loss of everyone I know." Some elders and families have difficulty discussing feelings and may unknowingly project their own emotional pain to others. COTAs can help by being available as nonjudgmental listeners, fostering creative expression of feelings, and encouraging dying people to leave a gift of themselves to loved ones. Rose was grieving the loss of not seeing her granddaughter grow up and the COTA encouraged her to write letters. Rose put together a treasure box of letters, photographs, and advice to her granddaughter, leaving behind a gift. COTAs also can help by acknowledging emotional pain and saying some words of encouragement in a caring manner. The COTA should consider the elder's spirituality as impacting the daily occupations of the elder. Christansen states "the inclusion of a spiritual dimension acknowledges a person's sense of self and his or her beliefs about power, control and meaning of life because these are formed internally and influenced by environmental forces" (Christansen, p. 9, 1997). Accepting an elder's religious beliefs or spirituality in a nonjudgmental manner is important to help the elder address his or her concerns and needs. Referral to a chaplain or other spiritual advisor often is appropriate.

Fear of Dying

Some elders may be fearful of dying, such as the person who said, "I don't know how to die because I've never died before." COTAs can assure elders that they have some control over the dying process. Facing the unknown is much more frightening than knowing the possibilities ahead. The assurance that they have some control helps. This control can be expressed through writing one's own obituary or requesting the company of family members or a spiritual counselor at the time of death. Some elders even seem to control the time of death to coincide with a significant anniversary, arrival of a loved one, or resolution of an issue. By the time dying people enter a hospice program, they have often, but not always, dealt with the fear of death. Almost all deaths that occur in a hospice are peaceful. The elder's perception of death is important. As Alice's condition declined, she asked a family member, "Am I dying?" The family member shared changes she noticed that were occurring and confirmed that she was proceeding into the active dying state. Alice closed her eyes for several minutes and when she opened them asked, "If I'm dying why are you still here?" It is important for the COTA to convey to the elder and family members that death occurs in different manners and over different periods (Table 26-2). Elders in hospice occasionally die when the COTA is present, because their condition can change rapidly. The COTA can facilitate a peaceful death. The COTA can help families and caregivers understand the importance of their roles as death nears. COTAs can convey to caregivers the importance of telling elders who are dying that they are appreciated and loved. The COTA also should recognize the need for the elder and his or her family to be the primary people in this situation and, therefore, take a background role. A person's dying may not be easy, but it is a part of living and is as important and valuable as any experience in life. It can be a rich and meaningful process for individuals and their families. Rando (1984) emphasizes the need for the family to be present at the time of death if possible. Individuals who have been keeping vigil but are not present at the actual moment of death often feel guilty afterward.

COMMUNICATING WITH THE DYING PERSON

When working with dying people, COTAs must have effective **communication** skills (Box 26-1). Kubler-Ross (1974) suggests that dying people communicate in three languages: their native language, nonverbal language, and symbolic verbal language. An elder's native language is clearly stated verbally and often conveys a literal meaning. Nonverbal language is communicated through obvious behaviors such as gestures, actions, and drawings. Symbolic verbal language conveys a message that transcends its literal meaning (Rando, 1984).

Attending behaviors signify that COTAs are listening to clients. These behaviors include eye contact, attentive body language, and verbal following (Rando, 1984). Minimizing the physical distance between speaker and listener is important. COTAs should maintain a relaxed position, lean forward, or kneel to be at the speaker's eye level. Verbal following is another way for COTAs to communicate attentiveness. This may be accomplished by summarizing or reflecting on elders' comments. The dying person may be talking to someone you cannot see. Accept the elder's reality. There is much we do not know.

Communication may be possible with low responsive dying elders (that is, those in a coma). The elder's response may be a subtle facial movement or a slight

TABLE 26-2

Signs of Impending Death

Signs	Comfort measures
Circulation	
Feet, arms, and legs feel cool to touch	Keep client warm with blankets or hot water bottle
Skin may become pale, cool, and covered with perspiration	Avoid using electric blankets
Skin of hands, arms, feet, and legs deepen in color and develop a mottled appearance	
Other areas of body become dusky or pale	
Metabolism	
Periods of sleep increase during the day	Plan to be with client during alert periods or at night, when the presence of a familiar person might be comforting
Waking the client from sleep is increasingly difficult	
Elder seems confused about time, place, and people	Mention your name, the date, and time when talking with the elder
Increased restlessness occurs	Use a calm and confident tone of voice when speaking
Anxiety, fear, and loneliness increase at night	Cool, moist washcloths applied to head, face, and body may relieve effects of dehydration
Need for food and drink decreases	
Secretions	
Oral mucus increases and collects in the back of throat ("death rattle")	Use a cool mist humidifier to increase room humidity
Increased secretions result from decreased fluid intake and inability to cough up saliva	Provide ice chips and sips of fluid through straw
Respirations	
Breathing pattern is irregular, may be rapid or shallow or very slow with snoring-like sound	Elevate head and shoulders to make breathing easier
Short periods of no breathing (10 to 60 seconds) may occur (Cheyne-Stokes respirations)	
Elimination	
Patient may have difficulty emptying bladder	Contact nurse; catheter may be needed
Elder loses control (incontinence) of bladder and bowel	Keep skin clean and dry
Urine darkens and decreases in amount	Put layers of disposable pads between the elder and mattress
	Consult nurse regarding hygiene techniques for cleanliness and catheter (urinary bladder tubing) care
Senses	
Facial muscles relax	Talk to the patient; provide comfort
Vision decreases in clarity and becomes dim or blurred	Never assume elder cannot hear
Hearing is usually the last sense to decrease	Continue to touch and speak to elder as reassurance of your presence
	Give good mouth care
	May need to remove dentures
	Leave indirect light on (candles are helpful)

Modified from Legacy Visiting Nurse Association. (2002). *Hospice program patient/family information hospice care* (p. 21-23). Portland, OR.

movement of the finger. One grandfather was actively dying while propped up in bed. He appeared unresponsive as his daughter sat next to him on the bed with her arm around him. Each time she mentioned a grandchild, he raised his left hand and wrist as if praising or blessing his grandchildren.

OCCUPATIONAL THERAPY INTERVENTION AND CAREGIVER TRAINING

Caregiver training is an important safety factor. **Caregivers** should be educated to follow through with the OT interventions. The challenges and responsibilities of caring for dying people can be emotionally and

BOX 26-1

Guidelines for Effective Communication

1. Keep speech simple and concise. Avoid wordiness.
2. Avoid medical jargon; it may alienate or confuse some people.
3. Use open-ended questions to provide opportunities for stating opinions.
4. Do not be judgmental; keep an open mind.
5. Allow time for elders to speak. This may take longer for those who are in poor health.
6. Do not interrupt or finish sentences.
7. Do not give too much information in one visit, because none will be retained. Give demonstrations during teaching and provide both verbal and written instructions. Adapt them for visual difficulties as needed.
8. Allow comfortable periods of silence.
9. Do not argue with elders about the way they perceive their condition. Unrealistic views may represent a defense mechanism necessary until the elder is able to face reality.
10. Talk to clients and include them in all conversations at which they are present. Do not talk exclusively to caregivers, even when the client is in a coma.
11. Be aware of decreased energy levels, and leave before clients become too tired.
12. Provide appropriate touch, such as holding a hand, if the elder permits it.
13. Respect **cultural differences** in communication.
14. Help elders write if they are unable to speak. Use alphabet boards, prewritten messages, computers, and even eye blinks as methods of communication.
15. Encourage elders to express important thoughts.
16. Encourage caregivers to let the dying person know that they, the caregivers, will be all right after the death.
17. Consider safety factors if a nonverbal person is left alone. A prerecorded message near the telephone could alert others to an emergency.

physically draining. The caregiver may also be sleep deprived.

During the progression of a terminal illness, major demands are placed on significant others. The transition from living to dying rarely is smooth. Sometimes, dying people lead normal lives with minimal changes. At other times, symptoms may severely curtail any semblance of a normal life. In either case, dying people wish to be treated as they were before their illness, despite the increasing assistance needed from caregivers (S. Park, 1991, unpublished manuscript).

Sometimes, caregivers do too much for dying people out of concern or guilt, leaving them weaker, with decreased self-esteem. Other caregivers deny the decreasing abilities of dying people and expect them to do more than they are capable of doing. Most caregivers, however, are realistic. COTAs can help caregivers understand the need for dying people to participate in meaningful activities and remain active within physical limits.

Some resources are available to help caregivers live a more balanced life. COTAs can refer them to the volunteer coordinator for help. Elders in certified Medicare hospice programs are eligible for respite care in a Medicare-approved facility, such as a hospice facility, hospital, or nursing home (Medicare Hospice Benefits, 2002).

COTAs should not impose their values on dying people and their families. Their support and willingness to learn from dying people and their caregivers can improve the quality of care they deliver. Some caregivers find touch comforting; hospice workers often hug caregivers when this is acceptable. COTAs also can help caregivers understand that laughing and having a sense of humor are acceptable. The therapeutic use of self is essential when working in hospice care. COTAs should receive thorough training in working with caregivers (Table 26-3).

CONSIDERATIONS FOR WORKING IN HOSPICE

COTAs who are interested in working in a hospice may consider the following questions:

1. Have you ever been around someone who is terminally ill? By being around someone who is terminally ill, you can better understand the feelings of elders and family members.
2. Have you ever experienced the death of a loved one, including pets? Experiencing the death of someone held dear helps you to understand the depth of caregivers' grief.

TABLE 26-3

Strategies for Training Certified Occupational Therapy Assistants to Work with Caregivers

Caregiver	COTA intervention
Help with physical aspects of care	Teach good body mechanics, safe transfer, and energy conservation techniques
Help in assisting with personal care	Teach provision of personal care by simple methods that involve energy conservation and maintain the elder's dignity Obtain needed adaptive equipment and teach safe use Arrange for removal of adaptive equipment late
Help with caregiver's psychosocial needs	Allow the caregiver to express emotion Encourage input in treatment planning Facilitate a realistic view of the abilities of everyone involved Encourage balance of life roles Offer therapeutic touch if the caregiver permits this Suggest additional counseling support
Help with resources	Explore availability of support from family, friends, church, and social groups Access resources in the community
Help with spiritual needs	Allow expression of spiritual beliefs and accept differences Suggest spiritual support from members of caregiver's religious community
Help with preparing for the person's death	Discuss and educate caregivers about signs and symptoms of impending death Help caregivers obtain closure Suggest ways to make the environment meaningful Review procedures to follow at the time of death
Support after death	Listen and be supportive Attend funeral or memorial service if possible

COTA, certified occupational therapy assistant.

3. How did you handle this death? If handling a personal loss was extremely difficult and time consuming, dealing with the many losses that occur in hospice settings can be overwhelming.
4. What helps you relieve stress in your life? OT stresses the importance of maintaining balance in life. Exercising, engaging in creative activities, and networking with other team members can help to relieve stress associated with this type of work.
5. What are your own spiritual views about death? Are you familiar with and willing to accept other religious and cultural views? As a health care provider, the COTA must accept people exactly as they are—physically, emotionally, culturally, and spiritually. This acceptance increases the comfort of clients and decreases their anxiety.

BENEFITS OF WORKING IN HOSPICE

COTAs who choose to work in hospice may find that there are both personal and professional rewards.

A qualitative study that examined the experiences of therapists working in Palliative/Hospice care in Alberta, Canada, found a personal/professional connection from each participant. The following themes emerged: satisfaction, hardship, coping, spirituality, and growth (Prochnau et al., 2003).

Satisfaction was identified as appreciation expressed by elders, their families, and other members of the treatment team. All of them developed reciprocal relationships with each other. A COTA working with an elder was practicing transfer training, and afterwards the family gave the COTA a basket of home grown strawberries from their garden in appreciation of the care provided. Satisfaction also can come from members of the team when the team members acknowledge the quality of care given.

Enduring hardships and difficulties also were identified as factors contributing to personal/professional growth. Coping with grief and occasionally multiple deaths can be emotionally draining. A COTA may grieve for possible losses within his or her own circle of family and friends when the situation does not truly exist. A sense of urgency and working quickly, because time is limited, can help the COTA to develop skills that require creativity and the ability to respond to elders needs immediately. There is satisfaction and growth in being able to overcome difficulties that arise.

The ability to cope with loss was another area of personal/professional growth. COTAs working in hospice may encounter loss on a regular basis. COTAs need to find ways to cope with losses. A variety of coping strategies such as meeting other members of the team to debrief and keeping a journal can release pent up feelings related to losses. Other self-nurturing tasks may include exercise, creative activities, and relaxation techniques. A sense of closure of the loss may be necessary. Time limitations may not allow the COTA to attend a memorial service, but developing a personal expression of a celebration of the elder's life may be helpful. Lighting a candle or planting flowers to honor the elder are examples of closure.

Spirituality was another important area of growth. COTAs working in hospice may find themselves with a greater insight of what is important in life. The "little things" are more appreciated. They may realize that death is part of life and become more comfortable working with dying elders.

The final identified area of growth was developing a deeper understanding of self and others. COTAs may experience an increased appreciation of family and friends as a result of working with dying persons.

The unique benefits of working in hospice can provide a COTA with a rewarding experience. The personal and professional connection are woven together and become impossible to separate.

CONCLUSION

COTAs interested in working in hospice settings should have a holistic background so that they can address physical, psychosocial, and spiritual needs of the elder. An understanding of terminal illness and the progression of disease is essential for COTAs to understand the elder's condition, make appropriate changes in treatment, and recognize the point at which the elder is actively dying. COTAs must be able to accept people and their beliefs about dying without being judgmental. Effective interpersonal communication skills are vital when interacting with families, elders, and hospice team members. Active listening promotes growth.

CASE STUDY

Vivian was a lively woman with a great sense of humor and a quick wit. She enjoyed being with others, especially family members. Vivian was living independently when she was diagnosed with ovarian cancer. She continued living alone until she was physically unable to care for herself. At that time, she moved to her daughter's home in another state. This new home was warm, accepting, and busy. Vivian's presence made this a delightful four-generation

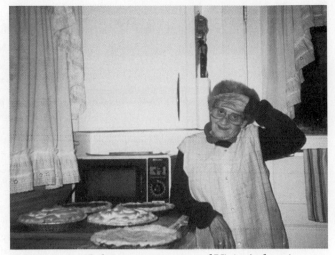

FIGURE 26-1   Baking pies was one of Vivian's favorite activities. (Courtesy Sue Byers-Connon, Mt. Hood Community College, Gresham, OR.)

home. Another daughter and her family, including a great-grandson, lived nearby.

Throughout her life Vivian was very active. She worked in a neighborhood tavern for 30 years. Her many interests included playing billiards, reading, listening to music, going to movies, playing cards, and working crossword puzzles. Baking was her specialty, and she delighted her family with lemon meringue pies (Fig. 26-1).

When her condition worsened, Vivian was referred to hospice by her oncologist. The hospice team, including the COTA, worked with Vivian. The role of the COTA was to provide necessary equipment for safety and comfort. A tub transfer bench was installed, and Vivian and her family were taught safe transfers. Other adaptations included a safety frame on the toilet and later a bedside commode. A trapeze was placed over the bed. A portable device that allowed moving Vivian in bed was designed and fabricated. A baby monitor was used as a communication system. After meeting these initial needs, the COTA concentrated on enhancing Vivian's life.

Scheduling rest periods between activities conserved Vivian's declining energy. The most necessary or desired activities were chosen in order of importance. Relaxation tapes helped to alleviate her pain. Listening to these tapes led Vivian to express an interest in music. She particularly enjoyed tapes of popular music from the 1940s. Her family often heard her over the communication system singing as she listened to the music.

A special bond existed between Vivian and her 3-year-old great-grandson, who lived in the home. He would eat breakfast with her and then climb on her hospital bed and cuddle with her (Fig. 26-2). This special relationship was mutually rewarding and engendered in the child a respect for elders regardless of their physical or mental status.

Vivian was an active participant in family activities. She helped with cooking and preparing meals. The entire family read aloud together and played cards and board games. Vivian rewrote and organized recipe cards, including humorous notes to be found later by her daughter. She ate meals with the family, and when getting out of bed became difficult for her,

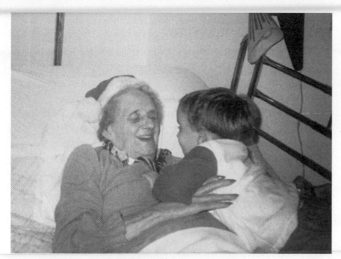

FIGURE **26-2**   A special bond existed between Vivian and her 3-year-old great-grandson. (Courtesy Sue Byers-Connon, Mt. Hood Community College, Gresham, OR.)

the family ate meals in her room. Keeping in touch with family and friends in other states was important to her, and she frequently wrote letters and made phone calls.

The family shared caregiving responsibilities, including shopping, helping with personal care, running errands, arranging respite care, preparing meals, and helping with household chores. Vivian's room was cheery, with family photographs on the walls. A bird feeder was placed outside the window. Frequently used items such as her tape recorder were close at hand on a bedside table. The family brought in fresh flowers from the yard. She operated the television by remote control to watch her favorite programs. As time passed and her condition declined, she was unable to participate in activities. She requested that her door remain open so she could hear the laughter and conversation of family members. She died with her family at her side.

■ CASE STUDY QUESTIONS

1 Considering Vivian's case, what was the role of the COTA in working with Vivian?
2 How can COTAs make life as normal as possible for elders in hospice, as illustrated by the case study?
3 What are some specific examples of ways to encourage participation in these activities, as illustrated by the case study?
4 What are some suggestions that COTAs can make to the family to enhance the environment, and how was this done in the case study?

■ **C**HAPTER **R**EVIEW **Q**UESTIONS

1 How could an elder benefit from a hospice program?
2 What previous experience should COTAs have before considering hospice work?
3 Define the roles of the following members of the hospice team: physical therapist, nurse, physician, dietitian, bereavement counselor.

4 Discuss two losses a dying person may experience.
5 Describe physical pain and emotional and spiritual pain.
6 List 10 effective ways to communicate with dying patients and their families.
7 What are five differences between rehabilitation and a hospice approach to treatment?

■ **E**XERCISE

The purpose of this exercise is to enhance sensitivity. Find a partner and ask him or her to lie on the floor looking up. Stand nearby and start a conversation, continuing for 5 minutes. Observe body language, and ask about your partner's feelings. How can you use this exercise with clients in a hospice? Reverse positions with your partner, and repeat the exercise.

REFERENCES

Albom, M. (1997). *Tuesdays with Morrie.* New York: Broadway Books.

American Occupational Therapy Association. (1998). Occupational therapy and hospice (statement). *American Journal of Occupational Therapy, 52*(10), 872-873.

American Occupational Therapy Association. (1999). Guide for supervision of occupational therapy personnel in the delivery of occupational therapy services. *American Journal of Occupational Therapy, 53*(10), 592-594.

American Occupational Therapy Association. (2002). Occupational therapy practice framework: Domain and process. *American Journal of Occupational Therapy, 56,* 609-639.

Brown, P. (1984). The growth of the hospice movement: A role for occupational therapy. *Occupational Therapy in Health Care, 1,* 119-128.

Carr, W. F. (1995). Spiritual pain and healing in the hospice. *America, 173*(4), 26.

Christiansen, C. (1997). Acknowledging a spiritual dimension in occupational therapy practice. *American Journal of Occupational Therapy, 51,* 169-172.

Cusick, A., Lawler, R., & Swain, M. (1987). Chemotherapy, cancer, and the quality of life: An occupational therapy approach. *Austr Occup Ther J, 34,* 105-113.

Dawson, S. (1982). The role of occupational therapy in palliative care. *Austr Occup Ther J, 28*(3), 119-124.

Duggleby, W. (2002). The language of pain at the end of life. *Pain Management Nursing, 3*(4), 154-160.

Flanigan, K. (1982). The art of the possible: Occupational therapy in terminal care. *British Journal of Occupational Therapy, 45,* 274-276.

Hamilton, M., & Reid, H. (Eds.). (1980). *A hospice handbook: A new way to care for the dying.* Grand Rapids, MI: William B. Eerdmans.

Hospice Task Force. (1987). *Guidelines for occupational therapy services in hospice.* Rockville, MD: The American Occupational Therapy Association.

Kubler-Ross, E. (1974). The language of dying. *Journal of Clinical Child Psychology, 3,* 22-24.

Legacy Visiting Nurse Association Patient. (2002). *Family information for hospice care.* Portland, OR: VNA Hospice Team.

National Hospice and Palliative Care Organization. (1995). *The hospice philosophy.* Arlington, VA: The Organization.

Parad, H. J., & Caplin, G. (1960). A framework for studying families in crisis. *Social Work, 5,* 3-15.

Pizzi, M. (1983). Occupational therapy in hospice care. *American Journal of Occupational Therapy, 36,* 597-598.

Prochneau, C., Liu, L., & Bowman, J. (2003). Personal-professional connections in palliative care occupational therapy. *American Journal of Occupational Therapy, 57*(2), 196–204.

Rando, T. A. (1984). *Grief, dying and death: Clinical intervention for caregivers.* Champaign, IL: Research Press.

Saunders, D. C. (1988). *St. Christopher's in celebration: Twenty-one years at Britain's first modern hospice.* London: Hodder & Stoughton.

Thiers, N. (1993). Hospice care helping bring life full circle. *OT Week, 7*(36), 14-15.

Tigges, K. N., & Marcil, W. M. (1988). Maximizing quality of life for the housebound patient: Specialized ramp allows accessibility to outdoors. *American Journal of Hospice Care, 3,* 21-23.

Tigges, K. N., Sherman, L. M., & Sherwin, F. S. (1984). Perspectives on the pain of the hospice patient: The roles of the occupational therapist and physician. *Occupational Therapy Health Care, 3,* 55-68.

U.S. Department of Health and Human Services Centers (DHHS). (2002). Centers for Medicare and Medicaid Services. Medicare Hospice Benefits.

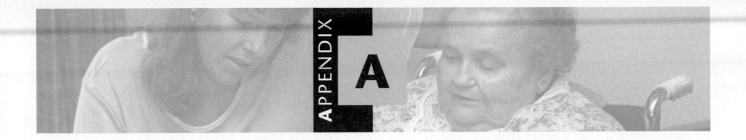

Resources

RESTRAINT REDUCTION RESOURCES
Chairs

Adirondack chairs (estate chairs). Manufactured by Rubbermaid. Available from outdoor furniture stores.

Alternating Systems

Sentry II Wireless Attendant Station
MRW World, Inc.
15 Central Way, Suite 313
Kirkland, WA 98033
(206) 826-6299, FAX: (208) 889-9779
Developed to meet special needs of foster care and assisted living settings, the call/alerting system requires no wiring to install and is simply plugged in. Basic attendant console handles up to eight residents. Cost of transmitters varies with type. The system is flexible: in addition to call/alerting exit from each room, a bedside beam sensor and a perimeter alert bracelet unit that alarms exit for only the individual wearing the bracelet also are available.

Baby Nursery Monitors

Available from Fisher-Price and other companies; nursery monitors allow caregivers to hear whether someone is moving about or calling for assistance.

Personal Alarms

Bed-Check
Bed-Check
4408 S. Harvard #A
Tulsa, OK 74135
(800) 523-7956
Chair Sentinel
Powderhorn Industries
931 N. Park Ave.
P.O. Box 1443
Monrose, CO 81402
(800) 336-1414

This releasable wheelchair seatbelt emits an alarm when it is unfastened.
Code Alert
RF Technologies, Inc.
3720 N. 124th St.
Milwaukee, WI 35221
(800) 669-9946, FAX: (414) 466-1506
Mugger Stopper
Safety Technology International, Inc.
2306 Airport Rd.
Waterford, MI 48327
(800) 888-4784
This device must be adapted to use as position-change alarm.

Personal Alarm

Radio Shack
Check phone directory for nearest outlet. This device must be adapted.
Posey Sitter
Posey Co.
5635 Peck Rd.
Arcadia, CA 91006-0020
(800) 44-POSE or (818) 443-3143
TABS Mobility Monitor
WanderGuard, Inc.
941 "O" St., Suite 205
Lincoln, NE 88501
(800) 824-2996, FAX: (402) 475-2281

Signs

Stopper Kit
Clock Medical
P.O. Box 620
Winfield, KS 67156
(800) 527-0049
This kit includes "stop" and "do not enter" signs, as well as mesh strips to put across doors.

Other Adaptations

Posey Grip
See phone and address under Posey Sitter above.

Scoot Gard
Designed for use in boats and recreational vehicles, this material is washable, with antimicrobial properties to inhibit bacteria and mildew. It is available in many stores.

Foam/Cushions

Armrest (padded flipaway)
Therafin Corp.
1974 Wolf Rd.
Mokena, IL 60448
(708) 479-7300, FAX: (708) 479-1515, order line (800) 843-7234

Cheese Leaner Cushion
Clock Medical Supply
118-124 E. 9th
Winfieki, KS 67156
(800) 527-0049
This cushion prevents lateral slumping in wheelchairs, recliners, and gerichairs.

Foam elevation inserts
Fred Sammons
P.O. Box 32
Brookfield, IL 60513
(800) 323-5547, FAX: (800) 547-4333.
For use with trough BK-6462-02.

Inflatable seat cushions
Roho
P.O. Box 658
Belleview, IL 62222
(800) 851-3449, FAX: (618) 277-6518

Ultra-Form Wedge Cushion
American Health Systems, Inc.
P.O. Box 26688
Greenville, SC 29616-1588
(800) 234-6655
This wedge-shaped cushion prevents sliding in addition to preventing pressure relief. Call local representative for estimate.

Varalite Chair Cushion
Cascade Designs, Inc.
4000 1st Ave. S.
Seattle, WA 98134
(800) 527-1527, FAX: (206) 467-9421
This lightweight cushion/seating system comes with firm or soft base with two to four self-inflating modular cushions that compensate precisely for posture deviation.

Firm Wheelchair Seats

Drop seats (hardware)
Adaptive Engineering Lab, Inc.
4430 Russell Rd. 2S-3
Mukilteo, WA 97275-5018
(800) 327-6080

Walkers

Next Step & Rover
Noble Motion, Inc.
P.O. Box 5366
58T1 Center Ave.
Pittsburgh, PA 15206
(800) 234-9235
This 4-wheeled, 8-inch, solid tire walker is equipped with hand brakes. Additional accessories are available.

Ultimate Walker (formerly Merry Walker)
Direct Supply
6761 N. Industrial Rd.
Milwaukee, WI 53223
(800) 634-7328
This adjustable wheeled walking frame made with PVC pipe allows wheeling in standing or sitting positions. It is useful for elders who stand unsteadily or are unsafely mobile on their own.

Printed Material

Christenson, M. (1990). *Aging in the designed environment.* Bingham, NY: Hawthorne Press.
This book provides detailed information on ways to adapt the physical environment to compensate for sensory changes associated with aging, enhance independence in the home, and redesign long-term care facilities. This is an excellent resource for modifying the environment.

Rader, J. (1990). *Individualized dementia care: Creative, compassionate approaches.* New York: Springer Publishing.
(212) 431-4370.

Robinson, A., Spencer, B., & White, L. (1989). *Understanding difficult behaviors: Some practical suggestions for coping with Alzheimer's disease and related illness.* Ann Arbor, MI: The Alzheimer's Program.
The Alzheimer's Program
P.O. Box 981337
Ann Arbor, MI 45198
(313) 487-2335
Written for professional and family caregivers, this book explains the causes of behaviors such as wandering, resistance, incontinence, and agitation. Problem-solving strategies for managing behaviors also are suggested.

Unite the Elderly
The Kendal Corp.
P.O. Box 100
Kennett Square, PA 19348
This newsletter on restraint reduction is available on request.

RESOURCES TO ASSIST THE OLDER DRIVER
General

The Handicapped Driver's Mobility Guide
American Automobile Association
Traffic Safety Department
1000 AAA Dr.
Heathrow, FL 32746
Provides state-by-state listing of driver evaluation programs and vehicle modification vendors.

Drivers 55 Plus: Test Your Own Performance
Self-rating form of questions, facts, and suggestions for safe driving. Available from:
American Automobile Association Foundation for Traffic Safety
1730 "M" St., N.W., Suite 401
Washington, DC 20036
Also offers other publications and videos related to the older driver, as well as general information related to driving.

Older Driving Skills Assessment and
Resource Guide
American Association of Retired Persons
601 E. St., N.W.
Washington, DC 20049

Association of Driver Educators for the Disabled
(ADED)
P.O. Box 49
Edgerton, WI 53534
(608) 884-8833
Provides information related to drivers with disabilities, such as information on Driving Rehabilitation Specialists and others in the fields of driver education and transportation equipment modification and educational conferences.

Architectural and Transportation Barriers
Compliance Board
1331 "F" St., N.W., Suite 1000
Washington, DC 20004-1111
(202) 272-5434
Issues accessibility guidelines for the ADA; ensures compliance with standards issued under the Architectural Barriers Act of 1968.

Equipment for Hearing-Impaired Drivers

HARC Mercantile, Ltd.
1111 W. Centre
P.O. Box 3055
Portage, MI 49024

Source for Key Holders and Door Openers

Sammons Preston
P.O. Box 5071
Bolingbrook, IL 60440-5071
(800) 323-5547

North Coast Medical
Functional Solutions Online Catalog
187 Stauffer Blvd.
San Jose, CA 95125-1042
(800) 235-7054

HEARING DEFICITS

Information on hearing aids that may assist certified occupational therapy assistants and elders is available through AARP (American Association for Retired Persons), *The Consumers Guide to Hearing Aids*, # D1777.
AARP
P.O. Box 22796
Long Beach, CA 90801-5796

LOW VISION

American Foundation for the Blind
11 Penn Plaza, Suite 300
New York, NY 10011
www.afb.org
The Lighthouse National Center for Vision and Aging
800 Second Ave.
New York, NY 10017
(800) 829-0500/TTY (212) 821-9713
www.lighthouse.org
Lighthouse is an organization that provides vision rehabilitation services, education, research, and advocacy for persons with visual impairments. The website provides information on rehabilitation services, courses, conferences, publications for practitioners, a newsletter, information on advocacy, product information, and vision resources.

National Library for the Blind and Physically Handicapped
Library of Congress
101 Independence Ave, S.E.
Washington, DC 20542
(800) 424-8567, TDD (202) 707-0744
http://www.loc.gov/nls
This is a free service that provides books and magazines in recorded format.

Independent Living Aids
200 Robinson Ln.
Jericho, NY 11753
(800) 537-2118
www.independentliving.com
This is one of many catalog companies that supply nonprescription low vision aids such as magnifiers, computer software, kitchen appliance adaptations, personal care items, Braille products, games, and hobbies for persons with visual impairment.

The Brain Injury Visual Assessment Battery for Adults by Mary Warren
This book may be ordered through:
Visabilities Rehabilitation Services, Inc.

210 Lorna Square, # 208
Birmingham, AL 35216
(888) 752-4364
www.visabilities.com

Besides instructions for administration of the test, this manual provides a thorough background on various types of visual impairment and guidelines for interpretation of test results. It also includes sections on treatment planning with suggestions for appropriate activities. The battery may be used with both low vision and neurovisual impairments.

New York Times/Large Type Weekly (Mail Only)
New York Times Company
Large Print Edition
329 W. 43rd St
New York, NY 10036

Reader's Digest Large Type Edition
Reader's Digest Association
P.O. Box 7744
Red Oak, IA 51591-0774

Guideposts
Guideposts Association, Inc.
16 E. 34th St.
New York, NY 10016

CONTINENCE RESOURCES

National Kidney and Urologic Diseases Information Clearinghouse
(800) 891-5390
American Foundation for Urologic Disease
(800) 242-2383
Simon Foundation for Continence
(800) 237-4666
National Association for Continence
(800) 252-3337

FAMILY AND CAREGIVERS

Publications

Many practical, hands-on guidebooks and personal accounts for family and professional caregiver are available. Many books are written in an easy-to-read style that is user-friendly and nontechnical, presenting key information on caregiver concerns. Of particular interests are books that assist the caregiver in learning ways to keep clients engaged through meaningful activities, preventing caregiver burnout, and coping with wandering and other difficult behaviors. Books that offer personal accounts written by patients experiencing dementia assist us in gaining empathy for our patients and family members.

Carroll, D. (1989). *When your loved one has Alzheimer's disease*. New York: Times Books.
Carter, R., & Golant, S. (1994). *Helping yourself help others*. New York: Times Books.

Cohen, D., & Eisdorfer, C. (1986). *Loss of self: A family resource for the care of Alzheimer's disease and related disorders*. New York: WW Norton & Company.
Dolan, M. J. (1992). *How to care for aging parents and still have a life of your own*. New York: Mulholland Press.
Greenberg, V. E. (1989). *Your best is good enough: Aging parents and your emotions*. Philadelphia: Lexington Books.
Greenberg, V. E. (1994). *Children of a certain age: Adults and their aging parents*. Philadelphia: Lexington Books.
Faloon, I., Boyd, J., & McGill, C. (1984). *Family care of schizophrenia*. New York: Guilford Press.
Friel, D. (1993). *Living in the labyrinth: A personal journey through the maze of Alzheimer's disease*. New York: Bantam, Doubleday, Dell.
Mace, N. L., & Rabins, P. V. (1981). *The 36-hour day*. Baltimore, MD: Johns Hopkins.
Morris, A., & Hunt, G. (1994). *A part of daily life*. Bethesda, MD: The American Occupational Therapy Association. (Includes a video and resource booklet.)
New York City Alzheimer's Resource Center. (1985). *Caring: A guide to managing the Alzheimer's patient at home*. New York: The Center.
Oakley, F. (1993). *Understanding the ABC's of Alzheimer's disease: A guide for caregivers*. Rockville, MD: American Occupational Therapy Association.
Reisburg, B. (1983). *A guide to Alzheimer's disease for families, spouses and friends*. New York: Free Press.
Sheridan, C. (1987). *Failure-free activities for the Alzheimer's patient: A guidebook for caregivers*. San Francisco, CA: Cottage Books. (Available in Spanish, Japanese, and Dutch translations.)
Susik, D. H. (1995). *Hiring home caregivers: The family guide to in-home elder care*. New York: Impact Books.
Torrey, E. F. (1988). *Surviving schizophrenia: A family manual* (revised edition). New York: Harper & Row.

Pamphlets

Intimacy with arthritis: Answers to the most commonly asked questions.
Arthritis Today. Available from the Arthritis Foundation.
P.O. Box 7669
Atlanta, GA 30357-0669
www.arthritis.org
Sex after total joint replacement. Available from Media Partners.
PO Box 1268
Duluth, GA 30097
Phone (678) 475-9988.
www.mediapartnersinc.com
Together again: Our guide to intimacy after stroke. Available from the American Stroke Association.

7272 Greenville Ave.
Dallas, TX 75231
Phone (888) 478-7653
www.strokeassociation.org
Sex and heart disease. Available from the American Heart Association.
7272 Greenville Ave.
Dallas, TX 75231
(800) 242-8721
www.americanheart.org

Support Groups and Referrals

Alzheimer's Association

The Alzheimer's Association has an impressive network of more than 200 chapters and 1500 support groups nationwide. Many major cities have local chapters of the Alzheimer's Association. It was founded in 1980 by family caregivers and provides programs and services to assist families in their communities. Information on Alzheimer's disease, current research, patient care, and assistance for caregivers is available. Support groups allow families to share their experiences in an emotionally supportive environment. The association has practical suggestions, educational handouts, pamphlets, videos, and publications to assist families and caregivers. The Alzheimer's Association has a website with information on the association, its local chapters, caregiving (which includes some online publications), public policy, and upcoming conferences and events devoted to Alzheimer's disease and related disorders. To locate a chapter near you, contact the national office at:

Alzheimer's Association
225 N. Michigan Ave.
Suite 1700
Chicago, IL 60611-7633
www.alz.org
24-hour information and chapter referral: (800) 272-3900, TDD: (312) 335-8882

American Academy of Ophthalmology

The American Academy of Ophthalmology offers information about the National Eye Care Project and referrals for free or low-cost eye care for financially disadvantaged older adults.

P.O. Box 7424
San Francisco, CA 94120-7424
(415) 561-8500
www.aao.org

American Association of Homes and Services for the Aging

The American Association of Homes and Services for the Aging offers a brochure on the selection of a nursing home or assisted living facility that can be obtained free of charge by writing the association at:

American Association of Homes and Services for the Aging

2519 Connecticut Ave. N.W.
Washington, DC 20008
(202) 783-2242
www.aahsa.org

American Association of Retired Persons (AARP)

The AARP organization provides caregivers with a resource kit when they write for item #D15267 at:

AARP
601 E St., N.W.
Washington, DC 20049
(800) 424-3410
www.aarp.org

American Dietetic Association

The American Dietetic Association offers free information and publications by mail:

American Dietetic Association
120 S. Riverdale Plaza, Suite 2000
Chicago, IL 60606-6995
(800) 877-1600

Area Agencies on Aging (AAA)

These agencies are local offices that can direct family or professional caregivers to sources of help for elders with limited incomes. Resources include subsidized housing, food stamps, Supplemental Security Income, Medicaid, and the Qualified Medicare Beneficiary program. Family members may be eligible for services provided through the AAA, including home health aide services, transportation, home-delivered meals, assistance with chores, home repair, and legal aid. It also provides a registry of home care workers for hire and information on home care agencies and volunteer groups that provide various services. This agency may also provide an assessment of the elder's needs. AAA also can provide information on senior center and adult day care programs and assist in arranging respite care. The national office can provide the numbers of local Agencies on Aging.

AAA
927 15th St., N.W., 6th floor
Washington, DC 20005
(202) 296-8130
www.n4a.org

Children of Aging Parents (CAPS)

CAPS serves as a national clearinghouse for caregivers, matching existing support groups to individuals looking for groups on a national level. CAPS has developed a national directory of caregiver support groups and private geriatric care managers. It also offers community education programs and assists caregivers in gaining access to community resources. Peer counseling, manuals, and materials are available through this organization. Programs sponsored by CAPS include workshops and seminars for caregivers and professionals; inservice training programs for health care agencies; educational presentations and consultations for programs and services to elders;

and an annual conference for caregivers and professionals. For more information, contact this organization at:

1609 Woodbourne Rd., Suite 302A
Levittown, PA 19057-1511
(800) 227-7294
www.caps4caregivers.org

AHA Stroke Connection

The AHA Stroke Connection network links stroke survivors, family members, and professionals. It promotes the development of support groups and provides information and educational materials about stroke.

AHA Stroke Connection
7272 Greenville Ave.
Dallas, TX 75231-4596
(800) 553-6321
www.strokeassociation.org

National Academy of Elder Law Attorneys

The National Academy of Elder Law Attorneys offers a free brochure on selecting an elder law attorney.

1604 N. Country Club Rd.
Tucson, AZ 85716
(520) 881-4005

National Alliance for the Mentally Ill (NAMI)

NAMI provides grassroots self-help, support, and advocacy.

2107 Wilson Blvd., Suite 300
Arlington, VA 22201-3042
(703) 524-7600

National Association of Professional Geriatric Care Managers

1604 N. Country Club Rd
Tucson, AZ 85716-3102
(520) 881-8008
www.nccnhr.org

National Citizens Coalition for Nursing Home Reform

1424 16 St., N.W, Suite 202
Washington, DC 20036
(202) 332-2276

National Consumers' League

The National Consumers' League provides information about medigap insurance and long-term care services.

1701 K St., N.W., Suite 1200
Washington, DC 20006
(202) 835-0747

National Institute of Mental Health (NIMH)

NIMH provides free publications for professionals and the general public on various topics related to mental illness. Information can be gained through:

Office of Communications
6001 Executive Blvd.
Rm. 8184, msc 9663
Bethesda, MD 20892-9663
(301) 443-4513, or toll free: (866) 615-6464

National Institute of Neurological Disorders and Stroke

Fact sheets, current reports, and brochures on neurologic disorders are available by writing the Office of Scientific and Health Reports.

Office of Scientific and Health Reports
Bldg. 31, Rm. 8A16
9000 Rockville Pike
Bethesda, MD 20892
(301) 496-5751
www.nindhs.nih.gov

Alliance for Retired Americans

888 16th St., N.W., Suite 520
Washington, DC 20006
(202) 974-8222, or toll free: (888) 373-6497
www.retiredamericans.org

Stroke Connection of the American Heart Association

The Stroke Connection maintains a listing of more than 1000 stroke support groups across the nation for referral to stroke survivors, their families, caregivers, and interested professionals and will provide information and referral. *Stroke Connection* magazine offers a forum for stroke survivors and their families to share information about coping with stroke. This association offers additional publications of stroke-related books, videos, and literature for purchase.

Stroke Connection of the American Heart Association
7272 Greenville Ave.
Dallas, TX 75231
(888) 478-7653
www.strokeassociation.org

United Seniors Health Cooperative

A list of publications are available from this organization on topics of importance to older consumers, including insurance and Medicare, nursing home selection, finances, caregiving, and health.

409 3rd St., S.W.
Washington, DC 20024
(202) 479-6973
www.unitedseniorshealth.org

World Wide Web Resources

CHAPTER 1: AGING TRENDS AND CONCEPTS

http://www.agingstats.gov/

Contains current aging statistics in *Older Americans 2000: Key indicators of well-being.*

http://www.siu.edu/offices/iii/

Provides information and many links on intergenerational activities (from the Illinois Intergenerational Initiative).

http://www.nlm.nih.gov/medlineplus/dementia.html

Provides a variety of health-related topics where information can be accessed.

http://research.aarp.org/general/profile97.html #Figure6

Graph indicating the percentage of older Americans who need help with activities of daily living based on data from national survey conducted in 1992.

http://www.cdc.gov/nchs/data/agingtrends/04nursin.pdf

A report examining the characteristics of U.S. nursing home residents from 1985 to 1997. The report examines the emerging trends to help those concerned make effective policy and programming decisions that impact the elderly population.

http://www.seniorresource.com/ageinpl.htm#ageinpltop

Topics relating to aging in place. Resources to help the elderly secure necessary support services in response to changing needs so that they may remain in their present residences for as long as possible.

http://www.aarp.org/bulletin/departments/2001/long_term/1205_longterm_1.html

Article published in the *AARP Bulletin*, December 2001, examining aspects of long-term care insurance. The article is informative and well written.

http://www.cdc.gov/nchs/releases/01facts/olderame.htm

National Center for Health Statistics provides information about aging activities, longitudinal studies, and other topics relating to the health of older Americans.

CHAPTER 2: SOCIAL AND BIOLOGICAL THEORIES OF AGING

www.aoa.gov

A division of the Department of Health and Human Services, the Administration on Aging website discusses a variety of topics of interest to older Americans. This is a general interest publication.

http://www.nia.nih.gov/

Website for The National Institute on Aging (NIA), part of the National Institutes of Health. It was established in 1974 for the purpose of promoting a scientific understanding of the nature of aging and to provide leadership in aging research, training, health information dissemination, and other programs relevant to aging and older people.

http://www.asaging.org/

Website for the American Society on Aging, a nonprofit organization committed to enhancing the knowledge and skills of those working with older adults and their families.

http://www.agingresearch.org/

Alliance for Aging Research, a nonprofit organization dedicated to supporting and accelerating the pace of medical discoveries to improve the human experience of aging and health. The website is easy to access and the articles are well written.

http://www.psychtreatment.com/geriatric_psychology.htm

"Growing Old in the United States," an article on geriatric psychology.

http://www.medicine.uiowa.edu/uhs/DRL/viewsub.cfm?CatID=Spe&SubID=1.0

Library of videotapes on aging.

http://www.surgeongeneral.gov/library/mentalhealth/toc.html#chapter5

"Older Adults and Mental Health'" is part of a larger work by the Public Health Service on mental health in the United States.

http://www.valenciaforum.com/Keynotes/pb.html

"New Frontiers in the Future of Aging: From Successful Aging of the Young Old to the Dilemmas of the Fourth Age" is a lecture given by Paul B. Baltes and Jacqui Smith of the Max Planck Institute for Human Development, Berlin, Germany.

CHAPTER 3: AGING PROCESS

http://www.e-geriatric.net/

This site talks about physical and mental changes related to normal aging.

http://www.innovitaresearch.org/index.html

Innovita Research Foundation website is intended for readers who want to review information about aging in general, as well as information about research on the molecular level. The points of emphasis are: to recognize the main problems of aging, to reduce aging factors, and to discover how aging is influenced by our genetic composition and lifestyle.

http://www.demko.com/m020116b.htm

"Ethics of Anti-Aging Medicine Questioned" is a brief review of many factors impacting the field of antiaging medicine.

http://www.ncbi.nlm.nih.gov/entrez/query.fcgi?holding=npg&cmd=Retrieve&db=PubMed&list_uids=12044939&dopt=Abstract

Large genome rearrangements as a primary cause of aging. This is a technical publication.

http://todaysseniorsnetwork.com/Brain%20changes.htm

"Age-Related Changes in the Brain's White Matter Affect Cognitive Function in Old Age" is a synopsis of the actual study.

http://www.apa.org/journals/pag/press_releases/march_2003/pag181140.html

Full text of the article, "Age-Related Changes in the Brain's White Matter Affect Cognitive Function in Old Age."

http://www.infoaging.org/b-neuro-home.html

How Does the Brain Change with Age? This is a general interest publication that is well written.

http://www.eurekalert.org/pub_releases/2003-05/nioa-nsi050203.php

Review of a new study matching genetic influences and cognitive impairment in rats.

http://www.healthandage.com/html/min/afar/content/other6_1.htm

Neurobiology and aging information center.

http://www.merck.com/pubs/mm_geriatrics/sec7/ch48.htm

"Aging and the Musculoskeletal System." This is Chapter 48 of the *Merck Manual of Geriatrics*.

http://health.discovery.com/diseasesandcond/encyclopedia/499.html

Encyclopedia site containing information about changes that occur in the bones, joints, and muscles because of aging.

CHAPTER 4: PSYCHOSOCIAL ASPECTS OF AGING

http://www.cdc.gov/nchs/agingact.htm

This website has a variety of studies and reports related to health and aging issues and many links to other aging sites.

CHAPTER 5: AGING WELL: HEALTH PROMOTION AND DISEASE PREVENTION

http://www.cdc.gov/cancer/nbccedp/info-cc.htm

This website provides cervical cancer information.

http://www.healthypeople.gov/

Healthy People 2010, a publication by the U.S. Department of Health and Human Services. Contains articles about and links to reliable health information. It is intended for the general public.

http://www.doh.wa.gov

This is the website for the Washington State Department of Health.

http://www.agingstats.gov/chartbook2000/default.htm

This site provides a report titled, "Older Americans 2000: Key Indicators of Well-Being," which is published by the Federal Interagency Forum on Aging-Related Statistics.

http://www.nlm.nih.gov/medlineplus/dementia.html

MedLine Plus provides answers to questions on health-related topics and links to relevant sites.

http://www.healthfinder.gov/Scripts/SearchContext.asp?topic=598&page=14

Health Finder provides information on health-related topics for all ages.

http://www.agingstats.gov/chartbook2000/slides.html

This is a PowerPoint presentation of statistics on aging found in "Older Americans 2000: Key Indicators of Well-Being," by the Federal Interagency Forum on Aging-Related Statistics.

http://www.medlina.com/geriatrics.htm

This site provides answers to questions and links to sites related to aging and geriatric health.

http://www.nih.gov/nia

National Institute on Aging website provides information on aging, research, health information, and a plethora of information related to elders.

CHAPTER 6: PUBLIC POLICY

http://capwiz.com/aota/issues/alert/?alertid=1097601

Clearinghouse for issues and legislation affecting health care for seniors.

http://cms.hhs.gov/medicaid/mds20/qifacman.pdf

Website accessing the *Facility Guide for Nursing Home Quality Indicators*, a technical manual reporting on key factors affecting quality of nursing home care.

http://www.agingsociety.org/agingsociety/publications/public_policy/index.html

Public Policy and Aging Report, a quarterly publication of the National Academy on an Aging Society, explores policy issues generated by the aging of American society.

http://www.cms.hhs.gov/medicaid/mover.asp

This website describes Medicare, Medicaid, SCHIP, HIPAA, and CLIA programs. This section describes the various aspects of the Medicaid program and is designed to be used by the general public.

http://www.medicare.gov/Publications/Pubs/pdf/10050.pdf

Website to an annual governmental publication describing Medicare benefits.

http://cms.hhs.gov/manuals/108_pim/pim83c06.asp

This website describes Medicare, Medicaid, SCHIP, HIPAA, and CLIA programs. It is technical in nature and guidelines are described for specific Medicare services.

http://www.hcanys.org/dementia/AlzheimerScully4-1.PDF

Statement 4/1/2002, by Tom Scully, Administrator of the Centers for Medicare and Medicaid Services, on therapy coverage for patients with Alzheimer's disease.

http://www.cms.hhs.gov/medlearn/refsnf.asp

This website describes Medicare, Medicaid, SCHIP, HIPAA, and CLIA programs. It is written for skilled nursing facilities as a reference guide for billing and payment systems.

http://www.cms.hhs.gov/medicaid/managedcare

This website describes Medicare, Medicaid, SCHIP, HIPAA, and CLIA programs. This section deals with Medicare Managed Care issues.

http://www.cms.hhs.gov/oasis/intguide.pdf

This website describes Medicare, Medicaid, SCHIP, HIPAA, and CLIA programs. It is a technical publication defining statutes and regulations regarding home health agencies.

http://www.cms.hhs.gov/manuals/12_snf/sn201.asp

This website describes Medicare, Medicaid, SCHIP, HIPAA, and CLIA programs. It deals with coverage of services for skilled nursing facilities.

http://www.cms.hhs.gov/oasis/hhregs.asp

This website describes Medicare, Medicaid, SCHIP, HIPAA, and CLIA programs. It provides explanations of and links to regulations supporting policy and technical information found in the OASIS website.

http://www.cms.hhs.gov/providers/hhapps/default.asp

This website describes Medicare, Medicaid, SCHIP, HIPAA, and CLIA programs. It contains useful information for understanding and implementing the payment system for home health agencies as of 7/3/2000.

http://www.medicare.gov/Basics/WhatIs.asp#PartA

Publication by the Department of Health and Human Services, "The Official U.S. Government Site for People with Medicare," provides a simple explanation of Medicare basics. It is also available in Chinese and Spanish.

http://cms.hhs.gov/providers/snfpps/fr12ma98.pdf

Published in the *Federal Register*, this is the final ruling on the "Prospective Payment System and Consolidated Billing for Skilled Nursing Facilities" in 1998.

CHAPTER 8: PRACTICE SETTINGS

http://www.cdc.gov/nchs/agingact.htm

This website is provided by the U.S. Department of Health and Human Services and has many links related to working with elders.

http://publish.uwo.ca/~shobson/scenario4.html

This website has a case study with suggestions for Occupational Therapy intervention.

http://www.aoa.dhhs.gov/NAIC/Notes/nursinghomes.html

This website from the Administration on Aging Center for Communication Services discusses nursing homes in depth and contains links to all aspects of elder care.

http://www.usc.edu/isd/locations/science/gerontology/MLA/mlabib_sex.html

This website has an extensive bibliography on sexuality and aging compiled by the Medical Library Association.

CHAPTER 9: CULTURAL DIVERSITY OF THE AGING POPULATION

http://www.aoa.gov/NAIC/Notes/diversityaging.html

The Administration on Aging website has beneficial information related to aging. It is very easy to use and contains many links to information on cultural and racial diversity and aging.

CHAPTER 10: ETHICAL ASPECTS IN THE WORK WITH ELDERS

http://www.aoa.gov/eldfam/Elder_Rights/Elder_Rights.asp

Administration on Aging website provides information and links to resources geared to protecting the rights of seniors.

http://www.elderabusecenter.org/

This website has resources that provide information regarding abuse, such as recognizing elder abuse, reporting abuse, institutional abuse, research, and conferences available on elder abuse.

http://www.senioranswers.org/Pages/elderabuse.htm

The Colorado Gerontological Society website provides answers to many questions including legal issues, Medicare, Power of Attorney, and many others.

CHAPTER 11: WORKING WITH FAMILIES AND CAREGIVERS

http://www.aoa.gov/eldfam/For_Caregivers/For_Caregivers.asp

Administration on Aging website provides information for caregivers, including family support, caregiver resources, and various types of information for caregivers. Information also is available in Spanish, French, Italian, and other languages.

http://www.co.rock.wi.us/departments/Aging/caregiver_support.htm

The National Family Caregiver Support Program (NFCSP) is described, as well as the basic services this program provides. NFCSP was developed by the Administration on Aging.

www.elderabusecenter.org

This is the website for The National Center on Elder Abuse (NCEA), a national organization to promote understanding and action on elder abuse, neglect, and exploitation.

http://www.elderabusecenter.org/pdf/publication/ethics.pdf

A consensus statement by the National Association of Adult Protective Services Administrators regarding ethical treatment of elders.

CHAPTER 12: ADDRESSING SEXUALITY WITH ELDERS

http://www.nia.nih.gov/health/agepages/sexuality.htm

This website offers information on sexuality later in life.

http://research.aarp.org/health/mmsexsurvey_1.html

Results of the "Modern Maturity Sexuality Survey" by AARP completed in 1999.

http://www.aarp.org/mmaturity/sept_oct99/greatsex.html

Another review of the "Modern Maturity Sexuality Survey" conducted by AARP in 1999.

CHAPTER 13: USE OF MEDICATIONS WITH ELDERS

http://www.generationsjournal.org/gen-24-4/guide.html

Journal article about medications and aging.

http://www.fda.gov/oc/olderpersons/default.htm

U.S. Food and Drug Administration site, which contains information for older people on a wide range of health issues, including arthritis, cancer, health fraud, and nutrition.

CHAPTER 14: CONSIDERATIONS OF MOBILITY

http://www.aoa.gov/eldfam/Housing/Housing.asp

The section of the AOA website dealing with housing issues and elderly Americans.

http://www.nih.gov/nia

Home page for the National Institute on Aging. Easy access to resources on elder mobility issues.

http://www.aging-parents-and-elder-care.com/Pages/Checklists/Elderly_Drivers.html

This website contains information on elderly drivers.

http://www.cdc.gov/ncipc/duip/spotlite/falls.htm

Centers for Disease Control (CDC) website on fall prevention; contains many hints.

http://www.temple.edu/older_adult/

Temple University offers many resources with their fall prevention project.

http://www.ute.kendal.org/

This site called Untie the Elderly contains information on restraint reduction.

CHAPTER 15: WORKING WITH ELDERS WITH VISION IMPAIRMENTS

http://www.eyesight.org/

Macular degeneration foundation contains information about research.

http://www.macular.org/

The American Macular Degeneration Foundation contains latest research, information, and links to help those with macular degeneration.

http://www.glaucomafoundation.org/

The Glaucoma foundation contains information and resources regarding glaucoma.

http://eckerd.healthcite.com/HealthReview/p2033.html

This is a general information site about cataracts.

http://www.nei.nih.gov/health/lowvision/resources.htm

This website, from the National Eye Institute, contains resources on low vision.

CHAPTER 16: WORKING WITH ELDERS WHO HAVE HEARING IMPAIRMENTS

http://www.asaging.org/at/at-235/IF_Vision_Hearing.cfm

Article in *Aging Today* titled "Vision and Hearing Loss Get Overdue Attention."

CHAPTER 17: STRATEGIES TO MAINTAIN CONTINENCE

http://www.health.gov.au/acc/continence/

The website for the National Continence Management Strategy is practical, informative, and written for the general public.

CHAPTER 18: DYSPHASIA AND OTHER EATING AND NUTRITIONAL CONCERNS WITH ELDERS

www.therubins.com

A website for senior citizens and those who care about them.

http://www.ssc.wisc.edu/aging/robbins.htm

Article about dysphasia from the University of Madison Institute on Aging.

http://www.stroke.org.uk/

This website, from the Stroke Association, contains information on dysphasia.

http://www.dysphagia.com/

This excellent website contains many resources about dysphasia.

CHAPTER 19: WORKING WITH ELDERS WHO HAVE CEREBROVASCULAR ACCIDENTS

http://www.strokeassociation.org/presenter.jhtml? identifier=1200037

The American Stroke Association website has two focuses. The first focus is a review of the effects of a stroke and methods of dealing with a cerebrovascular accident. The second focus is a more technical review of journal articles on the subject intended for professionals in the field. "Together Again: Our Guide to Intimacy after Stroke" is available from the American Stroke Association.

http://www.ahcpr.gov/research/aug97/ra3.htm

Article on the elderly in long-term care and functional stroke recovery.

CHAPTER 20: WORKING WITH ELDERS WHO HAVE DEMENTIA AND ALZHEIMER'S DISEASE

http://www.alz.org/

Website for the Alzheimer's Association. This national association provides many resources dealing with the issue of Alzheimer's disease.

http://www.aoa.gov/eldfam/Healthy_Lifestyles/ Mental_Health/Mental_Health_alz.asp

Administration on Aging website providing information and links to associations dealing with Alzheimer's Disease.

http://www.alzheimers.org

Alzheimer's Disease education and referral center provides current information and resources from the U.S. Government's National Institute on Aging.

CHAPTER 21: WORKING WITH ELDERS WHO HAVE PSYCHIATRIC CONDITIONS

http://www.aoa.gov/eldfam/Health_Lifestyles/Mental_ Health/Mental_Health.asp

The Administration on Aging website has information on Mental Health and Older Adults.

http://www.nlm.nih.gov/medlineplus/mentalhealthand behavior.html

Medline Plus provides information on behaviors associated with mental health.

http://www.cdc.gov/ncipc/factsheets/suifacts.htm

This website provides facts regarding suicide.

http://www.surgeongeneral.gov/library/mentalhealth/ toc.html#chapter5

"Older Adults and Mental Health" is part of a larger work by the Public Health Service on mental health in the United States.

CHAPTER 22: WORKING WITH ELDERS WHO HAVE ORTHOPEDIC CONDITIONS

http://www.methodisthealth.com/Ortho/painexer.htm

Methodist Health Center in Texas offers suggestions for exercises for persons with muscle, joint, and bone pain.

www.cdc.gov/aging/health_issues.htm

CDC website contains much information about health in general and is not solely devoted to seniors. It contains many links to other elder sites and is written for the general public.

http://www.niams.nih.gov/hi/topics/osteoporosis/ opbkgr.htm

National Institute of Arthritis and Musculoskeletal and Skin Diseases provides good information on osteoporosis and many links to other sites.

CHAPTER 23: WORKING WITH ELDERS WHO HAVE CARDIOVASCULAR CONDITIONS

http://www.americanheart.org/

American Heart Association website with information on warning signs, heart disease, and healthy lifestyle, as well as a link to the American Stroke Association. *Sex and Heart Disease* is available from the American Heart Association.

http://www.cdc.gov/nccdphp/overview.htm

CDC page on chronic diseases and disease prevention.

CHAPTER 24: WORKING WITH ELDERS WHO HAVE PULMONARY CONDITIONS

http://www.aaaai.org/patients/seniorsandasthma/ hurdles.stm

Article on asthma in elders.

http://www.aoa.gov/eldfam/Healthy_Lifestyles/Asthma/ asthma.asp

This website has good information about asthma and seniors and contains many links to access a variety of information.

http://www.lungusa.org/

Home page for the American Lung Association. This site provides information on many lung conditions.

CHAPTER 25: WORKING WITH ELDERS WHO HAVE ONCOLOGIC CONDITIONS

http://www.cancer.com/

This website contains information about different cancers.

http://www.health.gov.au/nhmrc/publications/synopses/ cp61syn.htm

Australian publication developed by the National Breast Cancer Center's Psychosocial Working Group to provide information to the treatment team to help in supportive care for women with breast cancer.

http://www.cancer.gov/cancerinfo/wyntk/colon-and-rectum

Information about detection, symptoms, diagnosis, and treatment of colon and rectal cancer from the National Cancer Institute.

http://www.ncoa.org/

This website for the National Council on the Aging is wide-ranging and informative.

http://www.cancerindex.org/clinks8a.htm

Information about psychosocial and emotional issues for those dealing with cancer.

http://www.cancer.org/docroot/home/index.asp

This site is the home page for the American Cancer Society. It is extensive in nature and is an excellent resource.

CHAPTER 26: WORKING WITH ELDERS IN HOSPICE

http://www.nhpco.org/
The National Hospice and Palliative Care website is an excellent resource.

http://www.wellworks.org/rka_hospice.html
A Resource Kit on Aging: Healthcare and Hospice by Wellness Works of Montgomery County, Maryland.

http://www.hospicenet.org/html/medicare.html
A website for the general public, Hospice Net is an independent, nonprofit organization working exclusively through the Internet. It contains good information and many links to a variety of information.

http://www.elderweb.com/default.php?PageID=1940
Informative website related to end-of-life care.

http://www.growthhouse.org
This is an independent association dealing with improving the quality of end-of-life care. It contains many links to a variety of information.

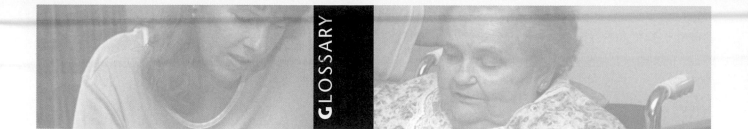

Glossary

acalculia A form of aphasia characterized by the inability to solve simple mathematic calculations.

acetylcholine A neurotransmitter substance widely distributed in body tissues with the primary function of mediating synaptic activity of the nervous system and skeletal muscles.

acute Beginning abruptly with marked intensity or sharpness, then subsiding after a relatively short period.

amyloid Combining form: starch of polysaccharide nature or origin.

angina Spasmodic choking or suffocative pain; currently used almost exclusively to denote angina pectoris.

angioplasty The reconstruction of blood vessels damaged by disease or injury.

ankylosing spondylitis A chronic inflammatory disease of unknown origin that first affects the spine and adjacent structures and commonly progresses to cause eventual fusion of the involved joints.

anosognosia An abnormal condition characterized by a real or feigned inability to perceive a defect, especially paralysis, on one side of the body; possibly attributable to a lesion in the right parietal lobe of the brain.

anoxia An abnormal condition characterized by a lack of oxygen.

antecedent Something that comes before something else; a precursor.

anticholinergic Agents pertaining to the blockade of acetylcholine receptors that result in the inhibition of the transmission of parasympathetic nerve impulses.

antihistamines Any substance capable of reducing the physiologic and pharmacologic effects of histamine, including a wide variety of drugs that block histamine receptors. Many such drugs are readily available as nonprescription medications for the management of allergies.

antioxidant A chemical or other agent that inhibits or retards oxidation of a substance to which it is added.

arrhythmias Variations from the normal rhythm, especially of the heartbeat.

atrophy A wasting or diminution of size or physiologic activity in a part of the body because of disease or other influences.

axis I Psychiatric disorder usually diagnosed in infancy, childhood, or adolescence, excluding mental retardation.

axis II Psychiatric personality disorder and mental retardation.

benzodiazepines A group of psychotropic agents, including tranquilizers, prescribed in the treatment of insomnia and to alleviate anxiety.

bradycardia A circulatory condition in which the myocardium contracts steadily, but at a rate of less than 60 contractions a minute.

bronchiole A small airway of the respiratory system extending from the bronchi into the lobes of the lung.

calcification The accumulation of calcium salts in tissues.

cataract A progressive condition of the lens of the eye characterized by loss of transparency.

catastrophic Sudden downturn; a pattern of medical and nursing care that involves intensive, highly technical life support care of an acutely ill or severely traumatized patient.

chronic Developing slowly and persisting for a long time, often for the remainder of the individual's lifetime.

cochlea A conic, bony structure of the inner ear, perforated by numerous apertures for passage of the cochlear division of the acoustic nerve.

cohort A collection or sampling of individuals who share common characteristics such as individuals of the same age or sex.

collagen A protein consisting of bundles of tiny reticular fibrils that combine to form the white, glistening, inelastic fibers of the tendons, the ligaments, and the fascia.

contralateral Affecting or originating in the opposite side of a point of reference, such as a point on the body.

contrast sensitivity The ability to distinguish the borders of objects as they degrade in contrast from their backgrounds.

cyanosis Bluish discoloration of the skin and mucous membranes caused by an excess of deoxygenated hemoglobin in the blood or a structural defect in the hemoglobin molecule.

cytology The study of cells, including their formation, origin, structure, function, biochemical activities, and pathology.

cytoxic chemotherapy Any pharmacologic compound that inhibits the proliferation of cells within the body.

D

decubitus ulcer Stage III Stage characterized by broken skin, loss of skin, full thickness of skin, possible damage to subcutaneous tissues, and possible serous or bloody drainage.

decubitus ulcer Stage IV Stage characterized by formation of a deep, crater-like ulcer, loss of the full thickness of skin, and destruction of subcutaneous tissues; exposure of fascia connective tissue, bone, or muscle underlying the ulcer, causing possible damage; an inflammation, sore, or ulcer over a bony prominence.

deleterious Harmful or dangerous.

detrusor urinae muscle A complex of longitudinal fibers that form the external layer of the muscular coat of the bladder.

diabetic retinopathy A disorder of retinal blood vessels characterized by microaneurysms, hemorrhage, exudates, and the formation of new vessels and connective tissue.

diaphragmatic breathing A type of breathing exercise that patients are taught to promote more effective aeration of the lungs; movement of the diaphragm downward during inhalation and upward with exhalation.

diplopia Double vision.

DNA Deoxyribonucleic acid: a large nucleic acid molecule found principally in the chromosomes of the nucleus of a cell that carries genetic information.

dopamine A naturally occurring sympathetic nervous system neurotransmitter that is the precurser of norepineprine.

DRG Diagnosis-related group; a group of patients classified for measuring delivery of care in a medical facility; used to determine Medicare payments for inpatient care.

durable power of attorney for health A document that designates an agent or proxy to make health care decisions for a patient who is unable to do so.

dyspnea A shortness of breath or a difficulty in breathing that may be caused by certain heart conditions, strenuous exercise, or anxiety.

E

eccentric viewing A technique in which the person views objects by directing his or her gaze to an area just adjacent to the target object to compensate for a scotoma involving the fovea or macula. This position allows the desired target to be focused on a healthy area of retina.

edema The abnormal accumulation of fluid in interstitial spaces of tissues, such as in the pericardial sac, intrapleural space, peritoneal cavity, and joint capsules.

elastin A protein that forms the principal substance of yellow elastic fibers of tissue.

embolus A foreign object, a quantity of air or gas, a bit of tissue or tumor, or a piece of thrombus that circulates in the bloodstream until it becomes lodged in a vessel.

endocarditis An abnormal condition that affects the endocardium and the heart valves and is characterized by lesions caused by a variety of diseases.

erosion The wearing away or gradual destruction of a mucosal or epidermal surface as a result of inflammation, injury, or other effects; usually marked by the appearance of an ulcer.

esthesia Sensitivity or feeling.

exertional dyspnea Shortness of breath during exertion or exercise.

expectoration The ejection of mucus, sputum, or fluids from the trachea and lungs by coughing or spitting.

G

gastrostomy Surgical creation of an artificial opening into the stomach through the abdominal wall; performed to feed a patient who has cancer of the esophagus or tracheoesophageal fistula, or one who is expected to be unconscious for a long period.

glaucoma An abnormal condition of increased pressure inside the eyeball, often leading to damage to tissues of the eye and vision loss if untreated.

glomerular filtration The renal process whereby fluid in the blood is filtered across the capillaries of the glomerulus and into the urinary space of the Bowman's capsule.

glycogen A polysaccharide that is the major carbohydrate stored in animal cells.

gracilis The most superficial of the five medial femoral muscles.

H

health care proxy A person designated to make health care decisions for a patient who has become incapacitated.

hemi-inattention (also referred to as hemi-neglect, neglect syndrome, unilateral neglect syndrome) A disregard or lack of attention for one side of a person's visual space. Inattention to the left visual space is much more common than inattention to the right.

hemiparesis (hemiplegia) Paralysis of only one side of the body.

hemorrhage An escape of blood from the blood vessels.

heterotopic ossification A nonmalignant overgrowth of bone, frequently occurring after a fracture, that is sometimes confused with certain bone tumors when visualized on X-ray film.

hypercalcemia Greater than normal amounts of calcium in the blood, most often resulting from excessive bone resorption and release of calcium, as occurs in hyperparathyroidism, metastic tumors of bone, Paget's disease, and osteoporosis.

hyperesthesia An extreme sensitivity of one of the body's sense organs, such as pain or touch receptors of the skin.

hyperglycemia A greater than normal amount of glucose in hyperparathyroidism blood.

hypertonicity Excessive tone, tension, or activity.

hypotonicity Pertaining to lower or lessened tone or tension in any body structure, as in paralysis.

I

IADL Instrumental activities of daily living, including health management community living skills, safety management, and home management.

intermediary A Blue Cross plan, private insurance company, or public or private agency selected by health care providers to pay claims under Medicare.

intrinsic Originating from or situated within an organ or tissue.

ipsilateral Pertaining to the same side of the body.

irradiation Exposure to any form of radiant energy such as heat, light, and x-ray.

J

jejunostomy A surgical procedure to create an artificial opening to the jejunum through the abdominal wall.

L

Lewy bodies Concentric spheres found inside vacuoles in midbrain and brainstem neurons in patients with idiopathic parkinsonism, Alzheimer's disease, and other neurodegenerative conditions.

lumen A cavity or channel within any organ or structure of the body.

M

macular degeneration A progressive deterioration of the macula of the retina and choroid of the eye.

malabsorption syndrome A complex of syndromes resulting from disorders in the intestinal absorption of nutrients, characterized by anorexia, weight loss, abdominal bloating, muscle cramps, bone pain, and steatorrhea.

motor planning The ability to plan and execute coordinated movement.

mucopurulent Characteristic of a combination of mucus and pus.

mucosa Mucous membrane.

Myelosuppression The inhibition of the process of production of blood cells and platelets in the bone marrow.

N

nasogastric tube Any tube passed into the stomach through the nose.

neurons Functional cells of the nervous system.

O

oculomotor control The ability to move the eyes together in a coordinated fashion.

ombudsman A person who investigates and mediates patients' problems and complaints regarding hospital services.

opacification Making something opaque.

orthopnea An abnormal condition in which a person must sit or stand to breathe deeply or comfortably; usually accompanies cardiac and respiratory conditions.

orthostatic hypertension Abnormally low blood pressure occurring when an individual assumes a standing posture; also called postural hypotension.

ossification The development of bone.

osteoarthritis A form of arthritis in which one or many joints undergo degenerative changes, including subchondral bony sclerosis, loss of articular cartilage, and proliferation of bone and cartilage in the joint, forming osteophytes.

osteomalacia An abnormal condition of the lamellar bone characterized by a loss of calcification of the matrix, resulting in softening of the bone, accompanied by weakness, fracture, pain, anorexia, and weight loss.

P

palliative Therapy designed to relieve or reduce intensity of uncomfortable symptoms, but not to produce a cure.

parenteral nutrition The administration of nutrients by a route other than through the alimentary canal, such as subcutaneously, intravenously, intramuscularly, and intradermally.

Parkinson's disease A slowly progressive, degenerative, neurologic disorder.

paroxysmal nocturnal dyspnea A sudden onset of shortness of breath while sleeping.

pharynx A tubular structure in the throat about 13 cm in length that extends from the base of the skull to the esophagus and is situated just in front of the cervical vertebrae.

Pick's disease A form of presenile dementia occurring in middle age that produces neurotic behavior and the slow disintegration of intellect, personality, and emotions.

polyuria The excretion of an abnormally large quantity of urine.

presbycusis A loss of hearing sensitivity and speech intelligibility associated with aging.

psychodynamics The study of the forces that motivate behavior.

R

RNA Ribonucleic acid; a nucleic acid found in both the nucleus and the cytoplasm of cells that transmits genetic instructions from the nucleus to the cytoplasm.

S

scotoma An area of the retina where vision is depressed or absent.

sedative hypnotics A drug that reversibly depresses the activity of the central nervous system, used chiefly to induce sleep and to allay anxiety.

semi-Fowler's position Placement of the patient in an inclined position, with the upper half of the body raised by elevating the head of the bed approximately 30 degrees.

senile Pertaining to or characteristic of old age or the process of aging, especially the physical or mental deterioration accompanying aging.

sinusitis An inflammation of one or more paranasal sinuses.

stent A compound used in making dental impressions and medical molds.

strabismus A condition in which an eye is deviated from its normal position and is not aligned with the other eye.

subacute Somewhat acute; between acute and chronic.

subluxation A partial abnormal separation of the articular services of a joint.

supraglottic swallow Coordinated muscular contractions of swallowing in the region of the mouth and pharynx.

syncope A brief lapse in consciousness caused by transient cerebral hypoxia.

synovium Synovial membrane; the inner layer of an articular capsule surrounding a freely movable joint.

T

thrombophlebitis Inflammation of a vein, often accompanied by formation of a clot.

thrombotic stroke Obstruction by the thrombus of the blood supply to the brain, causing a cerebrovascular accident.

thrombus An aggregation of platelets, fibrin, clotting factors, and the cellular elements of the blood attached to the interior wall of a vein or artery.

trachea A nearly cylindrical tube in the neck composed of cartilage and membrane that extends from the larynx at the level of the sixth cervical vertebra to the fifth thoracic vertebra, where it divides into two bronchi.

tracheobronchial tree An anatomic complex including the trachea, bronchi, and bronchial tubes that conveys air to and from the lungs and is a primary structure in respiration.

U

urodynamic The study of the hydrology and mechanics of urinary bladder filling and emptying.

utilitarianism A doctrine stating that the purpose of all action should be to bring about the greatest happiness for the greatest number of people and that value is determined by utility; often applied in the distribution of health care resources, such as in decisions regarding the expenditure of public funds for health services.

V

Valsalva maneuver Any forced expiratory effort against a closed airway, such as when an individual holds the breath and tightens the muscles in a concerted, strenuous effort to move a heavy object or change position in bed.

valvular heart disease An acquired or congenital disorder of a cardiac valve characterized by stenosis and obstructed by valvular degeneration and regurgitation of blood.

visual acuity The clearness or sharpness of vision, typically measured in Snellen equivalents, such as 20/20.

visual field The visual surround that can be seen when one looks straight ahead.

vital capacity A measurement of the amount of air that can be expelled at the normal rate of exhalation after a maximum inspiration; represents the greatest possible breathing capacity.

Definitions from Anderson, K. N., Anderson, L. E., & Glanze, W. D. (1994). *Mosby's medical, nursing, and allied health dictionary* (4th edition). St. Louis: Mosby; Miller, B. F., & Keane, C. (Eds.). *Encyclopedia and dictionary of medicine, nursing, and allied health* (5th edition). Philadelphia: WB Saunders; *Taber's cyclopedic medical dictionary* (17th edition). (1993). Philadelphia: FA Davis; Miller, B. F., & Keane, C. (Eds.). (1987). *Saunder's encyclopedia and dictionary of medicine, nursing, and allied health* (4th edition). Philadelphia: WB Saunders; McDonough, J. T. (Ed.). (1994). *Stedman's concise medical dictionary* (2nd edition). Baltimore, MD: Williams & Wilkins; The American Psychiatric Association. *Diagnostic and statistical manual of mental disorders* (4th edition). Washington, DC: The Association.

Index